M000210026

A COLONIAL LEXICON

BODY, COMMODITY, TEXT

Studies of Objectifying Practice

A series edited by

Arjun Appadurai,

Jean Comaroff, and

Judith Farquhar

A COLONIAL LEXICON

Of Birth Ritual, Medicalization, and

Mobility in the Congo

NANCY ROSE HUNT

Duke University Press

Durham & London

1999

This book is made possible in part
by an award from the University of Michigan Publication
Subvention Program
funded by the Office of the Vice President
for Research, the College of Literature, Science,
and the Arts; and the International Institute.

Typeset in Minion by Keystone Typesetting, Inc.
Library of Congress Cataloging-in-Publication
Data appear on the last printed
page of this book.

2nd printing, 2006

CONTENTS

ILLUSTRATIONS

Figures

Maps

ABBREVIATIONS

AA	Archives Africaines, Brussels
ARSC	Académie Royale des Sciences Coloniales
ARSOM	Académie Royale des Sciences d'Outre-Mer
ASBMT	*Annales de la Société Belge de la Médecine Tropicale*
BMS	Baptist Missionary Society
BMSA	Baptist Missionary Society Archives, Regent's Park College, Oxford
CFL	Chemins de Fer du Congo Supérieur aux Grands Lacs Africains
CMC	Congo Missionary Conference
DD	Dorothy Daniel
DPO	District Pastor's Office, Yakusu
ECZ	Eglise du Christ au Zaïre
FOMULAC	Fondation Médicale de l'Université de Louvain au Congo
FBEI	Fonds du Bien-Etre Indigène
FOREAMI	Fonds Reine Elisabeth pour l'Assistance Médicale aux Indigènes du Congo Belge
HCB	Huileries du Congo Belge
IJAHS	*International Journal of African Historical Studies*
IMT	Institute of Tropical Medicine, Antwerp
INEAC	Institut pour l'Etude Agronomique du Congo Belge
IRCB	Institut Royal Colonial Belge
JFC	John F. Carrington
KADOC	Katholiek Documentatie en Onderzoekcentrum, Leuven
Ling.	Lingala
Lok.	Lokele
MDO	Medical School Director's Office, Yakusu

MPR	Mouvement Populaire de la Révolution
MRAC	Musée Royal de l'Afrique Centrale (Africa-Museum), Tervuren
PL	Phyllis Lofts
SANRU	Santé Rurale or Projet des Soins de Santé Primaires en Milieu Rural (USAID-sponsored Rural Primary Health Care Project)
SGB	Stanley G. Browne
Sw.	Swahili (Kingwana)
TBA	traditional birth attendant
TRSTMH	*Transactions of the Royal Society of Tropical Medicine and Hygiene*
UNAZA	Université Nationale du Zaïre
USAID	United States Agency for International Development
USIA	United States Information Agency
WBB	Winifred Browne Burke
YQN	*Yakusu Quarterly Notes*

ACKNOWLEDGMENTS

I don't know how others do it, but I do it through memories of places, homes, meals, laughter. The places that have served as temporary homes since I began the project that became this book easily tops fifty. And these homes only include those where I slept, not the tables where I ate meals, read sources, drank conversation, and shared my ideas, stories, news, images, and chapters. Only through these memories of places can I begin to remember all those who helped me fathom, cast, and end this study, from its earliest conjurings in Yakusu, Madison, central Illinois, Bujumbura, even Hyde Park to its vexed and last casting out as "that dear book caught with *lokwamisa*" in Tucson, Brussels, and Ann Arbor. The succession of spatial memories takes in all my mentors and coaches, friends and family, research assistants and guides, healers and midwives, and not least those who made me laugh when I was sick or uninspired, told me stories, invited me to be present as they gave birth, loaned me vehicles, photocopied and posted documents, sang songs, told stories, transcribed tapes, paddled me and my bicycle, took me in, sent me out again, and read and reread drafts.

My greatest debt remains to the people of Yainyongo-Romée and Yakusu, as well as all my friends, informants, and assistants from Kisangani to Basoko and Opala in the country I knew as Zaire. I owe special thanks to my first family in Zaire, the BaTula, especially Mama Tula Sophie for being my first and last tutor, guide, and informant, and her son, Tula Rogier, for his work in transcribing interviews; Yainyongo's three midwives, Mama Lisongomi, Mama Sila, and Shangazi Angelani; Tata Alikuwa and his kin, notably Bibi Bilefu Mari-Jeanne, who embraced me as a *moseka wa Bokoto* (a girl of the Bokoto house); and Pesapesa. The Yakusu mission also took me in and helped me out in a myriad of important ways; I especially thank Pastor Batondo, Drs. Chris and Mairi

Burnett, Pam Bryan, Susan Chalmers, Angela and Tim Hinchcliffe, Annie Horsfall, Kelekele, Papa Lokangu, Lombale-Botowato, and Mota Moya.

Tata Tula and Tata Alikuwa have died since I left Yakusu and Yainyongo-Romée in 1990. Most everyone whom I knew then is certainly hungry now, unless they left for England and Scotland when the Baptist Missionary Society (BMS) evacuated missionaries from Yakusu in 1991. The BaTula left for Kisangani after Tata died. Last I knew, Mama Tula had arthritis and was having trouble walking, and Rogier had gone off seeking diamonds. How have they experienced the presence of Serb mercenaries, refugees, Kabila's and now Wamba-dia-Wamba's men in their midst? I have had no letters since these latest rounds of war and tribulation, flight and death began. That those alive are praying and cursing, including about my expected but delayed and redelayed return to their homes and lives, this I know. That the history of childbearing in this book needs at least one more, post-1990 chapter, this I still hope to do. Now, from here, I have little more to offer than this completion, their stories, memories, and names in print. May this book of a *lokasa*, in some manner, reach them and honor them and amuse them. Their trust and imaginations and care made it possible. My debts are forever.

Professor Sabakinu Kivilu welcomed me to Kinshasa and gave important advice, as did Professors Kalala Nkudi, Mulyumba wa Mamba Itongwa, and Yamvu Makasu in Kisangani. Frère Jerry of Kisangani's Catholic Procure gave me precious advice. Dani Frank, Toni Gierlandt, Marie Lechat, and Jean-Luc Vellut made Brussels possible. I concluded my fieldwork traveling in England, meeting former Yakusu missionaries as a guest in their homes. This book would not be the same without the documentation, photographs, and recollections that Mali Browne, Winifred Browne Burke, Nora Carrington, Dorothy Daniel, Mary Fagg, David and Gillian Lofts, and Margaret Pitt so generously shared with me. I thank them, and also Jo McGregor for the use of her car. I also thank John Sinclair of Roseville, Minnesota, who made papers of A. G. Mill available to me by post and who shared his own manuscript about Mill with me.

I am grateful for the generous funding that made the original research possible: a Fulbright-Hays Doctoral Dissertation Fellowship; an International Doctoral Research Fellowship from the Joint Committee on African Studies of the American Council of Learned Societies and the Social Science Research Council; an American Fellowship from the American Association of University Women; a Woodrow Wilson Research Grant in Women's Studies; a grant from the Institute of Intercultural Studies; a Belgian American Educational Foundation Fellowship; a University Fellowship from the University of Wisconsin—Madison's Graduate School; and a Bernadotte E. Schmitt Grant for Research in the History of Europe, Africa, and Asia from the American Historical Association. I owe a large debt to the University of Arizona's College of Social and Behavioral Sciences, the Vice President for Research, the Social and Behavioral Sciences Research Institute, the Women's Studies Advisory Committee, and especially my colleagues in the Department of History for generous research support, leaves, and inspiration during my five years of teaching there. I also am grateful to the University of Michigan's Office of the Vice-President for Research for a book subvention award, which was supplemented by generous funds from the Departments of History and of Obstetrics and Gynecology. I especially thank Tim Johnson and Rebecca Scott; this was only a small part in how they welcomed me to Ann Arbor.

Archivists, curators, and librarians in Madison, Evanston, Tucson, London, Oxford, Brussels, Tervuren, Antwerp, Kinshasa, Kisangani, Yakusu, and Louvain-la-Neuve were first-rate, generous, and kind. I am grateful to the staffs of the History Department at the University of Lubumbashi; the Baptist Missionary Society, Didcott; the Angus Library, Regent's Park College, Oxford; the Archives Africaines, Brussels; the Ethnographic and Historical Sections of the Musée Royal de l'Afrique Centrale (Africa-Museum), Tervuren; the African Library, Brussels; the Institute of Tropical Medicine, Antwerp; Katholiek Documentatie en Onderzoekcentrum (KADOC), Leuven; Centre Aequatoria, Bamanya, Congo; the Herskovits Library, Northwestern University; and Memorial Library, University of Wisconsin—Madison. I owe special thanks to F. Bontinck, Mme Dekais, Els De Palmenaer, Ed Duesterhoeft, David Henige, Susan Mills, P. Maréchal, Françoise Morimont, G. Roelants, Mette Sheyne, Gustaaf Verswijver, Boris Wastiau, and Honoré Vinck of these institutions.

Patricia Hayes inspired me to think about the photographs and images in new ways, and David Lofts generously and enthusiastically had reproductions made of a whole set of them from the papers of Phyllis Lofts. Lest they be read as mere illustrations rather than juxtaposed signs, a few comments on the diverse archives from which they were extracted are in order here. Few colonial doctors included photographs in the qualifying reports preserved at the Institute of Tropical Medicine in Antwerp, but G. Fronville included a couple dozen of removed tumors and chalk-marked patient bodies in his report on surgery in Elisabethville. None captures the social context of teaching, the social realities of colonial medicine, as does the one of an open-air autopsy included here; it speaks to the kind of masculine bravado that shaped the practice of tropical medicine on the ground and in qualifying reports back to authorities in the metropole.

In contrast to Fronville's use of photographs as intrepid proof are the two sets of cherished photographs that I stumbled on in the living rooms of former Yakusu missionaries in England. Nora Carrington found some envelopes of photographs scattered around her home in Salisbury and told me to choose those that interested me, just please to return them to her when I was done. These were her memories; many were of her beloved John, almost all of people she knew and esteemed. I first saw nine of the photographs included here in the home of David Lofts, nephew of Phyllis Lofts. My first introduction to Phyllis Lofts was from Phyllis Martin, the central African historian, who told me one day in Brazzaville to go find out about this Yakusu missionary nurse because she had grown up on her stories of the Congo, and without them she might never have traveled from Scotland to Africa. I knew, then, that I was seeing a collection of mementos (including the piece of wood from the sacred tree of cruelty that became the hospital benches) that Lofts had shown to children as she regaled them with memories of leopards, Bolau, and Yakusu. Very different archives these were, therefore, than those of a tropical surgeon. Even though there was a surgery scene among Lofts's papers, it was quite in line with all my other clues about missionary mirth and precious moments, all suitable for public consumption.

These missionary discoveries came after I was in the field. Before I went, I visited the Musée Royal de l'Afrique Centrale's (MRAC) Historical Section's photo archive at a time when they would give you free reign of the file drawers of Congopresse and other gifts classified by subject. Thus it was that I was able to see the extent and range of postwar propaganda on maternity care for Congolese, and the interwar—likely Union Minière—propaganda on maternities for Europeans. The discovery of the Mbumbulu comic strip and the centrality of maternity wards and bicycles came at about the same time at the Royal Library in Brussels. Semiotics was here to stay. The do-and-don't Congolese imaged messages date back to my Bujumbura days, when I discovered a spare copy of the Swahili edition of this booklet in a *foyer social* ("social home") closet. I located the do-do messages for Belgians in Madison, when the African Studies Program blessed me with some funds for slide reproduction.

In Tucson, Doug Weiner inspired me to take on the semiotics of postage stamps and coins, and I found about forty hygiene postage stamps in all, and incredibly easily besides, once I found my way to Brussels's stamp shop district a few years ago. One of my last stops was MRAC's Ethnographic Section as I sought out axheads and lances, first the objects themselves, and then images of Lobanga, Lokele chiefs, lances, and iron bridewealth. "Money," "bridewealth," and especially "Lokele": these were my key terms in this colonial ethnographic archive. And Poof!—out popped Lobanga and his colleagues in a set of photographs attributed to the provincial governor of the time, A. de Meulemeester.

I am grateful to many persons and institutions for the invitations to present portions of what became *A Colonial Lexicon* in stimulating settings over the years. I especially thank Terence Ranger for the invitation to try out my work on colonial humor at the African History Seminar, St. Antony's College, Oxford, in 1991; David William Cohen for the first opportunity to present my work on postcolonial debris and childbearing at the 1993 Institute on "The Politics of Reproduction and Fertility Control," Program on International Cooperation in Africa, Northwestern University; Charles Becker, Mamadou Diouf, and Jean-Pierre Dozon for the chance to present new work on colonial gynecology and STDS to a CODESRIA and ORSTOM conference on "The Social sciences and AIDS in Africa," Saly Portudal, Senegal, 1996; and Filip De Boeck and René Devisch for the opportunity to dig deeper into the history of currencies and wealth in preparation for their conference on money in central Africa, Katholieke Universiteit Leuven, Leuven in 1996. Karen Tranberg Hansen's invitation to write more on domesticity arrived before I went to the field and shaped my research immeasurably. Although substantially reworked via Christmas, humor, and surgery, portions of chapter 3 appeared earlier as "Colonial Fairy Tales and the Knife and Fork Doctrine in the Heart of Africa" in Hansen's anthology, *African Encounters with Domesticity* (Rutgers University Press, 1992). Several paragraphs of my "Letter-Writing, Nursing Men and Bicycles in the Belgian Congo: Notes towards the Social Identity of a Colonial Category" appeared earlier in *Paths toward the Past: African Historical Essays in Honor of Jan Vansina*, edited by Robert Harms et al. (African Studies Association Press, 1994).

Professor Osumaka Likaka of Wayne State University and Matthieu Yangambi of Providence, Rhode Island, made the Lokele text translations possible. Likaka was also a generous friend, comrade, and willing "native" after the fact and by telephone. I owe my Swahili to Magdalena Hauner and Chacha Nyaigotti-Chacha, my Kingwana to Asa Hale and Mama Tula, and my Lokele to the late John Carrington, Likaka, and Mama Tula. Beth Kangas, Moto Moya, Bonnie Ruder, Keith Shear, Rogier Tula, Sarah Womack, and especially Tristine Smart were fabulous research assistants.

A Colonial Lexicon began as a dissertation project at the University of Wisconsin—Madison. Jan Vansina assigned H. Sutton Smith's *Yakusu* in a course, and if he had not, I might never have known about the place. He also wrote me wonderful letters while I was away in strange lands, and by return mail, no less. And when I came back to Madison, he answered all kinds of questions about crocodiles, rainbows, and Belgian nuns, at length and often by phone. He saved me from many an error, led me to countless sources, and let me do what I wanted, at the same time that he told me, astutely, what was problematic and what to do next. I am ever grateful to him, and for his imagination, generosity, and criticisms. Steve Feierman introduced me to symbolic anthropology and sent me on a research chase about birth spacing that led me to this topic. He also helped me design my field research and has been there as an important reader and friend at several critical junctures. Ann Stoler introduced me to the anthropology of colonialism and more recently of Ann Arbor; she told me to publish from day one in Madison and inspired me to write "Le bébé en brousse." Judy Leavitt introduced me to the history of childbirth and obstetrics and made many important suggestions. Harold Cook, David Henige, and Michael Schatzberg were also excellent critical readers of *Negotiated Colonialism*.

Some may know how much I owe them. Quite a few probably do not. Thus my wish for an exhaustive listing here. But I desist, knowing all too well that I will seem to get the order wrong, forget obvious names, never end. My major readers, editors, and critics though, let them be named and blessed. There would quite simply be no book without the readings, comments, and ideas of (and dispatched materials from) Karen Anderson, Mark Auslander, Jennifer Beinart, Bilusa, Tim Burke, Catherine Burns, Barney Cohn, Jean Comaroff, John Comaroff, Guido Convents, Anna Davin, Suzanne Desan, René Devisch, Paul Farmer, Gillian Feeley-Harnik, Bruce Fetter, Deborah Gaitskell, Peter Geschiere, Jonnie Glassman, Donna Guy, Asa Hale, Eugenia Herbert, Douglas Holmes, Sharon Hutchinson, John Janzen, Diana Jeater, Bogumil Jewsiewicki, Deborah Kallman, Ivan Karp, Pier Larson, Michel Lechat, Osumaka Likaka, Helma Lucker, Maryinez Lyons, Janet MacGaffey, Kristen Mann, Achille Mbembe, Henrietta Moore, Mark Nichter, Christine Obbo, Tshonga Onyumbe, Hélène Pagezy, Hermann Rebel, Diane Russell, Meg St. John, Cathy Skidmore-Hess, Carl Strikwerda, Peg Strobel, Jan Thal, Megan Vaughan, Benoît Verhaegen, Luise White, Ann Whitehead, and Aziza Etembala Zana.

For reading and providing comments on the entire manuscript in one of the many versions that became *A Colonial Lexicon,* I am forever grateful to Laura Briggs, Fred Cooper, Joel Howell, Timothy R. B. Johnson, Phyllis Martin, Vinh-Kim Nguyen, Lyn Schumaker, Tristine Smart, Jan Thal, Lynn Thomas, and Jean-Luc Vellut. I could not have done it without them! For reading chapters, I thank David William Cohen, Sue Crane, Joan Dayan, Doug Holmes, Kali Israel, Paul Landau, E. S. Atieno Odhiambo, and David Schoenbrun.

I am also grateful to the three anonymous readers who read the manuscript for Duke University Press; the two who first read this study in its dissertation form brilliantly elucidated the challenges of revising for me and made them seem worthwhile. So, too, did my old friend and generous, patient ally Ken Wissoker, Hyde Park course guide, South Woodlawn coffee brewer, bookstore shopping consultant, latterly turned smashing editor, and video shrine visitor. His suggestions, as always, bolstered and inspired.

David William Cohen asked me a question in an SSRC interview that influenced a fair amount of what I did in the field. I owe thanks to Grey Osterud for her warmth, imagination, generosity, and editing talent; she provided brilliant readings of each chapter and assisted immeasurably with my final revisions. My family was baffled, though ever supportive. Joan Dayan and Jean-Luc Vellut were wonderful readers and remain the dearest of friends.

Huge thanks, then, to all my wry accomplices and kin, colleagues and students, some mentioned by name here, some not. Many more hover in the notes and interview list that follow. The excesses and flaws are mine.

INTRODUCTION

"I know how difficult it is to get hold of native bones, let alone female pelves," a colonial missionary doctor commented in 1938. Dr. Albert Cook had developed a pioneering maternity care program in Uganda with his wife Katharine and, like other doctors practicing in British East Africa, was interested in obstructed labor among African women. A colleague had challenged Cook's view that the high incidence of such obstruction was due to the flat shape of African women's pelvic bones, itself a result of their having carried heavy loads on their heads as children. The argument became an occasion for the two doctors to share stories about their attempts, "fired by anatomical zeal," to dig up African skeletons.

According to Dr. J. P. Mitchell, "an investigation entailing the acquisition of the pelves of women who died from obstructed labour is not easy and takes time." Cook admired Mitchell's success in unearthing five women's pelvises some of which were featured as a photographic frontispiece to the *East African Medical Journal* issue where their exchange was recorded. Dr. Mitchell had carefully supervised the women's burial in and excavation from the Kampala hospital graveyard, and he later acquired seven other women's pelvises for comparative purposes. Yet his colleagues questioned whether the total number of twelve pelvises was scientifically adequate. Dr. R. Y. Stones called for further investigation and more pelvic bones in eugenic terms: "As the nation becomes more advanced it is hoped this most important investigation will be permitted: the more intelligent coming to see it as a necessity for the future welfare of the race."[1]

Dr. Cook recalled his experience during the Nubian Mutiny in 1897, when his "native boy" claimed he was sick to avoid digging up skeletons.

I might have accepted the excuse, but unfortunately for him, I overheard him saying to his friends that if the Mazungu [white man] liked to emulate a hyaena, he would not join in. As we were under military discipline, I laid him down, and gave him a half a dozen of the best for insubordination, and attained my object with the help of a native Christian teacher, and procured an interesting skeleton, but even forty years later it is not an easy thing to do.[2]

This book lies at the juncture of this kind of evidence about colonial violence, medical research, and bodies in Africa. Such a source does not tell us as much as we would like to know about how colonized subjects interpreted the fixations and intrusions of colonial doctors. Yet to treat Cook's anecdote as a discursive representation of colonial disciplining of the body alone would render unintelligible the social action contained in this tale of colonial doctors searching for pelvic bones, an ill domestic servant, and a compliant "native Christian teacher." The harsh economy of colonial power is bared. The servant said he was too sick to dig up the dead, and the doctor whipped him for feigning sickness. Dr. Cook had greater social power, but the insubordinate "native boy" mocked and accused with an animal metaphor expressed behind the doctor's back. Also present in Cook's tale, however, was a "more intelligent" native. This Christian teacher's mediating action remains unclear, as it likely was to Dr. Cook. But the source flags how basic a *middle figure* was to colonial representation and violence; this book argues that such middle figures were also central to processes of translation in a colonial therapeutic economy.

This history seeks to mine such "tales of colonial folly,"[3] while conceding limits as to how far one can read interpretations of the colonized into and out of such an account. It tests these bounds nevertheless, by reading and listening to ethnographic, spoken, and Congolese-authored sources, and by vying with (as with Cook's anecdote) chronic narrative shapes, geographies, and closures in Africanist colonial histories.[4]

This study's central focus is ex-Zaire, the vast central African country formerly known as the Belgian Congo.[5] It, too, had Protestant missionaries among its colonial doctors and safe childbearing among its hygiene goals.[6] The Congo was known as the Congo Free State from 1885 until 1908, an empire evoked by Joseph Conrad in 1899 as the "heart of darkness."[7] This period, when the Congo was King Leopold II's private colony, became notorious for "red rubber," a brutal system of forced rubber collection and severed Congolese hands. When the Belgian parliament assumed control in 1908, the colony became the Belgian Congo. After independence in 1960, the new nation-state was called the Republic (later, the Democratic Republic) of the Congo until 1971, when Mobutu Sese Seko, who assumed power in 1965, changed the name to Zaire. In May 1997, after leading a new generation of rebels in a war that brought down the Mobutu regime, Laurent Kabila, the new head of state, renamed the country the Democratic Republic of Congo.

This study primarily dates from the 1920s, a decade during which medicalization[8] at the British Baptist mission station of Yakusu coincided with colonial panic about depopulation and a falling birthrate in the Belgian Congo at large. Depopulation was central to controversies over the human repercussions of red rubber atrocities and sleeping sickness in Leopold's Free State; by the 1920s, industrial labor requirements ignited a new round of outcries from mining companies and state authorities alike. Yakusu and its environs are the primary setting of this history. George Grenfell and other missionaries of the London-based Baptist Missionary Society (BMS) founded Yakusu on the Upper Congo River, in the Leopoldian land they knew as "Congoland," in 1896. The Free State period in the Upper Congo region was marked by struggle and war among the new colonial military forces and Zanzibari overlords, who initially entered the region in search of ivory and slaves about the time of Henry Morton Stanley's epic journey downriver in 1877. The Zanzibari period resides in local social memory as the first of two colonialisms. Likewise, this history of reproductive idioms and practice begins during this first period of foreign rule. It concludes in the same setting with postcolonial birth routines in 1989–90, and considers them as forms of remembering during a postcolonial period of "scattered hegemonies" in the Congo and beyond.[9]

No sub-Saharan African colonial regime took greater pride in relocating African childbearing to clinical settings than the Belgian Congo. When Raymond Buell toured Africa in 1925, he noted that the state-supported efforts of the Church Missionary Society in Uganda (the Lady Croyndon Training School and rural maternity centers founded by Dr. and Mrs. Cook)[10] "lead the continent in this type of work." Buell also praised maternity care efforts in Tanganyika and French West Africa, and criticized Kenya for its "underdevelopment of maternity work."[11] The Belgian Congo had only just begun to organize maternity care as Buell traveled. He mentioned the colony's midwife training schools and that was all. By 1940, however, Belgian colonial authorities were boasting that the Congo possessed a network of *maternités*, orphanages, and ante- and postnatal clinics that surpassed "in number and importance" those of any other African colony.[12]

In 1935, it was estimated that about 1 percent of Congolese deliveries were medically supervised.[13] By 1952, official claims had increased that figure to 28 percent,[14] and in 1958, the colonial information agency announced that some 43 percent of Congolese babies had been delivered under biomedical supervision.[15] The Belgian Congo had the most extensive medical infrastructure in

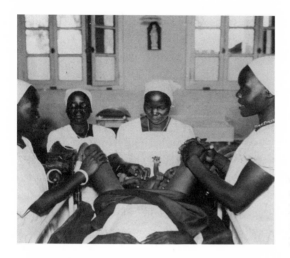

A delivery at an FBEI-constructed maternity, Hôpital Demba, Kasai, 1957. (Courtesy of KADOC, Leuven, Belgium.)

post–World War II Africa. The numbers of medically assisted Congolese births soared from 71,813 in 1947, to 110,000 in 1952, to 189,383 in 1956.[16] A massive program of construction, funded by the parastatal charity Fonds du Bien-Etre Indigène (FBEI), accompanied this postwar expansion. By 1958, every administrative territory, ranging from 50,000 to 150,000 inhabitants each, was equipped with a medical center, a surgical section, a maternity ward, and prenatal and infant welfare facilities.[17]

These numbers suggest the sweep of this Belgian colonial natalism, this reproductive policy intent on increasing the birthrate, hospitalizing deliveries, and reducing neonatal mortality. Yet medicalizing childbirth in the Belgian Congo was never simply about public health, nor was its pronatalism simply about "babies and the state."[18] Colonial employers used Catholic missionary routines to mark birth with bonuses, inscription books, and baby scales, long before there was money to fund the massive construction of maternity wards.[19] Natalist policy began as early as 1903, when a Congo Free State circular authorized territorial chiefs to give rations to pregnant or nursing wives of state workers. In 1910, Province Orientale authorities were exempting fathers of more than four from taxation, and Catholic missionaries in the city of Stanleyville were giving birth bonuses to city families with many children.[20] By 1935, one colonial doctor thought that Congolese women should be made to declare each pregnancy: "given the passivity of the native," he argued, "such a measure would be perfectly applicable."[21] His proposal, though never realized, suggests how desires to increase the birthrate and medicalize motherhood became enmeshed in the growth of bureaucratic state forms and *la paperasserie* of colonized life. The safe childbirth preoccupation was equaled, if not prefigured, by bureaucratic formulas of counting and inscribing birth. In Belgian colonial Africa, maternities and the census went hand in hand.[22]

When I began this study, my purpose was to understand why medicalized motherhood and childbearing became so prominent an agenda in the Belgian Congo. I also wanted to know why Congolese women complied with colonial desires in such great numbers, and *if* they did so with the ease—and, in Foucault's words, the "docile bodies"—that colonial documents imply. For a social and cultural historian of Africa, trained in a period when the shapes of colonial anthropology were laid bare and when bounded African worlds were no more, the question of what the unit of analysis should be was not obvious. The choice of Yakusu began as a likely counterpoint to medicalized maternity for workers' wives as practiced by the Congo's most important mining company, Union Minière du Haut-Katanga.[23] Yakusu, a British Baptist medical mission with a training school for midwives established in 1929, easily proved contrapuntal to this celebrated and aggressive program of imposed medicalization inside mining compounds. Yet Yakusu was not anomalous either, exempt from prevailing

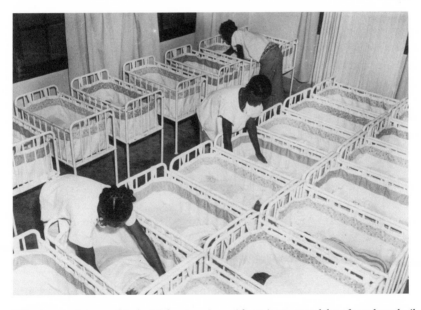

"The large mining and industrial enterprises with an important labor force have built their own hospitals, schools, maternities, etc. A nursery at the maternity of the Fondation Symétain at Kalima," Maniema district, Kivu province. Congopresse caption and photograph by H. Goldstein, ca. 1955. (Courtesy of MRAC, Historical Section [CID no. 72.44/7, inv. no. 56.32.34]. Courtesy of Africa-Museum, Tervuren, Belgium.)

maternalist trends in this Catholic-oriented colony. Yakusu's "foreign," evangelical missionaries invited the signs of Belgian royal favor. Its doctors became officially recognized sanitary agents in a plantation sector of the Upper Congo from the 1920s on, responsible for hygiene surveillance and touring in an area as large as 10,000 square miles. This history demonstrates how the Belgian colonial desire to enumerate and increase its subject population influenced the development of missionary medicine—and obstetrics—in Yakusu's district. In becoming state-associated doctors, Yakusu's medical missionaries became agents of a hygienic form of "indirect rule." (The ambivalence with which colonial authorities let significant powers devolve to these foreign missionaries makes this term accurate, even though it strains conventional definitions of indirect rule in colonial Africa as the necessary, but fraught, intermediary rule of African chiefs or "native authorities.") In turn, Yakusu received substantial subsidies for its medical mission and its doctors' evangelical work. Belgian colonial hygiene was pronatalist, marked by social hygiene movements influential in Belgium and elsewhere at the time.[24] Interwar Catholic social eugenics proved significant in the way maternity care, increasingly the object of colonial perquisites, acquired prominence on this British, Protestant mission station.

This microhistory is intended to contribute to the historiographies of medicine, missions, and gender in the Congo.[25] Yet it would be an error to confine its disclosures to the boundaries of this colony turned nation-state.[26] This study conjoins a Catholic-associated, pronatalist colonial state intent on medical, bodily, and demographic control, a British Baptist mission society engaged in evangelization, and a global profession of specialists in tropical medicine. Yakusu was a pocket of Protestant colonialism set down within a Catholic-oriented, colonial, and increasingly global, public health field. A corollary, a historical ethnography of a state maternity hospital operated by European nuns, is suggested here, even if a full rendering must await another study. Thus this history of the translation of biomedicine within Belgian colonial Africa sits within—as it contains traces of—local, metropolitan, colonial, and denominational frames. Likewise, as a historical ethnography of British Baptist, Belgian, *and* global colonizing processes in and near Yakusu, it is a microhistory of a hybrid colonial situation.

In the 1950s, British social anthropologist J. Clyde Mitchell studied a colonial dance form called *kalela*, developed and performed by Africans living in the mining areas of the Congolese and Rhodesian Copperbelts during the post-World War II period. The presence in kalela of a medical doctor and a "nursing sister" as two of the three character types posing as Europeans (the third was a king) is testimony to how colonial health care became embedded in African social imaginaries. Mitchell saw kalela in 1959 as "a sort of pantomime of the

social structure of the local European community . . . *as the Africans saw it.*"
Terence Ranger read kalela as satire in 1975.[27] In the 1990s, some scholars might
hedge with the word *mimesis,* in order to amplify the ambiguity of these pos-
tures and disrupt any analytic presumptions of defiance. Regardless, kalela
reminds us that how Africans represent(ed) colonial medicine among themselves and perform(ed) it for diverse publics remains a difficult subject to
discern. The way Africans routinely negotiate therapeutic economies within
postcolonial Africa, as they move with their kin among healing possibilities,
is well-known. What is not clear is the historical process whereby colonial-
derived forms of biomedicine may have come to reside, in John Janzen's words,
as a "separate therapy system in public consciousness."[28] A central argument
here is that these processes were mediated by the new colonial categories of
middle figures and the "entangled objects" of their work.[29]

The record shows that Africans have often read colonial doctors, hospitals,
and diseases with sinister metaphors. Influenza in 1918–19 was called "bom-
bom" by many in Tanganyika because the coughing reminded them of cannons
and the epidemic seemed to suggest a divine judgment on Europeans for making war.[30] Africans often used idioms of sorcery, power, and eating. European
medicines were strong yet dangerous because they contained stolen human
blood, they said, and tinned food was made from the bodies of the colonized.[31]
In the Congo, Africans imaged the Yakusu hospital as a tinned food production
site, and female bodies were imbricated within these representations.

Women's health care tended to be either neglected[32] or narrowly defined in
colonial Africa. If mission-organized antenatal care programs "defined women
as producers of Christian babies,"[33] mining companies that pushed obstetric
care on Congolese women defined miners' wives as producers of workers. The
eugenic reductionism of such formulations, though explicit in colonial discourse, warrants careful scrutiny. Some scholars have portrayed colonial maternal health care as a benevolent counterpoint to the coercive medical care
insisted on by colonial states and companies for men. The "devoted, effective, firm, and courteous" work of Protestant-trained midwives, for example,
emerges as an exception within Bernard Hours's ethnography of contemporary
Cameroon; he shows that most popular "representations" of public health since
independence suggest that citizens image the postcolonial state as a vector of
witchcraft, as an "*Etat sorcier.*"[34] Some have asserted that colonial obstetrics was
more readily accepted and actively sought than other forms of biomedical care,
especially among an emergent African middle class.[35] Others have depicted
midwifery programs as evidence of social control.[36] The problem is that arguments anchored in visions of either eugenically motivated social control or a
soft, female exception to the terrors of colonial medicine *conceal* local forms of
meaning-making. We need to know how middle figures and their subaltern

"others"—their "lows"—translated and debated biomedicine in Africa, and what elements were subject to struggle.

Rank among colonized subjects was nuanced and context-specific, malleable and contested; rank collapsed when middles identified as subaltern, aligning themselves with those whom they more often named as their "lows," as un-civilized *basenji*. I prefer the more subjective locution of "lows" (indeed, "their 'lows'"), rather than "subaltern," because it reminds us that claiming middle rank required naming a low. Thus, it suggests the insidiousness of acceding to colonial civilizing hierarchies, since their internalization necessitated their pro-jection; this more subjective term for colonial identity also insists on the sus-ceptibility of these rankings to social upset and transgression.

The gender of medical practitioners affected attendance at maternity clinics in Africa, a continent where nurses tended to be male until after World War II.[37] Age mattered, too. Some Ugandan women actively avoided maternity centers managed by pairs of young, unmarried African women trained in the Cooks' mission-operated school. I doubt that cost and fears of imprecation were the only reasons why.[38] Asking girls to handle the blood of childbirth would have transgressed living rationalities and habitus. In the Anglo-Egyptian Sudan, two British nurses organized a state maternity program for training and certifying midwives, although it appears to have owed its success to their inclusion of older, already practicing midwives and their cautiousness about violating local bodily manners.[39] When Kongo women gave birth to twins in maternity clinics in the lower Congo, twin cult initiates gathered to perform necessary customs.[40] Shambaa peasants demanded midwifery programs from the colonial Tan-ganyikan state in the late 1940s.[41] Yet how colonized men and women inter-preted what went on in maternity clinics affected their eagerness to attend. Some Kaguru men and women refused to have their babies born in Native Authority maternity clinics in Tanganyika because afterbirths were not turned over to the parturient's kin for disposal; they feared hospital attendants might bewitch mother and child.[42] Likewise, the clinic-organized disposal of placentas in Dar es Salaam meant Zaramo women avoided maternity births in this city.[43]

Maternity hospitals and clinics were—and remain—sites of debate and nego-tiation, translation and mistranslation, in Africa. Men and women challenged and transfigured the health care that they received through complex social processes of struggle, bargaining, and compromise. Colonial negotiation was occasionally succinct in time, visible in performance, and distinctly adversarial in form. More often it was less tangible, involving complex social processes of tentative navigation, secrecy and mischief, and theft and laughter. This study attends to how colonial medicine impinged on a *local* therapeutic and political economy in Belgian colonial Africa, and how *local* Congolese in the Yakusu region differentially translated and reshaped the opportunities that colonial

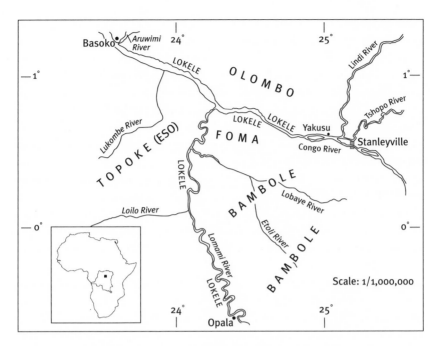

Region of Ya-prefaced villages, indicating river names and colonial-derived ethnic terms. With small map showing location of this map within the Congo and Africa.

medicine offered according to preexisting logic and emerging formulas of authority and prestige.

A word about the word *local*. If a specific ethnic designator is appropriate, I use it. When it is not, I refer collectively to whatever mixture of Lokele, BaMbole, Foma, Olombo, and Topoke (Eso) people is appropriate, after 1885, as "local Congolese" (and from 1966 as "local Zairians"). The expression is not meant as a new euphemism for "the natives" or "*les indigènes.*" Rather, I want to remind readers that there was considerable fluidity and border crossing among these colonial-designated "tribes"; and that they were subjects and citizens of states at least from 1885. Thus, Congolese and then Zairian is more specific, and less colonial in a discursive sense, than African. They also were not just any Congolese; there was historical and cultural specificity to this *local* world, however tangled it became in more global—colonial, national, denominational, and cold war—frames.

Notions of birth and delivery resonate throughout this study. Childbirth, in its literal sense, motivated the original lines of research. It was a logical theme for the Belgian Congo and remains a little-studied topic in African history.[44] As much as medicalization became a form of colony building in the Congo, it became a medium of church building at Yakusu. A key part of the argument concerns the centrality of intimacies and female bodies to imperial violences, fragilities, and chronologies. The Belgian Congo's hygienic modality of colonial power is revealed as distinctly maternalist, enumerative, and positive in its eugenics, unlike other imperial regimes whose sexual and bodily fixations were more obviously directed at eradication, whether to end bodily and genital practices such as *sati* and female circumcision, or to halt signs of colonial degeneration such as miscegenation and venereal disease.[45] The eugenic modality[46] of Belgian colonial power—concentrated on Congolese sexuality, fertility, childbearing, and mothering—influenced the expression of medicalized maternity in Yakusu's district. How this influence happened as social process is central to this study. Thus, we must ask who performed, narrated, and subverted this mixture, how and with what objects, and why. Yet this book argues that powerful cultural representations—signs and narratives—interpolated social process at every turn. It contends that African histories need semiotics as much as they need sociologies. A history of delivery episodes within the mission's maternity ward completes this mode of literary, historical analysis.

To contextualize the significance of these deliveries as routines and transactions, stories and memories, the book's scope is much wider than colonial childbearing and obstetrics alone. A history of mission domesticity proved important in shaping this book. The Baptist missionaries occasionally take center stage. A biblical sense of deliverance animated their undertakings, from daily investments in converts and medical trainees to their renderings of struggles over medicine, healing, and childbearing. Mission domesticity and medicalization were animated by and mediated through local Congolese reproductive codes. Idioms of food, fattening, and fertility were as integral to these mediations as they remain to body disposition and everyday practice in the Yakusu region. In order to bring a history of Congolese *meaning-making* to the core of analysis, the notion of birth work used here embraces the emergence and social reproduction of new colonial middle figures—evangelical teachers, nursing men, and midwives—who were key to the alteration of bodily practice and to the creolization and transcoding that were necessarily involved.[47]

The work entailed in the birth and birthing of these "evolving" (*évoluant*) social actors was simultaneously a method devised from above, a colonial-devised delivery of sorts, and a semiautonomous process of creative expression and brokered negotiations as these men and women labored, bearing new "hybrid" identities. It is through their presentation and performance of (a shared) self, through their writings and recollections, that it is possible to glimpse some of the mediation that was involved. Missionaries often exit from view, therefore, while the larger (and "lower") Congolese populace appears as audience, sometimes adversarial, to this kind of colonial delivery. The source material likewise alternates among missionary literary sources, texts in Lokele authored by Yakusu-trained evangelists and nurses, and memories (whether spoken, told, or shown) collected in Mobutu's Zaire. A tale-telling genre of local social memory suggestive of Congolese popular imagination in the region is central; so are memories inscribed in the landscape and on the body. Each stream of evidence is vital to grasping the Congolese meaning-making that intervened in this history of hygiene and birth work, displacing the linearity of colonial evangelical plans for domesticating and reproducing a Yakusu-centered realm.

Georges Dupré has described colonialism as the destruction of an order. Kwame Anthony Appiah imagines instead "an essentially shallow penetration by the colonizer," noting the enduring "cognitive and moral conceptions" still at play in postcolonial Africa's streets. These ideas are not mutually exclusive, especially if one moves analytically from Appiah's "topology of inside and outside" to a formulation of multiple architectures of morality and imagination. The dismantling of African social, therapeutic, and natalist orders by colonial medicine did not preclude new building and rebuilding, nor did it bar the sometimes concealed labor of colonial syncretisms.[48]

That colonizing processes involved violence and negotiation, dismantling and refiguration, is my premise. That childbirth was an arena of colonial bargaining and strife, translation and mixtures, is a starting point of analysis here, not the conclusion. The central questions concern *the terms* of struggle and negotiation, not only *what* these terms were, not only *how* these terms entered and continue to enter into memory and performance, but *why* these terms were the lexicon of debate. The lexicon was both more capacious and specific than birthing and bodies. I seek a history of moral imagination and "a science of the concrete."[49] I take inspiration from Claude Lévi-Strauss's ideas about historical knowledge and lived practice being rooted in a "logic of the concrete" that works with the "remains and debris of events." It is, he tells us, "a logic whose terms consist of odds and ends left over from psychological or historical processes and are, like these, devoid of necessity." Such a logic produces a "system" that "is always *lived.*" This lived language, in "constantly being drawn in by history," is "a grammar fated to degenerate into a lexicon." It is precisely this transformation of language into lexical "odds and ends," "remains and debris," (of *langue* into *parole*), that I seek to revalue as historical processes of meaning-making, of lexical mischief and debate.[50]

Michel de Certeau provided an important revision of Lévi-Strauss's notion of *bricolage* with his "procedures of everyday creativity" and "making do," while cautioning against a focusing on "lexical units," on "*what* is used, not the *ways* of using.*" He assumed, however, with his emphasis on contemporary consumer consumption, that "*what* is used" is "imposed on everyone by production." Such a formulation falls apart when it meets a colonial context like the Congo, where what is used—the concrete items of a lexicon, of a lived vocabulary and speech of remains and debris—is not necessarily imposed or worker-produced.[51] Indeed, as much as I use the notion of *a lexicon* to focus attention on the social life of objects and their complex cultural entanglements as differentially signifying symbols and commodities in colonial and postcolonial histories, I also retain a sense of *a colonial lexicon* as a vocabulary list open to abstract, bodily, and spiritual phenomena. This lexicon necessarily consisted of words in multiple codes—in Lokele, Swahili, Lingala, French, and English—which were alive as speech in a context of language and colonial power, a context of complex hierarchies and differential translations. Furthermore, I have not forgotten that a lexicon may signify simply a compendium, condensation, or sketch, as all attempts at writing history certainly are.

The lexicon of argument, borrowing, and mixture in the Yakusu region included (and includes) everyday colonial things—such as knives, soap, bicycles, and yaws—as well as elements from an abiding local moral imagination—such as crocodiles, placentas, food, and *fala*. The instant, "parachuted" hierarchies of colonial life assured that access to newer, imported elements was uneven. Such asymmetry was integral to the challenging and refashioning of moralities and imaginations that ensued. Tracing these processes of "colonial mutation,"[52] in part a history of social conflict and negotiation over the meaning and use of these objects, brings to the fore the central action of those subjects who had privileged access to colonial words and things.[53] These authoring subjects, the emerging *évolués* or hybrid middle figures—the teachers, nursing men, and midwives of this study—helped beget a new creolized lexicon in the interwar period in keeping with the concrete, contradictory modernity they imagined as theirs.

The word *hybrid* is used advisedly and in a heterodox manner. Rather than attempting to empty biological meaning out of the term, as some postcolonial theorists in "nonessentialist" desire would have it, the intent here is to garner the natalist connotations of hybrid[54] so as to clarify the metaphorical implications of colonizing projects broadly concerned with parturition and a middle category. The emerging "middles"[55] of Yakusuland, the social category I alternately label as hybrid, were leading translators. As hierarchically distinct readers and writers of colonial syncretisms, they were central midwives of colonial mutations. Yet they could never control the circulation and remaking of the *terms,* neither the concrete objects nor the moral metaphors of an emerging, moving lexicon at play, a local historical process that might be called, following Johannes Fabian, the poetics of colonial lexical borrowing.[56] Thus, as much as there were new hybrid big men (and a few, less big, big women) who authored and transcoded, they were not the only subjects living and performing in translation. Translation was a necessary condition of colonial life, a social practice of one and all.[57]

"Moi, je suis né à la maternité. Mais, toi, tu suis né à la case." I had only arrived in Zaire a few days before and was still in the capital city of Kinshasa when a prominent Zairian newspaper editor shared this verbal jest with me: "*Me*, I was born in a maternity ward. But, *you*, you were born in a hut." "All right, then, Mademoiselle Historian," this postcolonial évolué seemed to challenge at a United States Information Agency–sponsored dinner welcoming me, their Fulbright scholar, to the country. "You have come here to understand who welcomed and who evaded maternity births in the colonial period. Well, then, please tell me why it is, among my friends—Zaire's intellectuals, including historians not unlike you—that we tease each other in these terms?" This verbal taunt is part of a yet-to-be-studied repertoire of rejoinders and jests that belong to the popular verbal culture of the postcolonial Congo's intelligentsia. It suggests a jockeying for prestige through no less conspicuous a Belgian African colonial sign than a maternity ward, a symbol of the reproductive benefits of urban life and hygienic civilities, as these men toy with the meaning, the distinction, of being born in a hospital, rather than in a village onto a banana leaf.

Such jockeying has a history. Consider the words of an évolué in 1950, printed in a widely circulated Congolese journal of the time: "We must no longer tolerate the attitude of certain of our compatriots who prefer to give birth on the ground while our cities are endowed with maternity wards equipped with all modern scientific equipment."[58] Maternity wards joined bicycles and sewing machines as markers of social class, as the signs of rising, middle status in Belgian colonial Africa. This postcolonial quip suggests the continuing salience of maternity ward as metaphor late into Mobutu's regime, even as it poses questions about how to filter history through a knowledge of social practice and memory gained during a research period in postcolonial Zaire, in Mobutu's land.

Soon after this dinner, I left Kinshasa's offices for my field sites on the Upper Congo River, finding an odd mixture of remnants from Baptist mission domesticity, Zairian "authenticity," and colonial hygiene installations. (Mobutu decreed "authenticity" as an integral part of state party policy and national identity in 1973. *Authenticité* dictated that men should no longer wear Western suits and ties, women should no longer wear miniskirts and trousers, and all Euro-

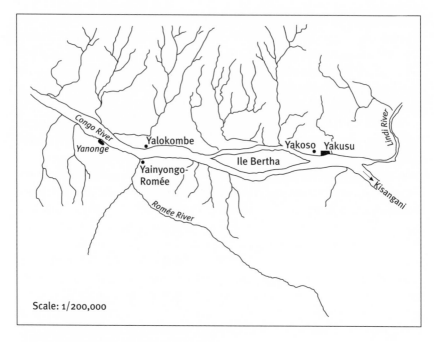

Area of field research along the Congo River.

pean or Christian names should be replaced by "authentic," Congolese ones.)
At first I lived at Yakusu, in a brick house of former English midwife missionaries. Eventually, I settled for five months in a small, remote riverain village
where popular midwifery was still active. During my first weeks in the Upper
Congo, I made a tour with two Zairian male nurses, a Scottish missionary
nurse-midwife, and the Land Rover driver. All worked at the Yakusu hospital.
We visited rural health dispensaries established by this Baptist mission in the
1920s. They were still operating as church-affiliated rural health centers, though
they had been recently incorporated into a primary health care scheme known
as Santé Rurale or Projet des Soins de Santé Primaires en Milieu Rural (SANRU),
which was centered in Kinshasa. We journeyed for about ten days, through the
forest by Land Rover and along the river by canoe, visiting over half a dozen
such health centers and staying in the homes of Zairian Baptist pastors. I took
in hand-embroidered doilies on chairs and old, military-uniformed, pre-
"authenticity" Mobutu photographs hung on walls.

An ecstatic line of ululating women greeted the Land Rover of nurses along
the road as we approached one Topoke (Eso) village. At most stops, greetings
were more muted, sometimes uninterested. In most locations, church women

fed us fine meals of turtle or monkey or antelope. I discovered that these hygiene tours were also a postal delivery service. Suddenly, the driver would stop in a village and hand over letters, or we would be stopped on the road to collect more. There was a large pile of mail by the time we returned to Yakusu. The driver and nurses bought forest products as we traveled, staple crops found more cheaply away from the city and forest meats, foods so difficult to obtain back at Yakusu that they were delicacies there. Meanwhile, serious, dedicated work went on as these Yakusu nurses met with local nurses and church health committees, inspected account books, sold drugs, and held clinic sessions for referral cases. Often the meetings were after dark by lantern light. Discussion could be heated, with loud voices interjected by laughter. Real issues were being decided: the salary of a health center nurse, the cost of drugs, whether a dispensary could purchase one or two thermometers when there were only four available for eight dispensaries. People were working out appropriate relations among the village church, dispensary, and nurse, and the Yakusu-centered SANRU zone in an era of self-financing produced by structural adjustment–inspired public health schemes emanating from Kinshasa, Washington, D.C., and Geneva.

The witty nurse who specialized in eye cases offered a running commentary as we traveled. A young Lokele man born on the Lomami River, he had come to the Yakusu mission for all his schooling. He had never left. His specialization meant that he had a ready, waiting clientele in the villages through which we passed. "Things are not stolen in Zaire," he announced one day, "they are displaced." Another day, he asked if I knew that bicycles in Zaire usually have no brakes, and explained that the people riding them are not afraid.

One day, we drove from Bandu, passing ex-Elisabetha first, an old Lever Company site of urban, "extra-customary" tawdriness where there were contemporary popular paintings, an old Mobutu official pose, and Zairian agricultural promotions hung up as knickknacks on the wall. We left this less composed, more nationalist, entrepreneurial "authenticity" for Lingungu. It was about a sixty-kilometer ride through thick Topoke forest. There were few villages and a long stretch of horrific road. We slid dangerously in and out of holes and mud, and over an old wooden bridge across a large flowing stream. Then we had to walk across the bridge, positioning the few remaining loose wooden slats to fit the width of the Land Rover's tires. A twenty-minute downpour coincided with some perilous, frantic accelerating through mud and water. Further on it was dry again. There were few people on foot as we drove along, although occasionally there were cyclists or women with heavy loads hanging on their backs from their strapped, bent heads. A well-dressed man came along, all in black. He wore a muted Mobutu suit or *abacost*[59] and leather shoes, and

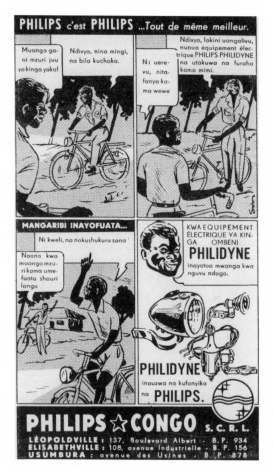

A typical bicycle advertisement of the 1950s in cartoon form from Philips Congo. From *Nos Images,* Sw. ed., 1955. (Courtesy of the Bibliothèque Royale, Brussels, Belgium.)

had a black briefcase in hand. He, too, had reason to traverse the forest. No one in the Land Rover seemed to see any incongruity in his walking along this broken road in Mobutu's land. How to understand what in my eyes seemed an oddity, I wondered, the out-of-sorts manufactured "authenticity," the abacost-suited, briefcased "big man" with no wheels on these spent roads, but obviously with somewhere to go? I did not know at the time to ask why this postcolonial "big man" was not riding a bicycle.

Except for the few occasions when I boarded a missionary or planter's Land Rover, such was my own means of transport in Upper Zaire. I also walked plenty and moved by canoe, and when I was ready to move away from mission life, I put my bicycle in a canoe and headed about fifteen miles downriver to a remote village, inaccessible by car. Bicycles became a theme of my stay in the village as they were in the semiotics of colonial life.[60] Old men would tell me how they used to own bicycles. There were even two or three per household, they would say. The subject of bicycles evoked nostalgia and regret for the good times of late colonialism, when imported objects had been abundant and many village men had been wage laborers, especially for a rubber plantation company called Belgika. The want of bicycles was the best way to illustrate to a white lady researcher, never mind local youth who could not remember the days of many bicycles,[61] the deprivation and hunger of today.

Although Yainyongo-Romée, the village where I was settled, was sited on a river, most of the people lived by what they produced from the forest. Most identified themselves as "BaMbole," the Mbole people.[62] The prefix *ba-* signifies a plural personal pronoun; I retain it to preserve the flavor of local speech forms and code mixing, as in "*ba-missionaires*" ("the missionaries") or "Ba-Stanley" (Belgian colonials). The village residents are farmers and trappers who also mud-fished in low-lying streams, harvested palm trees for oil, and gathered caterpillars, mushrooms, herbs, forest vines, and medicines. A few households had many oil palms. A few self-identified as Lokele and relied more on fishing as a livelihood. Whether oil palms or a canoe and nets were their capital,

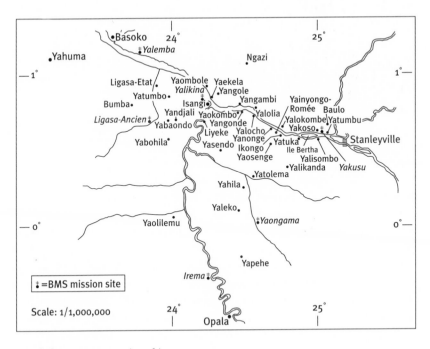

Local place-names mentioned in text.

these two kinds of households tended to be better off than the rest; they had something substantial to sell. There are fruit trees in the area, many likely planted by the Zanzibari-associated traders who had once lived there. Occasionally, women would have enough tangerines or avocados to fill a few baskets and find a space in a canoe heading upriver to the Kisangani market, a good day's distance away. Filling a canoe full of forest rope (used for house construction) or cassava was another activity, not likely to be achieved more than twice a year. Only two items considered essential required cash: soap and salt. Most people most of the time were subsisting by farming, trapping, gathering, and pressing palm oil, infrequently buying a little fish.

My second day living in Yainyongo-Roméé, I noted the presence of a bicycle: "The nurse from a SANRU post just passed with his Red Cross helper, his scale, and *kilo*[63] record book strapped to the back of his bicycle. They had been to a nearby village today for their monthly kilo there." Since arriving in the Yakusu district, I had been located in what United States Agency for International Development (USAID) officers in Kinshasa called a SANRU primary health care zone. SANRU was a USAID-sponsored Primary Rural Health Care Project created in 1981 in conjunction with the Zairian government and the Protestant Church (ECZ) of Zaire. When SANRU officers discussed the accomplishments of their sixty-seven rural health zones, they emphasized "safe motherhood" initiatives.[64] "Health for all in Zaire" was the going SANRU slogan, encoded in promotional literature with an image of a male nurse holding a baby. Alternatively, another slogan on SANRU document covers—"All forward toward health for all"—accompanied an image of a group of people walking up a hill and passing by a rural dispensary as they moved toward the year 2000. The walkers included a Mobutiste party man in "authenticity" dress bearing the same party torch, as well as international aid representatives, Zairians pushing bicycles, abacost-suited big men bearing walking sticks, academicians wearing cap and gown, and pregnant women. The Zairian map had been divided into 306 health zones, and a typical zone was supposed to comprise 100,000 people and 20 health centers. SANRU diagrams showed how such an ideal primary health care zone was to operate with arrows linking a central reference hospital, satellite health centers, rural village health development committees, and retooled "traditional birth attendants" (TBAS).[65]

An early inkling that there was something off-kilter with these neat SANRU diagrams came quickly, during some of my first visits to villages within the Yakusu "zone." I stayed, for example, in one village with an old colonial health center building and maternity ward, still bearing a colonial Fonds du Bien-Etre Indigène plaque, though operating in 1989 as a SANRU center. One midwife, who local people named with the French word *accoucheuse,* told me about her

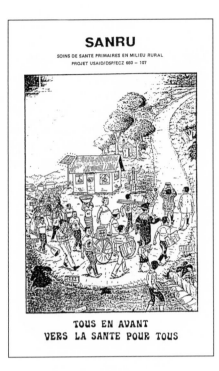

SANRU

SOINS DE SANTE PRIMAIRES EN MILIEU RURAL
PROJET USAID/DSP/ECZ 660 – 107

TOUS EN AVANT
VERS LA SANTE POUR TOUS

"Tous en avant vers la santé pour tous"
(All forward toward health for all).
SANRU graphic. From a SANRU
brochure, Kinshasa, ca. 1989.

work in the SANRU maternity ward. She was delivering about four babies a month at the time. Many more were being born, she told me. Another midwife, referenced by the Lokele word *mbotesa* (popular midwives with no clinical or TBA training), came around as I talked with this accoucheuse. The mbotesa said that she no longer practiced her craft. The accoucheuse indicated that sometimes people were fined for giving birth outside the dispensary. Yet it was not clear who, nor by whom. At one point she said it was "people of the state," but she didn't know precisely who. "Yes, it was soldiers," she later said. She also said that a health center birth cost 800 zaires; a "difficult" birth (involving an episiotomy or prolonged labor) cost 1,200 zaires. But if a woman gave birth at home and came for a birth certificate afterward, it cost 500 zaires (about one dollar at the time). She was troubled that women did not give birth at the dispensary, where her husband also worked as a nurse. Later, when the accoucheuse was not around, the mbotesa whispered to me about "state troubles." She said that it was the dispensary nurse who had told her threateningly that she should not assist women in childbirth anymore. It took away his money, the mbotesa explained. She was worried that the nurse would cause trouble, and then *l'Etat*—"the state"—would, too. "Soldiers will come and lock

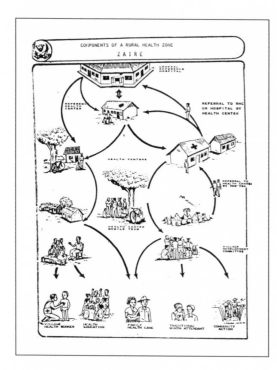

"Components of a Rural Health Zone, Zaire." SANRU graphic, 1985. Note the bicycles. From USAID, *Santé pour tous: SANRU II, Projets de Soins de Santé Primaires en Milieu Rural*, 11.

her up," another woman explained. I wanted to know: "When had these troubles begun? How many years ago?" The mbotesa asked the local pastor's wife a question. The answer came back first in years, the number of years since independence in 1960. But there was also reference to the word *vita*, suggesting that the tumultuous Simba rebellion period of 1964–66 known locally as the "war" would be a significant chronological marker in a history of this "second economy" of public health care that was emerging before my eyes.[66]

Studying postcolonial objects and routines became as integral to my historical field method as collecting postcolonial words. The postcolonial testimony I collected in the field—primarily in Yainyongo-Romée, although also in Yakoso, Yakusu, and Kisangani—alternated between statements like, "I went to give birth at the hospital because otherwise they would have fined my husband or thrown him in jail," and "I went because it was a holiday with beds, and they gave my baby clothes and soap." The first kind of statement, when elaborated, includes a cluster of ideas about coercive forms of state power and the need to give birth in a hospital in order to have the newborn inscribed in the identity book of the father. The second statement was not easily unpacked from the kind of postcolonial nostalgia that my presence tended to elicit about the sorely missed time when state and mission hospitals provided health care, often free, and gave away clothes, food, and soap. The contradictions in postcolonial testimony and the ironies in postcolonial routine need to be seen in terms of how colonial subjects ascribed meaning to papers, among other objects, and how they translated and continue to negotiate a mixed social reality of coercive and alluring messages.

My research began with simple questions. Who is giving birth where, and why? Yet the questions yielded convoluted itineraries quite at odds with the SANRU image of the harmonious state promoting health for all through simple circuits linking village committees and village-based "traditional birth attendants" to reference hospitals. In the village fifteen miles downriver from Yakusu, where I went to live, women tended to give birth at home with mbotesa; the woman would thank her midwife with a bar of soap, and her husband would cross the river to purchase a birth certificate under-the-table from the male nurse who operated a local rural health center. This postcolonial routine not only suggested a flourishing informal economy in birthing;[67] it also raised questions about the concrete colonial elements embedded in these routines. By tracing the same objects among the concreteness and vagaries of European- and Congolese-authored literary sources, this study highlights the social lives of things, and the contradictions and ironies of postcolonial Zairian memory and practice.

Distance was one factor in this local decision making. To reach a health facility from Yainyongo-Romée in 1989, people had to either cross the river in a canoe to Yalokombe or walk through the forest to Yanonge. Either journey took about an hour. The availability of birth certificates by postpartum purchase was another factor. In many rural health centers and urban clinics, it was possible to quietly buy birth certificates from hospital staff. The historical shards embedded in these routines were colonial elements—soap and papers—and these objects and the paths by which they circulated guided this study. What people *do* and the objects and commodities that people *use* have been privileged as much as, if not more than, what people *voice* and *recall*. As Michel de Certeau tells us, the "creativity" in practices of consumption and appropriation tend to flourish "at the very point where practice ceases to have its own language."[68] Birth certificates and soap remain key lexemes in local practice surrounding fertility, childbearing, and bodily flow.[69] Tracing these objects and procedures within the colonial record as well as postcolonial memory and practice imparts a sense of how Congolese continue to consume and digest their mired history.

Hygiene, hospital life, and birth work at Yakusu disclose the numerous relations of asymmetry that coexisted within a colonial culture, yielding the sociological complexity and multiple mixtures of a colonial situation. Asymmetry existed not only among "white helmets and black skins,"[70] but also along national, religious, ethnic, generational, and gender lines. Many who lived in and near Yakusu figure in the story: doctors, midwives, and ritual specialists, Baptist evangelists and Catholic state agents and planters, and Congolese river (Lokele) and forest (BaMbole) peoples—some Christian, and many not.[71]

This book draws on European archives and literary sources, especially British Baptist missionary articles and letters, though colonial novels, memoirs, cartoons, didactic literature, and photographs were mined, too. The interpretation of these sources is based on knowledge and interview data gained during a fourteen-month period of fieldwork in and near Yakusu in 1989–90. I divided my time between Yakusu and the remote riverain village of Yainyongo-Romée of some thirty-five households where popular midwifery remained active. I lived there, as the chief told me I should, in the home of the oldest person in the village. Tata Alikuwa once worked as a Yakusu teacher and was still clutching his ragged Lokele Bible from time to time. I did not wear a helmet or sell Bibles, but sometimes it seemed that I might as well have. I did bandage some wounds, distribute some aspirin, and give and receive gifts. Zairians constructed me alternately as their latest colonial patron, redeemer, and taskmaster, as their most recent Mademoiselle, mosquito net and papers in tow. These constructions were not incorrect, even if some of the village residents also incorporated me as their *lichecha:* their special, protected, pampered child. My bicycle, questions, and laughter occasionally jarred expectations, yet jarring was not my method. A good part of my method became to study how I—in their eyes, through their categories, and by my presence and gestures—reenacted as I evoked memories of the colonial, becoming a part of, as I played a part within, the complex social field I was trying to study. Didn't my arrival in this village with tape recorder, cassettes, Lux soap, and batteries galore represent some latest twist on global cultural flows?[72] The more I attended to the politics and meaning of my work in a postcolonial era of United States Information Agency (USIA)-sponsored research, in a USAID-sponsored public health setting, the more I understood the urgency for a history of the continuing formation—and deformation—of abiding local categories.

If the objects, words, and performances of this postcolonial present became important, so did the representations and routines of my textual sources. So, too, did my postfield realization that Christmas, as described in missionary writings and performed in Mobutu's Zaire, offered a parallel performance of domesticity and missionization in which were imbricated the same kinds of objects and performances I had begun studying as hygiene and childbearing. Perhaps no ritual was more socially reproductive of colonial evangelism and domesticity, and open to colonial "hybridization" (in both the Bakhtinian and postcolonial senses of the word), than this holiday celebrating the birth of Christ. Yet Christmas was not just emblematic of colonized domesticity. Like hospital childbearing, this special day was a routine, if shifting, performance, and embedded within it were things. Tracking Christmas as history and ritual meant simultaneously tracing the ingredients of soap and baby clothes and the colonial evangelical transaction of gift giving through time, from the Christmas presents that missionaries gave to their domestic servants in the early-twentieth century, to the wide-scale Christmas distribution of soap to baby clinic–attending mothers in the 1950s, to Christmas as debris in 1989.

The discovery of the oral virtually *as* African history in the 1950s translated into a disparagement of European sources until the 1980s, when they were revalued as "discourse." I have tried to disrupt the unspoken Africanist episte-mology of colonial historical methodologies, which I condense with the phrase, "to Africa for voices, to Europe for texts." This logic took me to Europe to read what the Congo's "colonizers" had written and to Africa to listen to (and tape-record) the "postcolonized" speak. But I soon sensed that it might be fruitful to mix up continental contributions with source material in new ways.[73] After my "fieldwork" proper, I spent six weeks in England tracking down the spoken words of "postmissionaries" as forms of remembering, followed by a summer and then some at taking in Lokele-language texts written by some of Yakusu's middle figures. As a result of these mixtures, I treat missionary texts as in-scribed forms of oral tradition and use postcolonial routines as historical evi-dence. I have also labored over the concrete objects mentioned in missionary sources in order to reconstruct chronological series of episodes, objects, and uses, and thus, changes in the representations contained and transactions re-ported in these dated, minutiae-filled texts. Finally, this book argues that oral evidence should not be flattened by transcription, but heard and rendered as complex performances marked in significant ways by the concrete historical research situations under which they were collected.

I once imagined this as a study of "negotiated colonialism." I still draw on the term *negotiation* in the classic sense of adversarial parties bargaining over con-tested ground, of mediation, arbitration, and sometimes even compromise. And I still invite a processual, performative connotation for negotiating—as in traveling, making a turn, veering—as is appropriate for rendering a situation of everyday "making do" with its uncontainable meanings, chronic misunder-standings, and laughter. Both dimensions remain important for a historical ethnography of a colonial situation. The term *middles* took me to translation, even though middles proved as multiple as the languages and codes used by "lows," translation being the domain of none alone. In the end, I aim to show that neither negotiation nor translation are over or complete, even though both know bounds. Local Zairians continued to use and rework colonial elements every day, even while they mediated and mocked my queries. The result is not a seamless narrative or single story. This is not an epic of *colonial encounter.* Rather, the method is to attend to *multiple* and *sequential* meetings from a (post)colonial situation as transactions, exchanges, routines, yet to mine them as lived tales and suggestive fables, with all the import and concreteness of social action, improvisation, and fanciful vision that such mining implies.

A Colonial Lexicon begins with a history of crocodile medicines and a male reproductive ritual known as *libeli,* and the challenges to mission practice and medicalization at Yakusu that were expressed in its performance. This two-chapter segment situates the historical and cultural context into which the missionaries inserted themselves and out of which the first generations of Baptist Congolese middle figures negotiated their emergence as initiated men and mission "boys." Gender and reproduction were prominent themes to libeli and the historical struggles that were central to its timing. These chapters argue that a study of colonial medicine and childbearing at Yakusu from the 1920s cannot be separated out from earlier conflicts over wealth, violence, and thera-peutic practice in the Zanzibari and Free State periods. The first chapter, "Croc-odiles and Wealth," concerns libeli and crocodiles as history and memory prior to the 1920s. It probes the importance of water spirits, crocodiles, and iron monies among the Ya-lancers of this region; the domestication of local idioms by the Zanzibari traders and planters who arrived in the 1870s; the chronologi-cal and visceral memories of these "BaTambatamba," who bathed with croco-diles, and ate, cut, and enslaved men and women; and the complex rivalries over wealth and erasures of red rubber cruelties in this British Baptist, "free zone" border region of the Congo Free State. The second chapter, "Doctors and Airplanes," continues this history of the Yakusu church; it explores its newly medicalized complicities with the Belgian Congo regime from the 1920s, and the work of translation and negotiation of its evangelical teachers and nurses. Conflicts over libeli in 1924 are considered in light of the new medical and communication technologies of the interwar period: letter writing, sleeping sickness research, yaws injections, surgery, and missionary-organized croco-dile killing.

These first two chapters comprise a single segment of analysis, framed by a 1934 popular metaphor comparing human-killing crocodiles with airplanes. Missionary "boy" paradigms insinuate their way into this exegesis of a local lexical pairing. But evangelical domesticity proper—that is, idealized mission-ary framings of middle or "boy" figures—is reserved for the third chapter, "Dining and Surgery." Yakusu was not an isolated foreign mission station, peripheral to the interests of the colonial state. Nor were the intermittent visits by Belgian royals inconsequential to the formation of a British Baptist imaginary of everyday colonial life. Chapter 3 elaborates the mission setting of Yakusu, and contends that colonial hygiene was mixed up with domesticity in complex ways. The chapter explores the career trajectories of Yakusu-trained Congolese Baptists; the organization of domestic and nursing labor on the mission station; and the gender asymmetries of "boy" careers. The contradictions and paradoxes of these asymmetrical "boy" framings are explored in missionary humor, colonial evangelical origin parables, topsy-turvy Christmas festivities, and "boy" memories.

"Dining and Surgery" owes its title to the efficacy of the missionary "boy" paradigm: domestic "boys" indeed became surgical assistants at Yakusu. But the chapter's title also flags a popular pairing about the eating and cutting activities of colonizing Europeans. Chapter 4 takes up this dining = surgery metaphor by examining a popular genre of cannibal-autopsy tales known as *tokwakwa* in relation to histories and memories of colonial violence and medicalization during the interwar period. It details the growth of a network of rural health dispensaries overseen by the Yakusu medical mission and operated by its Congolese nurses, and demonstrates the development of strong ties among Yakusu's British Baptist medical missionaries, state medical authorities, and the plantation companies in the district. The chapter draws on two distinctive sources—the printed Lokele-language letters of Congolese mission evangelists and tokwakwa tales—to consider the social effects of colonial medicine as it combined with new forms of a fast, mobile modernity during these critical interwar decades. Finally, "Nurses and Bicycles" introduces a counterpoint to the pervasive dining = surgery analysis of medicalization, mobility, and colonial rule; all Congolese were privy to this diagnosis, I argue, but middles also had access to dreams about heroic surgery and the vocation's seductive and style-setting objects: bicycles.

Thus, if the first pair of chapters consider crocodiles = airplanes and the second pair probe dining = surgery, chapters 5 and 6 also comprise a pair. A third pair about a third pair they are, and this local pairing is birth = death. This pair begins with a history of midwifery and childbearing at Yakusu; "Babies and Forceps" explores social and cultural obstacles, bodily troubles, and embodied memories surrounding medicalized childbirth at Yakusu. "Colonial Maternities" (chapter 6) considers the birth ritual at Yakusu within a series of larger natalist frames—global, Belgian, and Belgian African—before turning to Protestant, Catholic, and Belgian colonial medical cultures and their implications for local Congolese natalist practice in Yakusu's district in the post–World War II period. Medicalized childbearing was never irrevocably imposed, yet it had unforeseen consequences on local fertility and birthing practices. Colonial obstetrics began in the Congo with Congolese men and women who sought help in emergencies. Yet as maternity care became an important colonywide objective in the 1930s and a colonywide reality in the 1950s, it increasingly embraced efforts to count numbers of births and reward those taking place in clinical settings.

The final pair of chapters extend the meanings of the three local metaphors that frame the histories and vocabularies of *A Colonial Lexicon*. "Debris" moves forward in time to 1989–90; it is an extended exegesis of leftover colonial objects and their procedures of consumption within birth routines as practiced in postcolonial, post-Simba Upper Zaire. "Departures" is a mixture of conclusion and exit points, recollections and farewells. Birth may be death, but whether diagnosis or passage, this process is and always will be storied. "Departures," therefore, diagnoses a lexicon and passes in stories, too.

1 CROCODILES AND WEALTH

Crocodiles had "for many months been taking steady toll of men, women, and children" on the Upper Congo River not far from Yakusu. Dr. C. C. Chesterman described the terror in the *Yakusu Quarterly Notes* (*YQN*) in October 1933: "Never in living memory have attacks been so frequent and escapes so few." The crocodile killings suggested "special interventions of Providence," he added. Some rumored that somebody had "engaged the brutes in his service" to seize the Lokele from their canoes. Others thought that "large sums of money have been collected and offered and accepted in order to buy off this malevolence." One day, the hospital's hunter, Lofoli, shot one of these crocodiles, and its skin was mounted at the hospital "as a trophy and a nine days wonder for the curious." Local Congolese nicknamed the crocodile *Avion*. There was a historical specificity to this moral metaphor comparing an airplane with a human-eating water creature. Chesterman sensed the significance of this connection: he teased that local people were "putting two and two together and making five as usual," pointing out that the "saurian supremacy" coincided with the first routine schedule of flights to the nearby city of Stanleyville.[1]

The crocodile attacks continued, and Chesterman sought more trophies. The next time that the doctor went out on medical tour by boat along the Congo River, he added Lofoli to the party. They were about sixty miles downriver from Yakusu and opposite Yaokombo, a BMS chapel and dispensary site, where a Yakusu-trained nurse called Likenyule worked, when Lofoli shot another crocodile. Yakusu's senior missionary woman, Edith Millman, reported the incident in a private letter: "A big, fierce man-eating crocodile has been picking off men, boys, women, and girls. Our hunter went down and shot it. Great rejoicing. Sixty miles away from us, but these people are our neighbors."[2] The triumphant party was greeted by "surging, dancing crowds," echoed Chesterman. He had the dead creature towed to Yaokombo. The next day was Sunday, and one reward for Dr. Chesterman's new trophy was an extra-crowded, open-air service where he read the names of the twenty-two crocodile victims who had died: "No need to ring the Church bell. From up and down and across the river and from the forest towns they came to mock, and stayed to pray." That evening, there seemed to be little question about who owned the crocodile. The gun had been the doctor's, and he sold off the meat. The butchering, however, was not so simple. When some men gathered to cut up the meat, Chesterman observed: "The butcher band hesitated at the water's edge, itching to get at the meat, yet fearing the penalty, till an old wizened fellow stepped forward. 'I am nearly in the grave' he said. 'What matter if I get it?'" What was "it," this "penalty" to which Chesterman referred? It was fala. Yet the doctor did not write this Lokele word. He translated for his British readers instead: "there lurks the fear of a mutilating disease (tertiary yaws) from contact with the crocodile."[3]

In 1934, the Yakusu mission was over forty years old, the Yakusu church about thirty years old, and the Yakusu medical school and hospital some ten. I begin amid mission history, therefore, with this complex bundle of transactions that Dr. Chesterman narrated as a baffling, enchanting story about the meaning of crocodiles. Chesterman, like all Yakusu missionaries, would have read "Lest We Should Waddle," an early conversation between a Yakusu missionary and a man called Saili, which was prominently interposed in H. Sutton Smith's circa 1911 book, *Yakusu, the Very Heart of Africa.*

"What are they doing there?"

"Buying meat, white man."

"What meat, Saili?"

"Crocodile's meat."

"Where did they get it from?"

"Oh, the owner of the hut there caught it in the night up the Lindi."

"Oh, let me see the head, Saili?"

"No, you can't see that."

"Why not?"

"Because it is all covered up."

"Well, you can uncover it to show it to me."

"No, we daren't do that, for if its eye sees us we are afraid that our legs will get like the crocodile's, and we shall all waddle."

"Well, what will you do with it?"

"Oh, when all the flesh is sold the man who found it will call all his friends round and he will provide plantain and fish, and we shall have a feast."

"But what about the crocodile's head?"

"Oh, that is put in a big pot and boiled, and boiled; then it is ground into a powder, and when a man is caught stealing or doing anything of that kind, he has to take some of this medicine to prove by the result whether he is the culprit or not."

"And does nothing happen to those who eat the flesh?"

"No, because during the feast the man who found it goes round with a twig in his hand, and strikes with it the arms and legs of his friends so that they may not get bandy-legged."[4]

This conversation suggests that a specific event with implications for wealth and knowledge—the killing of a crocodile—prompted a ritual of medicine making, feasting, and flagellation. It also explains the ambivalent character of crocodiles, menacing yet necessary for poison-ordeal medicines. The poison used in such judicial procedures would derive its capacity to discern and judge from its consecrated character, its very derivation in spirit substance. The substance, in this Lokele case, was pulverized crocodile head. The conversation might well be an early rendition of a libeli-associated feast, translated into innocent, cryptic language for one of Yakusu's first missionaries. Crocodiles were also important in libeli medicines; after being in the forest for a week, initiates would have a mixture of medicines called *bote* rubbed into incisions in their backs. Bote consisted of crocodile bones, along with several kinds of lizards, millipedes, and a snakelike creature called *litutandiya*, which means water spirit.[5]

Nothing disturbed Yakusu's missionaries more than the supposed flagellation, sumptuous feasting, and deceit of libeli.[6] A dramatic series of events in the life of a village and often a district, libeli lasted for three or four months as male youth learned a secret language, took special oaths, and became scarred with special medicines. Libeli was simultaneously a rite of male initiation, social reproduction, and healing, a rite of composition and recomposition of—perhaps even alienation from—wealth. Adolescent boys, their already initiated male guides—known in Lokele as "mothers"—and elders withdrew into a small forest rich in medicinal plants for traumatic bodily trials, gestures of giving wealth to ancestral spirits, and fattening feasts. Symbolic replication was intricately reproductive in imagery, as men and boys metaphorically mimed phases of childbearing and female seclusion. In its ritual form and vocabulary, libeli simulated female reproduction and the dangers of childbearing. Yakusu's missionaries reductively regarded it as a masculine farce to deceive women. They were quick to notice that women were imaged as sources of pollution during libeli, but were also used as food producers and cooks. Libeli also involved composing, distributing, and consuming food and other goods of wealth.[7]

Bodily flagellation and scarring during libeli transmitted authority to invoke its power in word and gesture, in missionary words, to pop *lilwa*. This menacing, cursing movement of the hand and arm, like the gash on the back that conferred the right to make this aural, piercing gesture, was an expression of cutting lilwa.[8]

Embedded in the English doctor's published account—and in a letter published by Yaokombo's nurse, Likenyule—was an anonymous, elliptical refrain, compendious of popular moral review, equating crocodiles with airplanes. Some complex understanding of the mischief of colonial magic and terror, of what Michael Taussig has called "magical mimesis on the colonial frontier,"[9] inhered in this metaphor. The coupling compared new human-controlled crocodiles or *ndimo*—murdering men transformed into crocodiles—with the new, equally lethal rainbows of the skies, airplanes. This was, after all, a Congolese world of leopard-men and crocodile-men,[10] a world where people made power and won battles through magic and feasting, through poisoning stomachs and blocking wombs, and through killing and making medicines from body parts. Was the killing of a crocodile intended to kill an enemy ndimo and make medicines from his body? This seems likely. Certain is the fact that Chesterman's quest was to prove that the crocodile was just a crocodile, not a sorcerer's agent metamorphosed into one.

Chesterman's goal was not only to kill the "real" crocodile, but also to slay fala and libeli beliefs. His logic of surgery and surrogacy, of cutting out malignancies and inserting substitutes (such as church services and yaws injections), was mechanical. He wished to kill the demon of "superstition," and replace it with Christianity and medicine. Such brittle formulations survive only if we imagine this history as a colonial encounter of Europe confronting Africa, "moderns" confronting "traditionals." It is not enough to reverse these terms to say that the colonized confronted their colonizers. Congolese drew on a repertoire of metaphors and practices in flexible, creative, and differential ways. They asserted their control, at least symbolically, over the objects that these new colonizers carried—papers, monies, airplanes, shots—as they forged relationships that served them in their new situations. Colonialism also produced violence, conflict, and excess; its multiple translators often struggled over their ingredients and their meanings.

Chesterman's narrow surgical formula of the-doc-kills-the-croc has a violent history in BMS–Free State complicities and erasures. His narrative is not unrelated to what has become an iconic site of imperial lies, of brutes exterminating so-called brutes in the name of civilization, of colonial racist and sexual fantasies gone mad in darkness. Nowhere perhaps illustrates better than King Leopold's Congo Free State what Taussig has termed a "colonial mirror of production," that is, "the mimicry by the colonizer of the savagery imputed to the savage." Henry Morton Stanley and King Leopold's lie of a Free State, this quintessential colonial negativity, produced—and was reproduced in—Joseph Conrad's *Heart of Darkness*, E. D. Morel's *Red Rubber*, and Roger Casement's beleaguered diary entries: "Poor frail, self-seeking vexed mortality dust to dust—ashes to ashes—where then are the kindly heart the pitiless thought together vanished."[11] It was also produced and reproduced in and near Yakusu's district, boosting the missionary premium put on enchanting stories.

"Red rubber" and the bodily violences that accompanied it certainly cried out for cults of healing, yet we must not romanticize libeli, either as the reproduction of tradition or as colonial rebellion. Similarly, we cannot romanticize nonmedicalized, nonhospitalized childbearing as "natural" or "traditional," as a shared experience of communal sisterhood. Libeli was not about preservation or community; those terms would be too inertial, that model too flat. Nor did libeli equal resistance. To see the situation in those terms would be to adopt the egocentric missionary model of a Dr. Chesterman. Libeli, like birth, was about danger and death, and it could be a violent, traumatic process for those who underwent it. It made boys men, able to kill and mutable, capable of transforming themselves into likenesses of spirits from the forest and water, likenesses of leopards and crocodiles. Libeli gave birth—gave new form and power—to men through a wrenching experience, not unlike being pushed and ripped out of a blocked birth canal. Wars and rivalries produced libeli, and those who claimed power and followers worked through pushing and cutting, marking and mutilating, through violent birthing.

A history of libeli opens up layers of memories associated with a water goddess named Ndiya and a rainbow counterpart known as Bonama in a region where crocodiles were key to healing and harming, cutting and cursing. Libeli takes us to the core of the ambivalent meanings surrounding human metamorphosis—whether in cutting, birthing, or eating—in a region where sorcery powers have long been morally imagined as capable of transforming humans into violent leopards, crocodiles, and invisible, hardworking slaves. This tangle of meanings is much more than a parallel symbolic realm that will, in turn, help us understand the realm of childbirth. Rather, a history of libeli provides the best introduction to the extraordinary social turbulence in this region from at least the time when the Zanzibari first began raiding for ivory and slaves during the 1870s through multiple colonial violences of conquest, red rubber, forced labor, taxation, hyperinflation, and medicalization. This history is also essential if we are to give proper weight to the bloated heroics and reductive platitudes of the obtrusive, if ever earnest, missionaries of this study.

Their willful ignorance and infringements contributed to producing the seemingly "docile bodies" of Yakusu and its vicinity. Studying libeli reveals aspects of reproductive ritual and body marking that are critical for understanding a history of birth work and medicalized childbearing in this colonial situation. As Nurse Gladys Owen recalled, when she first arrived in 1923, having "a woman patient was almost unheard of & I myself was never called out to a midwifery case." By 1929, a hospital was nearly completed, and Owen was wondering why local people were agreeing to hospital births and autopsies for the first time.[12] This simultaneity in assent is uncanny. What produced this shift toward docile bodies cannot be understood, however, through a history of colonial biopower alone. Studying male reproductive ritual will yield broad insight into the meanings of birth work by men and women, providing essential context for understanding the history of medicalized childbearing in the Yakusu region from the 1920s on. It will broaden our focus from reproduction narrowly defined in demographic and medical terms as fecundity and the birth of children, to social and cultural reproduction. It will also shift our analytic entry point from colonial eugenics to a local therapeutic economy. In the context of the violence and afflictions in the Congo at the turn of the century, a future hardly seemed assured. Reproduction of offspring and a patrimony, of libeli and social memory, was at risk. A history of libeli demonstrates how historical subjects, both individual and collective, reproduced themselves differentially in the face of this aggression. This reproduction was neither homogeneous nor unified; it involved social division and struggle, violence and creativity; and it produced colonial evangelical middle figures who dared to imagine libeli big men and their followers as a world of uncivilized, pagan "lows."

This chapter and the following one consider how crocodiles figure in libeli as history and as therapeutic form. Yakusu missionaries observed public aspects of libeli on four occasions: twice before the founding of the Yakusu church, in 1900 and 1902, and twice afterward, in 1910 and 1924, when these performances were tumultuous for the church. Chesterman's version of events in 1934 contains a vocabulary of crocodiles and lilwa that was part of debate, conflict, and competition among missionaries and local Congolese from at least the turn of the century. This chapter traces this vocabulary in history and ritual through 1910, and situates libeli in the historical context of raiding, conquest, and violence before and after the arrival of the first missionaries in 1895. Chesterman also combined this older vocabulary of lilwa and crocodiles with another set of ingredients—airplanes, doctors, nurses, fala (tertiary yaws), and a hospital hunter bearing a gun—suggesting the newly medicalized, mobile, and fast modernity that emerged during the interwar period. The second chapter turns to this new, hybrid, and often divisive lexicon of the 1920s and 1930s. Together, these two chapters comprise a history of struggles over wealth and youth between the new church and Lokele elders. These struggles began over new forms of generating and composing wealth, of marking the body (clothing) and inscription (papers). They metamorphosed by the 1920s into competition over the signs and practices of missionary medicine.[13]

These chapters have two purposes. One is to use this mischievous crocodile = airplane metaphor of the 1930s to immerse us in such doubling and shattering of meanings in the concrete, missionized world of Yakusu's district in the Belgian Congo; and then to trace these elements so deployed (crocodiles, airplanes, guns, doctors, and the like) in the memories and histories of this same little mission world as it hovered over and combined with the violences of Leopold's Free State in the Romée-Stanley Falls stretch of the former "Arab Zone." This first purpose is about creating a context for a history of wombs and docile—and not so docile—bodies in the Congo.

The second aim of these chapters is to shake readers out of any temptation to reduce a womb to a uterus. Taussig suggests that the womb is "the mimetic organ par excellence, mysteriously underscoring in the submerged and constant body of the mother the dual meaning of reproduction as birthing and reproduction as replication."[14] These chapters are intended to dislodge conventional models—whether obstetric, colonial, missionary, feminist, epidemiological, or "development"—about what it means to medicalize childbearing, to relocate this perilous event, packed with meanings about death and reproduction, to a colonial space of confinement and surgery. We need the context of this male reproductive and power-making ritual, centered on symbolic wombs and produced in and through histories of struggle and violence, to plunge us into the thick of meanings yet to come, a history of women's wombs and medicine in the Free State's child, the Belgian Congo.

Lilwa, Lances, and Mobile Medicines

Libeli remained a dangerous, if not forbidden, subject in postcolonial Zaire. Some people in and near Yakusu simply refused to speak about it. Protestants who gathered for church meetings and song in 1989 sang: "Don't mix me in the affairs of libeli because those people of libeli are going to curse me."[15] Some were afraid to talk about libeli. Others wanted money for their knowledge. Tata Bafoya Bamanga declared, "libeli is trouble," and then hesitated to speak. "Pay first!" the old man began again, explaining: "We say a man after entering, he cannot express the matter of libeli. . . . There in the village, they would hear. They would come to make way at my place, my house here of leaves; they would destroy it. They would hit me. They would say to me, 'You, white man, you, are you going to sell lilwa? For what reason?'" Bafoya was the only man who mentioned the 1910 round of libeli called *falanga*. Memory was shallow for most; they only recalled the round of 1924, the last time that there was a visible Lokele performance. Bafoya said: "But then the whites of the mission arrived here and that one, Chesterman, he forbade it." Those at a remove from Yakusu recalled that the state, rather than the mission, had decided libeli was too dangerous and should be stopped.[16]

Memory was marked by a grammar of equivalences. People translated by comparison. "Libeli was like school." "Libeli was our *université*." "Libeli was like *kalasi*," or classes. In short, *this* was like *that*. These doublets speak to historical and symbolic processes of substitution that belie equivalence. *This* and *that* were no more simultaneous in universal historical time than they were in local Lokele time and place. Rather, *this* succeeded and replaced *that*. These two chapters reconstruct the historical formation of this grammar, this seeming doubling up of experience that created new openings and closed others down. They also recover the processes of translation, history making, and remembering that were—and are still—involved.[17]

How was libeli enacted and experienced through time? Consider first the data of John F. Carrington; this missionary took an interest in libeli in the 1940s, two decades after the last visible performance of this healing ritual. A literate, Protestant Lokele man gave him a list of local names for each cycle of libeli since its beginnings. The list suggests that there were eleven rounds of libeli since its introduction toward the end of the eighteenth or the beginning of the nineteenth century. The names imply that each round of libeli was provoked by tumultuous events. One round carried the name of "famine." Two others, also of the nineteenth century, were named after types of bodily decoration: armbands and brass bracelets. In 1888, the first cycle for which Carrington proposed a date, libeli was known by the local name for a steamboat. I focus on the rounds of 1900–1902 and 1910. Each carried the names of forms of money. The first of these was remembered as *bolaya*, a name that signified a European object, specifically a new model of *shoka* (Sw.) or axhead fabricated in Europe to resemble and succeed local axheads as monetary registers. Then in 1910, libeli was called falanga or francs, after the new colonial currency introduced in this region during that year.[18]

This chronology of libeli names suggests that historical shifts in forms of wealth, exchange, and distinction, occurrences with implications for social and symbolic hierarchies, coincided with—if they did not produce—a libeli performance. Although libeli was a reproductive ritual, each round was also a unique, historically produced political performance of restructuring authority over and wealth *in* youth, launched by Lokele chiefs and elders. Conjunctures between a material, structural shift in wealth and a simultaneous unhinging of the symbolics of wealth and value seem to have roused each performance.

How old were lilwa and libeli in this region of Ya-prefaced villages where the Lokele live? The word *lilwa* was in active use when Henry Morton Stanley traveled downriver in 1877. He heard "*nyama!* lilwa!" as he passed by Yakoso.[19] This cry of warrior imprecation declared might and rancor, even war. As one man told me, "A person who said to you, 'lilwa!' . . . he was saying, 'Get your spear!' " When Stanley journeyed down this stretch of the river, he and his companion, Pocock, appeared as provocative spirits associated with a frightening water creature: "It is said that long ago a couple of white spirits came from the forest and drifted down river in a large canoe." And about that time, "a frightful phantom vomiting forth fire had been reported to have been seen travelling up stream."[20]

Yet cutting lilwa long predated Stanley. Lances, lilwa initiation rites, and Ya-prefaced toponyms were among the features that farmers, trappers, and fishermen speaking Soan (western Bantu) languages brought to this Upper Congo region.[21] Throughout this area, people used special groves of primary forest for life cycle and healing ceremonies. These clusters of tall trees behind villages, which were called *fobe* (in singular, *lobe*), were likely as old as settlement in this Ya-prefaced region. By the mid-1940s, so much forest behind villages had been cleared for farming and lumber from Isangi to Stanleyville that European passengers aboard river steamers could easily spot the special groves.[22] Yakoso's lobe was destroyed in the 1930s; people told me that it had happened when a colonial officer nicknamed Mupendakula ("He likes to eat") insisted that Lokele cultivate fields.

Carrington's key Lokele informant defined libeli as "a rite of the Lokele, Foma, Olombo and Topoke peoples . . . which we call lilwá." One Foma man identified lilwa to me as "the father" of all the BaMbole, Topoke, Olombo (Turumbu), and Lokele: "He, that one, he begat all people." I asked: "So at one time did Lilwa live? Was he a person?" He replied: "Normally, he was a person." I persisted: "So is there a story of Lilwa, of where he was born and what he did?" "Now that was the story of Adam and Eve," he responded; "that Lilwa, if you follow that one completely, it would go up to the time of Adam and Eve." This man explained that lilwa was as old as "the beginning of the world."[23] Another man insisted that it was the esoteric lilwa language, learned by libeli initiates, that served to unite the Ya-prefaced houses and villages that the historical experience of colonialism had divided into distinct tribes: "They founded a language, yes, one *grammaire*, one traditional language of the country. They were speaking. The BaMbole were saying it, the Lokele were saying it, that one language—the Turumbu, the Foma, yes all the tribes around here. . . . The Foma, BaMbole, Turumbu, Lokele founded one lilwa language."[24]

Memories of lilwa and libeli have been mediated through biblical origin stories, but they also aspire to a notion of a collective, pan-ethnic identity. A Lokele oral tradition tells of a time when all Lokele and many of their neighbors, too, lived together somewhere to the north of Yangambi in a place called Isiko, where the water spirit Ndiya lived in a pond. There were so many blacksmiths that Isiko buzzed with the sound of their work. One day, wearied by the constant clatter of the smiths at work, Ndiya became so cross that the earth moved. The landslide killed many, and the rest fled. They moved in groups toward the south, each led by a *kumi* or leader. While some big men stopped with their followers in the forest north of the river, some pushed up the Congo as far as Yakoso, and others passed to the south of the river, entering what is now known as BaMbole forest. Some groups came winding back to the river in later movements.[25]

The ethnic designator Lokele seems to be of late-nineteenth-century vintage. People say the BaTambatamba (Zanzibari) named them Lokele. Before, those who led nomadic lives in their canoes were simply known as the BaLiande, or people of the river.[26] Others, who settled in larger riverain villages with distinct sections or *houses*,[27] were BaLokombe or townspeople. Like their forest neighbors, neither the river people nor the townspeople recognized a single, common ancestor. We have only a hazy picture of commercial and social relations prior to the arrival of the BaTambatamba in the 1870s and 1880s, which led to a profound reconfiguration of wealth and power. A far-flung network of trade was in place by the nineteenth century. The people who lived on the banks of the Congo between the confluences of the Lindi and Aruwimi relied on fishing and trade; so, too, did those who lived along the Lomami. These hunters of the water depended on those now known as BaMbole—the forest hunters, trappers, and farmers who lived south of the river—for bananas, meat, and copper items, and on Olombo—those who lived north of the river—for cassava, canoes, drums, and fishing net thread. The riverain people sold fish, pottery, salt, palm oil, and objects made of iron.

Thus, forest and river people had long had distinct economic activities and complex relations of exchange in wealth. Wealth is a key word in these chapters and this book, as it must be for historians of central Africa. I follow Claude Meillassoux (and more recently Jane Guyer) in arguing that people compose wealth in persons (by attracting and acquiring wives, followers, dependents, and slaves), things (whether in food or human-made tools and charms, condensed things of knowledge), and knowledge (whether in practical skills, such as farming, or in spirit-mediating knowledge, such as iron working or making medicines).[28] Jan Vansina has called the people of this region Ya-lancers; they encompass not only Lokele but their forest neighbors, indeed all those who also live in villages that begin with the prefix Ya. Their lances included remarkable spearheads called *ngbele* (Lok.) or *linganda* (Sw.), five to six feet long, made of

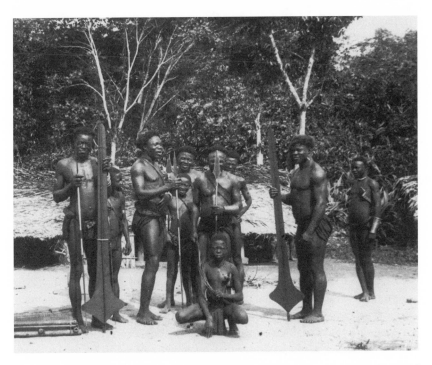

"Eso men and their big money." Iron linganda or ngbele lances in an Eso (Topoke) social setting, ca. 1901. (Courtesy of MRAC, Ethnographic Section [EPH 11715]. Courtesy of Africa-Museum, Tervuren, Belgium.)

iron, perhaps by the Olombo, and beautifully etched. A. Hingston Quiggin noted in his 1949 study of "primitive money" that these "gigantic" ngbele were among "the most spectacular" of Africa's iron currencies and, thus, "figure so conspicuously in museums."[29] Some Topoke (Eso) called these lances *ndoa*, the Lokele word for marriage. Thirty ngbele used to buy a male slave; forty to fifty were needed for a female, though a purchaser might have to go up to one hundred.[30]

These Ya-lancers—the Lokele, BaMbole, Topoke (Eso), Olombo (Turumbu), and Foma—saw themselves as collectively distinct from *batshuaka*, proximate strangers such as the BaManga (Mba), BaKomo (Komo), and Bali, who spoke languages. Each Ya-prefaced village and village section carries an ancestral eponym, such as Yakoso, the people of Koso; and each has its own traditions of movements and separations. Yet the villages of a district, like the houses of a village, are often linked in public social memory as father and sons. The mobility of the fishing traders in canoes gave them more access to wealth as they sought out new goods and gained trading access to new areas. In moving up the

Lindi and down the Lomami and Congo Rivers during the nineteenth century, they carried and adopted things, ideas, and women, especially giving brides in return for the right to trade with these people, some of whom practiced mambela initiation rites.[31] Marriage forms were multiple and hierarchical. While some women became gifts—as *likenja* wives—to initiate trading relations and settle disputes, there was an ancient word for servile dependent: *bokoa.*

Libeli resembled mambela, a Bali scarification, flagellation, and initiation ceremony with a *ndiya*-like water spirit called Maduali; indeed, a 1904 colonial description compared the two, at a time when the colonials spelled the Lokele variant Diloa. Vansina notes that mambela linked Bali villages into a district, and big men used the ceremonies to mobilize power and expand their hegemony. Lokele men told John Carrington in the 1940s that libeli came from their Mba neighbors to the northeast, where some Lokele houses were trading, battling, and giving and receiving women during the nineteenth century. Carrington also wondered about the similarity between the words *libeli* and *nebeli.*[32] My hunch is that Lokele living west of Isangi in what became the Yaokanja Lokele district mixed lilwa and mambela forms from the north and *nkumu*-related lilwa from the south and west with a new name, libeli, as rising Yaokanja big men consolidated their power around new nebeli medicines that they brought back from trade, battles, and alliances up the Lindi. This process likely began in the early nineteenth century as new forms of power and raiding for people and ivory shook the Azande and Mangbetu regions to the north, and intensified as Tippu Tip's ilk swept north and west of Stanley Falls along the Aruwimi, Lindi, and Congo Rivers during the 1870s and 1880s. Curtis Keim, following Evans-Pritchard, associates the origins and spread of nebeli among the Mangbetu and Azande in the 1850s with the dislocations of slave raiding and colonialism in the nineteenth and twentieth centuries. A group of fishermen on the Uele seem to have been the first owners of nebeli medicines, and these nebeli specialists introduced the medicines elsewhere, forming nebeli associations as they went. The resemblance between the words libeli and nebeli would not be so intriguing if the chronologies and capacities for a rebellious, anti-colonial character did not so closely coincide. Nebeli was also associated with the dangers of waters and a water/rainbow spirit known as *kilima.*[33] Just as the turbulence of nineteenth- and twentieth-century colonialisms led to ritual and medicinal innovation in nearby regions, lilwa and libeli changed over time.[34]

Blurred States and Visceral Memories

By the 1850s, Zanzibari traders from the Swahili coast of East Africa were moving into central Africa, as far as Nyangwe on the Lualaba River, in search of ivory for a world market. During the mid-1870s, Tippu Tip made an expedition from Zanzibar, backed by 50,000 Maria Teresa dollars in Indian capital, and established headquarters at Kasongo. Backed by the Omani Arabs of Zanzibar and their Indian financiers, he pushed the ivory, gun, and slave frontiers further into the center of the continent. He became the dominant trader and warlord in the region. European explorers and missionaries soon followed. Stanley met Tippu Tip in 1876, and could not have made his journey down the Lualaba from Nyangwe to Stanley Falls and beyond the following year without Tippu Tip and the workers he provided. After taking immense quantities of ivory back to Zanzibar in 1881, Tippu Tip returned to the Lualaba and moved on to Stanley Falls (Kisangani), dispatching twenty caravans from there into neighboring districts to search for ivory. These caravans traveled up the Lindi and along the Aruwimi Rivers, reaching beyond the Bali people who practiced mambela and into nebeli territory. By 1888, his men had bases at Yambuya and Banalia along the Aruwimi, and they were making alliances with chiefs along the Upper Uele. Raiding small villages produced captives and ivory. Some people turned over ivory to redeem captives; some captives became porters, carrying tusks to markets east of Lake Tanganyika; and others became trusted soldiers, house servants, blacksmiths, and the loyal leaders of trading parties. Some female captives became the concubines of the Zanzibari who settled in the region; other brides were gifts. The major permanent Zanzibari settlements in central Africa—and Romée was one of them—were distinguished by substantial dwellings and well-organized plantations worked by slave labor cultivating rice, citrus fruits, and avocados, all new crops to the region. David Northup has argued that these plantation slaves had to be replenished often because "they were worked hard, fed little, and most died off within a year."[35]

Stanley noticed the change to which the Lokele region had been subject when he returned in 1883 at the behest of King Leopold II; he saw fettered, naked bodies and upturned canoes.[36] The "Arabs" had strong garrisons at many riverain villages, including Yanonge, Yalokombe, Yatuka, Yakoso, and especially the important Zanzibari slave plantation site near the confluence of the Romée River. (The local name for the river is Lome; the shift to the Europeanized spelling of Romée certainly carried imperial meanings.) Delcommune noted the contrast between populous Lokele towns on the Congo, including "Yakussu," and the ones emptied of women and children on the Lomami.[37]

Baruti Lokomba has argued that it was the BaTambatamba who first coined the term *Lokele* for these fishing people of the Upper Congo because they had reached a zone where paddlers, who worked in crews as large as forty per canoe, sang the expression "*kelekele*" as a frequent refrain in their paddling songs. The word *lokele* refers to a special, exceedingly rare kind of mollusk with a smooth, glossy shell and glistening colors, associated, as its name *lokele lya ndiya* implies, with the water spirit. So exceptional was a lokele shell, such a beautiful sign of wealth and good fortune from Ndiya, that a fisherman so lucky to find one would exclaim joy with the cry "kelekele." This same term became the equivalent of thank you in Lokele. A song about Ndiya was part of libeli, as was learning about the importance of a lokele shell for making peace and alliances. BaTambatamba also learned to cut deals and share blood from incisions with big canoe owners in lokele shell-based treaties.[38]

Thus, these Zanzibari conquerors succeeded in domesticating local idioms and making alliances with big men, who profited from their association with the traders and used these ties to assert dominance over their own and neighboring peoples. Some Lokele were raid victims. Others avoided enslavement by working as *voluntaires,* allied soldiers with guns, who "went to get slaves for the BaTambatamba."[39] The BaTambatamba would have found Lokele big men, especially those who owned large canoes and controlled access to paddlers, useful. Such alliances are remembered as marriages between a BaTambatamba leader and a local chief's daughter. Some Lokele—like Topoke big men, Wagenia fishermen at the Falls, and specialized Komo elephant hunters—found it advantageous to become subordinate allies of the BaTambatamba, while most forest dwellers were unable to do so. These trappers and farmers were more subject to slave raiding than Lokele were.

These Zanzibari intruders, usually labeled "Arabs" by Europeans, were known by local people as BaTambatamba after the heavy gait with which they tread. So, too, are they remembered today.[40] People also used the terms BaArabe and BaNgwana to distinguish those presumed to have more East Coast credentials as Zanzibari from those assumed to be their imitators, subordinates, and followers. People told me that the BaTambatamba were BaKusu (Kusu) of Maniema; in colonial terms, this made them "Arabisés." The presumptions about difference in these social categories concerned how much "pure" Arab blood people had, whether their lives had begun in Zanzibar or the central African interior (Maniema), and who were leaders and who followers. These categories were fluid and overlapping; these identities could be claimed, hurled as insults, and denied.

The oppositions of civilized/savage and high/low, therefore, were not new to Leopoldian rule in this "Arab Zone"; they were part of the fluid Zanzibari repertoire of domination and incorporation of followers in the central African hinterland, where a man who professed to be Muslim and wore a *kanzu* could aspire to be of *bangwana* status—well-bred and civilized, though not necessarily of freeborn status. The new state agents and BMS missionaries were eager to designate the slavery of this recent past as evil incarnate, though they were unwilling and unable to comprehend the speech of this deeper local history at

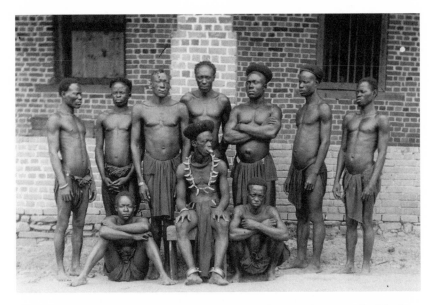

"Group of Lokele types from the village of Yafungas," 1898. This is a colonial ethno-graphic photograph, suggesting a big man with dependents and followers from this pe-riod. (Courtesy of MRAC, Ethnographic Section [cliché 798; EPH 2056]. Courtesy of Africa-Museum, Tervuren, Belgium.)

work. Paradoxically, they saw the "Arabisés" as more civilized than the typical indigène.

Many remembered the BaTambatamba in chronological terms, as the first of two colonialisms, separated by a war at Romée. "First the BaTambatamba colonized us. Then the Belgians colonized us," was a common refrain. Or: "They liked to colonize us, the Ba-Congolais of Province Orientale. But then the whites made war, and it was no longer possible for them to colonize us." Those who attended Yakusu mission schools contrasted the time of BaTam-batamba with that of "Ba-Stanley" and "ba-missionaires": "The war of BaTam-batamba was trouble. . . . They liked to kill Lokele. . . . So the time when whites came, these Ba-Stanley, they came to remove Lokele from BaTambatamba en-slavement."[41] There was indeed a "war"—the battle of the so-called Arab War of 1892–94—at Romée, a riverain base of "small forts" about twelve miles down-river from Yakoso (the village next to which the BMS mission post of Yakusu was later located). The Belgians defeated the BaTambatamba in a lively battle on May 22, 1893. According to colonial military historians, Belgian forces took Romée "tree by tree, house by house" as they overcame those "barricaded behind immense palisades." The "Arabs" tried to flee, but "a large number were massacred in the pursuit by natives not even one of whom had been seen during the whole affair, but who, during the pursuit, arrived to share the spoils." The official war booty included "2000 prisoners, ivory, splendid knives, guns, three Winchesters, six piston guns, sheep, goats, and chickens by the bulk."[42]

This clean break between periods, marked by the heroic Arab War and its decisive battle at Romée, is exactly how history was taught in schools in Belgium and the Congo. This clear periodization is also how Yakusu's missionaries wanted to see history. Yet they had stumbled into a complicated world whose idioms Zanzibari conquerors had succeeded in domesticating in their own interests; it was equally a world that Belgian forces were still busy pacifying and copying by domesticating these "Arabisés" as more civilized than local "basenji" (uncivilized, pagan, savages).

The first BMS missionaries arrived at Yakusu in 1895 with visions of a Cape-to-Cairo railroad in mind. The attraction of the riverain site lay in its proximity to the promised future capital of central Africa, its association with "Arab" slavery, and its seemingly rich potential for Christian deliverance. Yakusu was near the center of this old Lokele-BaTambatamba trading zone, and the Zanzibari lingua franca, Swahili (or Kingwana), was well entrenched. This region was appealing to BMS missionaries precisely because it had been so effectively colonized, and it promised to provide easy access to the many "tribes" along the Congo, Lomami, and Lindi. George Grenfell remarked that the rice plantations of this region made it "the 'land of promise' of the Congo" for his BMS and the Free State alike. "The Government is counting upon the rice crops of the Falls District of the State—we have already sent a reserve stock of it to Wathen Station (1100 miles away) to meet the recurring short seasons in that neighbourhood, & the Government is sending quantities to their Nile Station some 500 miles in the other direction." Grenfell also valued the "considerable native population" and "the very important Arab settlements" in 1898.

> Within a radius of twelve miles . . . we must have several thousands of these so called Arabs, and among them all, and also among their numerous dependents, education and a primitive civilization are at such a premium as to make the district a marvelous contrast to any other on the Congo— one realises at once that he is entering upon quite a different sphere . . . he finds the banks of river lined with magnificent plantations, carefully built clay houses, and comparatively well dressed people.[43]

Grenfell concluded that "there is no district where there is such an evident tendency in favour of civilisation or where there is a more marked breaking away from the old order of things." He admired those who had profited from collaborating with the Zanzibari; the Lokele, he noted, were "a particularly fine race. . . . [T]heir undoubtedly superior moral code explains the advantage they enjoy in the matter of physique and vitality." Yet in the same breath, he argued that this was the " 'Psychological moment' for entering upon great enterprises in the 'Arab Zone' . . . to take part in the moulding of the future of the long oppressed tribes which in this neighbourhood are just being freed from the Arab yoke."[44]

Deliverance from "Arab" raiders became a guiding idiom at Yakusu. Unable to persuade Lokele boys to work for them at first, these BMS missionaries attracted BaTambatamba victims of Mba and Olombo origins instead. They also imported Basoko and Bangala, who had skills learned at BMS mission stations downriver. The diffidence of Lokele may have been tied to the rhythms, prestige, and social organization of fishing.[45] Part of the reluctance was certainly due to their economic superiority in the region. The "boys" who gathered around the mission station from its founding in 1896 were, the missionaries realized, from subordinated rather than dominant groups. Those who sold Mr. W. H. White roofing leaves, for instance, were keen to purchase this first BMS missionary's supply of cassava bread. They were hungry after having only just moved away from "the 'Arabs of the great town of Rome' a few months before."[46] Some may have been ordered as sons or clients to go to Yakusu in search of knowledge or wages. Some may have been clients of the newcomer chief, Saidi, who moved his "prosperous village" upriver to Yakoso at "the request of the white man" just as the mission was established. Missionaries reasoned that they wanted to "obtain protection" during a time when the "Arab was still a terror in the land."[47]

Still others sought new patrons in the missionaries. Some, like Salamo, were the products of missionary ransoming. Mission Congolese were still talking about Salamo in 1989. She was born about 1881 in a Foma forest village about fifty miles downriver from the future site of Yakusu; her name was Lifoka or "Lucky One." One night when she was very small, slave hunters surrounded her village. They had captured a man from a riverside town and forced him to show them the path through the forest to the village. There, they set homes on fire, killed those who resisted, and seized and bound the rest. Lifoka's father and uncle were away hunting, but she and her mother were taken with the slave gang to the riverbank. They then traveled upriver to Stanley Falls and beyond by canoe, many of which were loaded with ivory for a long overland journey eastward. Lifoka's mother disappeared along this route. Missionary sources suggest that while nearing this new Free State post, however, the caravan leaders panicked when a company of newly trained Force Publique soldiers approached. Lifoka was among the smaller children who were hastily sold to European traders at the Falls. She learned to speak Swahili from the workers with whom she lived, and was given a Swahili name, Salamo. In 1890, when she was nine or ten, two BMS missionary couples, the Darbys and the Harrisons, came upriver and met the Belgian trader in whose household Salamo lived. He had bought several girls from the Zanzibari, and he let the Darbys take—or buy—eight of them. Salamo became the nursemaid for the Darbys' baby, living with them at Bolobo for three years, before becoming Edith Stapleton's "house girl" in 1893.[48] We will meet Salamo again in chapter 3.

The first young scholars were anguished by their "incompleteness." They could not give the missionary teacher the names of their "parents, town or tribe," and bore "the stigma of slave."[49] The raid memories of several ex-slave converts were intertwined with leopard attacks. When BaTambatamba raided Litoi's village, for example, a leopard chased after his mother, and she dropped her son in flight. Lamed by this injury, Litoi became a Yakusu-trained teacher; his daughter, Malia Winnie, became a mission midwife (whom we will meet later in chapter 5).[50] In another case, a young child named Sulila was stolen from her home far up the Lomami, and made to frighten away birds from rice fields by pulling at a cord stretched across them day after day until, "beaten and bruised, deaf in one ear from a blow," she passed into mission hands. She became a "house girl" in Mrs. Millman's home and nurse to Neli, the daughter of Salamo, before marrying the teacher-evangelist Baluti.

Sulila's passage into mission life is not without interest. Salamo and her husband, Lotoba, had been visiting Badjoko at Yanonge, the only Congolese *chef de poste* in the Congo Free State. Badjoko introduced these Yakusu Christians to a man named Bolombi, who "had secured"—bought—the slave girl Sulila from some "Arab slave traders." Bolombi gave—sold?—Sulila to Salamo and Lotoba, and she worked as Salamo's child's nurse.[51] What the missionaries presented as "redemption" from captivity and enslavement might have appeared, to those subject to such transactions, as moving from one form of subordination to another. Salamo's transition from redeemed slave to the position of a mistress who converted a slave into a house servant is suggestive of how profoundly intertwined the Yakusu mission and continuing BaTambatamba-Lokele slave traffic had become. Salamo herself had moved from slave to domestic servant to as near to kin as a Congolese convert could become at Yakusu; but nothing kept, indeed everything encouraged, this icon of missionary redemption from finding a new Salamo for Yakusu in Sulila. Sulila's conveyance into Salamo's hands is significant for another reason: the role of Badjoko as intermediary. His part dates this slave ransoming to at least as late as 1900, thus fifteen years into Free State rule, while it underlines the tight ties between the Yakusu mission and this anomalous Congolese man serving in a state role usually reserved for whites. Badjoko was an official rubber tax collector.

Thus, mission-authored slave redemption narratives had powerful effects on local forms of remembering. People living at Yakusu in 1989 often relayed history to me through a string of proper names featured in mission lessons. A common mnemonic string ran from Tippu Tib and the BaTambatamba, to Stanley and Livingstone, and then to the ba-missionaires and Salamo. David Livingstone was a figure of mission instruction and iconography, no matter that he never came near the place and died well before the founding of Yakusu. Likewise, postcolonial memories of two distinct colonialisms follow mission fantasies and state pretexts about a clear break between these two closely enmeshed periods; they suppress the fact that the break was not distinct at all. From 1886, the Free State was making agreements with Zanzibari for workers and offering commissions to its Belgian agents for "redeemed slaves" that could be used as soldiers; one military officer, Captain Nicholas Tobback, bought and freed some 2,000 such slave-soldiers at Stanley Falls alone. Military campaigns produced large numbers of captives, who were then declared liberated as state soldiers and missionary "orphans." Catholic missionaries were actively involved in ransoming slaves, and turning them into converts and workers; BMS missionaries were too.[52]

The war that was supposed to throw out the "Arabs" became an occasion to join in the predatory, raiding economy, while locating forced labor for the colonial army and public works projects. Congo Free State authorities allowed, even encouraged, these Arabisés to stay in the region after the war. When Yakusu's missionaries arrived, therefore, the stretch of the Congo between the Lindi and Lomami was still colored by, and partly still in the possession of, these "Arabs," who appear as shadowy figures in H. Sutton Smith's romantic history of the Yakusu mission's first years. A "salient" of "Mohammedism," stretching some thirty miles into Lokele terrain, was part of early missionary impressions. Smith contrasted the "native chief" observed on "parade" in a huge canoe full of "painted warriors" with "decorous" Arabs reclining under canoe awnings in long white tunics as their "neatly-dressed domestic slaves" paddled "to the accompaniment of harsh, discordant cries."[53] These BaTambatamba, meanwhile, became major rice planters along the river as the new colonial economy in rubber pressed in from all sides.

This blurring between the two colonialisms was precisely what E. J. Glave documented as he traveled down the river in 1895. The rubber economy was already in full swing, though state authorities depended on the raiding and slaving methods of their predecessors, the "Arabs."[54] Before long, similar arguments became part of E. D. Morel's anti–"red rubber" campaign, though he pressed that in the question of comparative "ethics of Arab *versus* Leopoldian slave raiding and trading," Free State methods were far worse:

One could assert and demonstrate abundantly that the raids upon villages by Congo officials and troops, to seize recruits and labourers ... to capture women ... to punish and terrorise communities short in their supply of rubber, raids in the course of which massacres wholesale and atrocities unspeakable are the habitual accompaniments, constitute proceedings indistinguishable from the raiding of Arab bands. One could prove—did not one feel that the reader is already sick with proof—that the "Congo Free State" in its basic claims, practices, and methods is primarily a huge slave-owning and slave-raiding corporation, and that compared with the cold diabolicism of its policy, Arab excesses extending over an infinitely smaller area were tame.[55]

In the district embracing Romée and Yakusu, we can see this blurring of periods—including the missionary erasure of "red rubber"—more concretely. A *chefferie arabisée* was created for these planters; in 1910, they numbered about 10,000 with their "dependents" and produced hundreds of tons of rice a year. After Leopold's infamous 1891 secret decree, which produced a state monopoly over the products of most of the colony, the riverain area including Yakusu was declared a "free zone," exempt from this decree. Yet red rubber was not far away. Badjoko, formerly Captain Tobback's domestic servant, had been granted honorary European status due to his heroic role in intelligence during the Arab War. He was acting as chef de poste at Yanonge and is remembered as the one who brutally imposed the rubber regime in the nearby BaMbole forest. The Lomami Company was ferocious along the Upper Lomami. In 1904, Grenfell commented: "The diminished population of the Upper Lomami is doubtless due to the Arab raiders who had it practically 'all their way' between '85 & '93." Again we find chronological blurring and erasure of Free State responsibility, though his very next sentence admitted human flight: "I am told there are more people in these parts than there appears to be—the visits of the tax-gatherer resulting in the river-side villages being abandoned for the less accessible interior."[56]

Perhaps Yakusu's missionaries did not see any direct evidence of red rubber atrocities, but they could not miss Badjoko. They gave him clerks, and he arranged for Salamo to find Sulila. Nor could they miss the BaTambatamba. The BaTambatamba went to the mission store regularly to buy imported products and sell rice, beans, onions, fowl, and ducks. Yakusu's missionaries were not in a position to be critical; they relied on these planters for their food staples.[57] Nor were they exceptional. Not being critical was official BMS policy until after Morel had made "red rubber" a cause célèbre in Britain and the United States.

Local memories of the BaTambatamba were not always chronological; domination was inscribed in bodies and engraved on the landscape. In 1989, people at Yainyongo also remembered the BaTambatamba period as a time when women did not give birth, human blood flowed, and strangers looking for the new wealth of elephant ivory controlled and bathed with crocodiles. People from deep in the BaMbole and Topoke forests were enslaved and brought to Romée: "One white Arab, he got them to come look for elephant ivory. They came because of an elephant *opération* and to colonize us." When I asked to go to the site of the 1892 battle, Romée (now the village of Yainyongo-Romée), my guides insisted on taking me to see the tiny waterfall that trickles from the bank of stone into the Congo, just down from the Romée confluence. They named it for its sound—"wa wa wa"—conspicuous from any passing canoe. This "wa wa wa" waterfall is remembered as a place where human blood once flowed regularly, wa-wa-wa-ing its way into the mighty river. It is remembered as the place where BaTambatamba would kill sick and unruly slaves: "They were cutting the throats of those slaves who couldn't work any more carrying loads."[58] This form of remembering is spatial and bodily. Other memories were equally visceral: "The WaTambatamba were eating us like meat. . . . The BaTambatamba pierced our ears. They locked our mouths with bolts. They cut our throats. They ate us."[59] Only men came and they married after they arrived: "They were marrying beautiful girls. They would chain you. They would dress them very nice. They would become BaTambatamba." They especially seized "our beautiful girls in *bowai* and in *wale,*" that is, the female periods of seclusion—and skin-clarifying—following marriage and childbearing. "They were white, *pe pe pe!* They were abducting them; if she was in wale, had given birth to a child, they would kill the child. They would take Mama because she was again white."[60]

Another spatial memory was the swimming hole where these colonizing traders used to bathe. My guides also insisted on taking me to see this nearly dried-up pool of water located along the forest path between Yanonge and Yainyongo. This swimming hole used to be full of crocodiles, alternately called *chunusi* (mermaids) and ndimo (sorcerers of the water or crocodile-men). The BaTambatamba would swim and bathe in this human-made "pit" to express their power, but no one else could because of the dangerous, invisible crocodiles kept in this pool. Only BaTambatamba could bathe there without being eaten. This slippage from crocodile to water phantom to mermaid to Mami-wata makes sense; a set of cosmological ideas surrounding water spirits and their celestial counterparts, alternately known as ndiya and *bonama,* were at play. People told me that persons can change into ndimo, a kind of bad, witch-like, water creature, living for years beneath the water; they considered ndimo to be more of a charm, controlled by a living person, than the contemporary mermaid figure of Mamiwata, known to entice with watches and drown chil-

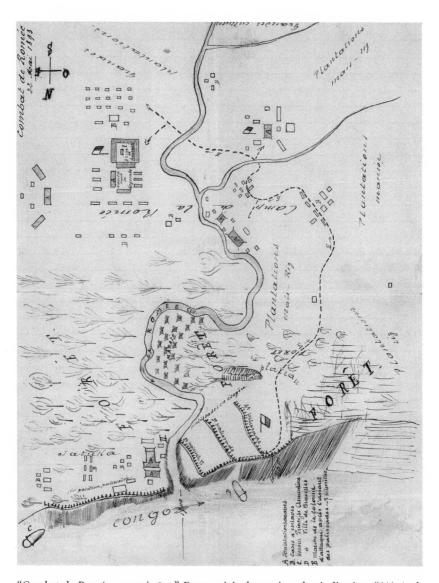

"Combat de Romée, 22 mai 1893." From original map in color indicating: "(A) Arab dwellings, (B) Slave huts, (C) Steamer Princesse Clémentine, (D) Steamer Ville de Bruxelles, and (E) March of the attack column after the assault of the palisades—7 kilometers." Also designates immense rice, corn, and cassava plantations; the houses and "seraglio" of Kayembe in the "Camp de la Romée"; marshes, a plateau, and a scratched-in area between them that coincides well with the forested area where people showed me the former BaTambatamba swimming hole. The "wa wa wa" waterfall flowed at about the point at which the column march line moves inland. Also identifies the slave dwellings along the river where Yainyongo-Romée is now located as Yatuka. From the Fivé Papers. (Courtesy of MRAC, Historical Section. Courtesy of Africa-Museum, Tervuren, Belgium.)

dren.[61] This slippage among terms expressed the liminality of these creatures, associated with land and water and, perhaps, with an ancient set of ideas about the water spirit, Ndiya, and her rainbowlike counterpart, Bonama. Bonama is known to lurk in the river, block rain and stomachs, and maintain a warlike relationship with its celestial shadow, the rainbow. The sight of Bonama, like the sight of a crocodile's head, is especially dangerous for children.[62]

Thus the BaTambatamba period is remembered through spatial and visceral memories about blood and hangings, being eaten, about crocodiles and crocodile-men (ndimo). But these memories cannot be dated with precision. One man told me it was Kayumba who put crocodiles in the swimming pit, and he was not appointed chief of the chefferie arabisée until 1913. Others spoke about Badjoko as if he had the same powers as the BaTambatamba. They talked about his control over many medicines near water and ndimo: "I heard that his family knew many medicines. . . . Badjoko, if he stood here near the river, sometimes he made something with medicines [and water]. He would go downriver with this water. There, he put these animals of the water."[63] Others slipped into memories of a colonial official nicknamed "He-likes-to-eat" (Mupendakula), who we will meet again in chapter 4. Thus, the most visceral memories, those rooted in bodies and in places, which carry terrifying resonances of symbolic power, seem to bespeak a time not of the BaTambatamba alone, but of the colonial regime that was built on its foundations. These memories and the symbols that they invoke suggest a profound continuity between these two colonialisms, that of BaTambatamba hegemony and of Free State cruelties, and underline the significance of the British Baptist Chesterman's attempt to appropriate power over crocodiles and libeli.

Bolaya, 1900–1902

By the time Yakusu's missionaries first noticed libeli in 1900, they were surrounded by "crowds of Lokele boys from various villages" who had "linked themselves on to the new power, the white man's power." As the "temporary booths" for libeli went up in the forest, several boys fled to the mission for protection. These young scholars, who could be "easily distinguished" by "their bright red fez caps, dark blue vests, and baggy breaches," did not want to miss class.[64]

The missionaries did not know what libeli was. They assumed that "reverencing something" was better than "reverencing nothing," even though they did not want to lose "our boys" to libeli. One night when these youth gathered for song and prayer, Mr. Millman advised them that they did not have to join libeli. The boys proceeded to join in chanting the forbidden curse word *lilwa* in a "restive," "cheeky" spirit. The men of neighboring, downriver Yakoso were irate at this "mockery of their oracle." Yakoso's chief, Saidi, demanded that each boy pay twenty axheads—the iron money of the time—as a fine. He also sent a man up to Yakusu whose cheek was eaten away by fala to demonstrate the consequences of a lilwa curse. The three missionary men admitted the mocking was wrong, but they sent the elders away without any axheads and warned them "that if they cursed any of our boys . . . they would be seized and sent up to the State for punishment."[65] The old men, furious, threatened to send thirty Lokele men up to Yakusu to tie these three Englishmen up with rope. This spectacle never happened, and libeli went on.

Soon, "village followed the example of village" and "the whole tribe was possessed." Towns were almost empty for six to eight weeks, except for women, who were so busy cooking large amounts of food that they seemed in missionary eyes like slaves and victims of theft: "Several women were lightened of their market burden and dared not protest." The missionaries wanted to visit the proceedings "in the bush," but changed their minds when one station workman, who wandered near the lobe, was "badly mauled." When the newly initiated began to emerge daily from the forest to parade and dance in their libeli regalia, missionaries observed them "marching in single file . . . guided and guarded by their instructors, who frequently popped the 'lilwa' at supposed hostile observers." All the "acolytes" wore "drooping crowns of verdure" with "their bodies fantastically marked with many stripes of clay." With slow, "mincing steps, they passed from square to square. . . . Very obvious was the pleasure of the old men at this brave show."[66]

Despite their offers of protection, the missionaries kept few of their youthful clients from entering libeli in 1900; and those who returned to the station for school and work a year later seemed "insolent and unemployable."[67] In 1902, "great hoards of fish were being dried" for two more months of "the huge feasts" of libeli. Yakusu's missionaries watched as all their workers again broke their contracts: "Away they went, and we were left without a cook."[68] One missionary explained that old Lokele men felt alarmed by "how eagerly the young folk were sitting at our feet to learn." These libeli organizers were determined this time "not to let a single boy slip through their fingers." Virtually the "whole tribe between the Lindi and the Lomami"[69]—thus the entire Yaokanja district—entered the "secret society" of libeli. "All other work was suspended, the women working like slaves to find whatever food was demanded by the 'society,' and we were scowled at whenever we went near."[70]

Although in 1902, as in 1900, they offered to protect "our boys" who refused to enter libeli, Yakusu's missionaries did not condemn or try to stop it. They learned about some libeli practices in 1900 and 1902, but they were powerless to

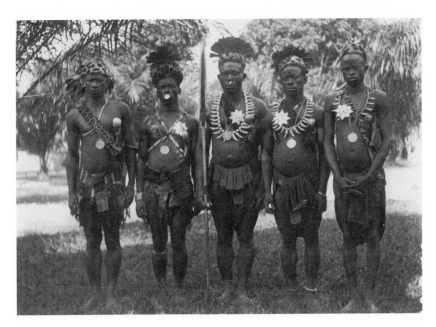

"Five principal Lokele chiefs," Stanleyville, ca. 1910. Chief Lobanga is in the center. It is unclear if these are only Yaokanja Lokele chiefs, or if the Yawembe chiefs are included, too. Photograph by A. de Meulemeester. (Courtesy of MRAC, Ethnographic Section [APH, neg. 10320]. Courtesy of Africa-Museum, Tervuren, Belgium.)

prevent their "boys" from becoming initiates. There was, after all, still no Yakusu church. After two months had passed, libeli of 1902 was over. So, too, was the social "discomfiture," and the loss of labor and influence that it had represented. The "boys" slowly came back to school, and eventually "all the chief men came along and begged us to be friends again."[71] Missionaries interpreted libeli and its scorn as a reaction against them, but it seems to have been something more. Boys were leaving Yakusu and coming back as initiated men. Despite missionaries' determination to divide people along civilized/savage, Christian/pagan lines, these early mission-aligned Congolese figures were finding ways to cross these categories, defy these divides, and keep patrons in two worlds, proving that it was possible to be both a mission "boy" and a libeli initiate. They were, in short, becoming the middle figures of their period. The vulnerable missionaries could threaten to send libeli organizers up to the state, but they needed workers, followers, and food.

The missionaries bent to the rhythms of libeli and worked to empty it of political danger by labeling it farce. They called it a "system of 'make-believe,'" "apparently farcical rather than sinful."[72] The missionaries learned that newly initiated young men were forbidden from even glimpsing a woman, whether a "maiden of nine summers" or a missionary; they used the word "laughable" for this unrecognizable masculinity.[73] At the one moment that libeli did seem menacing, they refused to pay Saidi's fines and imagined that Free State authorities would intervene if their "boys" were harmed by lilwa curses. Besides, they were accustomed to periodic loss of their "boys." They lost workers not only to libeli, but also to forced labor requisitions for the new railroad company. The Chemins de Fer du Congo Supérieur aux Grands Lacs Africains (CFL) was established in 1902, and the 125-kilometer railroad south from Stanley Falls was completed in 1906. The governor sent instructions at one stage that boys in the Yakusu school belonging to three specified villages must return home because they were needed by their chiefs to paddle the canoes bringing limestone from the Aruwimi River to Stanleyville for new railway buildings. Chiefs were obliged to furnish laborers to the CFL, just as they had to furnish soldiers to the Force Publique; indeed, conscripts were also directed to railroad-building tasks. The CFL workyards along the Lualaba became a notorious headquarters of forced labor in the province. Some chiefs raided to meet their quotas of workers, arresting people at night, stealing their belongings, and taking them as prisoners to work on the railroad.[74]

The CFL railroad company at Stanley Falls, the major employer in the region, was also implicated in the naming of libeli of 1900–1902 as bolaya. Carrington translated bolaya as "European axe-heads used for currency." When Saidi tried to fine the missionaries, he had demanded iron axheads or shoka. New factory-produced bolaya axheads were issued by the CFL, which arranged to have these uniform shoka produced for it under industrial conditions and with an alloyed iron in Birmingham, England from about 1902. By using its own axheads to pay workers, the company succeeded in virtually supplanting the use of the more substantial, individually crafted and etched axheads that had long been produced locally. These shoka or *tondo* (Lok.) had long been crafted by ironsmiths and used in local trade; made of pure iron, they did not rust and could be reworked into a variety of forms. Instead, the new bolaya shoka became the regional money standard for trade and wage labor, including at Yakusu.[75]

Records of Yakusu's commercial dealings reveal the effects of the new railroad on shoka supply as well as the mission's dependence on "Arab" planters. By 1902, the missionaries were paying their workers and purchasing much local produce in axheads. They operated a "store" of "barter stock," imported goods that they exchanged for BaTambatamba rice and iron monies. Grenfell, writing in 1903, said that these hoe or ax blades were made in Kasongo of locally smelted iron: "All the smiths in the Stanley Falls district depend upon these in making axes, knives, spears, arrow-heads, etc., and households depend on them as a market currency. All of our Yakusu food for work-people and children is paid for with shokas—three bundles of plantain = one shoka—and without these we are in difficulties at once." When he was at Yakusu early in 1903, however, the mission's stock of shoka was running low, "but we thought the interruption of the supply was only temporary, and that the Arabs and others would soon be coming along as before to exchange their shokas for cotton goods, enamel ware, and such-like things which we import for exchange purposes." They soon learned, however, the shortage in money supply was instead due to the new railway, which was "absorbing all the supply, and the Government and traders are being compelled to import from Europe."[76]

Congolese still paid colonial taxes in labor contributions during these Free State years. For most, this meant the notorious labor tax in rubber, though Yakusu's missionaries reported that the Lokele paid theirs in fish and iron.[77] Yakusu was located in a special "free zone," however, as was the riverain district bordering the river between Isangi and Stanleyville. The mission station had become a "recognised halting-place" for large canoes and their crews of some thirty-five to forty paddlers traveling to the Falls by 1902, but its missionaries were no experts on tax requirements. "I think every town between here and Isanghi . . . must send a pretty strong contingent of canoes loaded with produce, such as palm oil, salt, etc., up to the Falls for sale or as *tribute*, once every three or four months," noted Mr. Smith. He had become acquainted with "several Lokele chiefs simply by the visits they pay here on their way to or from the Falls." Perhaps this "tribute" was the same as *bosombi*, the local word for state taxes; the comment suggests that social power and wealth were organized in and through Lokele chiefs during these years.[78]

The libeli of 1900–1902 known as bolaya, then, involved a contest between Lokele chiefs and elders and the agents of European colonialism—Free State officials, Yakusu's missionaries, and the CFL railroad company—over forms of wealth and power, as well as the loyalties and bodies of male youth. Bolaya, the new European-manufactured shoka, were supplanting locally crafted tondo. "Arab" planters were important commercial partners of the mission station, and Lokele chiefs who had collaborated with the BaTambatamba in slaving and trading had reasons for attempting to create and sustain partnerships with the BMS mission station as well. But when the British Baptists moved to assert control over male youths, initiating them into prayer meetings with frolic and song, Lokele chiefs moved to initiate young men into libeli. Elders and ancestral spirits linked initiates to their people in space, through the sacred lobe in the forest beyond the village, and in time, along and across generations. Libeli of 1902 was named after the social affliction that it acted to heal, bolaya, the new counterfeit axheads that were affecting the value of local iron monies, tondo

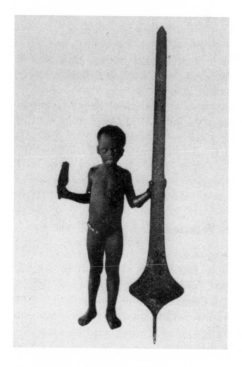

"Lokele Currency," Yakusu, ca. 1910. Congolese boy used to indicate the relative size of a shoka axhead and a linganda or ngbele lance. From H. Sutton Smith, *Yakusu, the Very Heart of Africa,* insert 18–19.

axheads and ngbele bridewealth lances alike. This healing process made boys men and recomposed wealth in the hands of local big men. While these mission followers tested the truths of lilwa curses one day, they also proclaimed with Lokele elders that mission "boys" could be Lokele men another. They effectively insisted that the competing powers of Baptist missionaries with papers and libeli organizers with crocodile curses coexisted, and that they required appeasing in this world marked by forced labor under slave conditions, mutilations and hangings of black bodies, and red rubber.

A New Church and Mitted Hands

Soon after libeli ended in 1902, Yakusu's missionaries baptized the first Congolese, founding the Yakusu church.[79] At the same time, youth led a "great wave of enthusiasm for the 'book' passing over the Lokele world." The new fervor for reading and writing seemed phenomenal: "Lads and lasses have paddled eighty miles to beg for a primer, or to buy an exercise book or pencil, or to secure a rough slab for a school seat."[80] The rewards of being a member, other than mission patronage, were in new kinds of healing, in baptism and communion, in learning to read and write, and in papers.

Routine church business, including discipline, also operated through papers; the inscription of a name on a paper or in a register took on powerful meanings. Members entered and were expelled from the church through the writing and crossing out of names in the *lokasa*, or register book, and a newly baptized member received a personal membership card. Indeed, papers were a defining symbol of the first Baptist missionaries for their Lokele neighbors. Whereas local drummers signaled all Europeans as "spirits of the forest," as "red as copper, spirit from the forest," or "white man evil spirit as bad as rain," drum messages distinguished Yakusu's missionaries as spirits from the forest "of the leaf which can be written on."[81] Forest leaves were ingredients in food, medicines, and charms, and the same Lokele words (*lokasa/kasa*) were used for books and papers. People used banana leaves as paper early in the twentieth century, and these kasa were magical to early mission followers. One man who had spent time at Yakusu as a boy kept the leaf on which a missionary had written as a special charm in his hut for years, an early missionary sermon tells.

In the Yakusu church, as in any Baptist community, members were involved in investigating and disciplining other members' misdeeds. The first recorded church meeting was in 1904. Seventeen people gathered to consider ten names for baptism on July 31. Seven days later, those chosen were baptized in the river; an evening communion service followed.[82] Banishment from communion and expulsion from the church became routine forms of discipline. Indeed, the minutes increasingly became a register of names, listing baptismal sponsors, those accepted for baptism, and those banned and excommunicated for various infractions. Violations of marriage rules and insufficient offerings to pay church teachers were frequent topics of discussion at meetings, though like all issues, they were reported in a brief, perfunctory fashion. Hemp (*basili*) smoking, a kind of dancing called *tosumbe,* and the wearing of camwood powder (*shele*)—all of which were features of libeli—were among the first markers that became subject to church regulation. New rules developed as circumstances arose, and the vocabulary for comprehending and disciplining custom became more elaborate, if not more refined. The lexicon of church regulation depended on the visibility of custom.[83]

The church minutes inscribe the imposition of new codes of behavior, as well as members alternating between partaking in communion and participating in "sinful" activities. Some cases resemble those in Baptist churches anywhere: the church banished members for adultery and expelled others for persisting in this offense; a missionary advised members that those who had participated in a wrestling match one Sunday could not take communion for two months; Bolongo was expelled for stealing some church offerings. In other cases, members were disciplined for locally specific offenses: basili smoking, tosumbe dancing, and shele body painting. Their names were effaced from the church lokasa until they changed, asked to reenter, and the members accepted. On October 5, 1907, sixty-eight members were banished for twelve reasons; forty-six of the sixty-eight had been smoking hemp. Hemp continued to be a problem, including among teachers and at church meetings. The use of camwood also continued, even though members who had their bodies painted with shele were barred from communion from 1908.[84] Although the missionaries understood these disciplinary proceedings as part of a struggle between "Christian" and "pagan" ways, the records suggest that a dynamic of back-and-forth movement between church communion and participation in communal rituals was a continuing feature of Yakusu life.

The collection of church offerings developed alongside a new culture of reading, writing, and publishing in "Lokeleland" (a missionary expression) from early in the century. Members contributed to the church in axheads or in-kind from at least 1905. These contributions, also called bosombi, became a frequent topic in church meetings from 1906. One teacher was expelled for stealing bosombi. The bigger problem was persuading people to give at all. In 1907, a missionary announced that bosombi giving would become a church requirement. Jean Baluti, an important BMS teacher, suggested on June 14 that village people be informed before the church adopted the new rule. Other church members objected to the amount required. Baluti appealed: "it would be better if church members . . . gather axe-heads, each according to his ability."[85] Part of the problem was the name: bosombi was also the term for state taxes. In June 1908, the church decided to change the name to *lifaefi*, a word derived from the verb to give. Yet at church meetings, there were complaints that lifaefi giving was still not felt as "a sign of love," as an important "effort in all the hearts of those of the Church."[86] But the bigger problem was a rupture in amicable relations between the BMS Yakusu mission and the Congo Free State, which had led to a tax in rubber being applied to the former protected riverain "free zone."

The Baptist Missionary Society became notorious for siding with King Leopold II and suppressing evidence about red rubber atrocities in the Congo Free State. Just as E. D. Morel's humanitarian campaign gained momentum in 1903, the London-based BMS secretary, Alfred Henry Baynes, gave a speech in Brussels, thanking the king for reducing the taxes owed by Protestant missions, and praising the success of his Free State. Baynes's speech created an uproar in the British press, especially as more evidence surfaced that George Grenfell and William Holman Bentley, as members of the king's sham Commission pour la Protection des Indigènes au Congo, were implicated in covering up Congolese cruelties. Baynes's speech also gave Morel more ammunition. He published three letters written by John Weeks, a BMS missionary at Monsembe, about the punitive severing of hands and the halving of the population in the Bangala area. Weeks wished to remain anonymous; he had already been reprimanded by Grenfell in 1898 for complaining to state authorities about abuses in his area. But he made it known that BMS missionaries on the ground did not see conditions as Baynes did.[87]

On October 19, 1903, several BMS missionaries witnessed atrocities at Yandjali, just below Isangi. If Yakusu's missionaries observed red rubber violations before 1905, they remained silent about them until public protests had forced a shift in BMS policy toward Leopold's Free State. When H. Sutton Smith published his book circa 1911, he noted that there had "not been wanting indications that west of Romée" Congolese had "been worried too much over the rubber tax" and "unscrupulous" state demands. He likely knew about the Yabohila massacre of September 8, 1905, which followed the murder of two European agents of the Lomami Company; one of the accused Topoke men was hung at Basoko in November. But when William Millman and W. H. Stapleton were interviewed by King Leopold's Commission of Inquiry in January 1905, they praised the Free State; as late as December 28, Millman was still acting as a public defender of the regime. But the tide was turning. When the commission's report, published in 1905, produced yet more damaging evidence, Morel managed to organize a series of anti–Free State meetings in Baptist churches throughout Britain for the first time; BMS missionaries home on furlough participated. By 1907, Baynes had retired, and his successor as BMS secretary was publicly objecting to Free State atrocities as even more revelations from BMS missionaries appeared.[88]

Some of these new disclosures may have been Millman's. In 1905, when Millman and Stapleton certified that there had been no atrocities in the Yakusu region, they may have been sheltered and naive, rather than consciously complicitous in covering up damaging evidence. By August 1906, Millman began writing letters to Roger Casement, the British consul who played a crucial role in investigating Free State violations in 1903. Central to Millman's revelations was Joseph Badjoko, the chef de poste at Yanonge and the Free State agent charged with tax collection in the area, the same Badjoko who helped the former slave Salamo acquire the slave girl Sulila.

Millman reported on a recent conversation with some Congolese living near Yanonge, "who had come complaining about some contempt shown them when paying their taxes at Yanonghi. . . . 'But I see nothing when I go about that is not right,'" Millman had protested, "'and, what is more, I have written a letter to the State saying that everybody is contented and has no complaint.'"

'Then,' said one, 'we are deceived, for you have lived among us and if you liked you could find out all things about us.'" A month before, they continued, fourteen people "had to eat and swallow some of their own rubber at Badjoko's orders, the stuff being cut small by the sentries, for coming with their baskets short in weight of rubber." One man reported that he "had seen men thrashed fifty and a hundred and more lashes by sentries working in relays. Such abuses had been going on "for years." Millman also shared some statistics he had collected on fatalities. Yaochwi village had been rated in 1904 as owing fifty baskets a month; there were only thirty responsible taxpayers left when the trader changed in February 1906, so the number of baskets owed became thirty. Between March and August, three of the thirty—two adult male collectors and one schoolboy—had died from accidents while collecting rubber. At Yaakaku, a village rated at forty-seven baskets, Baseko had died, while Lisambi had broken a thigh, and Megelema and Mandamba each a rib.[89]

Millman also described abuses in the "free trade zone" that stretched along the river from Stanley Falls to Isangi, including Yakusu, which was excluded from the state's monopoly over profits. Balembeko, chief of Yaolongo, a Foma village that had recently put up a schoolhouse and received a new teacher, advised Millman that he "must not be angry if the school attendance is small because they go away getting rubber and every month they spend nearly three weeks away from home." Balembeko explained that a man used to be able to fill a basket in three or four days, but "now hours and hours are spent walking about, climbing and creeping and clambering to get the stuff." Each of the three chiefs in the village were supposed to take ten two-kilo baskets of rubber to a white man named S. A. B. (Société Anonyme Belge), or Poli Poli, near the railroad; they received only one rubber-getting knife and one shoka in exchange for each basket. Millman continued:

> So the people had refused to go. Then one of the chiefs, named Bakom-bolotala, was sent down to Badjoko and put on the chain. The judge got to hear of it and was angry, reproved the agents concerned and set the chief free. But whilst he was in prison one of the other chiefs took charge and, failing to bring in the full dose of rubber of proper toughness and tenacity, was forced—at Stanleyville, this year—to eat some rubber chopped small. This man declared this before Kempton and myself. Also, two boys were forced to eat some white paint and one has since died.[90]

A man named Ilongosi from Yalikanda, "a day behind Yanonghi," had declared before Yakusu's missionaries that a *capita* (foreman) named Bangwani, who weighed and tested rubber in a receiving shed, reported Ilongosi and three other men to Badjoko for bringing in rubber with flaws in it. With Badjoko looking on, their rubber was cut into pieces "as big as a man's hand," and they were forced to eat this hand-sized shape, "each man his basketful, tearing it off in pieces with their teeth." Millman noted that Ilongosi "acted the whole proceeding before our eyes most dramatically." One of the four died on August 20; "the others reckon to have saved themselves by enemas," a therapeutic treatment still used to alleviate constipation and unbind blocked, sorcery-cursed stomachs and wombs.[91]

Cutting and consuming power, like eating rubber and cutting hands, were among the unspeakable scandals that produced Casement's beleaguered diary entries. Such cutting and eating also inspired a visit by Millman in 1906 or 1907 to a village opposite Isangi whose people had murdered a white man and his bodyguard, and whose women wrapped their hands in mittens made from this dead man's coat. The visit inspired a favorite missionary sermon about Yakusu healing. The sermon, preserved in notes likely written by Mr. W. H. Ford, began with the story of a man who had been abandoned to die on a nearby island in 1904.

> In 1904, two men were sent by Mokili [Mr. Millman] to make inquiries about evangelizing the district. Returned with a stranger in the canoe. Had a terrible gangrenous arm. "We found him left on an island . . . because you've taught us to help those in need we've brought him to you." No drugs but blue stove and very few instruments. Nauseating task to scrape the bad flesh away & clean the wound. No one would give the man house room. He slept in a corner of Mokili's dining room. After weeks & weeks of patient persistence the arm healed—big long scar left. Man learnt a few hymns—heard the gospel story & eventually left to go home.

In 1906 or 1907, when Mokili was 100 miles downriver at Yaekela, opposite the mouth of the Lomami, he tried to meet these people known for murdering a white man. The sermon notes explain that Millman had

> heard of savage tribe inland. Had killed a white govt officer & his body guard. Com[missaire] of Basoko had sent for Chief who had refused to come. So a Lt. & soldiers were sent. Found village empty. Set fire to a few houses. Was murdered on way back on forest path. Were cannibals. Women wore mittens from white man's coat. No one dared go near. Except for market days, announced by chiefs downriver, women went to exchange food at given spot.

Millman, I imagine on the trail of red rubber evidence, "felt the urge to try & contact these people," whose chief was called Alufulu, but his "boys" refused to accompany him.

At length after many refusals prevailed on 2 boys to show him the way. They went with him to the approaches of the village but refused to go further. Mokili proceeded alone—village deserted—evidently the alarm had been given of the approach of a white man & everyone had fled. Mokili called & called. No response. Very eerie. Mokili felt nervous, afraid if he turned he would run back. Determined to stay but could *not* go forward. Legs would not move. Sent up a prayer for strength and courage. Called 'gain then saw a man peep round from behind some houses. Called to him—man came near—had a badly scarred arm! The two men recognized each other & talked. The man called & others appeared.

Mokili tried to get the man to remember the hymn tunes he had learned years before, "but he had forgotten the words," so the missionary played his coronet and the man "began to *clap.*"

> Crowd increased. Chief came forward. . . . Talked. Then women appeared & soon were going round & round in ring clapping. . . . After some time Mokili walked away with promise to come again. Two lads still waiting in forest near the path. Amazed & thankful to see the White missionary safe & sound. So we joined an entry for the Gospel among the forest tribe of Yangole.[92]

The sermon is a parable about how the benevolence of healing the sick came to bear fruit years later as the healed man was miraculously rediscovered among a "savage tribe" of "cannibals," advancing the mission church. Yet it was also a parable, for British Baptists of the time, about the integrity of missionary work in the Congo, despite the ravages of Leopold's Free State. The meaning of these mittens may seem elusive now, although mitted hands certainly effaced fingers then. Did they look like part of a playful costume or like stumps at the ends of arms? Were these women protecting with hands or frightening with hands, in this darkest of imperial settings widely known for women hostages and rubber victims with dismembered hands? We cannot reconstruct the meaning of this gesture for these people moved to murder a white man. What is certain is that this sermon was a parable intended for Baptist congregations in Britain among whom it became impossible to talk about missionary work in the Free State without reckoning with Morel's accusations. It may describe a missionary victory over heathens, but the sermon also clearly distinguishes missionaries from retaliatory, village-burning state agents.

Why did Mokili feel "the urge" to contact these people, who had killed a Free State agent and his bodyguard? Millman had commented to Casement: "I could fill a book with horrors because of the connection we have. I never dreamed things were in such a state and the fact that the natives do not feel driven to strike somehow, I fancy dulls my own sense of the cruelty of it all." Yet he was still incredulous: "but surely the State cannot know." Thus, Millman was quietly making investigations and telling parables, though he confessed to Casement that he did not know what to do with his findings, feeling "restrained by his committee at home." He was still accepting invitations from Free State officials at Stanley Falls who were eager to court these loyal BMS missionaries; he feared taking "this matter home—it would be the last straw with our folks and provoke extravagance on either side"; though he was bothered to think that "our silence" would "lead the natives to think 'God's men' see no wrong in mean cruelties and oppression."[93]

In December 1906, Millman's good relations with Free State officials ended abruptly when Morel published a Millman letter in the official organ of the Congo Reform Association. The make-nice dinners were over. Free State authorities reacted quickly and punitively; in January 1907, they issued orders to fight the influence of these Protestants by introducing a rubber tax to profit the state into this "free zone." State police were assigned to villages, and Yakusu-trained teachers became involved in struggles against their authority. Balanachasemi, the church teacher in Yalikanda, was arrested in March 1908 during a police operation to insist on the new tax; he was imprisoned for planning a revolt against paying the new taxes.[94]

Saidi, chief of Yakusu, also found himself in trouble for backing the church in these contentious times. It was Saidi who had tried to collect a libeli fine in axheads from Yakusu's missionaries in 1900, though not long afterward, he was dining and sipping tea with them while looking at pictures in their copies of the *Wide World Magazine*. By 1908, Saidi, a man with seven wives, was "one of the most regular attendants at the services." He backed church measures against hemp smoking and palm wine drinking among his subjects, and he encouraged lifaefi giving as the new rubber tax system was applied. Fighting broke out when he also promoted a new house-building program along the riverfront of Yakoso town; a rival chief, Senga, had decided that it was "an opportune time for shaking off the yoke of the chief" whose allies were the missionaries. Millman stopped the battle, and sent the spears and shields to the state officer at Stanley Falls, but Saidi ended up in prison due to "serious charges against his reputation and loyalty."[95] In a context where the BMS Yakusu missionaries could no longer be counted on for their loyalty to the colonial state, chiefs and teachers, like Saidi and Balanachasemi, who were loyal church members and encouraged lifaefi giving, were outlaws.

In 1908, Millman wrote to Free State authorities asking that Yakusu teachers be exonerated from labor taxes. The reply was that they did not have to buy

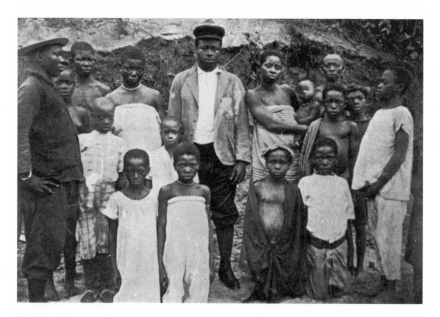

"Saidi and Family—as he sometimes appears," Yakoso, ca. 1910. From H. Sutton Smith, *Yakusu, the Very Heart of Africa*, insert 28–29.

workers' licenses if they were teaching in their own towns, but that they had to pay taxes "in francs or service or, where convenient and required by the official in charge of the district, in food stuffs at a fixed rate." Millman noted: "I don't know why they tax in francs when there are no francs."[96] As the crisis over inadequate church funds deepened in 1909, mission "scholars" stopped paying because they were "afraid of being suspected of sending money to Yakusu and of suffering the fate of chief Saidi." By the close of the year, the lifaefi collected would only pay fifty evangelical teachers, but eighty-nine were on the salary rolls. The missionaries threatened to cut the number of teachers; teachers complained that "Church members *were taxed* to the uttermost and could not give anymore." Their "storm of protests" went unheeded; the missionaries announced that anyone who skipped communion or did not pay lifaefi would be deleted from the church roll.[97] Soon there were francs, known as falanga. Soon, too, there was another round of libeli named after this new affliction to reproductive health; falanga began in March 1910. State police were stationed in Yakoso town at the time, keeping a lookout for Saidi, who had escaped from prison.[98] This round of libeli was also known, for the first time and among a new generation of middle figures—loyal Yakusu church members—as "sin."

Falanga

The new Belgian Congo regime placed new silver and nickel coins in circulation in 1910. Shoka axheads from Europe, the principal money since 1902, suddenly lost an important part of their value. There were at least three competing economies at that time. The first was the colonial economy, which forced Congolese to pay taxes in an individualized money form for the first time, as a "civilizing measure" intended to bring the notorious rubber tax system to a close. The second was the economy of the Baptist church of Yakusu, which required offerings from its members. Both of these were disturbed by the shift in monetary systems, as was the local therapeutic and political economy in the hands of the Lokele big men. The myriad, intricate relationships among these three economies were destabilized as well. The introduction of a divisible colonial currency and the obligation to pay taxes in falanga, rather than undermining this local therapeutic economy, seems to have sparked its dramatic expression. Libeli became a means to reappropriate wealth, to reassert the power of big men and elders, and to reattach male youth to their ancestral spirits and village patrons.

The economy of the Yakusu church was also upset. Devaluation and hyperinflation precipitated an economic crisis for Yakusu's missionaries: their stocks of shoka could no longer serve to pay their Congolese workers. It was difficult to collect church offerings from its members under conditions of insolvency. Finally, libeli itself created near famine conditions at this mission post because all their personnel, including their "boys" and cook, left for the forest, and for several months.

The change in the form of taxation that accompanied and, indeed, required the introduction of falanga had far-reaching ramifications. Before 1910, colonized subjects had to pay tax through labor, and this labor was calculated through the products of their labor, usually through quantities of rubber or fish. Moreover, taxation was collectivized. The chief of a village or a forest house would organize tens of paddlers to transport a gigantic canoe of fish to Stanley Falls, for example. Yakusu's missionaries used the word *tribute* for this colonial tax in the riverain "free zone" from Stanley Falls to Isangi; it was a coerced contribution between a local chief and the Free State.

When francs replaced axheads as money, individual taxation in this new currency form supplanted collective taxation in kind, effectively bringing the "red rubber" period to a close. Indeed, these changes in taxation and currency were part of a fundamental transformation, no less than the end of slavery as it had continued in a mixture of Zanzibari and European forms. In the Lokele region, there was a two-year lag between the end of Leopoldian rule and the advent of individualized taxation. The Belgian Congo's imposition of this new tax system and introduction of this official currency were, in fact, the most visible signs of the transition in the form of colonial rule to people living in this riverain and forest region. The new tax was calculated in francs and paid by each male aged thirteen and over; when a man paid his tax, he was given a metal token to wear around his neck.[99]

Church record keeping changed radically with three meetings in April 1910. For the first and only time in some thirty years of meeting minutes, the scribe wrote a detailed account of the proceedings. A notice went to press just before these meetings took place. The Lokele text began: "In all countries, native peoples have something like libeli." It declared that libeli was only for basenji, pagan, uncivilized people.

> When people leave the customs of basenji, they drop these things. We don't say they're bad. No. When frogs gather together on the river bank, they are not doing anything wrong. So too basenji have their ways. But for one who has started to leave the ways of basenji, who has for instance begun to learn to read and wear clothes, then if we see he wants to return to do former things, we should feel shame. . . . We urge you to look fixedly in front—don't look back again desiring to return to former things, like an animal that goes back to what it has vomited. . . .[100]

Frogs are wily and difficult to catch, and with their distended stomachs and tiny legs, they are unseemly and disproportionate. Someone with "the waist of a frog" is bloated, physically and morally. Thus, the frog was an apt comparison for those who feasted too much, ate vomit, slyly abandoned books and clothes for the waste of libeli, and would then want to leap back to church life again.

Church meetings were a form of disciplinary litigation, and the libeli proceedings in 1910 were characterized by fierce debate over knowledge, secrecy, and coercion, as well as spiritual truths. The missionaries insisted that church members who had entered libeli openly discuss its rituals, in violation of the oath of secrecy they had taken. A man named Bokanga explained that the church members from Yakoso who had entered libeli refused to attend the meeting in order to avoid speaking about it, even though they knew they were risking expulsion. He had overheard people say: "We will not go. We will not change in our hearts. The best is that he makes us leave the Church." He insisted that their refusal was "really refusal and not because the elders are coercing them." But the missionaries embraced the coercive power of the church. When Yakoso Bafoya inquired what was going to happen to church members who refused to renounce libeli, Millman declared that they would not be able to take communion again. Yakoso Bafoya pressed for a vote. All those who supported libeli raised their hands. The scribe took Millman's side and did not count the vote. He observed instead that the "white men are very angry to see that some are fooled by Satan." Millman announced that those "who want to meet with us in communion" must first agree to a set of new church rules in order for their names to be "written in the lokasa." Members must *not* go to the lobe to meet spirits, give *bieka* (food) to spirits, encourage others to enter libeli, or accept any libeli gifts. Finally, they must try to stop libeli. When the final meeting broke up, there was no prayer.[101]

The defection of mission "boys" provoked an intense debate about spiritual truths. Botuku, a Yalokombe teacher, had told Mr. Millman that he had to leave the school at Yakusu because his *nyango* (mother) was sick; he later claimed that his nyango had died. Bonyafala of Yafolo, H. Sutton Smith's domestic servant, had asked if he could enter libeli; Smith refused, but Bonyafala, "afraid of people," fled anyway. Mr. Smith explained that he had not wanted his "*boi*" to enter libeli: "I knew that there is no one here below who has received the power of *balimo* [spirits] above. The elders who respond that they have this power are liars." Libeli initiates, Smith continued, claim that "their lives were left in the hands of balimo long ago and that they will be renewed by these same balimo." The next day, returning to the issue of those who entered libeli but claimed to know nothing about it, Millman insisted that they "stop adoring these spirits [*balimo bale*] and to stop believing that those of libeli have seen balimo and stayed together with them in the lobe." Another missionary interjected: "We know that angels [*bakitomo*] of heaven are *belimo* [little spirits, or messengers]—those of God and Satan who do not come here below. However those that are here in the bodies of people, if they die, what are they?—balimo or belimo?" Yakoso Bafoya quipped: "They are balimo, and we do not know this matter of angels because we have never seen them."[102]

While the missionaries attempted to substitute bakitomo, or angels of God, for balimo, or ancestral spirits, Yakoso Bafoya's words focused on bieka and eating. He explained that during libeli a person took bieka to his paternal ancestral spirit, his *bolimo wa fafa*. He would leave this bieka there forever. "Suddenly when making a libeli visit," he concluded, "I will no longer see my fafa [his ancestor], but I send a lot of bieka so that he will eat." Bieka commonly means food, though its singular, *yeka*, means thing. Yakoso Bafoya specified that a bieka gift during libeli could consist of food or axheads. Either way, he stressed, the balimo consumed this wealth by "eating" it.[103]

Food and eating are too ubiquitous in central African expressions of wealth and power for us to be surprised that balimo and—or as—big men consumed wealth and power in edible and monetary forms during libeli. When falanga supplanted shoka as the local money of trade and wage labor, the newly minted coins replaced collective expressions of labor in rubber and fish as the currency of taxation. Falanga currency worked to cleave bieka as a single lexeme for wealth in things—whether in gift giving or gift eating, whether in axheads or food—into two forms that were neither interchangeable nor analogous. These were the distinctions that Yakoso Bafoya so carefully made in the 1910 church meeting, when he tallied up what libeli participants were giving to their balimo: "bieka in tondo or bieka of eating." The elders who invoked libeli in 1910 were struggling to forestall this cleavage, to reconstitute the political economy of gift giving, to restore the interchangeability of money, things, and food, and to retain their seniority in relationships constituted by the movement of wealth.

Lokele chiefs and elders felt the destabilizing effects of taxation in falanga most acutely. Big men had long controlled wealth in women and in the special, beautifully crafted iron lances that were used for bridewealth payments. As Yakusu's missionaries were well aware, a chief often made the payments in lances and other iron monies for a young man, thus binding the groom for life to the big man who advanced the money. The missionaries had long worried about the effects of polygamy and bridewealth on the capacity of young men to independently control when and who they would marry. There seemed to be a shortage of unmarried women, and in 1909, bridewealth cost what a "young man would earn in six or seven years as a labourer if he could save it all."[104] The shift to falanga thus eroded the control of Lokele big men over marriage, bridewealth, and young men, whether as sons, dependents, or slaves. The new, coined form of reckoning wealth gave young men who worked for wages unprecedented autonomy. Paying colonial taxes became a new "sign of manhood" and independence, intensifying generational tensions among youths and elders. "Wonder of wonders, these boys are anxious to pay and get the receipt cheque to wear and so be men."[105] As the individualized, monetary taxation system took hold, "Arabised slaves"—whether of BaTambatamba or local Lokele chiefs is unclear—arrived at mission stations on the Upper Congo seeking wage work to pay their taxes.[106]

The monetization of the local economy may have undermined slavery, but it also privileged "Arab" traders within the regional and state system of exchange. Long known as "born traders," these "auxiliaries of the whites" were benefiting from "very lucrative commercial operations." Since the new decrees were applied gradually, region by region, the "Arabs" purchased devalued shoka in one area, and then used them to buy animals and ivory in neighboring regions where the old currency was still in active circulation. They also profited from the fact that local people accepted only one of the new coins, the silver one-franc pieces engraved with the face of King Leopold II. They "generally refuse to admit the introduction of" other coins, the centimes made of nickel and five-franc pieces, which amounted to "obstinately refusing all divisible money." The

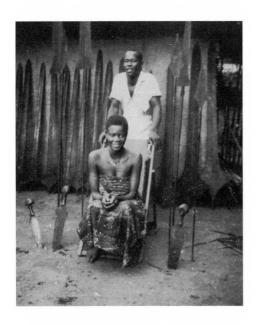

"Bridewealth." In an Eso household, ca. 1910. Several *linganda* lances lean against the structure in the back. (Courtesy of MRAC, Ethnographic Section [EPH 1768]. Courtesy of Africa-Museum, Tervuren, Belgium.)

Belgian tax collector explained that "for them this coin of silver, which they have welcomed, has an intrinsic value to which all others respond. It's a term of comparison. . . . Thus the native sometimes receives twenty nickel coins for a franc, sometimes ten, sometimes five."[107] While the residents of riverain and forest villages retained older, more concrete notions of value inherent in things, "Arab" traders embraced and took advantage of the new, more abstract notions of exchange value that operated differentially across geographical and political boundaries.

These "Arabs," therefore, continued to maintain considerable power into the Belgian Congo period. So, too, did Badjoko, who collected taxes for the Free State and then for the Belgian Congo. As Millman described in 1910:

> Badjoko is supreme judge in all matters not previously taken to the four or five officers of justice stationed at Stanleyville and even in some of these. . . . His authority below Yakusu right away to the Aruwimi district is beyond all appeal and so gets taxes fully paid, rubber amounts complete. He enforces a proper food supply to all his favourite white men when they pass through his districts. He has marital relations with the families of most of the powerful chiefs and has royal decorations.[108]

Central to the connections among almost all forms of power in the region, Badjoko had an authority that few others—whether Congolese chiefs, Belgian colonial officials, or British Baptist missionaries—could contradict.

The 1910 libeli performance identified as falanga was thus closely linked to the changes in wealth and its reckoning that accompanied the introduction of the new currency. Falanga posed a challenge to the capacity of chiefs and elders to compose power and wealth, to assert and maintain authority over young men, and to control the exchange of women. Through libeli, they reinserted themselves in the political economy of gifts and patronage, reconstituted young men's dependence on their "mothers" through their ritual passage to masculine adulthood, and mediated the relationships among households generated through marriage.

The advent of taxation in cash also had immediate and far-reaching implications for the church. Not only did the church have to manage the externally imposed and disruptive transition to a currency-based system of reckoning and exchange, but it had to compete with the state in the collection of wealth from its Congolese members. Furthermore, church offerings, like mission workers and "boys" themselves, became enmeshed in the generational and political conflicts that the new system precipitated within Lokele society; local chiefs like Saidi and Senga clashed over tax collection and church offerings as they vied for power. The mission at Yakusu was in a vulnerable position as the monetary system was transformed. It was deeply implicated in the exchange economy of axheads, foodstuffs, and import/export goods with BaTambatamba planters, Lokele chiefs, and forest villages; it employed domestic servants, laborers, and teachers; and it depended on "voluntary" contributions from local church members. Even at the mission dispensary, patients paid for services in bieka of things and bieka of eating, in axheads and in palm oil.[109] The missionaries realized that a divisible currency would be, in some respects, to their advantage. Axheads were an awkward form of payment for the small sums charged for medical care; during the first four months of 1910, the dispensary collected only two hundred shokas, an amount then equivalent to four British pounds. "The payments would have been more if we had had a better form of currency in which we could charge for medicines," remarked an article in the Yakusu Quarterly Notes.[110]

The mission had begun 1910 "in straitened financial circumstances" because the introduction of francs meant that the "old native money" suddenly lost its value. "The change has been so phenomenal and complete that our little balance in hand seems to be in immediate jeopardy," complained one missionary.[111] In 1909, the mission store held over 1,200 pounds' worth of imported goods, such as bentwood chairs, sewing machines, beads, and hair oil,[112] which it was accustomed to trade in return for shoka. When "Arab" planters, river traders, and forest chiefs lacked the francs to purchase these commodities, the British Baptists had to go without basic foodstuffs. With its flow of trade interrupted and worthless shoka left on its hands, the mission lacked cash to pay its employees.

Many mission workers—more underpaid and broke than usual; less able to keep up with their church lifaefi than ever—departed from their posts. Three teachers had grown "discouraged and went off fishing." Others resigned to marry: "the wife cannot put up with the irregular and perhaps uncertain food supply that is the lot of a teacher's wife," one man explained. The salaries of mission teachers, in particular, depended on the contributions of Congolese church members. "Unless every member pays his penny per week we cannot keep even the present number of teachers and evangelists," remarked the missionaries. Many church members had not been paying lifaefi regularly even before the economic crisis. The church was attempting to enforce the collection of lifaefi in 1910, just when the falanga round of libeli began; the same church minutes that forbade giving or receiving bieka in libeli record debates over making lifaefi compulsory. To make matters worse, in December 1910 the church required lifaefi payments to be made in the new falanga of the Belgian Congo because "the matter of axe-heads is terminated by Bula Matari," the widespread eponym for "the State."[113]

Libeli was an overarching form of authority among households, towns, and districts. It was also a form of discipline, of issuing commands about forms of wealth and property that should not be touched, backed by the force of a lilwa curse. A woman picked up a teacup and shook it with a threatening, "don't-you-dare-touch-this" gesture to illustrate the force and specificity of a dictate backed by a curse. A man picked up and shook my flashlight, which had been resting beside my tape recorder, to demonstrate the meaning of cutting lilwa. Libeli curses were unequivocal ways of saying "No!" to specific objects of imported, colonial-associated wealth. Its performance was a time when young men—whether strangers, slaves, or new mission clients—became incorporated as dependents and followers. It was also a time for exclusions, of things and people. In 1910, when the hated native-cum-state-official Badjoko asked to enter libeli, he was refused because he was not "Lokele."

In 1900–1902 and 1910, new social realities associated with social turbulence over wealth, money, and power created conditions that made elders and chiefs seek to regain control over youth, including those who wore new clothing, read books, served in missionary homes, taught girls and boys to read and write, and gave bieka to the church. The bounty and gesture of bieka giving alternated in a local moral imaginary with menacing phantoms of the water (ndiya and ndimo), sky (bonama), and forest. Stanley and Pocock, like all Europeans who followed them, were spirits of the forest. If the clatter of their arrival incited the calamitous Ndiya to vomit forth fire, Bula Matari's victory at the mouth of the Romée brought to a close a particular period of overrule when BaTambatamba raiding summoned the ravages of mother-killing, child-maiming leopards. But these strangers from afar—who walked everywhere with big, loud steps— invested their power in invisible, ndimo-like crocodiles that did not go away once the new missionary- and Stanley-associated leopards of colonialism arrived. These leopards, too, vied for power over crocodiles and reproductive wealth, other youth and tributary payments.

Libeli and Fertility

It is important to remember how much of libeli was about elders composing and consuming wealth as bieka, the cooked food or precious things that local women, middle-aged men known as mothers, and new initiates offered to their balimo. Most people who spoke to me about libeli lamented it as a lost institution. Libeli was a remembered enchantment, a lost authenticité: "Ahh!! True happiness . . . because it is tradition." This authentic happiness, men recalled, was about eating. Libeli was performed "in order to eat food and get things to eat," one man explained to me. "They were cooking. They were eating . . . men, old people. We, you see, we cooked. We cooked food to give to those children, so they would become people." This locution suggests that, in libeli, men assumed women's roles as cooks and fed boys to transform them into men, through a process that resembled the fattening of girls in *likiilo*, a puberty ritual that made them women.

Libeli seems to have been enacted mostly among men. Women were on the sidelines of the debate within and outside church meetings. Yet gender and fertility were central themes both in libeli itself and in the struggles over its performance. The church's critique of libeli, too, was profoundly gendered. To eradicate libeli implied major transformations of power relations between and among women and men: of who was cooking for whom and under what circumstances, and of who would have access to what knowledge. A history of colonial childbearing in and near Yakusu needs the context of libeli as history and reproductive practice in order to understand the implications of a form of biomedicine expressly focused on maternity and women. The parallels between female and male reproductive rituals will become clearer, and acquire more layered and historically specific meanings, in the chapters that follow. The lexicon common to both will be revealed as composed of symbolic, performative elements, deployed in struggle by the subjects of this history, and what seem now to be *parallels* between male and female rituals will be revealed as connections in social practice. This chapter concludes by comparing libeli and likiilo, and by considering the meaning of libeli as a therapeutic phenomenon.

Libeli was less a subject of my early queries than a point of entry. Men boasted to me about the scars on their backs. Men and women recalled the peppering of eyes and the esoteric language, and they knew that someone who broke libeli prohibitions would speak with an odd, nasal-sounding voice because of the severe facial disfiguration of fala. Since many were reluctant to speak about libeli, and since I imagined my subject as childbirth, I did not persist. I posed libeli as analogy. "Was there anything comparable to libeli for girls and women?" I asked many times during my first weeks. Over and over again, people said likiilo. Soon, I was asking about this female ritual instead.[114]

Women (and men) described likiilo as a time of eating, fattening, and dancing. "We would eat, and we would dance. Our fathers would decide it was time for likiilo, and they would build a special house where we would live. They would spoil us with food and food and food." Women would list the fish and meats that fathers would bring the girls in likiilo. "And from time to time"—at night, at special intervals, as the conclusion—"we would come out with our skin lightened, *peee!* and our bodies fattened. We would wear special body adornments of shele and *pemba* [kaolin], and carry special staffs also colored red and white and black, and dance to the admiration of young men looking for wives."[115] (Peee! is a high-toned sound that ends abruptly; it means clean, light, bright, perhaps "sharp and just right"; no one ever mentioned the purpose of likiilo or wale without it.)

Likiilo resembled other periods of seclusion in the female life cycle known as bowai and wale. Bowai, which continues to be practiced, follows marriage; wale follows childbirth. Ideally, bowai should extend until the wife's first pregnancy and end with her first wale, a seclusion period of one to three months. The longer a period of female seclusion is, the more prestige it carries. All three types of female seclusion were focused on bodily aesthetics and the health and wealth of food. Women described how they ate copiously, growing fat and beautiful in likiilo as their skin lightened and radiated. Some also boasted about the length of their bowai, which seems to have been practiced only for the first, more valuable wife. This distinction reflects seniority among wives, but it probably rests on a historical difference between "wives of the knife" and "wives of the shield," that is, wives produced through marital alliances "cut" with bridewealth and wives produced through war. The first type of marriage was backed by prestige wealth in the beautifully etched iron lances known as ngbele, which were given by the elder men of the house of the husband to the elders of the house of the wife. Bowai, though intended to protect and enhance fertility, was less important with a wife acquired in raiding or war because no investment in wealth and prestige went unfulfilled in the event that she failed to bear children.

Women also recalled likiilo in terms of "fathers"—elder men of the house—

who decided it was time for this special period and made an abundance of food available. The capacity to sponsor a plentiful likiilo for female kin expressed wealth and enterprise, and this capacity, like the capacity to provide bride-wealth for sons, was one of men rather than women, even though women were crucial to the extra cooking involved. Fathers were proud of an impressive likiilo, just as men were proud when they were able to give new wives and mothers lengthy, abundant bowai and wale. Once a girl had entered likiilo, a collective fattening of girls, she could be married. She was ready for bowai.

How were likiilo and libeli like each other? How was libeli performed? A description of libeli phases is in order. The following composite account is not a direct quotation; it closely follows William Millman's 1927 account, but also draws on pertinent details that a literate Congolese man wrote down for John Carrington in the mid-1940s.[116] This long, ethnographic summary contains several concrete elements that have been critical to this historical exegesis: the water spirit Ndiya, the disfigurements of fala, the lokele shell, libeli offerings of food or bieka, and the seclusion period called bowai.

Strange nocturnal voices and rapping coming from the forest would signal that balimo, ancestral spirits, were about to visit. Women could no longer cut their hair or eat certain foods. Household heads began to collect bark cloth, feather headdresses, and rattles. Men went to build a hut and fenced enclosure near the lobe, the cluster of sacred, medicinal trees in the forest. Each boy began to sleep at night with his nyango in his nyango's hut. These ritual sponsors ("mothers") were men who had taken part in one round of libeli since their own initiations. An initiated man shared food with his nyango for the rest of his life.

The boys first went near the lobe for an evening of intense dancing. After everyone was asleep, uncanny sounds of a crying, marching company could be heard approaching, then ceasing, then beating the ground again. These visiting balimo sounded like a herd of wandering chimpanzees. Back in the village, the sounds of slit drums told women to prepare food for these spirits from the dead. The nyango would carry this food into the forest during a special dance. They would not see the balimo, but when the nyango turned for a last look at their gifts, suddenly the food would be gone. One nyango returned to town to tell everyone that the spirits, having eaten, were ready to admit boys into libeli. Women could cut their hair again and eat the food that had been forbidden to them.

The boys began to sleep in the special forest hut, and early each morning at about three, they would hear the balimo dancing. One morning, the boys would be taken to the river for their last bath for three to four weeks.

The nyango would lead the naked boy back to the forest as he clutched onto his guide's waist belt. This imagery evoked umbilical cords. Birth could become death: balimo were at the edge of the path ready to kill those who dropped hold of the tie linking them to their mothers. Men carrying knives and scimitars, their faces daubed in white, passed by. Branches moved. Bundles of attacking sticks and stones fell. The nyango distributed sticks and told everyone to fight with all his might. He who was wounded was someone the spirits wished to kill.

Finally, the nyango and their children would reach a fenced forest clearing containing a large hut, obscured by pungent smoke. Eerie sounds of many spirits could be heard. The nyango told the initiates to lie down, put packets of pounded peppers into their eyes, and tied blindfolds of leaves and feathers around their heads. Then, with the boys again holding onto the waist cords of their nyango, everyone would push on in a double-column procession into the enclosure, passing through two smoky rows of balimo. These ancestral spirits shouted with scorn as they beat the boys with long wands or whips; fearsome shapes swarmed on all sides. He who dropped out or let go died. The nyango pulled the initiates into the hut. The initiates remained in the dark, closed hut until morning, while the balimo retired to the forest, and the nyango joined them for a feast. The initiates might overhear "scraps of a dialogue" about manhood or charms, but alone and still blindfolded, they were in agony. Some fainted from their burning eyes, the beatings, the smoke. Not until day came[117] did the boys receive honey and oil or pounded sugarcane to soothe their eyes. Thus, a major trial of libeli ended.

Men came from the village with more gifts of food and watched the boys march around the outside of the enclosure. The initiates could eat some of this food, though men also told them, "give this to the spirits." After eating, men smeared pounded charcoal mixed with palm oil on the boys' bodies and told them that the water spirit Ndiya had swallowed them. The boys returned to town singing the words, "he who goes into the lobe is no longer a child, he has become an adult."[118]

The next trial centered on cutting the boys' backs and rubbing medicines into the incisions. Another procession began. The initiates, once again blindfolded, held onto the cords of their nyango and shook rattles as they reentered the enclosure. Balimo beat the boys' feet again. Strange noises of chimpanzees and large birds reminded the boys that they were entering the dwellings of ancient balimo. To the sounds of drums beating and bull-roarers whirling, each boy found himself cut in the back. More grunts and screams from balimo, the "founders of their clans," reminded the initiates in whose presence they received these incisions. The nyango, wearing skirts of dried banana leaves, formed a circle around the initiates. Then men rubbed a consecrated medicine known as bote or *wete* into the wounds. The medicine, stored in a pot hidden near the base of a tree in the lobe, conferred bravery and cunning, and joined these young men to their ancestors. Bote was a mixture of calcined snake, lizard, millipede, crocodile bone, leopard skin, and skin from the body of an ancestor. This medicine had the power to ensure that he who broke a libeli prohibition or defied a lilwa curse would get fala. More teaching and oath taking began the next morning.[119] Initiates had to promise to continue to perform libeli, and never to kill chimpanzees, eagles, or a special snake. According to Millman, they also learned that elders impersonated spirits, and then had to promise never to divulge libeli as masquerade. With their bodies smeared with a thick layer of palm oil, the boys—now men—could not cut their hair, wash their bodies, or return to village life until their cuts healed.

After several weeks or even months, preparations for a series of village "exhibitions" would begin. The initiates' skin was rubbed with "coloured earth," their arms were encircled with feather bands and leaves, and their bodies were dressed in bark loincloths and blinding caps with drooping feathers and split leaves. No one could recognize the newly initiated men when they reentered the village. Holding rattles in one hand and wooden knives in the other, they were led out in the afternoon to dance. They repeated this public show every day for weeks, and each time, women gave them gifts of cooked food. The initiates also continued to receive training in the forest about preparing medicines and charms, including "the pill which gives bravery." They learned how to kill and use special animals, how to make warfare at night and on the river, how to conclude a treaty with a lokele shell, how to speak the esoteric libeli language, and how to make the menacing, popping gesture of cutting—or cursing with—lilwa. They learned by doing, and some of these lessons were further ordeals. They had to stage battles on land and water. They had to creep through a thorn heap, find a wild boar's head, and bite it like a dog. And they had to crawl under a tunnel of men until they reached a dead man's head, then throw it aside and swallow "the pill which gives bravery." More oath taking, dancing, feasting, and teaching followed these trials.

When the time finally came to return to the village, the initiates made a procession to the river for a ceremonial bath. They plunged into the water shouting, "Ho! No longer any taboos!" Their first month living back in the village was called bowai, a term that was usually used to describe a woman's postmarital protective seclusion—a special fertility-promoting period of being fattened, lightened, and pampered. The new men were not to go near any women until this month of bowai ended. Then libeli was over.[120]

Thus, libeli and likiilo were initiatory fertility rituals that prepared girls for marriage and childbearing and boys for marriage and war. While girls learned about the parallel between childbearing and war, birthing and dying, in the act of giving birth, libeli performed this metaphor in and through the bodies of boys. Their birth as men resembled the reproductive life cycle of women; the trials of libeli were patterned after the trials of womanhood.

During libeli, boys and their "mothers" presented food to spirits. They also feasted in the forest. Were boys bodies' fattened and lightened? It seems not. But their bodies endured and suffered; they were prepared, marked, tested. Libeli resembled childbearing. Boys were like newborns at first, led into the world by their nyango, to whom they were linked by a cord. Then they suffered and struggled with all their might, as a woman must to give birth. When libeli came to a close, the young men entered bowai. Thus, libeli was mimetic, simulating key episodes of the female life cycle and borrowing its vocabulary of nyango and bowai. It also inflicted bodily harm, cut in medicines, and allowed for seclusion and healing.[121] The early phases of libeli, when initiates had pepper burning in their eyes and underwent frightful blows to their bodies, echoed the central metaphor still used today to describe childbearing: birth is death. Everyone wants to keep the metaphor as metaphor, though the risks are always there. Responsibility for a birth that ends in life is attributed to the mother's strength in pushing her baby out of her body. If labor is prolonged, or if death threatens to become more than metaphor, her birth attendants hit her, jeering that she is weak and must push more strongly.

There was no flagellation or jeering of young women in likiilo. Rather, likiilo was a public display of prosperity and wealth, of future fertility. It ended with a procession of fattened, decorated, dancing girls ready for marriage and motherhood. Did likiilo involve medicines? No one told me so. But why would it not have? During this time of bodily preparation, girls learned new dances and had their bodies scarred in sensual patterns that were erotic to see and pleasant to have touched. The same word was used for each case of body cutting. *Ndotinya* means to cut, whether in cutting female scars, cutting skin to apply medicines, cutting an oath or a judicial decision, or ndotinya lilwa, that is, cutting libeli oaths in and through the crocodile-laced medicines smeared in incisions on initiates' backs.

How could a ritual practice that formed age-grades also resemble a healing cult or brotherhood? And how did libeli "heal"? Libeli embraced the marking of boys' bodies through the cutting of oaths and medicines, although the mixtures of medicine certainly changed over time. This marking and cutting made them men; libeli was indeed a boys' initiation. But key chiefs called each major, district-level performance of libeli in relation to specific historical circumstances of injury and affliction, of hunger and infertility. Such conditions made human hearts hot and heavy, and bodies sick and moribund. Chiefs called for a major drama to mend injuries, heal afflictions, and compose and reconstitute wealth and power. This reconstitution occurred in and through the marking of junior boys with cut-in medicines, an esoteric language, oath taking, and manhood. Libeli was a time of secret learning among men, boys, *and* ancestral spirits; of learning about rights and wrongs and medicines, about what should and should not be done, about the risks of having one's body eaten away by the calamity of fala. Moral and bodily violence to the possibility of reproduction—whether manifest in a famine, raiding slave traders, cruel red rubber tax collectors, or the loss of the wealth of dependents to alien patrons—were the kinds of afflictions that called for healing. Death necessitates birth. Such calamities necessitated giving birth to men, that is, pushing and guiding these boys through tortuous trials in which they withstood the turmoil of meeting enraged ancestral spirits who needed to be calmed and placated with gifts of wealth and food.

Keeping this age-grade-forming, reproductive *healing* analytically *distinct* from the narrow purview of biomedical (even evangelical medical) diagnosis and *curing* is our challenge. Only by imagining this extraordinary gulf can we begin to glimpse the narrowness of missionaries' interwar conceits about the easy substitutes of their Great Physician (Jesus as healer, hence doctor as evangelist) brand of colonial, sanitary mobility and evangelical hygiene. Just kill the crocodile, sell off the meat, and inject neosalvarsan? Such earnest missionary heroics have a violent history in BMS-Leopoldian complicities and erasures of red rubber, which this chapter has revealed in and through the intertwined histories of libeli performances and currency and taxation shifts from 1900 through 1910.

The challenge is to imagine the gulf between the history and poetics of libeli as performed on the Upper Congo and the obtuse interpretations of Yakusu's missionaries, who imagined libeli as a static article of culture, as farce, deceit, and theft. Further, it is to imagine libeli as history, as the work of healing and restoring, of recomposing wealth and power, and calming the anger of ancestors in the face of unspeakable violences and humiliations in Leopold's heart of darkness. Just as much as we cannot afford to romanticize these medical missionaries as well-meaning dispensers of charity and pity, books and drugs, we cannot afford to romanticize this Congolese form of healing either. We tend to associate the word *healing* with doing good, with making the sick well. This study cannot determine libeli's exact origins and mixtures, but it can clarify what we mean when we situate libeli among "rituals of healing and their brotherhoods," which Vansina, following Wauthier De Mahieu, defines as "the oldest pattern of ritual" in this region.[122] In this central African healing brotherhood, the word *ndotinya*—to cut, as in cutting a palaver, cutting a deal, cutting medicines, cutting oaths, and cutting skin—evokes the sharpness, danger, and ambivalence of medicines. Some cut-in medicines kill; some cut-in medicines heal. Some deaths kill; some deaths heal. This ambivalence is as basic to central African therapeutics as it was to Mobutu's thirty some years in power. In John Janzen's more measured words, medicines and charms in equatorial Africa are "possible purveyors of health care as well as sickness."[123] Goodness or evil never resides in a thing itself, in the medicine or the charm, the crocodile or the airplane. The moral imagination turns first to social relations, to the question of *who* not *what*, to whether this *who* is using the *what* to benefit you (whether for protection or in loyalty and respect) or using the *what* to hate, harm, kill. In either case, the *what* is the medicine—often the human-made crocodile or ndimo—at stake, and healing lies in the process of gaining control over this charm.

Libeli's healing worked through seizing power and control. It also worked through violence: for most, a patterned violence of subjugating and terrorizing followed by calm feasting, of burning hot peppers in the eyes followed by the cool soothing of pounded sugarcane or honey. Yet libeli was also a time of intense and violent struggles for power, a time to tame unruly boys and kill opponents. Local men and boys certainly understood that libeli was a time, like childbirth, when your enemies—bad, jealous people who steal body parts and harm and kill by cutting them as medicines—might eliminate you. Herein lies the full moral import of the symbolic parallel with childbirth. Childbirth was never natural on the Upper Congo. Nor was it just a cultural item, easy to pluck out or switch about. No wonder that Europeans who acted so bluntly could seem like enemies, keen to sterilize and disembowel.

The mission church's attempt to distinguish libeli-participating basenji from well-bred church members focused on clothes and books in 1910. Struggles over Saidi's siding with the church had begun at least two years before; H. Sutton Smith mentioned that a powerful "secret society" of women defied Chief Saidi's demands about clothing in 1908.[124] Women were afraid that wearing European clothes damaged fertility, and some refused to marry a man who wore a shirt and trousers.[125] Basenji is a local Swahili (Kingwana) term that also arrived in the region with the BaTambatamba; it means the uncouth, the uncivilized, and is used on the Swahili coast of East Africa to refer to the less-refined, non-

Muslim Africans of the interior. British Baptist missionaries and local African Christians remade the meaning of basenji, using the word to distinguish Christians from "heathens" or pagans.[126] In the first decade of the century, clothes were a significant marker of who was associated with the mission as opposed to basenji. Yakusu Christians were not the only persons to wear European clothes, however. Soldiers and state workers did, too. Indeed, the chiefs under Badjoko expressly forbade the wearing of such clothes. Millman noted that "in form" this rule was "a repudiation of white influence and culture," whereas "in practical effect it provided a rough and ready way of distinguishing people who could be conscripted on the spot for paddling one of Badjoko's men to his next destination or some such task, from those (natives in government employ) who could not."[127] During the same decade, the wearing of European clothes was regarded as dangerous for women.

> The native women and girls being, if anything, more susceptible to dread of the mysterious powers of the conservative dead are a formidable and persuasive influence against any change in general and against the adoption of body clothing in particular. It repeatedly happens that a young man getting on very well learning his trade of carpentry or brick laying or farming or printing or tailoring leaves us altogether saying that although all the presents and payments to the girls' parents and friends are made and the girl has declared her love toward him yet she cannot leave her people for him unless he leaves his place with the whites and becomes a "man" again and puts on native dress. She fears the offended spirits will vent their anger on her offspring.[128]

The new forms of wealth and social reproduction represented by the Yakusu church were mediated not only by new forms of feasting (communion) and clothing, but also by papers. Books and papers constituted a source of wealth and prestige that made teaching work attractive. From early in the twentieth century, Yakusu's missionaries found it "a never-ending source of wonder" that teachers would work for so little money. Yakusu teachers taught "to the tune of a little over a penny each per day," while workers who cut wood for steamers just above Stanley Falls "have house and garden free and good—and money to the value of about a shilling [a] day." In 1913, when teachers were making less than "station boys," one teacher earning six shoka a month (less than two francs) was offered five times his pay to work for the Catholics and ten times that to be the personal domestic of a state official. The "poorest paid workboy" at Yakusu could clothe himself better than a teacher in 1915.[129] Most teachers were bachelors in these years, and most left once they married in order to feed their families. Papers, more than axheads or coins, seem to have kept teachers working in the name of BMS Yakusu.

Millman noted that the missionaries' "only credit" with Badjoko "is because we provide good clerks for him." By 1908, Yakusu had twenty-one Lokele publications available for sale, and the first issue of a church "magazine in the native tongue," *Mboli ya Tengai,* appeared in October 1909.[130] *Mboli ya Tengai* was free for all church members and baptismal candidates who had paid their monthly offerings. Indeed, the same mission courier who collected lifaefi distributed the new magazine, which included a monthly calendar, a biblical text, elementary French lessons, and lists, by town, of baptismal candidates and church offerings.[131] Members who had been disciplined had to write letters seeking readmission from at least 1914: "Two wrote to express their shame and demand pardon from the church. Because of their letters they can take communion." And once a year, teacher-evangelists sent members' baptismal and lifaefi papers to Yakusu to "compare" them with the "grand book of lifaefi."[132] Access to books and letters and the talent of writing represented new capacities to mobilize wealth and power. As forest leaves, kasa were likened to charms and medicines, and some teachers began to equate such lisoo with school. Youth scrambled for books and papers in 1903; their children of the 1920s assumed that they belonged in school. By then, Dr. Chesterman was trying to spawn yet another grammar substituting shots for lisoo and tertiary yaws for fala.

In the 1900–1902 and 1910 rounds of libeli, medicines and scars were not part of the lexicon of mission and church debates. Balimo, bieka, lobe, and lokasa were key terms in 1910, when libeli coincided with a major restructuring of power as competing systems of wealth and social discipline—state taxation, church lifaefi, and libeli offerings—clashed. Wealth in women, control over marriage, and the meanings and purposes of money were involved. In 1910, the threat of being removed from the church lokasa, or membership list, became part of the incentive to return. Reinscription, Millman pointed out, preceded reentry to communion. A new culture of papers, reading, and writing was present in "Lokeleland" from early in the century. There were few references to *kanga,* religious specialists or healers, anywhere in these early church minutes. Though little attention was paid in 1910 to the relationship between libeli and the cutting of incisions on initiates' backs, references to lisoo (medicines) increased in church sources during the following years. Although the minutes contained occasional references to libeli confessions after 1910, there was little mention of lilwa or libeli again until 1924, when Yakusu's hospital was under construction. Missionary medicine—a complex, weighty bundle of novelties and mutations—represented a profoundly dislocating presence in "Lokeleland," capable of stirring libeli once again as gesture and effect.

2   DOCTORS AND AIRPLANES

We heard a lot about King Albert and now we have seen him and know he is real, all doubt has gone, but who has seen God? Why don't you send Him a letter seeing you can all read and write? Send him a letter, if you know where He is, and ask Him to stop people being sick and dying all the time.—Congolese retort, quoted in "native evangelists' " letter, *Yakusa Quarterly Notes,* 1930

During the 1900 round of libeli, the angry old men of Yakoso sent a fala-inflicted man up to the station, so that the missionaries and their defiant followers could see what someone suffering from a lilwa curse looked like. This man was a "loathsome sight, with no nose and part of one cheek eaten away," and "the disease was slowly marring the rest of the face."[1] In 1934, we saw, after Chesterman's crocodile was dead and displayed on Yaokombo's beach, the butcher band that gathered hesitated to cut up the meat, fearing the mutilating illness of fala. Chesterman translated this Lokele affliction in biomedical terms: "There lurks the fear of . . . tertiary yaws . . . from contact with the crocodile." Yaws is a contagious treponemal disease found in tropical and subtropical environments. Its first and second stages are characterized by joint and limb pains, skin lesions, and ulcerous eruptions. The tertiary stage, which tends to follow after a latent period of several years, can cause bone changes and permanent deformities; it is characterized by destructive ulcerations and bone lesions, joint lesions and nodules, and skin fissures and ulcers.[2] Local associations among crocodiles and fala were part of missionary knowledge from early in the century when Smith published "Lest We Should Waddle," a conversation about how someone afflicted by fala, with a waddling demeanor and textured skin, resembled a crocodile. Libeli oaths were consecrated by medicines containing crocodiles and other elements evocative of water spirits. By the early 1920s, when the capacity to diagnose and cure tertiary yaws and a desire to undermine libeli practice converged, the significance of this missionary knowledge changed. Millman clarified local associations in 1927: "The Native generally points to the head of a crocodile as the best illustration of the skin resulting from defiance of the *libeli* authority."[3]

Chesterman's junior colleague, Dr. Raymond Holmes, mentioned that Yakusu-trained nurses were skilled in saving the lives of crocodile victims; at the Yangonde dispensary, the Congolese nurse "had used a needle and suture to such good purpose" that a fisherman's "severe wounds from a crocodile's jaws" had nearly healed.[4] Nurse Likenyule of Yaokombo was absent from Chesterman's big-show version of events, in which the missionary doctor emerged as conquering hero, the killer of crocodiles and fala beliefs alike. But Likenyule wrote his own account and published it in the church magazine, *Mboli ya Tengai*. "Read my news," his story began.

> In 1933, we had a dispute on the side of our river about an animal known as crocodile. This animal was given the name Avion by the people of the village. People of our clan had an idea that this animal was sent by the hand of some people. They sought to kill the owner of the animal. The kanga suggested that they kill the owner of the animal, and the kanga of the Bangwana was given a lot of money for this matter because the people said that the animal had gone among their people in the place where they live. What do we say, we of the Church? God helps us in prayers to praise the hearts of the missionaries who have saved us from the customs of our ancestors. They have sent us our beloved friend, and by the generosity of God that friend came down and killed that animal. It is wonderful, give thanks to God for his generosity. . . . In 1934, the kanga came again to ask for 500 francs and said: "If it were not for me the animal would not have died because I took away the power of the animal. Without that, the animal could not have died with a gun, and I also made medicine to kill the owner of the animal." . . . Friends, don't stop praying because some of us in the Church are lost in customs and clinging to the ideas of kanga. . . . Friends, be courageous.[5]

Likenyule's account demonstrates that Chesterman intervened in a complex therapeutic economy with his desires and gun. It suggests that people were not convinced that Chesterman's gun had killed the crocodile after all. The problem had always been less the crocodile than the "owner of the animal," and to resolve it, they had engaged a BaTambatamba healer, a specialist in ndimo. He claimed to have made medicine, which in killing the human owner of this ndimo-crocodile, "took away the power of the animal." With-

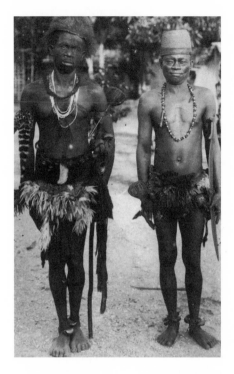

Two *kanga* in the Yakusu district,
ca. 1927. (Courtesy of David Lofts,
PL Papers, Barton-on-Sea, U.K.)

out his medicine and this death, the healer asserted, the doctor's gun would have been powerless. Nurse Likenyule evoked Chesterman as Christ himself in his alternative version of those "lost in customs and clinging to the ideas of kanga." His final words to the readers of *Mboli ya Tengai* were "Friends, be courageous." A history of libeli and reproduction needs to consider the emergence, writings, and social action—the "courage"—of mission-trained middle figures such as Nurse Likenyule. He was translator and buffer as he coped with the consequences of Chesterman's intervention for local wealth and knowledge.

The struggles over libeli were among young and old, Protestants and pagans, Europeans and Congolese from 1900; they were also contests *among* Congolese over power and appropriate reproductive and therapeutic practice. In 1910, the lexicon of debate concerned bieka, falanga, and clothing, even if within church meetings, the primary lexeme of attention was that of balimo. By 1924, new vocabulary—"pills of bravery,"[6] yaws injections, communion cups—was at play; new actors, *ba-infirmiers,* were involved. A decade after this last round of libeli, as Chesterman chased after his crocodile trophy, cutting lilwa was still alive, and public opinion likened murderous crocodiles to airplanes. The doctor was still

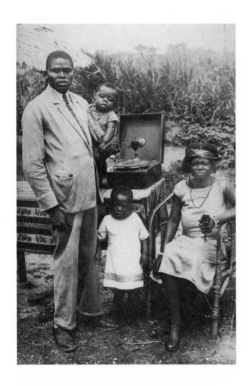

Likenyule with his phonograph and
family, as sent to Phyllis Lofts in
1933. (Courtesy of David Lofts,
PL Papers, Barton-on-Sea, U.K.)

trying to prove something about libeli and fears of its crocodile-related curse,
fala. The previous chapter began to demonstrate the significance of crocodiles.
This chapter continues this history of crocodiles by considering Chesterman's
purpose in killing one. It also turns to the other component in the 1934 metaphor, airplanes. More important, it continues the analysis of libeli contests
and colonial intrusions and violence begun in the last chapter. It examines the
links between missionary interventions and complicities and colonial medicine that developed during this period, contorting the beneficent meanings of
missionary medicine. It also introducing the preeminent mediating work of
Yakusu-trained teachers and nurses, who much more than Yakusu's missionaries shaped the vocabularies by which evangelical medicine came to be admired and understood. The chapter devotes particular attention to Chesterman's sleeping sickness research, the capacities of yaws injections, the letters of
Yakusu's teachers and nurses, and libeli of 1924.

Crocodiles and airplanes were significant things in the quickly metamor-
phosing 1920s' lexicon of mission life. On Christmas Day in 1922, a newcomer
missionary, W. H. Ennals, noted that there is a special tense in the Lokele
language "for things that are going on at the same time," and he thought it just

as well, "for things have a habit of 'happening profusely.'"[7] I turn to these profuse happenings now.

Medleys of the Early 1920s

Dr. and Mrs. Chesterman arrived at Yakusu on October 14, 1920. The doctor performed his first surgical operation in December. When he set his surgical gloves to boil on the cookhouse fire, two of his domestic servants saw a boiling soup of black human hands and imagined that the doctor was going to eat them. Waokwa and Yenga nearly ran away, but "furtively watched the operation through the hospital window" instead. Other local Congolese, too, became keen to watch the doctor perform what they called the "work of the knife."[8] This formative incident in Yakusu's medicalization of its mission activities reveals how strongly themes and symbols from the period of Free State terrors remained alive during the interwar period. Severed human hands, black and in the missionary's pot, resonated with global and local images of "red rubber" atrocities and cannibals in the Congo. The naming of surgery as "the work of the knife," a naming which Chesterman clearly welcomed, also indicates the links local Congolese people were able to make between lilwa cutting—both as a form of cursing an enemy and of achieving the prestige of libeli scars—and Chesterman's new style of colonial surgery. Chesterman's aim was to make the incident a transformative one, and so it was in the case of Victor Yenga, before long a nurse-in-training at the hospital. It was not so easy to dispel suspicions about the purposes of missionary and colonial medicine, especially given the way they so easily became intertwined with mortality, compulsion, and the work of the *chicotte* (whip) in Yakusu's district.

By the end of 1920, Chesterman had met with Dr. Grossule of the state medical service in Stanleyville, arranging for the Yakusu mission to take over a medical census area reaching between the Lindi and Romée Rivers. State funds paid for a new sleeping sickness *lazaret* (the Belgian colonial term for a center to quarantine those with this contagious disease) two miles below Yakusu. Chesterman began to experiment with a new drug provided under Rockefeller research funds, tryparsamide, leading to what he later called "resurrections" or "winning our way into the hearts of these people."[9] Within eighteen months of his arrival, Chesterman was teasingly calling the newly overhauled mission dispensary "Yakusu Hospital Ltd." Patients were coming from as far as 400 miles away to pay for injections and surgical scars, and to buy ointments, pills, and homemade soap.[10] It was during this same eighteen-month period that an airplane flew along the Upper Congo River on a mail run to Stanleyville for the first time. People were "spellbound till it was out of sight. . . . Old croakers said there would be a plague or a famine in the wake of this new apparition. Others were seized with fear and believed that to look on it meant death." The passage of these new "air-steamers that fly like birds" became a monthly event and created a "craze" of activity and discussion in the Yakusu region. While some older people "covered their heads that they might not see the new wonder," Mr. Mill explained, the "quick eyes of the native boys" began to reproduce the main features in model airplanes.

> It was only when one day the wonderful machine descended opposite Yakusu and then opposite Isangi that the craze got its full impetus. Multitudes crowded to the beach and little eyes drank in the details of observer's niche and Pilot's seat, engine and floats and most wonderful of all of the screw and its motion hitherto invisible. Then the mechanical part was added to the model. Old models were spiked on a log rod and supplied with a pith and palm leaf propeller which spun round in the wind. Little urchins formed the same device on a short stick and made it whiz as they ran with it against the wind. In market, on the road, by the hut door, and even in the Sunday School almost every boy carried a whirler.[11]

Congolese boys found it difficult to understand "what forces of nature were harnessed by the aeroplane except that it went by wind." Mill was surprised when some boys "mixed up the same idea" with his bicycle. One day, while busy putting air in his bike tires, this missionary overheard one of them say: "It also goes by wind."[12]

Yaws injections, like airplanes, closely followed the arrival of Yakusu's first doctor. In 1922, Chesterman received a large quantity of salvarsan to treat this "increasingly prevalent" treponemal disease.[13] By 1927, yaws had become central to Yakusu medical care. One doctor, K. W. Todd, called it the "one really common and disabling disease" in the district. Ennals, though not a doctor, sold neo-salvarsan injections while traveling on preaching and school inspection tours in 1923, a year when Chesterman was away on furlough. The "terrible suppurating sores" of yaws were "exceedingly common," Ennals noted, "though they 'respond almost like magic' to the injections." He drew crowds of people eager to pay the high price (two and a half to ten francs) for such a shot, and within ten days, he "had run quite out of this important line."

Ennals also assisted Yakusu's new doctor, F. G. Spear, with sleeping sickness inspection work during 1923. The work involved lining people up and checking their neck glands for enlargement: "This sounds very simple, 'parading the people before their doors' but it is fraught with all sorts of difficulties, and several times one saw the occupant in full plight [*sic*] from the scene of action."[14] Those found to be normal received a medical passport specifying the exam's date and results, and granting the person the right to travel. (Medical passports, key to sleeping sickness policy, became mandatory from 1910; all workers required them, as did those traveling on steamers and trains or crossing colonial borders.)[15] This kind of missionary labor was new. Not only had Mr. Ennals just arrived at Yakusu, but the contract whereby Yakusu's doctors served as state-approved hygiene agents charged with medical census and passport work was less than a year old. Mr. Mill had previously worked at a state lazaret; the new contract formalized missionary collaboration in this colony's sanitary regime.

Ennals thought that he would never forget the reaction of one man "when he received his coveted piece of paper": "this lusty native all painted with camwood powder and presenting a most gory appearance scrambled out from the eaves of the hut and brandishing his precious paper ran for the large drum which occupied a hut in the centre of the village, then laying his paper on the floor he excitedly beat out the message telling all and sundry that he had got his 'lokasa.'" A "witchdoctor," who "was smart enough to ask Doc 'as a brother in the profession' to give him a letter saying that he was a reliable doctor," also seemed "an interesting little personality." Spear gave the kanga a microscopic slide and bought "one of his mysterious rattles for a franc" instead of giving him a testimonial. Ennals and Spear did more than play tourist, even if they did find pleasure in their work: "I confess it was really rather good fun to have them all paraded outside to have their glands felt." When they arrived in the village of Yalikonda,

> it was easy to see that there were very special things in progress. Nearly everybody was painted in some weird style, in red or white. Many men had their feet painted bright red up to the ankles, some had daubs of white paint on one eye, others on the forehead. The hair of most of them was done in a most peculiar style. . . . Some of the wildest spirits were in the midst of a native dance, and they were wearing garlands of palm fronds . . . as the[y] danced round the three drums which were in the centre of the village.

What began as an adventure "undertaken as part of our work for the Government Medical Service" became a "strange medley of heathen ritual and scientific investigation." Ennals and Spear did not have time for Christian prayers or sermons, it seems, but Ennals concluded that the day had been a "battle for the Lord." After all, their state powers had given them a way to end this "native"— perhaps tosumbe—dancing: "We stopped all this and all the dancers had to form up into line to be examined."[16]

There were other medleys during Chesterman's absence in 1923. Mrs. Millman called Dr. Spear away from work one morning to go down to a "palaver" in Yakoso. The doctor returned to the hospital with a feverish boy who believed himself to be "the victim of a witch's malevolence." The boy accused an old man of making him ill; the old man became sick two days later and died on the third. The boy stayed in the hospital, got well, and began working as one of Yakusu's first nurses-in-training.[17] Another day, a man in a canoe rescued a fisherman who had been in the river pulling a net around to a bank when a crocodile seized him, tearing away flesh from his back and mangling his arm. He brought him to the hospital, where the patient was soon on the operating table, annoyed at Dr. Spear's stitches.

> "What is a man to die twice in one day? Twice in one day! Oh!" "There now" says the Doctor quietly "keep yourself calm, one place is finished all right" and he proceeds to draw together the edges of the next wound. It required some manipulation and several stitches. Snap! went a needle as the patient wriggled at the first puncture. A new needle was handed up and the work went on. "Not finished yet" calls the man, "Eyaya! Fancy sewing a man like a piece of cloth." Click! Another needle has gone. The Doctor sighs "That's the last of our curved ones; give me a straight one." The man on the table takes the next stab quietly, then bursts out laughing "Get a sewing machine Doctor. Get a sewing machine. O dear! what next will they do at men's bodies."[18]

The man's metaphor comparing surgery to mechanized sewing was part of the "appearance of bustle and activity" during the early 1920s. Sewing machines had been available at the mission's Barter Store earlier in the century, and Yakusu's missionaries were giving them as wedding gifts to their favorite Congolese girls from at least 1919. The hospital had tailors sewing nursing uniforms for a wage, and this crocodile victim perhaps had witnessed them at work. The missionaries found pleasure in his comparison, appropriating it into their repertoire of mirthful mission tales.[19]

Dr. Chesterman returned from furlough with his architect brother in 1924. The brother supervised the construction of an imposing hospital complex on the riverbank. Mechanical power, in the form of a semidiesel engine running on deep red palm oil, arrived in the same year. The engine fueled a circular saw, used to cut some of the timber that gangs of men were clearing from the forest to build the new hospital.[20] Rumors began to spread about the construction: "At one stage women passing to the market noticed the foundations of inner rooms, and suspicions were aroused that it was to be in there that the doctors would take their victims, cut them up and put them in tins for sale." No one passed by for weeks, Chesterman recalled. The hospital construction also "disturbed" local people, according to Nurse Phyllis Lofts, because a tree on the site, which BaTambatamba had used to hang disobedient slaves and those too old or infirm to be of value, was cut down. Lofts saved a piece of the tree among her memorabilia with a note explaining that local people called it a "sacred tree" and a "tree of cruelty." Chesterman arranged for three canoes to carry the tree trunk to a Stanleyville sawmill. The planks became the hospital's benches and tables.[21]

It was in this context of rapid, startling change—featuring airplanes, injections, and the sewing up of a crocodile victim—that the first visible performance of libeli in fourteen years began. It was soon after Chesterman returned in 1924. According to Ennals: "the old men of the Lokeles . . . are afraid that there having been no initiations into their spirit worship cult for many years, owing to Mission influence, that they will have no one to minister to their spirits when they die." As in 1910, the missionaries complained, "many of our boys have been forced in against their will."[22] Few "dared to disobey the call, or even wished to keep out of it, for to do so meant persecution and social ostracism." They also feared "the songs of the women who all refuse to marry a man who is an outcast." After five months had passed, in July 1924, men were only beginning to return from the forest: "there is nearly a famine in food stuffs." Yakusu's missionaries and church leaders met to discuss how to handle this "recrudescence of the tribal initiation ceremonies accompanied with orgies and deceptions denounced by the Church." They passed a resolution barring libeli participants from communion. Some 1,500 members were expelled at the time.[23]

A Doctor's "Healing Knife"?

What provoked libeli of 1924? Was it an expression of public opinion, a way to reclaim and uphold wealth in persons and things? When William Millman wrote his quasi-academic, ethnographic essay of 1927, he suggested that libeli was a last-ditch Lokele effort to rescue their society from the onslaught of colonialism. Other missionaries blamed the 1924 return to libeli on "a knowledge seeking official" who let "a few influential chiefs know that he thought it would be interesting to see some harmless customs of the past again." State authorities refused to help the Yakusu church suppress libeli in 1924.[24]

Wealth and its extraction in church offerings may have been involved. Church finance remained a frequent subject at meetings, and problems in paying teachers from offerings alone did not disappear. By the early 1920s, francs and centimes were everywhere in the Belgian Congo, and the former "glory of the Barter Store" at Yakusu was no more. Riverside churches were paying the salaries of their own teachers, as well as contributing to the salaries of those who worked in forest schools. Church offerings increased in 1920, and special cards were issued for this purpose. In 1922, this gift card had to indicate "paid up" for a member to take communion.[25] In 1923, a missionary named H. B. Parris made a special district tour to collect lifaefi; he noted, "nothing but the visit of the white missionary will make them bestir themselves." His timing, Parris also said, "might perhaps have been more happily chosen, for to be on the road at the same time as the annual State taxes are being enforced is not conducive to the best financial results."[26] Parris's lifaefi tour may have signi- fied political competition to Congolese chiefs and the Belgian agents to whom they reported.

The donations Mr. Parris received made clear the rival regional economy that the church represented. Tables, chairs, "iron spearheads" or linganda, chickens, paddles, baskets, a strip of leopard's skin, a cummerbund, an antique pair of European braces, and a Belgian flag were among the lifaefi that people gave Parris. The mission's Barter Store may have lost its glory, but the deck of the mission boat "began to look like a curiosity shop." The sundry gifts suggest that people wanted their gift cards, their entry tickets to communion, to be marked "paid up." They also demonstrate that bieka, whether in food or things, re- mained the lexicon of church offerings in the 1920s. If in falanga people were broke, in things they were not. By the end of 1923, however, many had still not contributed. They received word that they had "lapsed from membership."[27]

Who these lapsed members were is unclear. So is their reasoning. Did they not give because they could not, because they refused, or because they did not care enough to keep their memberships active? The early 1920s brought multi- ple changes to the Belgian Congo. The development of plantations near Yakusu was particularly significant for the mission church. Much of the BaMbole forest was being marked out as a plantation district for the first time, and road construction began to make this region remote from the river accessible by automobile. Baptist Congolese began to have less time for church activities, complaining that they had to clear roads and tidy villages for "the State." Some were pressed into forced labor in road building; others were recruited for paid jobs on plantations. Yangambi began as a rubber plantation; a white planter and his wife were living there with their four children in 1926.[28] European company agents buying palm nuts were visible in Yakusu's district from 1917 onward.[29] Early in 1926, Parris met "one of my old boys" and some Topoke (Eso) people at Basoko, the town at the confluence of the Aruwimi; the former student was "now a clerk in the HCB," the Huileries du Congo Belge, the Congo affiliate of the British-based soap manufacturer, Lever Brothers (later Unilever). These Topoke told Parris that "they had been decoyed from their homes for work at Basoko only to find that they were now to proceed to Kinshasa."[30]

Rubber became a plantation crop in some locations, as did coffee, cocoa, and palm, though the HCB encouraged palm collecting from existing groves until its own plantations were established.

State authorities were distributing palm nut presses and groundnut seed to local chiefs, who in turn were organizing labor to plant new crops, collect palm nuts, and produce oil from them. Palm oil concessions—purchasing and selling points at least; perhaps plantations, too—of the HCB were present in the district by 1923; an English-speaking West African from Accra was supervising labor at one of them. By 1926, the state was working on better allocating "the labour assets of the population," balancing the requirements of mineral and plantation companies in the colony; 7 percent of the Yakusu church's 2,140 male members were away working at "large labour centres."[31] By the close of the decade, mining prospectors were searching for diamonds in the area, and "thousands of natives" were "working in large groups and separated from their own folk," on nearby plantations and farther afield in the Kilo-Moto mining region.

Lokele generally received work as foremen and clerks, especially if they had received some education in Yakusu's schools; Olombo and other formerly en-slaved forest peoples were more likely to receive manual work. Lokele tended to return home to visit their towns with "pencils behind their ears and books in their hands." All workers were bringing back new signs of wealth and style during the 1920s, such as sun helmets, eyeglasses, secondhand clothing, mirrors, soap, and sewing supplies.[32] The imported "left-off winter garbs of soldiers and policemen and postmen" became a common form of dress. Missionaries esti-mated that local forms of body decoration such as "greasing, colouring, tattoo-ing, or carving the skin"—the staples of libeli—were "losing any esteem" in 1921.[33] Ennals and Spear observed otherwise during a medical tour in Yalikonda in 1923; white clay, camwood, and palm frond garlands were in active use there. Rather, a creolized calculus of value was at play during this critical decade of social and material change. Imported salt remained an important *matabish* (tip) and register of wealth; the mission's domestic workers reveled in names like Saboni (Soap) and Waokwa (Of Salt), and chiefs continued to wear monkey and leopard skin caps with plumes of red parrot feathers as well as leopard tooth necklaces, at least on special state occasions.[34]

The Yakusu church still forbade tosumbe dancing; its missionaries encour-aged more wholesome Maypole dancing during the mid-1920s instead.[35] Yet to-sumbe was not the only dance form forbidden as a "worldly practice" in the 1920s. Congolese had returned from First World War battles in Tanganyika dancing *kwaya*, and just a few years later, workers were coming home from company posts dancing new "jazz" steps. *Malinga* dancing from Kinshasa, accompanied by music made with "the clackety-clak" of "little wooden cas-

tanets," spread up the Congo and Lomami Rivers about 1929. In one missionary's words, malinga was "an imitation of the white man's jazz." Both kwaya and
malinga were, in missionary eyes, "immoral" and "obscene." The problem with
malinga, according to "the opinion of mature minds in the native Church," was
that although it seemed "harmless enough when danced by either sex separately," it was "highly objectionable for men and women to clasp one another
thus promiscuously in public." When Mr. and Mrs. Mill asked a Belgian company agent to help them suppress malinga dancing, he responded: "But you
have the Tango and the Charleston in England." The missionary couple replied
that "it is for those at home to protest there and for us to protest here and to
help a nation in the making." The Lomami Company generally cooperated with
the missionaries in prohibiting their Congolese employees from "dancing the
immoral dance on their concessions." But local chiefs proved better allies in the
struggle against these new, modern dances than either company or state agents,
Yakusu's missionaries discovered. One Congolese chief "had sworn by his father's spirit that no one should do it." Some chiefs imposed heavy fines, while
flogging—the giving of "stripes . . . in the Native Government Tribunal"—acted
as a "deterrent for future relapses."[36]

Chesterman attributed the 1924 outbreak of libeli to "the ever-tightening grip
of the State on the people, and the limitations to personal liberty and tribal
authority." He did not acknowledge the Yakusu mission's appreciation of, nor
the mission's continuing complicity with, this state's disciplinary labor and
hygiene regimes. Chesterman chose to mystify instead, while writing himself
into a narrative as a heroic Great Physician figure engaged in a colonial evangelical battle: "some said it was that the Devil was giving special attention to us
at close quarters; some say simply that the point where the Doctor puts his healing knife and stitches, there you must expect reaction before healing is done."[37]

By 1933, active membership was down to 3,000, "about half of normal membership." Active members attended services, gave "towards expenses," and were
"not known to be involved in any worldly practices." Three prominent church
leaders read relevant papers at a church meeting. Abalayama's talk was on
"Suggestions for Establishing Christian Marriage," Lititiyo spoke on "The Problem of Slack or Inactive Members," and Bufululu's paper was called "Notes on
Journeys Made to Visit Church Members Employed on Distant Plantations and
Concessions by Trading Companies."[38] In 1934, a missionary teacher named
K. C. Parkinson tallied the 500 "boys" who had entered Yakusu's school since
1929, noting that there were four things that a boy who had completed school
and gained a certificate could do. He could stay on at the station and learn a
skilled job such as printing; go to Stanleyville or a company post and get a job as
a clerk or foreman; join the ordinary teaching staff in the district at a low rate of

pay; or sit for the entrance exam to enter advanced training as a teacher or nurse. George Baluti, the son of Yakusu's senior Congolese pastor, had taken a new job at Yanonge, directing the loading and unloading of cargo for the Bamboli plantation company.[39] A teacher named Toleka and an "Elève Diplomé," Bofofe, were wearing BMS shirts with pride and holding services on the Upper Lomami near Opala in 1932 for "many of the plantation workers of the Lomami Company" who, like them, were "a long way from home."[40] Lokele-identified, BMS Christian communities became significant at Belgika, Lomami, and HCB (Unilever) company posts. Some endured into the 1950s: in 1952, Yakusu's missionary W. H. Ford commented on the "migratory and commercial traits in the Lokele character" after discovering "small colonies of people who have migrated from the villages around us here," who were practicing Protestants while working as "fisherman, traders, clerks, store-keepers, mechanics, and labourers" at riverain commercial and plantation centers at Lowa, Bumba (Alberta), and Lisala.[41]

Great Physicians

Yakusu students were increasingly spotted by Europeans in the Congo as potential reliable clerks and nurses for "big companies and plantations," and some of Yakusu's "hospital boys" were running rural dispensaries, some on company plantations, by the early 1930s.[42] Yaokombo was not a company dispensary, but Nurse Likenyule was one of these reliable, Yakusu-trained nurses. A decade and a half earlier, there were no Likenyules, unless we include the anonymous "lad of about fifteen" who helped Yakusu's first missionary nurse, Rose Gee, dress wounds.[43]

Missionary medicine was hardly new at Yakusu during the early 1920s, even though doctors were. An evangelical Great Physician idiom had long been part of activities at Yakusu, and at play in missionary deeds and parables; we saw the rewards of Millman's kind healing in chapter 1. Miss Gee saw about sixty patients a day in 1913. Many arrived wearing "hideous markings of whitish-brown clay" all over their bodies "to prevent the disease from attacking them." She held short services before treating patients, and other assistants—those she called "our Christian young men"—delivered speeches on the "Good Physician and His healing power."[44] Surgery was limited to scraping ulcers and, occasionally, extracting teeth. Anesthesia seems to have been unknown. Although pharmaceuticals and medical technologies remained limited in 1916, patients paid for drugs and clinical care at Yakusu, the only missionary dispensary within 500 miles.[45]

Trypanosomiasis had begun to sweep the district in 1903, and there was a state-operated sleeping sickness camp near Yakusu by 1910; this rudimentary isolation center was quarantining the sick, forcibly separating them from their homes and kin. Yakusu lost its first victim to the disease, Salamo, in 1911.[46] As the epidemic expanded throughout northeastern Congo, protocols and medicines for treating this "colonial disease"[47] came down to missionaries from state medical authorities. So did free drugs for treating it. From 1906, Yakusu's missionaries, like all Europeans, were obliged to try to protect their workers from the trypanosomiasis.[48] Many Congolese tried to escape the new hygienic policing, leading to even tighter controls over inspection. Medical passports certifying that a worker had been examined were required by 1912. Henceforth, uniformed Congolese soldiers or police were to be present during medical censusing work.[49]

Sleeping sickness treatment became an exception to the BMS tradition of charging fees for medical care; it also led to new, more coercive formulations in the Great Physician model of mission healing. Injections of the blinding arsenical compound called atoxyl, available in the Congo by 1906, were free but compulsory.[50] Mill took a three-month, state-qualifying course in tropical medicine in Brussels with an additional month of training in Leopoldville in 1914. When he returned to Yakusu with nine cases of medical supplies—including a microscope, balances, hypodermic needles, and atoxyl—he assumed responsibility for inspecting villages for sleeping sickness. Youth, eager to obtain the state papers certifying that they had been examined, "presented themselves" to Mill. Those who knew they were sick avoided him. Mill would have used the standard diagnostic techniques of his time, palpating cervical glands at the back of the neck and examining under a microscope blood samples taken from pricked fingers, lymph fluid aspirated with a syringe from swollen neck glands, and cerebral spinal fluid taken from the lower back by means of the painful procedure known as a lumbar puncture. Lumbar punctures were performed with such regularity and dispatch in the Congo that the procedure became a verb by 1904: "we lumbar-punctured."[51] Atoxyl, the only trypanocide available in the Congo until 1920, cured few in the early stage of the disease and had no effect on more advanced cases. The mortality was fearful; rumors that colonial doctors caused the disease and rounded up patients in "death camps" in order to eat them circulated widely during the final years of "red rubber," a time rife with rumors of being cut and eaten. The fact that sleeping sickness investigators were keen to perform autopsies did not help. One doctor commented in 1903, "we are told that we are believed to eat parts of those on whom we do autopsies, and to preserve other portions for the purpose of making medicine."[52] Patients understood, Mill said, that "few upon whom the needle is used live a year out." He did not entirely approve of state methods and mercenary worries; he knew that authorities feared a tax shortfall if many died, and that patients in the state's new "Isolation Island" were "prisoners while there." Yet he had been trained for the state-affiliated job and had his state-provided supplies, and he continued to assist at the island lazaret near Yakusu, where the forest had been cleared and "good Mud & grass houses" built for the quarantined receiving "free Medical treatment" there.[53]

There were continuities in labor and hygiene policy between the Free State and Belgian Congo regimes, just as there were continuities in Yakusu missionary complicity in state-organized economic and sanitary regimes between the 1910s and 1920s. The 1920s were distinctive, however, for the increased cooperation between state authorities and the newly medicalized mission station; this process meant new compromises with coercive state methods and an enlarged capacity for Yakusu's doctors to act as the state. Special mobile medical teams also began to operate in the 1920s, surveying whole regions and identifying and treating sleeping sickness patients in their villages. In Yakusu's district, Dr. Chesterman took on these duties as an officially recognized doctor (*médecin agréé*).

After Chesterman arrived in 1921, rounding up patients to inspect for sleeping sickness intensified. Mrs. Chesterman would spend "her time making friends with the women and children" during a medical tour, while the doctor would examine people "square by square weeding out the sleeping sickness patients."[54] The sleeping sickness patients who went mad while under treatment were bothersome for Chesterman; he ordered one to be chained by a long, heavy piece of iron in the station's timber storeroom in 1924. He injected this man, whose "naked body" had been "smeared all over with white chalk," with two doses of Twilight Sleep (a short-lived fashion in obstetric analgesia) to calm him from his "fiendish hilarity."[55] The use of chains and "lock-ups" with trypanosomiasis patients was common in the Congo during these years, even if detailed case records, like those Chesterman published, were not.[56]

Chesterman's first sleeping sickness patient at Yakusu was a sixteen-year-old girl named Lisoi. After a few months' treatment with tryparsamide, she returned to her village, where she was "bludgeoned" to death, Chesterman explained, "for having come for treatment to the white man" instead of a local kanga. One day during a medical census tour, Chesterman met the chief responsible for killing Lisoi. The chief was trying to hide two wives from the doctor's lumbar puncture work. Chesterman reminisced about this incident with his doctor-colleagues in tropical medicine in London in 1947: "I got my own back; it was still in those days permissible to use the chicotte, and the Chief got the benefit of it."[57] Chesterman did not need to use the word whip. British tropical doctors knew the meaning of the French word *chicotte*—a "fearful whip made of hippopotamus hide," often with a wooden handle, "with which the natives in all parts of the Congo are so familiar"—as well as Belgian colonial doctors did. Flogging was central to colonial discipline and abuses in the Congo. Chicotte had entered the English language during the humanitarian campaigns against "red rubber" in the Congo early in the twentieth century,[58] and painted images of its official colonial use remain a central catalyst for postcolonial social memory today. The history of the object, and its purposes of cutting skin and terrorizing, were older than Free State times in the eastern Congo; indeed, the use of hippo hide in whipping would have represented another continuity among the Zanzibari, Free State, and Belgian Congo periods for Congolese people.

Soldiers—and hippo-hide whips—became such a banal feature of sleeping sickness inspection tours that they tended to go unmentioned after 1912, when a circular first insisted that Congolese soldiers or police accompany all tours.[59] Yet Chesterman's language in London resembled that used by Uganda's Dr. Albert Cook some ten years earlier (in 1938), also before an audience of tropical medical specialists. Cook, when describing his 1897 difficulties with a "native boy" who refused to help procure human skeletons, had boasted of laying him down and giving him "a half a dozen of the best for insubordination." Each of these missionary doctors strayed far from Great Physician idioms in these scientific circles, where they spoke proudly—code switching into a register of imperial masculine bravado impossible in missionary magazines—that they acted as agents of colonial discipline, using flogging to punish those who dared to defy them. Chesterman had served as part of the medical corps in Serbia and the Middle East during World War I; he entered missionary service almost immediately afterward, at a time when colonial authorities throughout sub-Saharan Africa were reorganizing native medical services along new lines. Cook was of an earlier generation of colonial evangelical doctors in Africa who more directly combined conquest with medical work. Striking is the common language of imperial, violent masculinity used among such colonial doctors of different generations, who mixed together at tropical medicine meetings in metropolitan capitals.[60]

Chesterman tried to distance himself from state violence in 1921 when he insisted to missionary supporters that he did not travel with soldiers, though he was "working hand in hand with the state, and trying to impress that the authorities desire to act as a father, as well as a master."[61] Yet, to Chesterman, "father" and "master" were complementary terms, in the colonial Congo as in theology and the family; he endorsed a paternalistic construction of both the state and rubber plantations. Much like Dr. Cook during the Nubian Mutiny, Chesterman performed his tours as médecin agréé under military discipline. There may have been no soldiers, but colonial forms of corporal punishment were readily available. Mrs. Chesterman would be there perhaps, praying with women and children. Still, Chesterman carried census books, and hippo-hide whips were not far away.

In 1926, Chesterman reported that over 10,000 injections had been given to 700 patients. He also oversaw the state's sleeping sickness campaign in this region, including ordering the relocation of whole villages: "delinquents have been searched for, unhealthy villages removed and breeding places of the fly have been cleared." Although sleeping sickness inspections were obligatory on paper, wage workers (who were, by definition, men) were the privileged category subject to them in the Congo. Doctors and officials repeatedly complained about how difficult it was to examine women for sleeping sickness; they did not need medical passports like wage workers did, and they were more likely to hide at inspection time. Chesterman's published case data indicate, however, that over one-half of his tryparsamide research subjects were women and girls. Clinical care at Yakusu remained elective and strongly skewed toward male patients, at least until 1930. When a new wing was added to the Yakusu dispensary in 1916, Mr. Mill confessed, "How shall I justify myself when I say the wing which has been built is only for men?"[62] Men had always outnumbered women as patients of medical care at Yakusu, and they continued to do so at least through 1949. The number of female inpatients was as low as 14 percent in 1929 and never higher than 32 percent during the years 1921–29. A special women's ward was not opened until 1930, and even then, female patients represented only about one-third (35 percent) of all those treated. Further, the evidence suggests that these gender differentials among hospital patients were as equally skewed among boys and girls as they were among men and women.[63] But Chesterman was exceptionally effective in coercing women as well as men to undergo sleeping sickness investigation during his district inspection tours.

Women and girls may have avoided the mission hospital, but they were unable to elude lumbar punctures and blinding pharmaceuticals in Chesterman's district.[64] His clinical success was uneven, however. Chesterman's tryparsamide treatment records impressed specialists in tropical medicine at a London meeting of the Royal Society for Tropical Medicine and Hygiene. Yet some argued that the side effect of blindness that resulted in so many of his cases was "no trivial matter." Madness was a nuisance that was part of the course of the disease; blindness was not. One professor told him: "Certainly I, myself, would hesitate greatly before I deliberately ran the risk of making a patient blind."[65]

Fala, Crocodiles, and Yaws Injections

The same people who tried to run away from lumbar punctures and tryparsamide shots were eager to pay for salvarsan injections for fala. Not unlike the way in which missionaries and other colonial observers tended to gloss kanga as "witch doctor" (or *sorcier*), Chesterman glossed fala as "witchcraft" when he talked with doctors about yaws. In 1927, he noted that one of the most common bony lesions of tertiary yaws at Yakusu was antero-posterior bowing of the tibia. Local people called this bone curvature "matchet leg." Tropical medicine specialists often called it "boomerang leg."[66] Chesterman commented in 1947 that "the capriciousness of the onset of tertiary lesions has led some . . . to attribute this to witchcraft, and it is supposed to be the curse from the neglect of a certain taboo." He knew that according to local vocabularies, fala (Lok.) was distinct from syphilis or *kassende* (Sw.), which people associated with the arrival of the Zanzibari and the Swahili language in the nineteenth century; fala "had been with them from time immemorial."[67]

Ninety-five percent of all people contracted yaws before puberty, he estimated, though most only developed primary yaws in infancy.[68] Mothers understood that secondary manifestations often led to more serious tertiary ones, but that the extremely disfiguring fala—the later, more advanced form of the disease—did not always ensue. Chesterman explained that, consequently, "women had a great objection to bringing their children for treatment until the secondary granulomata were well developed"; they feared "driving the disease inwards." People had their own treatments for fala. According to Chesterman, during former times of "war and bloodshed . . . old women acted as ghouls, and went to the scenes of bloodshed and collected clotted blood and mixed it with palm oil, then applied this mixture to the lesions. It was said to be beneficial in healing them." This story, however embellished by Chesterman, resonates with the cure for yaws that Mill heard about in 1915; it "could be made from pounded bark mixed with a red stone which was supposed to be the coagulated blood of their dead ancestors petrified in the earth."[69] Consider John Janzen's words: "Control of the agent that contributes to chaos . . . is the therapy which leads to health."[70] The evidence suggests that blood was as important as crocodile in local medicines, and that violations such as slavery, war, sorcery, and murder were known to cause not only bloodshed and angry ancestral spirits but fala.

Though mothers may have hesitated to obtain salvarsan injections for their infants with primary lesions, older people with relapses of tertiary yaws eagerly paid for them. By the mid-1920s, 3,000 yaws patients a year received treatment within the Yakusu district.[71] About 1,000 of these had tertiary yaws, half of whom were treated at the hospital rather than rural sites. When Chesterman was touring in 1924, an old woman on the edge of a crowd gathered for his dispensary session hesitated out loud: " 'Shall I show him that ulcer on my ankle?' she asked. 'Can he really surpass Fala?' echoed another. 'Yes, he says that his needle can frighten it away,' responded a third person."[72] A grammar of substitution was suggested here. Hypodermic needles eradicated the curse of crocodile-associated fala, while replacing libeli scars formed by crocodile-composed medicines. Chesterman was working on a similar grammar about biomedical efficacy and the fallacy of fala during the libeli revival in 1924, and he was still honing it as he organized his crocodile killing in 1934. Thus, Chesterman's medicalized interpretation of how his "healing knife" provoked libeli in 1924 may not have been inaccurate, just as his notions of easy substitution had evident effects. Even though a more complex conjunction of signs and social realities was at play, Chesterman's success was partly due to the fact that his patients could interpolate the novel treatments he offered within local symbolic grammars. Chesterman's construction of therapeutic competition—his oppositional pairing of the healing knife of mission surgery with libeli—also guided missionary reactions to events.

The missionary campaign against libeli became an opportunity to claim the superiority of biomedicine, while also gaining greater knowledge of therapeutic and surgical aspects of libeli. The missionaries learned for the first time, for example, about the secrecy of "the hiding place of the 'medicine,' some of which was inserted into the wounds made in the back of each novice" and "acts fatally on themselves if they are disloyal to their oath in any detail."[73] The Belgian colonial state may have refused to help the British Baptist mission in suppressing libeli. But Chesterman, as médecin agréé, could pose as the state, and he "worked from within to hasten the exposure and discomfiture of the business." His goal was to undermine fears of and beliefs in fala: "We handled it by penetrating into its Holy Places in the course of our official Medical Inspection of the people, invoking all the curses imaginable on our helmeted heads. We exposed in every possible way the fallacy of the association between disobedience to it and a disfiguring disease which is very prevalent."[74]

Chesterman's intrusions into fala and libeli, into a lobe, expressed his will to violate, destroy, and extract; and they left their mark on social memory. Remember Tata Bafoya's words: "But then the whites of the mission arrived here and that one, Chesterman, he forbid libeli." People told me in 1989 that Chesterman had trampled in a territory of dangerous medicines when he had entered Yakoso's lobe. They claimed that he became sick and nearly died: "Even Chesterman, the medicines got him. . . . If there had not been shots—it was as if Chesterman wanted to get that sickness. . . . Because he entered, he entered. So we stabbed him with our knives. We stabbed him: 'Ah! That you die! Ah! That you die of this ailment, fala. That it gets you.'" Chesterman exploited this associational logic, this local metaphorical pairing of the symbolic knifing of a libeli curse and injections. When touring in 1924, he did not contradict local ideas about the power of salvarsan injections to frighten fala away. Social memory suggests how multiple grammars of substitution came into play. Thus, the counterpoint to the knife wound—the libeli curse—that could have killed Chesterman with fala was a hospital injection that the missionary claimed would cure the condition. This counterpoint was readily available: "Fala: thus ulcers. You see it in the eyes. You see it on the arms. Thus fala, the ulcer itself, that one. So, you come to the hospital; they give you a shot."[75] This pairing, like a series of others, was evident in people's memories. Libeli was about eating, everyone insisted. Here, too, Chesterman had rejoined appropriately. Tata Bafoya's memories slipped swiftly from images of knifing Chesterman in the lobe to images of the grand feasts of food, shot by mission hunters and cooked by Congolese women, that the doctor gave to the local people at Christmas time: "Ah!! Mama, at Noel time and *bonne année*, he would call us the old people of the village. 'I want, the old people should come, they should come, they should come.' You would see, he would get women, they would cook food, food, so much food you could not eat. . . . Three guns, four guns, sending to the forest."[76]

Yakusu's missionaries aimed to provide other substitutes for libeli during the 1920s. For example, they organized Boy Scout activities for Baptist youth, intended to be parallel to the age grading of libeli, and they promoted French as an esoteric language, parallel to the secret one learned by libeli initiates. Yakusu's newly trained Boy Scouts performed *Sir Robert Baden Powell's Story of the Meeting of Stanley and Livingstone* at Christmas in 1924. The mission play may have been removed from a libeli spectacle, and less enticing than grand feasts or man-making athletic games in the forest. Yet replacement was the objective, violent, inchoate removal the means.[77]

Confessions and Communion

The church decided in July 1924 that all libeli participants would be under discipline, "debarred from Communion" for the rest of the year. They could only receive communion again by making a public oath denouncing libeli as fraud. This measure was applied alongside another one that disciplined members for unpaid contributions. The "application of these two rules" affected 1,500 of the 4,000 church members, "a staggering figure." According to Millman, "more than a thousand men" came "under discipline either as initiates, sponsors or active supporters." Only 3 of over 300 teachers were among them.[78]

Such exclusions proved a slow but effective tactic. "One by one" during the coming year, "members made their public oaths condemning libeli, so they could take communion once again."[79] By 1926, "the enmity of the Libeli times" seemed to be "supplanted by goodwill and cordiality once more." In April 1927, there was a "rise" in the building of schools, with men constructing structures and women slopping in mud to complete the walls, so new teachers could be sent in. Yet only a quarter of the expelled members had returned to church membership by 1927, and Millman imagined "a large number of the rest may never return."[80]

One teacher who lost his job and membership due to participating in libeli turned to plantation work. He left this job later, however, and returned to teaching for the church after dreaming that a "messenger of the Lord" was calling. Two of "the latest and youngest recruits" among thirteen hospital workers and students "failed to make good their stand against" libeli. Some mission youth, instead, became nurses through refusing libeli. Mrs. Chesterman spotted Victor Yenga, the same "boy" whom she described running away from the doctor's soup of boiling cut-off human hands, "standing on our verandah, before his father and uncle, with tears streaming down his face, as he denounced them as traitors to the Lord." Shortly afterward, he became seriously ill. Kin gathered, offering to take him home and make medicine "that they might find out who had bewitched him." Yenga refused: "I believe in God, and I will stay with the white Doctor, whose wisdom surpasses all your witchcraft." He was soon in nurse training at the hospital.[81]

Stories told while confessing about libeli, like Yenga's refusal, turned on issues of medicine, illness, and therapeutic choice. "Seeking the wayward" was a process of eliciting—indeed, coercing—confessions. It was not enough to say, "we are repentant and we wish to rejoin the Church." Penitents were required to "renounce the cult for ever because it is based upon deceit." They had to state that they would "dare the curses" of fala and death, putting their trust in God alone. Men and boys were terrified: "Why do you make it difficult? Do you not love us any longer? . . . You know all about what happened. Let it be. Why try to force us to say things for which we should have to suffer?" No one could take communion or give offerings until his renunciations were complete. Many were unwilling or unable. By April 1925, only one-tenth of those who had left the church for libeli had confessed. When eight young men "from Libeli villages" arrived from a rubber plantation to make the necessary statement to Mrs. Millman one night, the last to confess suddenly balked: "Then I noticed that his face had grown ashen grey as if he were ill. I knew the symptoms, I had met them several times during the trip. The veins in his neck stood out and beads of perspiration began to form on his brow but he uttered no sound. At last when I had put two or three questions to him without avail he suddenly gasped out 'I cannot say it.' Then he walked away." Another young man did not get beyond the third question: " 'I feel very ill,' he said 'I think I must go to the hospital' and he struggled to the door."[82]

Middles and Papers: A New Scriptural Economy

In 1927, a church teacher named Daniel Yaliole complained of hypocrisy: "Some people come to the white men and say we have changed. We have given up our libeli. But those words are just lies, and they act like a dog, which after being washed with water to become neat, goes to sit down in the soil again." In 1935, another teacher criticized the superficiality of confessions, again in animal metaphors. The problem, B. Phillipe Falanga said, was that too many church members had not "vomited libeli." Dogs were returning to food previously refused. Wild pigs had washed their bodies, but were coming "back squirming in the dead black leaves on the bank of the river." Thus, some were renouncing libeli "in front of White Men, and later after repenting, when they go back to the village. . . . he will fear the eyes of the people and then he will take [cut] libeli again." Some "elders of the Church and some youth of the Church have . . . not abandoned eating the food and wealth of libeli, and if they hear that one of theirs in the Church has cut libeli, they will not make it known." Yaliole and Falanga published their criticisms in the Lokele-language church magazine, *Mboli ya Tengai*.[83] Chesterman did not create these animal metaphors, these images of washing and wallowing in dirt, of eating and vomiting. These poetics, this lexicon, these pairs had been present in BMS-trained teachers' vocabularies since at least 1916, when Yakusu-trained teachers, posted at district chapels and schools, began publishing letters in *Mboli ya Tengai*.

A new culture of papers, reading, and writing was present in "Lokeleland" from early in the century. This "magazine in the native tongue" first appeared in 1909; by 1923, *Mboli ya Tengai* (Church News) had a circulation of 300 to 400 and was "read nearly 100 miles along the Congo river." It continued to be published for the next fifty years. The teachers' letters published in the magazine reveal that their authors were usually Lokele strangers in the forest villages where they worked,[84] and their presence provoked rivalry and strife. Conflict especially erupted over *lisoo*, a Lokele word for medicine and charms. Lisoo, although not part of the lexicon of debate in church discussions about libeli in 1910, was a frequent subject in teachers' letters.[85] "If you do not have courage you cannot be a *boekesi*," or evangelical teacher, insisted Isamoiso, in 1916.

> Listen. Sunday I crossed the river to go teach at Binasilonga. On my way, one person who had lisoo spread them in the pathway so I would step over them. So I stepped over this medicine, saying in the name of Jesus Himself who is the Master of this work, "Nothing is going to happen to me." . . . Later the boekesi Isalombi sent me a message telling me to come again to Binasilonga because people were going to be hiding, waiting for me with medicines as I went on my way there. So I said, "Yes, those who have

hatred kill only the body. My spirit belongs to God." . . . The people of my village told me frequently to be careful and seek protection. And I told them that I have the power of God, the Lord.

Isamoiso knew how to read the placing of medicines in his pathway. He knew some village people were trying to kill him. Yet he also knew a new language centered on the separation of body and spirit, and was not afraid to plot a confrontation so as to assert the superior power of God. Another teacher, Tolanga, also arrived as a stranger in the village where he worked. At first people were afraid of him, until he "learned their language and continued very well to talk to them and to give them good thoughts." When young people started to come to Tolanga's school, their fathers said to him, "You, teacher, give our children lisoo." Tolanga responded: "No, in the work of God, there is no lisoo. The only lisoo is to come to School."[86]

Such queries and challenges prompted this boekesi to underline a new grammar equating lisoo with school in 1917, some three years before Yakusu's first doctor arrived. The equations I heard in 1989 were an extension of Tolanga's pairings. Younger men told me that they had not entered libeli because they went to school instead: "Libeli is like kalasi. Libeli was our université." One man explained that "children of kalasi" could not help me learn about libeli: "They just followed class." So were choices structured historically. Many youth left school for libeli in 1900, 1902, and 1910. Some did not in 1924; many others did. "I was going to class first and then I left to enter lilwa," noted one man. Another said that he didn't enter libeli "because, me, I was at class again. Others were entering. Us, the children of classes, we didn't like it [lilwa] anymore. We didn't like it because to go there to stay in the forest, the time of kalasi was passing."

Memories from this generation, who had all witnessed libeli in 1924 whether they had joined or refused to participate, were also medical in expression. One simply called it "trouble," before sharing memories of libeli medicines and the pepper rubbed in initiates' eyes. A man who at first refused to speak to me without payment declared: "Don't tell her the tradition of lilwa because there were very many medicines, many medicines." His refusal to speak weakened as he slid into memories about how libeli had crossed into the world of missionary medicine: "They came to the hospital: 'I have a sickness on my back.' 'It is a lilwa cut that one. This is the medicine of lilwa.' . . . Yes, very bad medicine. So you would see a child coming to the hospital: 'I have a sickness on the foot, all over the back.' . . . Hurting because you cut lilwa. So you said, 'Lilwa, lilwa, lilwa.' It isn't a small thing. It was a huge thing among the Lokele."[87]

Just as youth pressed for books and papers in 1903, many of their children, those who spoke with me in 1989, assumed that they belonged in school during the 1920s. Chesterman had arrived, too, and his work favored another grammar equating shots (and pills) with lisoo and yaws with fala. Such doublets—lisoo/school, libeli/kalasi, lisoo/lokasa, lilwa/shot, fala/shot, and fala/yaws—were not the only ones that formed, decomposed, reformed, and deformed in this colonial situation. Their elements were the "remains and debris" of history and practice. Local pagans, Protestants, and evangelists coupled these "odds and ends"[88] in unstable pairs, as metaphors and equations, but also as opposed terms and thus choices, as they made sense of and later remembered their unstable worlds and social identities.

A teacher named Lititiyo extended an especially complex field of pairs, substitutions, and preferences in a 1922 letter attacking kanga.

> Let us help people in the light of the truth. I am telling you this because when somebody among you is sick, you follow the kanga to get him to give the medicine, smearing the person with lisoo and a mixture of medicine which is in his horn because the mixture of medicine is not for one person. It is for many people. Thus there are many things which people give and receive to each other through blood. The kanga wants only to get wealth and does not fail to apply medicine through cuts in the skin whether it be those who suffer from Sleeping Sickness, Leprosy, or Tokoli. The very fact that the horn of the kanga is only one is not good. The kanga crushes the coal from the fire, crushing it into a black powder medicine, and asks the person to leave the medicine with him without going to the village, giving to other people theirs because he will use the same blood to treat another person. So this kanga of ours in this way will allow a good and a bad blood to mingle. He will introduce and take out the medicine from the kanga horn. I am not saying this out of nothing. I am saying it for a reason. First, the Lord's cup of Communion—each person drinks his own, each person drinks his own—it is not done this way for nothing. It has a reason. Another person does not leave his for another person.
>
> Why is it that the horns of Kanga and the medicine with which they treat people combine many bloods? And the kanga is not someone of the village. Come on! Be serious! He goes to treat people with only one horn and one medicine which is in the horn. As you can see, you People who found the light, you see with your own eyes. Don't allow yourself to accept the things of people who are in the darkness. We, who have found the light, we say that he should make for each his own medicine.
>
> When White Men treat a person and dirt gets in the blood, they don't use it again. But the kanga doesn't remove debris from the water.[89]

Although Lititiyo was a teacher rather than a nurse, he used medicalized language to critique kanga and their methods. In questioning the validity of lisoo, his language of substitution alternated between liturgical and biomedical practice. He opposed kanga with European doctors, and he opposed common horns for mixing blood and medicines with the individualized church cups for drinking the (lemonade-made)[90] blood of communion. His letter united the church's own symbolic ritual about food and blood with evangelical hygiene as parallel, linked forms of clean, hygienic practice, where people remained individuals before God and before White Men doctors and their assistants. These physicians and nurses, like all communion partakers, were superior to healers and clients depending on "only one horn and one medicine."

Lobanga and Lititiyo

In 1910, Yakusu's missionaries did not want to discuss libeli with pagan men and had no inkling that a *Tata,* a senior man or chief, could have a wide, libeli-calling authority. By late 1925, Yakusu's missionaries sought out their most important confession from the "biggest chief on the river," a man named Lobanga who was the key "champion" of libeli. Lobanga was the foremost Tata of libeli in 1924. His confession—a "storming of the citadel"—was a major turning point in this period of soliciting confessions and reconstituting the church; missionaries called it the "swan song" period of libeli. Lititiyo was the other prominent figure in missionary representations surrounding libeli during the 1920s. Generation and church membership distinguished these two men. Whereas Lobanga and libeli seemed "practically synonymous,"[91] Lititiyo became "one of our most trusted Lokele teachers" because he refused to be intimidated by libeli threats, and his "sterling character" and "influence kept his village from joining in the ceremonies."[92] While the libeli confession of greatest significance occurred in Lobanga's "big important town" of Yalocha, a major scene of "seeking the wayward" from libeli took place in "Lititiyo's town" of Yaokombo, a small village of only forty households, where by 1930 all the men except two were "monogamists" and the chief was attending the class for inquirers (those seeking baptism).[93]

Lobanga was, by the time he died in 1929, a "romantic and picturesque" figure in missionary eyes. He wore a leopard tooth in his upper lip, and had some 40 wives and over 140 children. He was one of the "old-time"[94] chiefs who had mobilized paddlers for the large canoes that shuttled goods up to Stanley Falls as trade items and tax payments early in the century, stopping at Yakusu on the way home. These chiefs were critical characters to the early mission recruitment of youth, as they sent sons and daughters, fictive children and dependents, to receive missionary educations.

Yalocha was on the mission map from early on. Lobanga never became a Christian, but H. Sutton Smith noted in 1901 that Yalocha, "ruled by a powerful chief," had "sent seven boys at different times to work for us, and attend school."[95] Colonial signs and objects came early to this village, which became strongly Baptist. Lokangu, one of the harshest critics of libeli in the 1910 church meetings we saw, also came from Yalocha. Village men took literate BMS school-girls as wives, and they had imported objects in their households. When a Yalocha boy claimed one of the first Yakusu-trained schoolgirls as his wife in 1902, Achaka was "whisked off" from the station so quickly that she was soon writing back a note in charcoal on a plantain leaf asking for her slate and pencil.[96] By the time Mr. Ennals spent a night in a Yalocha home in 1923, he observed rooms shut with European bolts and heard an old British bugle, which someone sounded at night as "the last post . . . followed by several others rather like it, the series lasting a minute or two." Ennals stayed in "a little house which was the abode of two brothers," where he noted:

> I have never seen a native house before that made any real attempt at furnishing, but this little seven foot square room was full of things. It had a four poster bed, carved, and adorned with a fine mosquito net which I was told cost 32 francs, a small table near the bed was decorated with a few of the tings [sic] a native delights to have, such as a few empty bottles, and some dining plates of various sizes and patterns. Truly my host was a rich man! The tables had cloths on, and there were pictures on the wall, but what I like best was a text painted to fit in with the stencil design on the whitewashed wall: "Gloire à Jesus Christ." This was really most surprising. But none the less pleasing.[97]

It is not clear what kind of bed Lobanga slept on, nor who owned this British bugle—likely debris carried back, like kwaya dancing, by Congolese porters and soldiers who served during the war in Tanganyika. But Lobanga thought that European clothes had ruined the morality of the young and always wore the clothes of a Lokele chief,[98] quite unlike Saidi of Yakoso, who was quick to don a European suit during the 1910s.

The fault line between Lobanga and Lititiyo was, in great part, one of dif-ferently constituted, staggered colonial modernities. Lobanga was born about 1859 and became chief at the age of thirty, at a time when the political economy of translation required a speaking knowledge of Swahili. Yakusu's missionaries of the 1920s were fond of stories about local chiefs' interactions with the Ba-Tambatamba. Some chiefs had quickly offered women as wives to form alli-ances with these new big men and then helped in hunting down people from the forest. Lobanga, in contrast, had refused to give up his daughters to these raiding intruders. Perhaps Lobanga authored this story of defiance and auton-omy to enhance his image in missionary eyes.[99] He did offer these new mission-

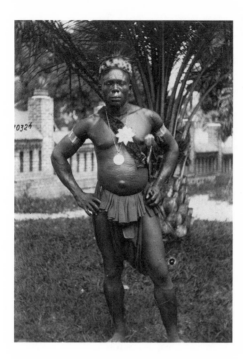

"Lokele chief." Lobanga, ca. 1910.
Photograph by A. de Meulemeester.
(Courtesy of MRAC, Ethnographic
Section [APH, neg. 10324]. Cour-
tesy of Africa-Museum, Tervuren,
Belgium.)

ary big men boys and girls for their "modern" schooling upriver. Whether they
understood it as such or not, this gesture of giving secured a form of alliance, though one in which he tried always to keep the upper hand. Lititiyo was
born about 1899, some forty years after Lobanga. Throughout Lititiyo's youth,
Lokele, evangelical language though it was, competed with Swahili as the lingua
franca of local colonial power. Lititiyo's modernity lay in his capacity to read
and write Lokele. In the early 1930s, he became not chief, but church pastor and
district overseer.[100]

The missionary vocabulary of representation for Lobanga was richer and less
hackneyed than it was for Lititiyo. This Lokele chief with a tooth in his lip
evoked the Zanzibari era. Edith Millman remembered when Lobanga had been
"reproved . . . for murder," for the "ritual death of three strangers on the death
of one of his wives." He was eager to display a box with a key, from which he
would remove a handkerchief to reveal a "beautiful case with a medal and a
letter from King Albert to our Lokele chief Lobanga." His life embraced relations with multiple colonialisms that had passed through the region, that of the
so-called "Arab Zone," that of Bula Matari and Bokota Ofi or Big Chief Albert
(who visited as prince in 1909, as king in 1928, and whose image was on colonial
coins from 1921), and that of Yakusu's missionaries and their steamer, books,

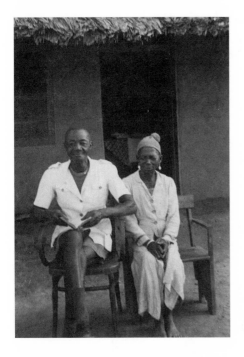

Lititiyo and his wife, ca. 1948.
(Courtesy of Nora Carrington,
JFC Papers, Salisbury, U.K.)

and surgeries. Lobanga may not have been a self-made big man, yet he was no simple colonial creation either.[101]

The missionary vocabulary for Lititiyo was more skeletal, even caricatured, perhaps explaining why he so easily became an important, abiding figure in missionary—oral and written—tradition. Lititiyo was a former cannibal in missionary lore, "who as a boy ate human flesh," but went on to become a leading teacher and pastor, responsible for a large church district. I first heard about Lititiyo from Annie Horsfall, a BMS missionary who had served in Kisangani since the 1970s. One day, she told me, just after William Millman had arrived at Yakusu (in 1898), he came down a path and saw Lititiyo walking along carrying a human arm in his hands. This tale had long been in print, and had perhaps been repeated in mission lessons and sermons as well. Lititiyo's own version, in a letter to Millman, went: "You, my dear master, found me a beast and made me a man to serve Christ." A Yakusu doctor, Stanley Browne, told the story in 1938 with Millman seeing Lititiyo "running away from a battle with a human arm he was going to cook and eat!"[102] This cannibal-to-pastor tale makes Lititiyo appear more as a missionary creation than as a self-authored man. Yet it was Lititiyo who, in 1922, adumbrated the complex grammar of substitution centered on the cleanliness and individualization of communion cups, whereby colonial hygiene and communion would replace local therapeutic practice.

Lititiyo's voice rarely emerged from the historical record again. When it did in 1934, Supervisor Lititiyo was pleading for a new communion plate because his had been stolen when he was in the hospital. Chesterman also made Lititiyo's village, Yaokombo, the stage for his crocodile show that year. Nurse Likenyule's dispensary had opened at Yaokombo in the early 1930s, even though the depression was in full swing locally and some company dispensaries were closing down. Yaokombo became a model of appropriate evangelical relations between chapel and dispensary, and Lititiyo's son became a nurse.[103]

Not only Lititiyo's life passed through hospitals. Indeed, if the fault line that distinguished Lititiyo from Lobanga was their generational difference in relation to libeli, Christianity, and colonial change in the region, what united them was a necessary, though different, relationship to medicalization. Lobanga would extravagantly display his wealth at the Yakusu hospital and ask for the most powerful injections available: " 'The needle is what I want,' said he, 'and I want one with strength, so I will give 100 francs for it.' "[104] He went up to Yakusu from Yalocha as a patient for a week just before New Year's Day in 1926, after spending "thousands of francs on native medicine men."[105] Indeed, the power of hospital medicines, not any desire to take communion, seems to have produced his memorable confession. Chesterman went down to Yalocha to wrest a libeli denunciation from this chief only two weeks after his hospital stay. "Give me power you white men," was Lobanga's plea to the doctor. He finally gave in on the deck of the *Grenfell* steamer in front of several "old church members." Chesterman insisted that this chief, who had called for libeli and cursed all who opposed it, at least give others open permission to confess with the words: "For ever and ever [I] denounce Libeli because of its deceit. I did not see the spirits in the forest only men of the town, and I don't fear the curse of disease because I trust God in all things." Lobanga broke into the words of a libeli song about guarding libeli secrets like one's own flesh, before Lobanga "cut short his song with the jerked-out words. 'Yes, deceit, all of it, tell him so.' "[106]

Lobanga had been "the incarnation of all that is heathen and reactionary in the district" before he confessed.[107] Yet he was deemed "a very courageous man this old-time chief with a great many good qualities and some very bad ones" once he did. In 1929, Mrs. Millman was back in Yalocha asking Lobanga for some of his daughters for their new boarding school: " 'How many do you want?' he enquires. 'Six,' I say. 'Choose,' says he." One of Lobanga's wives added a seventh daughter, along with her school fees, and Lobanga sent Mr. and Mrs. Millman a sixteen-pound fish before they departed on their steamer with his daughters and other girls collected along the river. The Millman's expeditions,

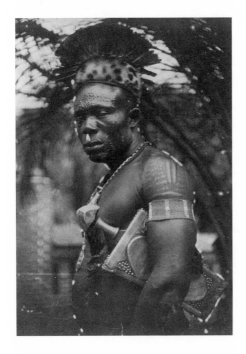

"Chief Lobanga (of the Lokele),"
ca. 1910. Photograph by A. de
Meulemeester. (Courtesy of MRAC,
Ethnographic Section [APH, neg.
137239]. Courtesy of Africa-Museum,
Tervuren, Belgium.)

gathering new young clients as they traveled, resembled long-standing forms of creating alliances in the region. Mrs. Millman obtusely concluded victory: "He is annoyed at the modern boy and girl but he is clever enough to realise that he is powerless to stem the tide."[108]

Within three months, this "incarnation of the Lokele tradition," the "last but one of the big chiefs of the early days," was dead. Lobanga died back at the Yakusu hospital as the rage of malinga dancing arrived in the district and markets were flooded with new goods, "from Bibles from the Mission to cigarettes and face powder which looks ghastly on a black face." Lobanga died in no less of a symbolically laden place than the hospital's operating table as a crowd of wives, kin, and other spectators observed: "Outside the windows of the operating room the crowd, usually so stoical and resigned burst into a mad frenzy and barely permitted us to compose the body before hurrying it off to his canoe." The crowd was angry, likely at the surgeon and the mission. There might have been "more than a few broken windows," Chesterman noted, if one of Lobanga's senior wives had not declared that he was "like melted palm oil, ready to be spilled if disturbed."[109]

Palm oil was—and remains—a staple of diet, healing, ritual, and medicines; its deep red color likens it to shele and blood, and in its congealed state, it is an excellent base for medicinal creams and salves. Palm oil balm is smeared on the bodies of those present at a birth to neutralize the blood of childbirth that can "kill eyes." The womb of a pregnant woman in labor is soothed and reddened with palm oil mixed with medicines, as were the bodies of libeli initiates. Missionaries learned quickly that palm oil made excellent ointment and accepted it as a form of dispensary payment in the early 1900s. Palm oil production and use changed enormously over the years. By the 1920s, palm was one of the major forest products of plantation companies being processed and used locally. This rich local food and symbolic medicinal blood, long produced in small amounts through artisanal talent and intensity, was suddenly seen in previously unimaginable quantities, and in easily convertible, easily spilled liquid form, ready to be bought and converted into commodities. Mechanized presses and palm oil trading stands became commonplace, and palm oil–based soap production and sale were beginning in the vicinity. Even Yakusu was finding new uses for melted palm oil, as a fuel for the mission's diesel engine and circular saw. The imaginative work of Lobanga's wife's metaphor, therefore, did much more than absolve Dr. Chesterman and calm the angry crowd. More than just her husband's body was "like melted palm oil, ready to be spilled if disturbed." She spoke to the instabilities and dislocations of these new social realities in concrete and figurative ways, through evoking her husband's corpse as powerful, though unsettled, spilled blood.

At that historical moment, Lititiyo was just gaining power, establishing a new form of chieflike yet church-born authority. Lititiyo was the son of a chief, but he had "long ago rejected the inheritance of Chief because it involved conforming to native superstitions and immoral practices." Lititiyo's right to inherit is less clear than is the missionary desire to co-opt a semblance of "traditional" authority in making Lititiyo a key church leader. In 1930, Lititiyo became the church's third ordained pastor and soon was appointed as "overseer" of the Yaokanja district, some fifty-seven villages between Yalikina and Yangonde. His public ordination was an occasion "to see our chiefs welcoming the messengers of God again." Lititiyo had some troubles in his new job as "general superintendent." Teachers and chiefs argued over the location of schools and teachers' homes. State-required roadwork and fieldwork were keeping some villages from building chapels. Some schools needed new registers. And Lititiyo had an accident on his bicycle one day while touring his villages, smashing his bike but escaping with few bruises.[110]

Lobanga's and Lititiyo's lives emerged and intersected in missionary representations at a historical juncture when forms of power and signs of modernity shifted significantly. It was not only Lobanga's person that died on April 5, 1929.[111] Lobanga's death signaled a passing of the seasonal and work rhythms necessary for—and the capacity to mobilize people as actors within—a stirring, prolonged, and visible performance of libeli. Libeli, a male reproductive ritual disassociated from circumcision among the Lokele, may only date to early in the nineteenth century. Yet ritual forms of mobilizing wealth and knowledge, tied to what Jan Vansina has called the "equatorial tradition" of big man power, seem to have died with Lobanga.[112] Wealth manifest in numbers of wives, dependents, and paddlers certainly did. Yet the evidence does not point to a complete eradication of libeli, either as a word or as a skin-cutting and wealth-gathering, therapeutic practice, nor of ancient associations linking ambivalent water creatures and crocodiles with affliction and ruin, luck and medicines. Rather, scarification seems to have become even more important as it carried greater symbolic load. There were no more grand male retreats to the forest or public spectacles marking the completion of such rituals. But people continued "cutting lilwa" and "eating" libeli wealth at least through the 1930s. Nor did the period of "heckling" BMS teachers, which followed libeli of 1924, cease after Lobanga's death. People continued to mock these new big men for monogamy, for low pay, for performing work that was unproductive in food and children, and for their "joke" of a god, who was not visible like King Albert was, and who was unable to end disease and death.[113]

Memory, Remains, School Essays

Libeli confessions continued until at least 1933, the year before Chesterman was distributing crocodile meat in Yaokombo. That day, he heard women chanting the word lilwa because this ndimo-like crocodile was at last dead, and he saw men afraid of getting fala from butchering it. Thus, libeli forms were still alive. Nor did debate disappear. Colonial evangelical medicine had become more influential and commonplace. Yet as the 1934 dispute between Nurse Likenyule and the angry kanga showed, Chesterman intervened in a complicated economy with his surgeries and gun. The exchange between the nurse and the healer was absent from Chesterman's version of events; he may well have been oblivious to it. Yet Nurse Likenyule—who later posed for photographs with his dress-wearing wife, a gramophone, and a flower-decorated table by his side— was acting as translator and interceptor as he coped with the fallout for local wealth and power of Chesterman's intercession.

A history of libeli, I have been arguing, needs to consider the emergence and social action of mission-trained middle figures like Likenyule. Whether they resisted libeli or not, they talked and eventually wrote about such practices. They named and translated as they spoke and wrote. At the turn of the century, these interlocutors were known as "boys," and some of them worked as mis-

sionaries' boi or domestic servants. By 1910, some had become evangelical
teachers, and by 1916, some of these teachers were published authors. By 1923,
the first nurses-in-training had joined the teachers as colonial middle figures,
and by the early 1930s, these evangelical nurses were writing and publishing,
too. Missionary narratives suggest that libeli was over forevermore by 1927,
whereas there is ample evidence that libeli as a form of cutting and applying
medicines—and likely as a form of authority, too—continued well into the
1930s.[114] Libeli remained a significant, condensed cultural marker within the
written discourse of Yakusu's Christian students and evangelical workers.

In 1930, Mr. Ford asked Yakusu schoolboys to write essays about libeli in
order to rehearse the church's critique of these practices. A certain line of
reasoning about libeli as fraud and a form of female oppression, evident in
firsthand missionary accounts by 1902, was reproduced over time, reemerging
in these Yakusu schoolboy essays in almost standardized form. Yet these students did not simply recapitulate the kinds of arguments that their missionary
teachers had taught them. Side by side with arguments about deception, du-
plicity, and women was an obsession that missionary observers hardly noticed.
These schoolboys wrote much less about medicines, about people continuing
to cut incisions and oaths, than about food, confirming libeli as an expression
of wealth and fertility resembling the fattening of female seclusion rituals.
These boys were jealous of libeli feasts.

Women's fears of the Yakusu hospital as a tinned food production site in 1924
were not unlike schoolboys' objections to libeli. The imagery in each was about
sinister, selfish forms of eating. One schoolboy, Bofeka, in an essay titled "News
about Libeli and Its Cheating," focused on why the older men sought to continue libeli: "Old men do not want libeli to end so they can continue to dupe
women and children and other people of far away." When strangers learned
about libeli and asked to be initiated, Bofeka continued, they would

> give payment to Lokele so that they . . . show them the way to do it: have
> ready certain fish and crabs, and go to the forest when your wives have
> cooked food to be given to the spirits, and go with those who want to be
> initiated into libeli into the forest, maybe 200 or 300 people, and put *biako*
> [peppers] in their ears and leave them with the biako from 8 o'clock until
> noon. At that time the spirits themselves will kill them. People who will
> not have biako in their ears will die, truly, truly. They should know that
> this biako biako are peppers which they will put in their eyes and put it in
> the nose. The Lokele will cheat their friends a lot.

The essays also suggested that libeli made "the lives of village women difficult."
Some of this difficulty related to authority: "the 'mothers' of libeli like it because libeli makes a woman take an oath binding her when she does certain

things." Another student, Bosolongo, clarified that if "women wanted to do some things which men don't want a woman to do or say, they will cut her, cursing her with libeli so she will stop."[115] Memories of women being punished for defying the authority of libeli were part of mission discourse. Mrs. Millman turned to an old woman at one of the mission's first tea parties and asked: " 'Do you forget when that poor girl was drowned, pushed under the water and held there by determined men because she had said lilwa which none but initiated men say?' 'No, I cannot forget,' " responded the old woman.[116]

Male youth and women were subject to the same authority, according to these boys writing school essays for Mr. Ford: "If you ask a youth for food and he refuses, then you will curse him with libeli and he will go get it. When women quarrel they will curse them with libeli and they will disperse. The elders have gone beyond the limits." Much of the difficulty involved exclusion from knowledge and food: "The food received there is a lot, and it is unlike the food of those who stay in the village, and the food in the village is really small." Jean Falanga explained: "People . . . want libeli so that they can eat a lot of food." Bosolongo restated: "People of the village and the 'mothers' will agree . . . that we want our children to be initiated in libeli to become fat." Bofofe echoed: "The matter of libeli and its purpose is this: some people eat food and lie to women saying the spirits are looking for food so that they can eat the food themselves. . . . The old people do not abandon libeli because they receive a lot of money and food." He then suggested that the authority of libeli extended beyond a performance: "Because if one is hungry, he will tell a woman that the spirits are asking for food from the house. So the woman will quickly cook food . . . quickly, quickly," cutting the banana paste with "raffia string."[117]

The texts alternate between two Lokele words for bounty: *bieto,* meaning wealth or money, and bieka, signifying things or food. Thus: "The 'mothers' of libeli . . . will eat a huge amount of bieka which they do not buy with their own bieto. And if they want to be given falanga which will help to buy yeka [things, pl. of bieka] in a *magasin* [store], he will receive it." Libeli, then, according to this Yakusu schoolboy grammar of 1931, was theft:

> We will come to take those who will be initiated and to receive things, and
> will say that if you don't pay us, we are going to kill your child. The parent
> of the child when he hears this, he will give them many, many, many, many
> things. This . . . is only to take things, thus to steal things. . . . Yes this is a
> matter of lying. . . . We, ourselves, we used to be cheating. Another person
> now has cheated us.[118]

These youths' concerns resemble those about Yakusu's hospital as a place where doctors would cut up stolen victims and produce tinned food. The historical conjuncture of the imaging of the Yakusu hospital as a human meat cannery and the revival of libeli expressed much more than a struggle over a doctor's "healing knife." Libeli was always an expression of struggle over control of natality and social reproduction, over bieka as a ritual substance integral to wealth as power in people and things. It was about power and wealth as food, the right and desire to eat copiously, the power and beauty of being "fat," including (latterly) "fat" in things bought in stores. Indeed, at play in the Congolese imaging of the hospital was an idiom of ingestion that posed a threat to women's fertility. If we take seriously these clues about food and power, we find not only stark terror in the face of imperial medicine, but also several tangled Congolese interpretations, some poetic and sardonic, about colonialism and forms of loss as new forms of social and medical surgery occurred in their midst. Key was a specific category of colonial middle figures, the Congolese Protestants who objected to libeli, who indeed emerged in large part through the struggles over its performance. They were not the only middles, and they certainly were not the only persons making and translating meaning. Yet teachers and nurses had access to new therapeutic media, such as shots and papers. Using these concrete things, they authored a vision of evangelical wealth and hygiene, and communicated it to new publics through their new scriptural economy.

Fat and Papers

During the late 1920s, many men and boys had confessed because they wanted to take communion again. But communion did not inspire Lobanga's confession; illness and surgery did. Indeed, the sociology of the libeli conflict of 1924—the perceived threat of the mission boi who were becoming ba-infirmiers and paying lifaefi—underlines the historical conjuncture of hospital construction and libeli revival. Meanwhile, as the moral metaphor of crocodile = airplane revealed, signs of a new, quick and mobile modernity became part of local social imaginaries in the interwar period. There was also a new naming of missionaries in this metaphor. The ba-missionaires were no longer just spirits of the forest with papers by 1934, but also rainbowlike spirits with control over new technologies, such as airplanes and injections, which were capable of healing crocodile-associated afflictions.

A history of colonial childbearing in and near Yakusu needs the context of libeli as history and reproductive practice to weigh the implications of biomedicine focused on maternity and women. Before turning to childbearing and maternities, the next chapter extends the sociology of the libeli conflict of 1924 as it introduces more explicitly another moral metaphor about mission life: dining = surgery. This comparison between dining and surgery was a corollary of mission routines in part responsible for forming the new Christian men and women of Yakusuland. Confrontations between nurses and kanga, and relationships among eating and fertility, will return as a major theme in chapter 4 as well.

Arguments in Yaokombo in 1934 took place among the doctor and a jeering crowd, the doctor and the old men, the nurse and the kanga. The doctor was making a point about fala and churchgoing, while the kanga clashed with the nurse about medicines and money. There was, by contrast, no nurse, nor even necessarily a church member, in the turn-of-the-century conversation between a missionary and Saili—likely Chief Saidi—about how to cut up a crocodile. Saile was acting as an interpreter explaining crocodile-related therapeutic practice to a missionary stranger. Social differentiation and relations of deference changed dramatically in the interim, as some Congolese became church members, teachers, nurses, and letter-writing men and women. In 1910, this middle category of privileged translators consisted of teachers and "boys" who lied to their missionary masters and defied them in church meetings. The imagery in Lokele texts focused on frogs, clothes, and reading in 1910; missionary knowledge of Congolese constructions of Christianity was limited to the fertility dangers of European dress. In 1924, scars mattered and libeli took on medical inflections.

As in 1910, libeli of 1924 may have been partially spurred on by an intensification in lifaefi collecting. Yet more than competition over money was involved. Rather, a profusion of unprecedented events converged: the coming of a medical doctor, surgical practice, airplanes, and yaws injections; the construction of a teaching hospital for training Congolese nurses; a rapidly changing political and therapeutic economy; even the surgical sewing up of a man whose flesh was torn by a crocodile. Together, these novelties posed a deep threat to those who organized libeli. Although there had been mission-sponsored healing and sleeping sickness investigations in the Yakusu district before 1921, missionary medicine at Yakusu had not previously been so tightly associated with state power and prerogatives. Nor had there been the kind of targeting of women that Chesterman achieved through his sleeping sickness research. The new hospital in 1924 was a tangible culmination of increasingly intrusive medical interventions. Its construction bred stories about sinister forms of eating, bodily excavation, and abuse of power. Clothes dropped out of the lexicon of debate, as airplanes came in. One woman was bludgeoned to death for going to the hospital, and rumors and patient statistics suggest that the Yakusu hospital posed a special danger for women, girls, and their fertility.[119] A mixture of admiration and terror about colonial medicine, technologies, and mobilities also animated the events of 1934.

Missionary interpretations of libeli concerned deception and female subjugation. Yet a libeli performance represented an assertion about wealth and authority, as well as the reckoning of this power. Indeed, studying libeli has enabled us to glimpse change in social differentiation and struggles within and over the Yakusu church. Other social clashes over hegemony and wealth, provoked by larger and less local shifts in the colonial political economy, were certainly also at play. Hence, perhaps, the recurring resonances about forms of money. Both the 1902 and 1910 rounds of libeli were named after new types of currency that had just entered local circulation. Even the 1924 round seems to have coincided with a local struggle over the alternative system of taxation that Yakusu church offerings represented.

The evidence reveals that libeli was an institution of Lokele—indeed Yaokanja—hegemony, perhaps concentrated in Lobanga's house in 1924. Still, libeli cannot be reduced to political or economic struggle. Integral to the rituals were mimetic ideas and practices concerning procreation, fertility, the body, social reproduction, and difference and likeness among men and women. These were equally questions about who should and could heal, about who should and could initiate, claim, and reproduce young men.

Crocodiles and their domestication, like boys and girls, were part of Yakusu's history long before Chesterman's quest of 1934. H. Sutton Smith's publication of "Lest We Should Waddle" was a first go. When the Belgian prince visited Yakusu for a special "pageant" in 1926, mission girls wore white drill dresses and knitted white puritan caps with small rosettes of black, yellow, and red, Belgium's national colors. "Hospital boys" followed in white drill tunics and khaki shorts. Congolese station women showed the prince crocheted doilies, lace for tea cloths, and trays that they had decorated with poker work patterns of young boys carrying dishes and "fishes swimming into a crocodile's mouth." Phyllis Lofts further domesticated crocodiles when she authored a "Yakusu alphabet" for *Yakusu Quarterly Notes* readers in 1930. Avenues, Boys, and Clinic began the series of rhymes; for instance, "B for the Boys, at work and at play, 'Boys will be Boys'—I expect you would say!" Exhibition, girls, hospital, instruction, journeys, Lokele, quinine, steamer, and umbrellas were among the words that this missionary nurse chose to capture the essence of Yakusu. Crocodiles were there, too, but not as an alphabet word: "R for River, so big and so wide, There are horrible crocodiles in its inside!" Lofts reserved the letter *C* "for the Clinic, for babies each week, For lovelier babies you'd have far to seek."[120] As Congolese on the Upper Congo compared crocodiles with airplanes in a moral metaphor about colonial power, clinics supplanted crocodiles in this cute missionary lexicon for British readers. Lititiyo's lexicon of 1922 was never hackneyed as he wrote out kanga horns and wrote in communion cups. Nor was that of Lobanga's wife. She likened her big-man husband, once dead under surgical lights, to spilled palm oil, before kin whisked his body away to a canoe, back to Yalocha, and propped it up in a chair under a canopy for final review.

3   DINING AND SURGERY

If any friend finds a difficulty about the pronunciation of Yakusu, make the name rhyme with Crusoe.—*Yakusu Quarterly Notes,* 1919

Strangers possess natives in a laugh.—Greg Dening, *Mr. Bligh's Bad Language,* 1992

In 1911, Rose Gee wrote about what happened when she came to Yakusu for the first time. After Yakusu's missionaries welcomed her at the riverbank where she had arrived by steamer, they made their way "escorted by a crowd of natives" to Mr. and Mrs. Millman's house. "Then followed what would appear to people in England a positive crime. The whole of the natives—dozens of them—flocked into the garden, up the steps, on the verandah, and stood in the doorway to watch us eat!"[1] Almost twenty years later, when a colonial official visited Yakusu, Mrs. Millman took him for a tour of the mission hospital. Colonel A. Bertrand was surprised to find a crowd of Congolese subjects gathered around the operating theater—a whitewashed room with open windows— watching the missionary doctor perform what was popularly called the "work of the knife." "Anybody can see these" operations, Mrs. Millman explained in a private letter. The colonial agent had turned white himself. " 'Let's go,' he says to me. . . . 'I can't stand to see him cut up.' " Mrs. Millman smiled and took Colonel Bertrand along to the school.[2]

These missionary-narrated anecdotes offer analogous missionary renderings of two everyday routines at Yakusu: dining and surgery. They allow us to peer in at the "imperial eyes"[3] of a European who, as newcomer and outsider, witnesses for the first time and with considerable astonishment these gatherings of colonized eyes gaping at missionary manners of order and precision, and huddling around tables with knives and prayer. Missionary eating and mission surgery

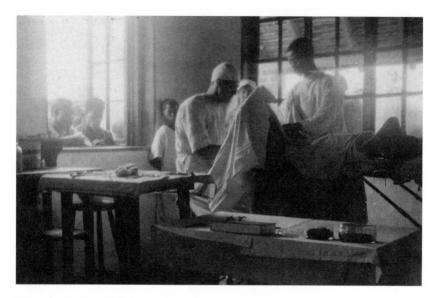

"An operation" at Yakusu, ca. 1926. (Courtesy of David Lofts, PL Papers, Barton-on-Sea, U.K.)

were kindred worlds in several senses. Each began with prayer. Mrs. Millman's smile reminds us that there was a missionary purpose to these performances: mission spectacle as object lesson. They also reveal "topsy-turvy"[4] colonial sight-seeing, the inversion and internalization of curiosity and visibility, of gaze and spectacle. Yakusu's missionaries performed. They did the cutting and the passing as they assembled around a table. Congolese watched from the outside, actively peering in through doors and windows. They participated as sightseers, witnesses. Most Congolese, that is. A small group were expressly part of the performance. These Congolese attended, assisting, serving, and following orders. These Congolese *scrubbed.* Soap, like knives, prayer, and "boys," linked these worlds. So, too, did a specific mission code nicknamed "the knife and fork doctrine" that found new practical meaning as this mission station underwent a medicalization of its activities in the 1920s.

Mission dining for local, public consumption was a pronounced aspect of mission life at Yakusu from early in the twentieth century. Congolese men and women (and boys and girls) appear in missionary vignettes as invited guests, domestic servants, enthralled spectators. The antinomy of cannibalism with knife-and-fork use was, as Norbert Elias has argued, central to Western bourgeois notions of civilization and domesticity.[5] Congoland as a cannibal land was also a popular convention of the day in European imaging. Just as cannibal stories sold books,[6] quaint tales of reformed cannibals eating with knives and forks resonated with cultural expectations of metropolitan mission supporters and patrons. Missionary-authored domesticity narratives were captivating, picturesque, and mirthful. Their display of burlesque and satirical elements grew more explicit over time. Deliverance joined domestication as linked themes in missionary anecdotes about girls. Indeed, girl stories were more labored and sober than the topsy-turvy confoundings of cannibals and cutlery in "boy" stories.

Colonial domesticity, as a discursive field and thus a realm of social practice, was often indistinguishable from colonial hygiene. This chapter begins to explore a first set of parallels and connections between dining and surgery, domestication and medicalization (the analysis is continued in the following chapter). Christmas meals, royal visits, tea parties, domestic service, and hospital work were integral to domesticating processes at Yakusu. "Boys" and "house girls"—like evangelical teachers, nurses, and midwives—were among the "not quite/ not white"[7] characters who assisted in these performances. One missionary-authored Yakusu origin fable is about a Congolese cannibal who became the church's first teacher and pastor. Another is about a slave who became Yakusu's first "house girl," Congolese mother, and translator. These hybridized, domesticated, gendered transformations—taming the savage, redeeming the slave—are explored in narrative and practice, in evangelical forms of remembering, and in domestic service and festive rituals at Yakusu. I also turn to memories of former Yakusu "boys" and "girls" about servant work. Domesticity narratives and racialized humor were common to Europeans in colonial and metropolitan contexts. They also figured in, while being betrayed and parodied by, these social and autobiographical forms of Congolese remembering.

Dining and surgery, though parallel in form, were not chronologically linked as realms of Congolese sight-seeing. Miss Gee and Colonel Bertrand's analogous experiences pointed to a time lag. Indeed, the focus of mission life at Yakusu shifted from dining to "the work of the knife" during the 1920s. Anesthesia seemed like a miracle: "She sleeps, she feels no pain." Relatives worried that a patient had died once under the effect of chloroform, a common anesthetic in the 1920s.[8] There was a screen just outside the theater window in 1924, but a nurse, Gladys Owen, often noticed "a black head peeping round the screen." Once she discovered someone spying through the keyhole. Chesterman began to allow a friend to enter in order to watch: "Such visitors are always tremendously excited not only at the operation but also at the doctor's theatre clothes."[9] By 1926, the new hospital was open, the screen was gone, and crowds were gathering to watch the most intriguing and readily available public spectacle at Yakusu, surgery. Chesterman noted:

We encourage this "gallery" as it helps show the countryside that there is less magic and more method in our madness than is generally supposed. The size and noise of the crowd varies according to the stage of the operation and we find that spectacular scenes attract and sanguinary ones repel, at least temporarily. The proverbial peace and quiet of an operating theatre is not for us. . . . [I]n all this cutting and dividing an entrance is being ministered to us not only beneath the black skins but deep into the affections and thought of our people.[10]

Dining as Domesticity

Christmas 1915 seemed "different from all the rest" for the missionaries at Yakusu. "Instead of monkey stew for Christmas dinner, we had roast beef for the first time in the history of the mission."[11] This news of domesticity achieved appeared in the pages of the *Yakusu Quarterly Notes,* sent to Baptist Mission Society supporters in England. Yakusu was founded twenty years earlier in what had long been imagined by Europeans as the "very heart of Africa."[12] Roast beef for Christmas dinner conjured an image of tamed, domesticated harmony, reversing the popular association of the Congo with "darkness," violence, and decay. Gothic imagery was not part of this evocation of a Congo Christmas: "The rose trees from England were flowering in our garden and the tables were gaily decorated."[13]

The popular evangelical missionary, Dan Crawford, called such efforts to re-create England in the Congo "a policy of make-believe . . . a loving fraud, but a hollow one."[14] Yakusu, "beautifully situated some forty feet above the water on the north bank of the Congo River," was known in Belgian colonial circles for its country cottages and rose gardens. It was located fifteen miles downriver from Stanleyville, "on the fringe of the great gloomy forest" made famous by Henry Morton Stanley. The station was within easy reach for touring visitors, who were eager to witness this English Protestant version of colonial domesticity. When William Roome wrote of his Congo travels in 1930, he depicted Yakusu as "a delightful 'home from home,' " and an opportunity "to enjoy the sight of a clean and well-spread table" for travelers "tramping through Africa."[15] When Prince Albert visited Yakusu and the Millmans's "comfortable home" in 1909, he remarked, "One would truly think one was in England." Everything reminded the Belgian prince of "those extra clean English cottages, with bright, congenial rooms, but decorated with all the knick-knacks, articles or pictures which take the occupants back home through the memories linking them there through these reminiscent fragments of the mother country." Nor was there any escaping the missionaries' pride in their work, the prince noted: "they made us see everything."[16]

The future king's tour became ritual as Yakusu came to be a regular visiting place for Belgian royalty touring the colony.[17] Mission choreography began well in advance. Mrs. Ennals recalled the weeks of anticipation as a godsend from "the realm of fairy tales and story books" that animated mission life. As these "middling class" British missionaries described the visits, they inscribed their lives as colonial fairy tales, where princes moored at the river beach, mounted the steps of Yakusu's "Dover Cliff," and toured the mission and its rose gardens. Rehearsals gave new meaning to the "policy of make-believe," and it was not a hollow fraud: "The day of the rehearsal was a great day, when Mokili and Mama"—Mr. and Mrs. Millman—"came round and 'pretended' to be the King and Queen, but after all that was only make believe and not the real thing. At last the great day came. . . ."[18]

Scenes of "the white people . . . at table" did not usually deserve mention in the *Yakusu Quarterly Notes*. It was when Congolese participated in mission dining rituals, when the policy of make-believe coincided with the "knife and fork doctrine," that the monkey-stew-to-roast-beef theme made good copy.[19] The knife-and-fork doctrine was an early-twentieth-century Protestant missionary nickname for the idea that introducing cutlery use was an efficient way to alter eating customs and domesticate the "savage" milieu of Congoland. Object lessons in using knives and forks were equally allegories about taming cannibals for an English evangelical reading public. Thus, the local chief Saidi "cut a pretty figure at the table" when Yakusu's missionaries invited him to eat with them in 1900: "He managed with his knife and fork very well, and behaved himself most becomingly." In 1916, Chief Bonjoma dined on the mission steamer at Yalikina: "We are having tea and our cannibal sits down and joins us." These stories were colorful, though chiefs were not part of educational goals in the same way that mission "boys" were. Accompanying "boys" illustrated for one and all another aspect of the knife-and-fork doctrine, while the chiefs whom these "boys" served were busy sampling missionary food. At Yafunga in 1915, for instance, the "boy" John featured as prominently as Chief Osinga: "We take our meal by the light of the brilliant moon. John has done wonders. There is soup and 'setu' (stew), pancakes and coffee. Osinga has had his European chair carried along and sits up straight and uncomfortable. He samples our fare, and the ivory disc bobs up and down."[20]

There were many Johns at Yakusu. As in much of colonial Africa, domestic servants tended to be male in the Belgian Congo. Regardless of age, they were referred to diminutively, as "boys." There was a feminizing aspect to making men domestics and calling them "boys," and this gender meaning—tamed sexuality—was useful. Yakusu students understood the common colonial meaning of "boy." In 1928, they wrote in class compositions: "White people are people who sit at a table to eat food . . . with forks and spoons, and they are constantly saying to their boy 'Never bring us dirty plates and spoons.' " Yet the semantics of "boy" at Yakusu extended beyond table server and personal servant.[21] In 1904, Mr. Stapleton noted that in a single month, four "deputations" had paddled some twenty miles "to beg" for a teacher: "We got them away three times with a few alphabet cards. . . . The fourth time they won and went off proudly, having secured the personal boy of one of the missionaries."[22]

The missionary conviction that they were working among former cannibals authorized domestic service at Yakusu as a form of "industrial education," itself a basic method among Protestant missionaries in the Congo: "If we simply train their minds we will have on our hands a grand company of 'big heads.' " Days at Yakusu were divided between classroom instruction and industrial training: "Some start in the printing shop, some do chair-making and cane work, others work for the white man in his house as his cook or his wash jack or his personal boy, or in his garden." The "industrial element" was to instill "practical Godliness" and "good, clean, healthy living." Learning domestic cleaning, bed making, and table serving would foster "better houses" and better "health and morals" in the Congo.[23] The knife-and-fork doctrine, therefore, linked dining to hygiene.

However controversial the issue of "European caricatures" and "puffed up" Congolese may have been, individual cleanliness and industry were of capital importance to Protestants. Eating with knives and forks and cleaning them with soap as an occupation were in keeping with such "self-reliance and individual responsibility . . . the keys to Protestant conceptions of the Christian society and the New African Man." Learning the "rudiments of 'kitchen cleanliness' " at Yakusu meant, as late as 1954, learning "orderliness, attention to detail, honesty in little things." Yet not everyone believed that a "decent little table, a plate or two, a spoon, knife, and fork," and a bolt of cloth were good ideas. Nor did all Protestant missionaries agree that Congolese should wear European clothes and stop eating with their hands from collective dishes. Some Catholic priests *discouraged* European plates and food early in the century in order "to counter the tendency toward pride or aping European manners."[24] Some evangelical missionaries in the Congo lamented colonial mimicry: " 'Ah! Europeanised!' say some." Others objected to Congolese "Dandies," who like urban minstrel figures, wore exaggerated, mismatched, flamboyant clothes. "The outcry should not be against European dress but against absurd European dress," one declared, revealing an anxiety not about duplication but about pantomime and parody. These Protestant missionaries repeated the tale of the "lad who appeared at church with a discarded corset worn proudly above his coat; and of the chief whose robe of special honour was a lady's night dress." Such transgressive, carnivalesque dressing suggested a loss of control—including control over humor.[25]

Cannibal island motifs, jungle songs, and minstrel shows increased in popularity among "respectable," middle- and lower-middle-class theater audiences in London at the height of British imperial expansion. Comic blackface acts became standard features of music hall bills. Michael Pickering has argued that this racialized, transgressive humor, where whites cross-dressed as blacks, contributed to forming imperial mentalities in Victorian and Edwardian England. Yet this assertion remains imprecise. Investigating how minstrelsy informed missionary ideas is not the aim here. I seek to understand how minstrel conventions of miming and clowning—with their "hidden desires and darker impulses"— entered into and were excluded from narrative and performance at Yakusu.[26]

Lantern Pictures and "Jollification"

Missionary dining endured as spectacle in the so-called "bush" much longer than at the central station of Yakusu. Indeed, staged dining was a counterpart sensation to magic lantern shows during missionary "itineration" tours from early in the century. What better way to gather a village chief and crowd for hymn singing and prayer than lantern pictures shown under a fig tree on the riverfront? In 1901, several "Arabs and their women" gathered for a "lantern display." In 1910, chiefs were requesting this form of entertainment for soldiers and state workers living in their midst. Evangelical services attracted large crowds in riverside towns early in the century when they "took the form of Lantern Services," and many wanted "to see the wonderful pictures."[27]

It was not unusual for "a couple of hundred people" to gather and watch "before and behind the sheet." If curiosity seemed endless during lantern shows, so did it during meals. Mrs. Ford described the scene when she and Mr. Ford stayed in a state rest house in 1927: "As we take our meals, dark smiling faces peep from behind trees and houses, coming slowly nearer till we are surrounded by a crowd which discusses all we eat, how we eat and with what we eat."[28] Mrs. Pugh noted that "a great audience assembled" during one meal in 1913: "many and varied were the comments." When table boy Kutukutu could no longer find a passage from the cook's fire to the dining table, "he drove them all off, with a stick and very impressive Lokele . . . drawing a wide circle round our chairs." He also threatened: "If anyone passes this barrier he will receive a wound: I Kutukutu say it!" Kutukutu continued to repeat this "formula" wherever the Pughs stayed, "although of course the children were always near enough to see all they wanted to." Mrs. Pugh concluded that it would be "cruel to deprive" these children "of such an innocent spectacle which affords so much pleasure." The meaning of children in this context is not clear, though Kutukutu's formula seems to have been designed to exclude those for whom missionary dining, and the laughter it aroused, was not "an innocent spectacle."[29]

Such exclusions applied less to the lantern services that followed dinner. And showing "the pictures of the night" was a postdinner affair for missionaries itinerating in the forest in the 1920s. Humor attracted: "A few pictures in lighter vein are always shewn first to secure attention, but our idea of humour is not theirs. Still the pictures serve their purpose."[30] From early in the century, "miscellaneous ones, both ludicrous and informing," preceded the "one dozen picked slides from the Life of Christ." By 1929, Yakusu lantern shows included fifty slides representing "the history of the world from Adam and Eve, through the Old and New Testament," to the coming of the first BMS steamer to the Congo. Attention-grabbing miscellany was no longer preface, but punctuation; "interspersed here and there" were pictures of India, zoological specimens "both prehistorical and modern," and a "ten little nigger boys" series.[31]

"Ten little nigger boys went out to dine; one choked his little self and then there were nine." Jan Pieterse has suggested that this imaged, counting rhyme was "a violent vanishing act" by which European children learned to count by "causing little blacks to disappear." And an Englishman, Frank J. Green, may well have written the rhyme, based on the earlier "Ten Little Injuns," in 1864. Regardless, the "Ten Little Niggers" became popular as a minstrel rag tune, children's rhyme, and illustrated storybook in Europe, North America, and beyond.[32] So popular was this humorous series of rhymed, racialized images that it passed almost unnoticed into Yakusu's missionaries' lexicon and, willy-nilly, into their lantern slide projections. How did Congolese spectators read the "ten little nigger boys" series: as innocent, ludicrous, informing, or violent? Congolese spectators *noticed*, and apparently they laughed. That much we know. We also know that BMS missionaries learned quickly how to get an audience for biblical images and how to keep one. Since the visual humor of the "Ten Little Niggers" resides in great part in its serial quality, the ten-slide series would have been well suited for the "ludicrous" spotlight technique used to keep a restless audience in place. Yet the "Ten Little Niggers" series was not the only "miscellany," and Yakusu's missionaries understood that "our idea of humour is not theirs." Unlike dining spectacles, where "nonchild" exclusions came into play for the very reason that "our idea of humour is not theirs," the "Ten Little Niggers" lantern slides apparently remained in missionary eyes "an innocent spectacle" for old and young alike.[33] We need no better example of minstrel humor being culturally reproduced at Yakusu than this counting rhyme and rag tune—unless it is the comic "topical [*sic*] ditty" that entered into an after-dinner missionary singsong at Christmas in 1938. This missionary-only "Christmas jollification" involved singing freshly written verses to the tune of a minstrel-derived, farcical Sunday school song, readily available in "wholesome" American songbooks as late as 1945. Yakusu's missionaries sang to the tune of "Darkies' Sunday School."

Young folks, old folks, everybody come,
Join the darkies' Sunday school, make yourself at home,
Please to check your chewing gum and razors at the door,
And you'll hear some Bible stories that you've never heard before. . . .

Salomi was a dancer and she danced before the king,
She wiggled and she wobbled and she shook most everything.
The king says to Salomi, "We'll have no scandal here."
"The hell we won't," Salomi said and kicked the chandelier.[34]

Did such Salomi-like figures, reminiscent of minstrelsy's sexualized, wild, Topsy characters, extend beyond the "hidden desires and dark impulses" of this missionary song at Yakusu? This will prove an important question.

Boy Elves

"Boys" and "house girls" had access to missionary households, and often lived in special enclosures in missionary backyards. A missionary home, an emblem pointing "to the Home above,"[35] was to act as "the greatest influence in building up the Christian home in Congo." It was also a concrete world where boys and girls could "see the husband treat his wife with affection; see them sit down together to their meals; read the Book and pray together,"[36] and learn domestic skills. Intimate evangelism began with surrogate children, many raised and bottle-fed in missionary homes from infancy. Thus: "if you had peeped in on us at dinner last night, you would have seen Ainaosongo on the Doctor's knee learning to whistle, and Batilangandi on my lap enjoying a banana. They were very happy, and we were 'at home.' "[37]

The missionary idiom was servant to God or shepherd to lost sheep. Yakusu "boys" (and "house girls") were to be privileged, trusted, domesticated Congolese who as the servants of God's servants resembled members of the family. Local patron-client idioms were also at play: "Adopting one of us as a 'Fafa,' the happy missionary so favoured has found himself shadowed by a willing servant."[38] Impulses for new patrons would have been strong, especially among those first Yakusu followers who had fled from Zanzibari-associated turbulence, raiding, and enslavement. Yakusu's missionaries were not unique in procuring orphans and redeemed slaves as a first generation of converts. Theirs was a classic method in Protestant and Catholic missions in the Congo.

Whimsical, caricatured biographical tales about mission Congolese were common in the station quarterly. They had simple plots with an elementary, earnest message that boasted: we "can take savages and make them saints."[39] A story in installments in the *Notes* of the 1940s, for example, narrated one "boy's" life as "Elf's Progress":

A dainty little black face and sharp ears and an erect little figure is dubbed "the Congo Elf" by the Missionary. He is too young to work but is the Cinderella of his brother in the kitchen. The Missionary releases him to go to school. . . . His eagerness to learn how to read leads him to seek short cuts, but he has to realize that only steady work brings success. . . . He is promoted to the kitchen as cook's helper. . . . Through a cycle accident Mrs. Mill had to lie on her back for six weeks . . . [and] he had taken her orders daily at the bedside and managed the kitchen and cooked the food and brought a cup of tea early in the morning all by himself. . . . He can add up figures in two columns but he does not just see what the 10s column means. . . . Mrs. Mill has promoted him to under-boy in the house cleaning and she says that she . . . finds he is very clever with his hands, can undo seams, and opens tins very well. He is still the tease he was, and teases the solemn boy about twice his size who helps in the house.[40]

We do not see the elf become teacher or nurse. Rather, a series of domestic service promotions within a missionary household—further inside the most intimate, domestic center of mission life—represented the spiritual and moral advancement of this "boy," tellingly called an elf.

When Mr. and Mrs. Millman had "a unique dinner party" on their veranda in 1922, the guests were Congolese "teacher-evangelists" serving in villages in the mission district. Their faces "literally shone with recent contact with soap and water" as they sat down for a three-course, British-inspired menu of roast meat with mint sauce, potatoes, peas, and rice. "Of course it *was* a little difficult to convey peas safely to their destination by means of a fork, when you have never done it before," the doctor's wife teased, "but with the assistance of a dessert spoon all went well." Mrs. Chesterman remarked that the dinner party must have been "an inspiration to our host and hostess," who had been at the mission station since its founding days in the 1890s. The Millmans "knew these men as they *used* to be—all ignorant savages, and some of them actually cannibals."[41]

The first time the choir "boys" and "girls" had a tea party in 1931, they joined the missionaries for biscuits and sardines over tea served in cups and saucers. The lady missionaries doubled as guests like their husbands, while teaching their Congolese girls about catering to company. Mrs. Millman described the tea party by distinguishing it from a savage yore. Symbols of home, order, and authority seemed to come to life with approval: "The cane chairs and the wooden tables quietly creaked 'Things are different.' The photographs of the King and Queen of Belgium smiled to each other from their high places on the wall and seemed to say 'Delightful.' "[42]

A variety of images, then, signified colonial domesticity at Yakusu: roast beef for Christmas dinner; the "not quite/not white" qualities of a domesticated savage; soaped faces, peas eaten with spoons, and a sardine tea party; and the observing Belgian king and queen, the state conveniently domesticated as approving father and mother, as the senior missionary couple themselves. Whatever the image, each rephrased an evolutionary theme—darkness-to-lightness, savagery-to-civilization, heathens-to-Christians, monkey-stew-to-roast-beef. Such mission social events reinforced the themes of creating home, domesticating the savage, making history. Royal visits, teas, and dinners were first representations of domesticity for those who performed them, before being re-represented as advancement when inscribed as enchanting narrative for the readers of the *Quarterly Notes*.[43]

Yakusu "boys" had names, and they made stories. They were the transforming/transformed jester figures of evangelical parables, like Bongamba, who began by impressing as "a likely boy" and soon was to be seen clothed and in a kitchen, cleaning "knives and forks for an occupation."[44] Boy Elves were—in sexual, gender, spatial, and vocational senses—liminal figures who began working in gardens or kitchens and progressed to dining rooms and bedrooms. Stapleton's anecdote exposed a typical trajectory: "boy" becomes teacher. It developed in a turn-of-the-century context, common in English-speaking missions in the Congo, where the first converts played multiple roles as missionaries' personal servants.[45] By the early 1930s, the more conspicuous elf trajectory was boy-becomes-nurse. Even early in the century, Mr. Smith commented: "In the house he was my head boy, in the dispensary my head assistant." By the late 1920s, visitors were asking: "Who then are these boys in similar clothes to the teachers?" They were first-year student nurses, and each one received a cup of rice a day as a "reward" for an hour's work sweeping the station after school. When medical student admission exams were in progress in 1935, Mrs. Millman noted: "I am losing my boy who can make cakes better than most white women. Mrs. Ennals her cook. Washjacks are turning their backs on big bags of dirty clothes and are looking longingly at the smart medicals in their uniforms." One former "boy" became known as the one "who when a boy was always breaking things" in Mrs. Millman's "pantry . . . and now wears the hospital uniform and is important."[46]

Good performance on the job, in the classroom, and in moral behavior was rewarded by greater responsibility in a missionary household and greater access to its interior rooms.[47] One had to be trusted to move inside. Such was the elf's progress. Moving up meant moving in. Thus did a student become "under-boy" in housecleaning. And moving in permitted moving out: a "boy" became teacher or nurse. By the 1920s, domestic service became a method of training male workers and their "house girl" counterparts for schools and dispensary outposts, thereby expanding the borders of Yakusu's domesticated, evangelized domain.

Yakusu's missionaries were not just evoking missionary homes as icons of evangelical domesticity. In Victorian and Edwardian England, the cult of domesticity and the glorification of Lady Bountifuls as supremely moral, philanthropic figures of salvation went with fantasies of housewives playing multiple roles—"at once employer, tutor and surrogate mother"[48]—in complex households with large, specialized staffs. Missionary housewives at Yakusu did not administer complex upper-class households like those they dreamed about in Britain. Yet these "middling class" wives of "not quite gentlemen"[49] backgrounds would have envied this upper-class world, and colonial life would have nourished class-crossing fantasy and nostalgic make-believe. One missionary boasted in 1924 that her servants were "able to sweep, dust and keep my whole house as clean and bright as any well staffed mansion in England."[50] Someone like Mrs. Millman was dealing on a daily basis with how to have meals served at her table, train a future nursing staff, and prepare girls as wives for future Congolese evangelists. She also had aspirations about bourgeois domesticity that were reaffirmed as "fairy tales" by Belgian royals who showed up to observe English domesticity in the colony from time to time.

Boy elf narratives are not revelatory of mood and metaphor alone. They tell of the social organization of domestic labor within missionary homes, and demonstrate the concrete historical bonds and crossings between the gendering of domestic service in missionary homes and sanitary labor in the hospital. Before Yakusu's missionaries identified *who* would make able medical assistants, they trained potential nurses as domestic servants in their homes. Once a so-called "boy" was, in their words, "kitchen-clean," he was ready for the hospital. Boy-becomes-nurse trajectories proved effective, and Yakusu's missionaries grew to depend on them. Of eighty-one students admitted for nurse training at the Yakusu hospital during the years 1935 to 1942, 58 percent had previously worked as "boys" in missionary homes.[51] Dining and surgery, then, were kindred worlds, *intellectually* linked in missionary thought by the knife-and-fork doctrine, and *practically* linked by a set of tangible, missionized, domesticated young men who moved *from* kitchens, dining rooms, and bedrooms *to* hospitals, operating theaters, and rural health centers.

The boy-to-nurse trajectory resembled, even drew on, the mid-nineteenth-century "closeness between good housekeeping and medical science," for especially prior to the professionalization of nursing, the line between domestic service and nursing was slight. This closeness fostered the gendering of nurses in Britain and much of Europe as female.[52] In most of colonial Africa, this gendering went topsy-turvy, to draw again on a Protestant missionary expres-

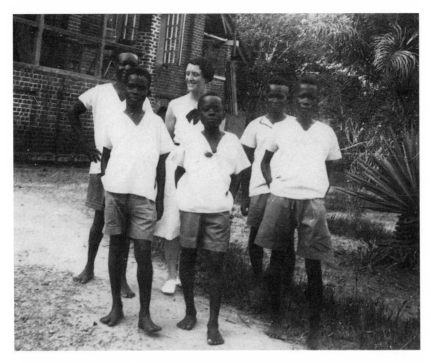

" 'Mama' & her boys," ca. 1942. Nora Carrington with her "boys" at Yakusu. (Courtesy of Nora Carrington, JFC Papers, Salisbury, U.K.)

sion in the Congo to which I will return. The trajectory began as an elaboration, as did all colonial medicine, of the primacy of European needs for domestic and nursing care.[53] The personal "boys" of turn-of-the-century tourists in the Congo doubled as their masters' quinine injectionists. A central aspect of the "boy" figure in Belgian colonial memoirs and novels was the sometimes thief who saved the life of his sick master.[54] Kathryn Hulme's *The Nun's Story,* about a Belgian nun who went to the Congo as a nurse (and took Audrey Hepburn and Peter Finch to Yakusu's adjacent leprosy camp in order to film the Congolese scenes of the Warner Brothers hit film of 1959!), shows the newcomer nun surprised to find "black boys were everywhere . . . working as clerks, typists, baby-sitters and practical nurses." She had never before seen a man "look upon nuns at their meals," nor imagined that "hospital boys" could be "as deft as women at the bed making and bandage rolling."[55]

Whatever the European colonial community seeking domestic service in the Congo—state agents, settlers, private tourists, Catholic nuns, or married Protestant missionary couples—the apparent inversion of roles as gender imaging moved between metropole and colony was, on one level, a matter of *who* was released from Congolese households for wage labor in European-operated clinics and hospitals. They were largely men and boys, not women and girls. Identifying a parallel between metropole and colony in servant-to-nurse trajectories, and especially its gender inversion on colonial terrain, implies that to understand why the category of native colonial nurse was gendered as male in much of Africa, we need to look more closely at representations of "boy" as diminutive, servile male. The subject will lead to relationships among topsy-turvy colonialisms, blackface rubrics, and in Mikhail Bakhtin's words, "Christmas laughter."[56]

"Boy" Humor

The distinction between colonial domesticity and colonial hygiene was blurred. Hygiene in the Belgian Congo became a colonywide enterprise to remake, sanitize, and discipline native space, homes, gender and sexual relations, and eating and elimination practices. It also became a standard feature of Congolese school instruction beginning in the early 1920s. Hygiene books taught men and boys how to create a home, avoid disease, and tell their wives to prepare food. Most contained a section on eating at a table with cutlery. Mr. and Mrs. Millman were among the first in the Congo to write a schoolbook on hygiene.[57]

The Yakusu evidence reveals neither negative eugenics nor a racialized discourse (which were both strongly pronounced since the 1880s in England) about eliminating the degenerate and unfit. Either finding would reflect parallels with metropolitan social hygiene movements and constructions of dangerous sexualities. Instead, hygiene at Yakusu suggests something much closer to colonial "sanitation and seeing," a privileging of "openness, visibility, ventilation, boundaries, and a particular spatial differentiation of activities." Yakusu's nonconformist missionaries were drawing on the pre-Darwinian language and social management visions of moral environmentalism, the early social medicine and associated female philanthropy of the mid–nineteenth century.[58] They were less obsessed with procreation than with personal cleanliness and moral habits—in a word, soap. The word *hygiene* came into use in early-nineteenth-century Europe as the novelty of bathing with soap remade the distinction between clean and dirty. Soap was not only for bodies, however. Among Protestants working in the Congo a century later, soap was both a "moral enterprise" and a worthy "commercial enterprise."[59] Bongamba, as we saw, was soon washing knives and forks for an occupation. Protestant missionaries' efforts to create literal and spiritual cleanliness were inspired less by the "dirty" color of Congolese skin than by Congolese eating practices. Nothing, to follow Elias again,

was more constitutive of European hygienic sensibilities, and the civilized/
noncivilized polarity that accompanied them, than the way fork use stood
conceptually opposed to cannibalism.[60]

Leonore Davidoff has shown that the Victorian preoccupation with domesticity and "rituals of order and cleanliness" were aspects of a new imaginary born of the industrial revolution. As new class divisions emerged within
English society, the polarity of working class versus middle (or upper) class
combined with a series of others: white/black, clean/dirty, lady/woman, home/
empire, masculine/feminine, urban/rural, public/private. These semantic polarities formed in and through bodies "were, partially at least, created in the
nursery."[61] The way missionaries assembled and rewrote these polarities within
evangelical parables is an important part of this inquiry. Yakusu parables—
whether sermons, anecdotes for British readers, or representations for those
mission Congolese who performed and reenacted them—were forms of remembering. Victor Yenga made it to the *Reader's Digest* as jester figure in such a
story. Salamo was a less well-traveled, though more enduring and somber
Yakusu heroine—quite distinct, as we will see, from Salomi of the "Darkies'
Sunday School" missionary carol.

Of all the early Yakusu slave converts subjected to BaTambatamba raids,
Salamo was the most well-known. Her story condensed this violent history as
redemption. As described in chapter 1, she was stolen from a village near the
mouth of the Lomami River when her "town had been burnt and looted by the
Arabs when she was quite a little child." Her person exchanged hands several
times before some BMS missionaries paid a ransom for her at Stanley Falls. She
was baptized at the downriver BMS station of Monsembi in 1895, where she
became the first "house girl" of BMS missionary, Edith Stapleton, later widowed
and remarried to Yakusu missionary, William Millman. Salamo's trajectory
included a trip home to England with Mr. and Mrs. Stapleton, before traveling
with them in 1897 to their new upriver assignment. As they approached Yakusu
by steamer, Salamo heard her native language for the first time in years: "A little
later, in a town very near to the station, she saw her own father again, and her
cup of joy was full."[62]

Before Salamo and the Stapletons arrived, Yakusu's missionaries were using
Kingwana to speak with local Congolese. Salamo helped the missionaries write
their first Lokele sermons, and taught and wrote the first Lokele hymns. She
also became a favorite icon of mission histories, sermons, class lessons, and
station plays, demonstrating how "God works out His purposes, using even an
Arab slave raid for the furtherance of His Kingdom."[63] Deliverance from slavery
was a central theme at Yakusu, and Salamo's story had the miraculous content
needed for a colonial evangelical parable. Mission Congolese learned in class

about this slave girl turned translator, evangelist, and mother, especially from the former Mrs. Stapleton, Mrs. Millman. The oldest Yakusu Protestants whom I met had never met this famed woman, who died of sleeping sickness in 1902. Yet they grew up singing hymns Salamo had written. During the "time of troubles," they explained, BaTambatamba went off with this girl, and not until Salamo returned did Lokele people accept the missionaries and their work. Salamo also reproduced. The *Yakusu Quarterly Notes* is full of story threads about her daughter and granddaughters, which together form a history of mission domesticity and social reproduction, centered at Mrs. Millman's— Mama Mokili's—home.[64]

Salamo was a solid, sober figure. There was nothing farcical, elflike, or sultry about her. Indeed, a Yakusu girl was less a jester than a flower.[65] Girls figured not as former cannibals, but as former slaves;[66] not as carnal, disorderly women, but almost ladies. The erstwhile cannibal boy became "boy," teacher, nurse; the redeemed slave victim became "house girl," wife, mother. Boy plots were integral to the cannibal humor of the knife-and-fork doctrine. Girl plots were neither funny nor topsy-turvy. Yakusu's origin parable about domesticated boys was based on a tale about Lititiyo, the Congolese pastor-to-be whom Mr. Millman first glimpsed with a human limb under his arm. Lititiyo, we saw, first became a church hero when he rejected libeli in 1924. The plot's extremes encapsulated the capacity to domesticate cannibals, and this missionary story was still traveling as lore in 1989.

Victor Yenga's plot assumed that savages possessed this capacity. When the Chestermans first arrived at Yakusu, the ten-year-old Yenga was lined up along with five other "boys" who were to help "run our house" in return for their schooling. As the Chestermans' "table boy," Yenga had been frightened, as described in chapter 2, by the sight of the doctor's surgical gloves boiling on the cookhouse fire in 1920, imagining them to be a cannibal's soup of human hands. Yenga was soon digging a chigger out of the doctor's foot, rejecting libeli, and turning to nurse training at the hospital instead. By 1931, Yenga was a prized "nurse-evangelist" at a village dispensary sixty miles away.

Yenga's early moves compressed a historical transition in colonial evangelism, the 1920s' intensification of social surgery that coincided with, perhaps even provoked, libeli in 1924. The Chestermans called Yenga (the Lokele word for Sunday) "Boy Sunday" as they authored his experiences into familiar simplifications. When Chesterman authored his 1947 "boy elf" story for the *Reader's Digest*, the title was "My Man Sunday: How a Congo Houseboy Became a Conqueror of the Dread Diseases that Ravaged His People." Man or Boy Sunday was an obvious reference to Man Friday, the savage who rescued Robinson Crusoe from cannibals and went on to become his faithful servant in Daniel

Defoe's 1719 novel. *Robinson Crusoe* was one of the most widely read stories of empire, and the Chestermans' Boy Sunday versions were some of its many "independent retellings" across Europe and its colonies.[67]

The literary strategy of "boy" stories was partly comic. Reducing Yenga to a "Man Sunday" figure engendered amused admiration. Hence, the *Reader's Digest* piece included the episode of comic reversal when the doctor's boiling surgeon's gloves became, in "native" eyes, a white cannibal's soup of simmering black hands. This colonial hygiene joke, mediated through stock European cannibal humor, moved in unexpected ways among metropole and colony, among missionary theaters and pantomimes, evangelical and popular publications, and the social memory of mission-affiliated men and women. I first heard the soup story in 1989 from the Yakusu printer, Papa Lokangu from Yalocha. He told it as a joke about basenji who, unlike him, "a mission man," had been afraid of the hospital, and the same cannibal soup tale became part of a historical pantomime staged by mission Congolese at Yakusu in the 1940s. The incident of comic reversal also found its way into a "pageant play" performed in London in 1951, commemorating fifty years of BMS medical missionary work at a time when Chesterman was the chief medical officer in the society's London offices. Chesterman said to a grinning Sunday in one scene: "No—you eat fish and bananas now, don't you? Much more tasty than men, I should think! . . . Go with Salt now and learn your tasks in this household."[68]

Also elaborated for the London audience was a missionary dining scene about the day Boy Sunday appeared from the kitchen, carrying a tray of dinner dishes and a small jar of bitter mint sauce. Sunday nearly poisoned the Chestermans to death by serving them a mint sauce that he had prepared in a jar previously used for "the drink for the table legs," a chemical used to keep ants from climbing up on the dining table. The scene ended as the Chestermans quickly took an emetic, as Boy Sunday peeked in, admiring the effects of "the white man's medicine." Like a blackface episode in a London music hall bill, this mint sauce scene offered comic relief. Colonial servant jokes were virtually by definition hygiene jokes, and this one was about a "boy" figure who with utter devotion and hygienic stupidity nearly killed his master.[69] This joke was a farcical elaboration of the cannibal humor implicit in the very notion of a "knife-and-fork doctrine." Yakusu's British missionaries, for all their evangelical earnestness and anti-Papal sentiments, laughed about many of the same things as the Belgian colonials among whom they lived. They drew from a common stock of minstrel-associated tropes in this situation where, despite enormous sociological and cultural complexity, they frequently split their worlds semantically into "white helmets and black skins."[70]

Africa, Patrick Brantlinger tells us, served "as a foil to Europe, a place of negations." The mirth of Yakusu's missionaries, and the way it alternately drew on the ribald cannibal humor of their day, suggests something more. Protestant missionary evangelists called the Congo (both the Congo Free State and its successor regime, the Belgian Congo) Congoland. They thought of it as a "topsy-turvy" place of mixed-up inversions and, in Dan Crawford's words, of "thinking black."[71] In 1930, a BMS Yakusu teacher wrote from the BaMbole forest to Chesterman: "Do you white men think that we blacks are men or animals that you do not send us an Infirmier here?" The doctor drew from a book written by a well-known Scottish missionary, Dan Crawford, *Thinking Black* (1912), a conspicuous example of colonial evangelical humor, when he commented on the teacher's question: "He can think white easier than we, perhaps, can think black."[72] Dan Crawford had worked "without a break for 22 years," as his subtitle proclaimed, in Congo's southeastern savannas; and his *Thinking Black* became a Yakusu missionary guide to humor and contradictory mixtures in Congoland. He spoke of the Congolese intellect as "a ray of intelligence" that "actually pierced the mists of the cannibal brain." He described Congolese cannibals who had "hurled clouds of arrows against Stanley's canoes" only to become Free State soldiers with "the veneer of the barracks, smart uniform and deadly Albinis only helping to hide the horrible man-eater wrapped up in this official envelope." He evoked a classic trope of cannibal humor when speaking of "the march of events" that "swept dozens of young Belgians into the cannibal pots" and of a "diabolic epicure" who "had his scouts out, catching strings of little boys and girls, all doomed to the pot, all reckoned titbits!" Yakusu's missionaries drew on the same repertoire when they narrated dining stories for their British reading public with, like Crawford, cannibals at their elbows telling them all.[73]

Jan Pieterse has suggested that the comic cliché of a European being boiled up in an African cooking pot coincided with conquest. He distinguishes this first era from a second of "new cannibal humour," which he does not anchor firmly in time: "Fear and loathing gave way to humour and the tone became lighter and ironic. . . . The point of the new cannibal humour is usually the contradiction of the savage gourmand. A savage, *therefore* a cannibal, but a cannibal with refined manners, with the attributes (chef's hat, implements) and attitude of European cuisine. . . . the icon of the colonized savage and of a pacified Africa."[74] Pieterse's distinction may resemble the contrast between Crawford's ribaldry and the mirth of Yakusu's missionaries. Yet it tells little about the use of colonial humor or about how earlier cannibal humor inspired those who veiled theirs more.

Crawford's words about topsy-turvy Congoland gave Yakusu's missionaries a sensibility that they, in turn, called "thinking black." Although for some post-1945 missionaries, "thinking black" was a way to express an appreciative, relativist attitude toward Congolese practice, their predecessors quoted Crawford's title while laughing at seemingly mixed-up, topsy-turvy Congolese ways. Several equated thinking black with thinking evil.[75] The range in colonial evangelical humor was wide. Missionaries at Yakusu knew colonial life as sometimes funny, even surreal, and this attitude facilitated their simplistic, self-entertaining appropriations of local figures and objects for bureaucratic, domestic, and parodic purposes. They seized on the capacity of slit drums to signal messages, for example, and converted one into the keeper of time and order at Yakusu. Every morning, the station slit drum signaled to Congolese that it was time to get up with the message: "wash your feet, wash your legs, wash your face, wash." We can see the humor in this now, even if sanitary wake-up calls were serious business then.

Yakusu's missionaries also used droll incidents to enliven sermons and initiate missionary newcomers. One treasured sermon told of the day some "savage" BaKomo women across the river asked Mrs. Millman to come visit. She was the first missionary to do so for several years, ever since the day a missionary man had been tied to a tree for tampering with a ritual drum. Mrs. Millman went alone. When her male colleagues who waited behind anxiously in Yakusu heard drumming from across the river, they feared for her safety, until they understood that it was only Mrs. Millman calling to say "bring in the laundry" because it was going to rain.[76] This is a quaint example of, in Greg Dening's words, "dramatic ironies in which the appropriation of the natives allowed the strangers to be entertained by themselves."[77]

Magic lantern humor reveals less quaint appropriations coupled with minstrelsy projections. Missionary elaborations of "boy elves" were burlesque in their reversals and reductions. Colonial jesting, of course, was not only a form of missionary distraction and amusement. Protestant missionaries in the Congo *used* humor as they fashioned colonial joking relationships. In 1909, one advised "Do cultivate humour for your health's sake, your colleagues' sake, and if you are married for your wife's sake." He added: "you must get the best of the shirker, and if you can do it with the laugh from the spectators so much the better." Missionaries argued about tone, purpose, and effect. The same missionary thought sarcasm was "a much better tool than temper." Another objected that, "The native takes wrong notions of sarcasm," which was "a very dangerous weapon" that "smarts and leaves sore places which are difficult to heal."[78] We saw this same spectrum in colonial laughter—as imperial self-entertainment, as disciplinary tool, as dangerous and sadistic weapon, as colonial theater (with alternately imperial and colonized spectators), as incorporated joking—in the multiple, caricatured retellings of Victor Yenga as Crusoe's Friday. The same range will remain significant as we turn to parody and the gendering of "boy" work in missionary narrative and postcolonial memory alike.

Boi Work as Parody

"Boy" work seemed prestigious early in the century. Yakusu's missionaries noted that boys felt a pleasant "pride in being able to say, 'I am Mokili's boy,' or 'I work the paka-paka (typewriter) of Kienge,' or 'I cook the food for Mama Ebongo.'"[79] Some, no doubt, were former slaves, honored to locate new patrons yielding access to a new social ladder. Domestic service arrangements at Yakusu made economic sense.[80] Hiring students was cheaper than hiring full-time servants. When questions arrived from troubled parishioners in England, Yakusu's missionaries would explain that youth, aged eight to fifteen, worked in their households as "part of the educational scheme. . . . But servants, in the sense that that term is understood at home, these boys and girls are not. . . . Here the rule obtains: one person one work! . . . Of course the missionary pays."[81]

By 1950, being a "house boy" was no longer prestigious. Pastor Batondo of Yakusu, born about 1939, told me proudly that he had never been a "boy." "The punishments" for work-related failures "were too severe," he said, mentioning expulsion from school. Caning, integral to Mrs. Millman's notions of proper child rearing, likely was to her "boy" rearing as well.[82] New colonial regulations established an upper age limit for students and a longer school day in about 1954. Dr. Browne bemoaned the changes because the hospital school could no longer screen future nurses through domestic service in the home: "Now knowledgeable lads are not even 'kitchen-clean' when they come to the wards and operating theater, and have to be 'house-trained' at great cost of time and patience and energy." "Boy" work and schooling had been simultaneous experiences, and a first career step for many. Most "boys" went on to become nurses, teachers, or printers for the church. Tata Tula became an important clerk. Pastor Lofolata became a teacher. Papa Boshanene went from "boy" work to infirmary work, both under the supervision of Browne. Papa Lokangu became mission printer. Other Yakusu "boys," in fact, worked as missionaries' main cooks and servants for years on end, never graduating from their afternoon schooling. In keeping with the new state rules, these men called "boys" had to leave school, disrupting the missionary "educational scheme" that had long provided cheap labor.[83]

The memories of most who had worked as "boys" were fraught with ambivalence, alternately marked by nostalgia, parody, and scorn. Prince Albert noted in 1909 that Mrs. Millman was "sour and dry." Papa Lokangu's recollections confirmed this royal impression, while mixing in flowers, mischief, and bustle. One day, Lokangu led me out on the riverbank lawn opposite the Millmans' home to the spot where every afternoon just before the sun set, all the missionaries would gather to sit on three beautiful wooden benches surrounded by flowers, as the Congo Belge flag flew above them.[84] He recalled the stairs leading to the Millman house, the demanding manner in which Mama Mokili gave orders, her piano playing, and her love of flowers. Only missionaries would gather "to talk," "to relax," he insisted, though a few servants would be there.

Thus did Lokangu insert his own social origins into his historical tour of the mission station. He had been born at Yakusu in 1918 to a church carpenter from Yalocha, who later became a teacher. Lokangu's own work as "boy" for Mrs. Millman began when he was nine. "I was working, working, working," he told me, then clarified the meaning of his reduplicative: "Me, I was a boi." He mimicked Mrs. Millman, embellishing his performance with the English words "all right" and the bending movements she made as she gave orders on tending her flowers. Lokangu also called her by her middle name, Rebecca, as if remembering how he and others used to mime Mr. Millman's voice. He also recalled gathering for mission choir rehearsals with Mrs. Millman, and drinking the "sulfa" and "tonic" available on these special days.

Mrs. Millman had many, many workers, including a cook, someone to iron clothes, someone to serve table, someone to sweep, and the like. Lokangu thought there would have been about ten at once. Those who worked changed often. When I asked Tata Bafoya if he had been the only worker for the Millmans in the early 1920s, he cried, "Ah! Ah! many people! . . . Every job was separate. . . . There were many parts." Mama Tula echoed, describing the minute division of labor: "Each person with his own job. One person just preparing the bed. . . . Each day he will come and do just this job here. . . . Another had the work of cooking the food. Another had the job of cutting trees." Bafoya's work was to sweep the Millman house; his older brother was the cook. Mrs. Millman called schoolboys from nearby Yakoso like himself, he said, to come plant cassava and sugarcane in the large, enclosed garden in her backyard.[85]

Most men who had associated with Yakusu's missionaries in the 1920s and 1930s, even in the 1940s, spoke to me proudly of these relationships in 1989. Several were sardonic when the subject of "boy" work arose. Lokangu said he liked "boy" work, though his animated, parodic performance of stooping down, working hard, and following orders showed how taxing and demeaning—at least retrospectively—the work had been. Papa Boshanene, Yakusu's aging pharmacist in 1989, began his mission career as the Brownes' garden "boy" some fifty years before. He did not mime. He remembered rewards.

"Sometimes they would give me five francs. Sometimes they would give me some sardines. Sometimes they gave me soap, sometimes sweet bananas."[86] The church pastor in the Olombo village of Yalolia recalled Mr. Ford coming to the Foma village where he was born, Bieti, in about 1936. Lofolata, then eleven, was eager to go to Yakusu's school. Ford saw him as bright, and Lofolata's father agreed he could go. The elderly, esteemed pastor described setting Ford's table and making his bed, while living in the *boyerie* structure next to the missionary's house. Yet Lofolata never used the word *boi*. The memories he shared with me were full of proud dignity, underlining the intimacy of his relations with Ford instead. He had traveled to both Kenya and Uganda with this missionary master and teacher, almost going with him as far as England.[87]

Most "boy" memories alternated among images of hard, minutely supervised labor; the meticulous, quirky habits of missionaries and their selfishness with food; affectionate nostalgia; and a moral economy that turned on irregular matabish (gifts or tips), often dished out as rewards for ethical conduct. "If you had a good heart, you would go sweep . . . for Mr. Millman," Bafoya explained, though "his Madami would come to test the heart of the person" by leaving money lying on the floor.

> You would take their blanket. You would shake the mattress. You would put it in the sun. And when it was time, you would put them back inside and spread their bed well. You would take this money they had left, and you would hide it. Another time you would say: "Madami, isn't that money that you left there." "Thank you, child, thank you." There would be a matabish. She would give you something saying, "Go." But if you were committing theft in the house of a white person: Impossible! You could not enter. You would have to go away. "We don't want thieving; theft is very bad."

At some point, Tata Bafoya's father forbade him from going to class and doing housework for the Millmans anymore; he "feared the white man liked me too much and would run off with me." Young Bafoya acquired libeli scars in 1924, perhaps at one and the same time (we met a Bafoya elder, Bafoya Yakoso, church rebel and libeli defender in 1910, in chapter 1).[88]

"Boy" recollections lacked the compression, linearity, and mirth of missionary-authored "boy elf" tales. Compare missionary representations of Joseph Tula with his own storytelling. Tula first appeared in the *Quarterly Notes* as the "master of ceremonies" at Yakusu's celebrated tea party of 1931. "Mr Ford filled the teapots from a never failing source; Mr Ennals fed the gramophone"; and Tula (whose name Mrs. Millman enjoyed translating as Mr. Electric Fish) "rose and blew a whistle" before unexpectedly asking four missionary men to rise and sing a song. Tula also helped a single woman missionary teacher, A. Wilkinson, train BaManga teachers in 1931. He spoke Swahili, assisted with evening lantern services, and rode a bicycle. By 1934, Tula was "the 'clerc' at Yakusu." According to another missionary, K. C. Parkinson, he was "a most efficient man to accompany you on a forest journey." Parkinson and Tula arrived at Yalilo "well ahead of our porters, cook boys, etc., who were not so lucky to have bicycles." Tula was "well acquainted" with the policeman who had sent someone to fetch the white man eggs, "as indeed he seemed to be with anyone of authority in any village, white men included." Tula improvised as he helped Parkinson to inspect schools, announcing in one village that he would give an extra speech "illustrated by the gramophone." In 1935, Mrs. Millman featured Tula and his difficult wife, Paulina, in a story about their first baby boy, "weak and puny, fretful and unlovely," soon covered with "loathsome sores." A baby girl was born to them dead, as was a third child. Tula, meanwhile, was "wonderful." He was "not quite usual" because he "came to us from the Rubber Plantation Island with a knowledge of reading and writing gained in one of our village schools." He had "a very pleasant respectful manner and could do what he was told." The "Rubber Plantation Island" was Ile Bertha or Yaolimela, the island opposite Yakusu, which the Belgika company made an important base for its rubber plantation operations. By 1952, Tula was church overseer at Bokuma, Belgika's "collecting post for rubber" on the opposite side of the river with striking "avenues of rubber trees." Tula was "a fine man" and "African Christian" because he was a much trusted capita (foreman) for Belgika, "a man of great religious zeal who uses his influential position to help the church." Some missionaries who went to visit Bokuma one Easter, stayed in Tula's home, where a small choir on his veranda welcomed them with song.[89]

In 1989, Tata Tula lived at Yakusu in a brick house just behind the hospital. A missionary took me to meet Tula, then the oldest mission man with deep Foma facial scars, who still rose a couple of times a day to signal station work schedules on the slit drum outside. His daughter-in-law became one of my most important teachers, assistants, and advisers; Tata Tula's grandson transcribed most of my tapes. Tula, I learned meanwhile, was a paradoxical figure in local social memory. Those who had previously worked for Belgika at Bokuma, including his kin at Yainyongo, remembered Tula, post capita for Belgika, as "a white man of trouble there." Tata Alikuwa also recalled Tula as the village teacher who encouraged him to go off to Yakusu for further schooling. When Alikuwa lost his job as church teacher because he took a second wife, he became a rubber collector at Bokuma. Tula, he reminisced, called roll, sent people to work in the forest, sent others to prison, while "he was just in his *bureau*." Tula was also harsh, and he "had a lot of things, everything, many things, yes, many things. If you saw his house, it was just like the house of a *muzungu*. He was a man there that one Tata Tula."[90] Others remembered Tula similarly, if more simply. The links in the common social logic that made Tula an ambivalent local icon went: He drove a car. People called him Monsieur. He was a "white man."

Tula's career did not have a linear, boy-to-teacher shape in either missionary representations, social memory, or for that matter, his own autobiography. Tula remembered being a "boy" twice, first for a Yakusu-trained Congolese teacher and later for the Millmans. His memories stretched back to his days as a young boy in a village way up the Romée and Lilele streams. When Seleki of Yatuka came to work as teacher there, the chief gave him a house to live in and girls wanted to cook for him. Tula just studied the sounds of letters during Seleki's first two weeks, and then began to read the first Lokele primer: "When you had finished that one, the missionaries would give you money, one franc. When you finished that you would get another book, the 'News of Jesus,' a big one that one." Soon Tula was assisting Seleki. When Seleki went to Yakusu for more schooling, Tula went with him. Each teacher came with "two children" cooks for the one month's training: "we were cooking them food there in that little, little house here. When their class was finished, they would come, and we would give them their food. . . . When the food was finished, the 'people of work' here, the children, would enter" class. At the end of the course, Tula received small amounts of clothes, pencils, and notebooks because "you went to teach back there to those who remained behind. You had now become their teacher since now you knew a little."

At the time, Tula was twelve. The missionaries sent him to teach in another village, paying him a franc with King Albert on its face once a month to pay his tax. The missionaries would say: "Go pay. We don't want our teachers to have troubles with the State." Other people planted fields to pay their taxes, Tula recalled: "Mine, it just came from the missionaries." One year, the missionaries let Tula return to Yakusu: "I just did the work of writing. They saw my penmanship was good. They said: 'you will stay as clerk.'" Soon afterward, Belgika agents asked Mr. Millman to send them "a good man who knows how to write the names of people." Tula signed a three-year contract at fourteen. He spent the first month building his house with the axes and machete provided by Belgika: "I pounded the mud in the house and my brothers came to help me." His job was to walk behind a bigger boss, a father of fourteen children named Liketa. Tula wrote the names of the "children" present at roll call and again in the forest, and marked down those who did not finish their work. On Saturdays, Tula gave five *makuta* each to these "children" who were clearing the forest for roads and fields of palms, coffee, rubber, and cocoa.

Tula wanted to marry when his contract ended. He returned to Yakusu first. The missionaries said to him: "Good, so you will stay. You will stay as a garden boy." So Tula went from house-owning plantation clerk to planting "those little, little fields which the missionary white men had." He also washed plates and attended class:

> When their food was prepared, they would call me, removing me from the garden. I would wash my hands. They would say: "Sit down because you will eat with this one, the one who cooks a little food. When we leave our plates, you will wash the plates." . . . Yes, when you had stayed there eight hours, the work would finish. The white people would finish eating. The bell would sound, *allez*, we would go to class.

Tula performed parodically when talking about his "boy" work during missionary meals. Their dining habits were peculiar: "Eight o'clock would come, they would get their little bell and they would play it '*nge, nge, nge, nge*' to call me." He would go stay by the cookstove while they were eating and "then the plates would come. They would give the plates to me. If a bone remained, me, I would eat it." Tula broke into laughter as he showed how he used to sneak leftovers once out of missionary view.

One day, Tata Tula returned to see his "fathers" in Yainyongo. He was ready to marry. When another letter from Belgika arrived at Yakusu, Tula returned to work as plantation clerk, this time recording the amount of rubber latex that workers had collected in their buckets—for some ten years' time. His father arrived one day with chickens and a goat to send to the household of the woman Tula wanted to marry—a girl from Yalokombe whose father worked for Belgika. Once wed, Tula sent his Lokele wife home to his Foma village for bowai, returning there himself each Saturday after receiving his pay. His female kin fed and fattened his secluded wife until her bowai was over; then they gave her plates and other gifts, and sent her to stay with her husband. Tula organized baptismal classes for his wife with Mama Mokili's help. His autobiography, like those of most local men and women, continued with the births and deaths of his infants. After his son was born, Tula "gave birth" to two babies who "died in the belly." Tula, less typically, said: "Me, I went to the doctor." He also bought false teeth for his sick son, after watching Dr. Chesterman remove the boy's sick teeth. Furthermore, Tula agreed that Chesterman could perform surgery on his wife, pregnant once again, while Tula was away training BaManga (Mba) teachers for the church.[91]

It is possible to detect a movement from dining to surgery in Tula's autobiography. But Tula did not move up, inside, and out as in "The Elf's Progress." His story was one of backs and forths and betweens. He moved from young village scholar to a "boy"-cook for his village teacher, from Yakusu scholar to village teacher to plantation clerk. Yet when Tula decided to move from Belgika roll caller to more Yakusu schooling, he was demoted to garden boy. After moving up to plate-washing duty, he became plantation clerk again, and also a Protestant husband and evangelist who accepted Chesterman's proposal of a cesarean section for his wife, never mind the removal of his son's decayed teeth. Tula's story is also about food. He cooked for Seleki and was soon a teacher himself. He took home his paychecks to fatten his wife in bowai. He secured power through food, and long before, he was plantation capita (foreman) and church overseer with storehouses of company food at his disposal.

Just as local idioms linking fertility and wealth, food and power, recurred in this colonial church-plus-company big man's story, so did discontinuities wrought by a specific colonial modernity combining biomedicine, mobility, and obstetrics. Tula cycled, lived in brick houses, drove a company car, bought false teeth, and consulted missionary doctors and heeded their surgical advice. His unusual career path, which broke with typical "boy" trajectories, began with inscription. The young Tula had exceptional penmanship. This fact, perhaps more than any other, initiated his anomalous vita. He remained the only Yakusu "boy" who moved up from garden boy, to cycling evangelist, to driving a Belgika automobile as a proud Congolese "Monsieur."

Tula moved in and out of multiple colonial worlds, glimpsing complex mission, state, and plantation complicities within and beyond his Foma, Belgika, and Yakusu homes. His autobiography reminds us that Yakusu was not an insular, uncontaminated world. In the 1890s, Yakusu's missionaries ransomed

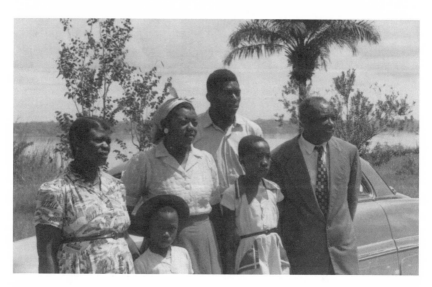

Tata Tula with his automobile and family, ca. 1957. (Courtesy of Nora Carrington, JFC Papers, Salisbury, U.K.)

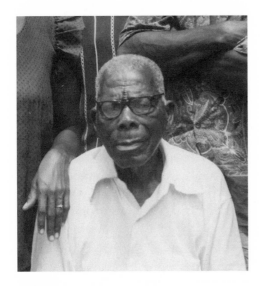

Tata Tula, Yakusu, 1990.
Photograph by author.

slave girls from traders at the Falls. In the 1920s, while encouraging Congolese teachers to have "boys," they gave the local plantation company their best scribe. By the 1930s, Tula was improvising, asking unprepared missionaries to sing at teas, and preaching by gramophone in itineration tours. Mrs. Millman caricatured Tula, by translating his name as Mr. Electric Fish in the *Yakusu Quarterly Notes*, but he became indispensable to Yakusu and Belgika alike. Indeed, in missionary and local Congolese eyes, it seemed Tula knew colonial spaces, persons, and things better than anyone else. By 1989, Belgika was long gone. So was the car. Tula was a respected mission elder dependent, drum signaler, and no more. He did not talk about his driving Monsieur days. Rather, Tula recounted "boy" stealth in the face of missionary dining habits with parody and glee. No other work provided such ready access to missionary habitus. No work was as demeaning or ironic, no memory more important now. Snitching a leftover bone was remembered with laughter—perhaps "broken laughters,"[92] yet with snickering, miming, and fond nostalgia nonetheless. Indeed, the laughter of "boy" memories is consonant with the kind of public fascination with missionary dining ritual that Rose Gee witnessed when a crowd gathered to watch her first meal at Yakusu.

Girls as Boys

When Mrs. Millman invited Congolese teacher-evangelists working in the mission district to dinner in 1922, her "house girls" served the men. When Belgian royals came to visit, a Congolese girl made special cakes "for the moment when we shall say 'Will Monseigneur honour us by taking a cup of tea and a cake made by this girl?' " Brown Mary was waiting for her, teapot in hand, when Princess Astrid arrived at the Millman house in 1933. The princess smiled when Mrs. Millman asked her to sit in the same chair that King Albert had used in 1928. " 'I want to ask you,' she said, 'Do you have girls to keep the house so beautiful or must you do it yourself?' " Mrs. Millman replied: " 'I have always had girls and even the flowers are arranged by them.' 'Today?' 'Yes, Princess.' 'And the girl prepared this tea?' 'Yes, Princess.' " The princess marveled: " 'I am very interested. It seems wonderful. Why is it not done everywhere?' "[93]

Princess Astrid's basic question was: Are "boys" girls at Yakusu? Girls *could* be "boys" at Yakusu, as former "boys" (both male and female) remembered. Girl trajectories also circulated through missionary dining rooms and bed-rooms. Yet, as Tula and Bafoya recollected, there were gender asymmetries in "boy" work in Mrs. Millman's house. Bafoya recalled Mama Mokili having fourteen girls. They entered her house to work, he said. Yet he remembered "*wa-boi*" putting food on the table and clearing afterward, while Mama's girls were "sitting. They were singing songs of God. They were dancing." He also recalled seeing the girls when the mission hunter would "give out meat—the girls their part. Us, boys, we had our part. Tons of food, you couldn't eat it all, my child, you couldn't eat it all. . . . Now again it is hunger." Tula did not remember huge quantities of food and he was more explicit about the favoring of girls: "If there were three white people, two would give the work of bringing the food to the table to the girls. They didn't like boys, just girls. . . . The boys, like me, would wash the plates."[94]

Mrs. Millman's career was largely dedicated to adopting young girls—many orphans, some placed by willing Christian parents—who lived in a special *lopangu* (enclosure) at the back of her house.[95] Salamo, as we saw earlier, was her first. In 1918, her "house girls" were learning how to crochet yokes in their frocks and how to make butter, flour, sugar, lace, and soap. Mama Mokili was the senior "White Mama." ("White Mama" was a missionary expression for a married missionary woman.)[96] The plots of her girl stories, like that about Salamo, tended to culminate in marriage and motherhood. The idioms were "weed becomes flower" or "orphan/slave becomes Christian wife." Marriages between former "house girls" and "house boys"—approved, if not in fact ar-ranged, by missionaries—were the crowning aspiration of mission endeavor.

Missionary ladies worked with girls, missionary men with boys. Yet domestic necessity meant that some missionary women ordered "boys" to make beds and serve tea. Missionary men, however, only supervised boys and never girls. The sexual anxieties that underlay these asymmetries became more pronounced over time. Mrs. Millman had long had a girls' home in her backyard, in keeping

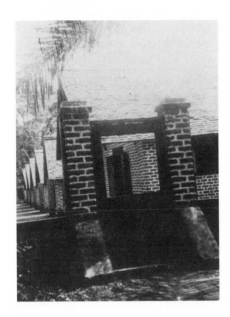

"The Fence," ca. 1929. (Courtesy of David Lofts, PL Papers, Barton-on-Sea, U.K.)

with the Protestant missionary suggestions of 1911 that "every lady missionary" in the Congo "take as many girls as possible into her home, with a view to winning them for Christ." Fears grew, however, that having girls work close to Congolese boys would endanger their honor: "if a married lady has boys she should not have girls as well." "Go softly. Be mothers to them," had been Mrs. Millman's reaction to this Protestant preference for instituting girls' boarding schools in the Congo in 1921. She feared crowded schedules and rigid institutional structures.[97]

When the Yakusu boarding home for girls was founded in 1928, it followed a recommended "home life" model, with a series of separate brick houses, each inhabited by seven or eight girls and with older girls as house mothers. A brick fence around the whole compound was supposed to guard the girls. The home of two missionary teachers closed the rectangle. These single women missionaries were the superintendents; they took over Mrs. Millman's former work. The new boarding home was called the "fence" (not unlike Mrs. Millman's lopangu), a term suggesting enclosure, boundary, blockade. The "fence" placed girls in a bounded space, safe from what might contaminate them: men and boys, "town girls" from nearby Yakoso, and "raw natives" or basenji.[98] Congolese women recalled it as a barricaded space with one door. You had to be inside this door by 6 P.M. each day or meet with punishment: caning.

Single women missionaries in the Congo had long been an issue of debate among BMS and other Protestant missionary societies. They would, it was feared, confound church teachings about marriage. They would be sexually and psychologically vulnerable. And they posed a threat to married missionary women: "Several single ladies located at a station may engage themselves in good works but someone's wife, through their presence, becomes a household drudge."[99] It would also be difficult to develop surrogate families for these women "relegated," in Mrs. Millman's words, "to the very straight jacket of the single woman." Issues of sexual asceticism and territoriality were involved. Since 1907, Protestant missionary recommendations advised on the appropriate activities, living arrangements, and companionship for single woman missionaries. They were to work only with children and women. They were to live together in pairs, preferably without male domestic servants, ensuring their distance from European and Congolese men *and* married missionary women.[100]

The arrival of "single ladies" made the development of a boarding school at Yakusu practical just as "the oversight of girls" became "one of the most important branches of single ladies' work" at BMS stations in the Congo.[101] Yakusu's "fence" for girls in training to be teachers and midwives simultaneously institutionalized "girls' work," protected girls from the apparent dangers of working beside boys, and in giving a home and surrogate family to single women missionaries, helped contain the tensions surrounding their arrival at Yakusu. As Congolese girls moved up and within a hierarchy of age and domestic service jobs inside Yakusu's new "fence," they became the "Mamas" of the younger girls in the individual houses. In local Congolese terms, this was not so unusual; they were becoming *cose,* the youthful maternal guardians of yet younger children. But the White Mamas at the head of the household were not Mamas at all. Each was a Mademoiselle.

Intimate evangelism had previously been cast in maternal and marital terms. Mrs. Millman's house of girls provided exposure to the supervising, caring Lady Bountiful figure and to her idealized, companionate marriage. The new "fence" strained these idioms. Congolese women's memories illuminate the new rigidities of hierarchy and control. When a girl became a "Mama," she effectively became a "boy," because it was then and only then that you entered into the big White Mamas' household and served at their table. The pinnacle of these movements was to be in charge of a Mademoiselle's bedroom. This promotion, associated with two new tasks, meant you were a Mama-girl ready for marriage. Mama Machuli Bolendela, who had lived in the "fence" while in midwife school, explained: "The one who was in the kitchen, she was already a Mama. When you entered there with those machines [kitchen appliances], you went into the house of the *Ba-Mademoiselle* to fix up their room, saying you were a Mama, ready to enter marriage." The first new duty was folding the missionaries' large sheets: "Enter, enter a Mademoiselle's bedroom to remove those bed

sheets, those huge, huge ones, could you do that!? Not until you were a Mama."
Machuli recalled hearing a Mademoiselle say: "You are a girl who will marry
soon, so you will clean up Mademoiselle's house there." The girls did not object.
"We just said: 'So this is to teach us work.' "

She spoke of the second task given to a Mama-girl who would marry soon in
terms of the effect of memory on routine.

> We didn't feel hungry. We didn't feel a single thing. We were carrying the
> shit of these Ba-Mademoiselle, throwing it away. We didn't do a single
> thing [to object]. . . . We were just saying: "So that's how it is. . . . These are
> just their customs." But after independence, up until today, Mademoiselle,
> those white buckets . . . even if someone brings water in one, I won't drink
> that water. I just remember, just knowing that that shit of those Ba-
> Mademoiselle is there each day. . . . I go to look for something else to drink
> water from. Not one of those buckets I was degraded by many years ago, as
> I regularly carried the droppings of Ba-Mademoiselle going to throw them
> in that *cabinet* there. Those Ba-Anglais truly aggrieved us, but we didn't
> brood over a thing then at all.[102]

This work of removing the lady missionaries' sanitary buckets was revolting
and degrading, she recalled, while stressing that, at the time, "we just felt fine,
that was all."

Machuli Bolendela's memories, however, were mixed with others about dining, food, and hunger, suggesting that the fence girls did brood and rebel.

> If you came late, they were already at the table, they were eating. You would
> get the smacks of Mademoiselle hitting you. And when people would come
> the next day from the *cité* to see why you had cried, Mademoiselle would
> say she was just teaching you not to come back to the fence at night. . . .
> They had their cupboard there of sardines, of everything and everything,
> every single thing. They could feel if the food filled them well or instead
> say: "Take this, throw it away." You felt hungry. . . . We would take it and
> hide it. We would go eat it. . . . If they asked us to bury a dead chicken, we
> would pretend to bury it. . . . Trouble! We were persecuted by those Ba-
> Anglais there. We ate *matembele* leaves before they were cooked because of
> hunger. . . . Trouble! They would call a missionary man to come to beat
> you, *eee!* You would feel *paa!* "I am dying, *eee!*" *Paa!* "I am dying, *eee!*"

She remembered that one Mademoiselle who worked at the hospital "loved"
the midwife students who lived in the fence. "Her heart was just to love people.
She didn't call us monkeys. She said: 'A person is a person, that's all.' " One day,
she called the midwife students to her house for a feast: "We went to eat there. If

you saw the faces of those other Ba-Mademoiselle. They were swelling, swelling up with anger—'*Nègres,* they can't eat food with us'—because Ba-Anglais are like that."

Yakusu's boarding home for girls may have resolved anxieties about sexuality and transgression by bounding unmarried women—English and Congolese—into one closed space. Yet Mrs. Millman's intimate tone did not survive in this fenced enclave of and for women. The girl students of the postwar period were locked in and forced to do servile "boy" work long after dining tasks had been supplanted by surgical ones among their male counterparts. These girls used sarcasm as armor and underwent violent blows in return. Local ideas about kindheartedness and generosity with food nourished their diagnoses of white women's greed "at table." Like Tula, though with more sarcasm and animation and at much greater length, Machuli reveled in performing amused memories of "boy" work while missionaries were dining:

> They finish eating. You come with another tray to show her. If she is full, if she is not full, she will take more, *teee,* it's finished. "That, that remains, go stash it in the cupboard." The meat stays in the cupboard, the *pommes de terre* stay in the cupboard. "Don't touch it!!!" . . . Eight o'clock at night, you come out of there to eat a small bit of cassava bread. And so we were mocking them. They were full. We were hungry. We were mocking them teee, until again they would take it out on our behinds.[103]

"Discipline is difficult to maintain," noted Mary Fagg, a missionary midwife, in 1953 after all but two of about eight midwife students went on strike. Fagg said her students rebelled after being "admonished for badly done work"; three had not returned to school, and these "upsets . . . call us to prayer."[104] Mama Machuli Georgine, who graduated as a midwife that year, remembered going on strike over inadequate food in the "fence": "One cup for three people and a little oil, one spoonful. So we made a strike, saying, 'We won't go to class again. We will go hide in the forest.' "[105] Machuli Bolendela, too, recalled hunger and anger leading to a strike. The "fence" students, obliged to serve the Mademoi-selle missionaries their meals and resenting that they did not share, said to themselves one day: "today we will make a German war like they made a long time ago there at Romée." They ran into the forest in the morning and were still there late in the afternoon cooking cassava greens: "We left those misses in the boarding school. We ran into the forest, we stayed there *tiii.* . . . But they were eating well." Ten girls in all—four from Yakoso and six from villages far away—stayed in the forest until Dr. Browne came to call them away from their "war of the Germans."[106] Bolendela remembered them crying, "We don't want to enter class. We won't work again!" They cried until Browne came and asked "each girl, one by one, if she wanted her *feuille de route*"—a colonial document for travel and relocation. Those "from very far away villages" did not want to "come from afar to die for nothing, not getting a diploma." These six replied to the doctor: " 'We want to enter class.' So we remained six only. Those four girls from Yakoso, they left [school]. . . . All of us had the strike."[107]

Leonore Davidoff argued that the "double exposure" of women, a legacy from classical culture and Christian theology, found new meaning in Victorian society. The polarity lady/woman became aligned with new divisions in domestic labor and "mixed with other polarities," such as white/black, familiar/foreign, and home/empire.[108] Who was "woman" and who "lady" in a colonial evangelical situation where boys were "boys" and future nurses, and girls were "boys" and future wives and mothers? How did the lady/woman polarity get mixed up and played out when a mission home became training ground for desired gender representations and identities? As in middle- and upper-class English homes, missionary women and doctors divided domestic (and nursing) tasks semantically according to these same polarities (clean/dirty, lady/woman, white/black, etc.). If making successful Congolese evangelists, nurses, and wives was the goal, who had to perform the defiling and hidden work of disposing of the "recurring by-products of daily life"—rubbish, fecal matter, urine, blood—that in English households almost always fell to female servants, and in the absence of servants, to wives?[109]

Who had disposed of fecal matter in Mrs. Millman's home? Certainly not her "house girls." Remember Tula's words: "They didn't like boys, just girls." Mrs. Millman positioned her "Brown Marys" too far along the continuum from dirt to cleanliness, from evil to goodness, with the woman/lady polarity cast along slave-victim/Christian-wife-and-mother lines. The senior "boys"—those long-standing domestic servants who went to school but never graduated to nursing, teaching, or technical work—were likely assigned this daily bucket duty.

Boys and girls in Mama Mokili's household were on different tracks. Boys moved from knives and forks (kitchens) to delivering bedside tea (bedrooms), and then they were ready for nursing and surgery in a hospital. Girls were trained with needles, irons, and teapots, in sewing, ironing, and entertaining, effectively moving from the less polluting, less degrading end of the scale of domestic jobs to the most prestigious (serving the queen a cup of tea).[110] These domestic tasks and trajectories, separated by gender in Mrs. Millman's household, became conflated in the girls' boarding home. The trajectories of "as-you-move-up-you-move-in" and "as-you-move-in-you-move-out" still operated, as did the "policy of make-believe." Everything operated by maternal idioms, yet no one was mother and no one was wife. The seemingly asexual, barren, sinister Mamiwata-like figures,[111] who were supposed to be like mothers but never were, guarded the sexuality of their Congolese counterparts every night by locking the one and only door to the compound as the sun set at 6 P.M. They disciplined the girls, often calling in a male missionary when flogging was due. Decorum was necessarily different for single lady missionaries. The bounding of "house girls" within the confines of a boarding "home" and the intended extension of a maternal idiom to single woman missionaries meant that these Ba-Mademoiselle became less Mamas than husbands (masters), and their Congolese servants less children than "boys." These ladies only trusted their most senior "boys"—Mama-girls—with their sheets and body wastes.[112]

The social geographies for girls and boys also diverged. Yakusu teachers had always been allowed, even encouraged, to have "boys" themselves. So, as we saw, began Tula's personal trajectory. When housing for nursing students opened in 1925, it was called a "little 'town,'" where they lived "two by two," with "one boy detailed for orderly duty" each week, "to be known as Le Garçon."[113] There was room, therefore, for colonial mimicry among these male nursing students, who proudly decorated their homes with flowers from the beds out front and rotated as "boy" among themselves. Girls also put flowers in their homes.[114] But girls had less leverage to mediate the forms of mimicry offered to them. Boys could be sent out alone to accept positions as stranger teachers and nurses at Yakusu outposts. Girls could not. They could only go as wives, sometimes wives doubling as teachers or midwives. Like their Mademoiselle counterparts, they were fenced in with other females while unmarried. Older girls acted as Mamas (masters) to younger girls, but their "home" became elaborated as a confined shelter, named after a customary lopangu, but made with colonial brick walls and a gate. Girls rebelled, and when they did, the idiom of rebellion was hunger and food.

Christmas Laughter

Christmas at Yakusu provides rich evidence about the performance of colonial evangelical humor. Why humor collected around Yakusu boys—and not girls—lies partly in a history of Christmas, too. Anthropologists have analyzed modern Christmas festivities as a structured, rhythmic ritual that like its medieval counterparts, transforms "a particular vision of everyday social life," through its "crucial relationship between lavishness and the domestic sphere," into a "sense of the exuberance and the transcending of ordinary life."[115] Roast beef in Congoland embodied this lavishness in 1915, as did Christmas puddings in 1905.[116] By 1911, "friends in England" or "'Home mission' workers"—some "working week by week for a good many months"—were sending dresses, toys, and other homemade gifts for "the house Boys and others, as well as prizes at the famous Christmas sports."[117] Christmas was the one holiday of the year. Collapsed within it were summer sports festivities with, by 1917, races, a greasy pole, and rice-eating competitions, as well as dramatic pantomimes, gift giving, prize winning, and a missionary Santa Claus. Yet as Lévi-Strauss has noted, "this modern festival" with "archaic characteristics" is "not just a *hoax* imposed by adults on children," but "a very onerous *transaction* between . . . two generations."[118] Missionaries and their metaphorical children performed Christmas transactions at Yakusu. At least two audiences, a metropolitan reading public and a local Congolese public, "read" Christmas events.

Congolese spectators were often participants, too. Consider, again, the Christmas of 1915. Missionaries alone did not eat this historic roast beef: "all our work-people helped to eat the meat and pronounced it very good."[119] Christmas dining at Yakusu was a double feast. The missionaries would eat separately during one meal, and then reverse roles with their "boys" in another. The first meal rarely warranted description; only private, sentimental letters reveal the energy devoted to preparing Christmas puddings.[120] A Christmas meal for station Congolese was as old as the first documented Christmas "feast" that Yakusu's missionaries offered to the stations' "schoolchildren" in 1889. The menu—goat soup, plantain, rice, "native bread root," and salt—"seemed sufficiently varied to satisfy all tastes," but the missionaries discovered that their plan violated local etiquette. In missionary words, while the "boys and men set to with a will as the steaming portions were served out," the girls refused to eat the "forbidden food" because they did not witness its "manner of cooking" and "promiscuous eating could never be approved." The missionaries gave the girls shoka instead to buy fish, bananas, and palm oil "that they might cook them apart. This they were nothing loth to do, and in their noisy way enjoyed their exclusion from the main body of feasters."[121]

These festive occasions continued to be for men and boys, as a photograph of a "Christmas feast" in 1909 suggests. Two missionary "waiters" stood above the fourteen young Congolese men gathered around a veranda dining table ready to eat stewed monkey and boiled rice. This Yakusu Christmas celebrated a particular notion of family as it clarified and inverted everyday habits. Indeed, the sober photo from 1909 is reminiscent of a scene from Charles Dickens's *Pickwick Papers,* when the Wardle family and their guests sat down to Christmas dinner with their servants in the kitchen. Yet by the early 1920s, this Yakusu holiday was closer to a carnivalesque Caribbean Christmas, where colonial plantation masters served their slaves.[122] Indeed, Yakusu's annual festive parties of the 1920s contained considerable, in Bakhtin's words, "Christmas laughter."[123]

Chesterman wrote of Christmas in "those warmer lands where children never grow up." On December 23, 1921, mission hunters returned with "Meat!

Meat! Meat! Hungry eyes fastened on it. Monkeys galore. A large wild pig. A few sheep. The butchers at work. Nothing uncommon or unclean." On Christmas Eve, the missionaries assembled on the Congo's banks in the afternoon: "Sumptuous tea in breezy shade. Ever increasing crowd. Much reminiscing of home and relations. Crowd getting more impatient." A "promenade" followed, and sports, games, races, and prize giving began. The missionaries gathered that evening around dining tables and sorted out garments, soap, schoolbags, and other gifts: "Estimation of merit of recipient. Adjustment of packet to same. A little pile for each member of the house staffs."[124]

In 1922, the topsy-turvy meal was for the "children of the house," those who did "daily work in the houses of the white people . . . though not those who work in the gardens." Both the "House boys and girls" came for this "real Christmas jollification" on the Millman veranda, as Mr. Ennals described:

We white people according to ancient custom did the waiting. This was really the amusing part, for we had been told beforehand by Mama [Mokili] to be as "silly as we could," it is very seldom that I get this sort of

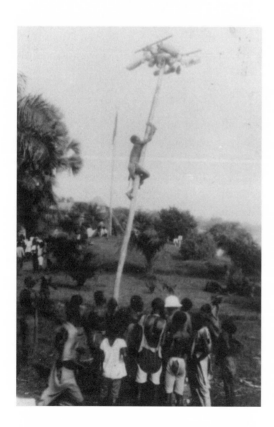

Greasy pole festivities at Christmas, ca. 1927. (Courtesy of David Lofts, PL Papers, Barton-on-Sea, U.K.)

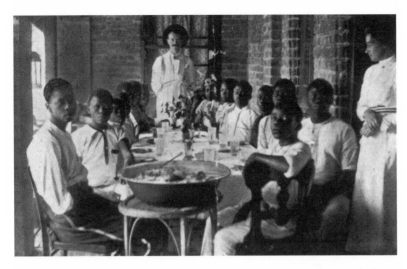

"A Christmas Feast, 1909." From H. Sutton Smith, *Yakusu, the Very Heart of Africa*, insert 84–85.

authority, so I availed myself of the freedom it allowed and the result was very interesting. The little people know the way waiters should behave at table so that it was much easier to do ridiculous things than to attempt to do things properly and fail. Some of the boys were on their dignity, and got very annoyed when one made some mistake, such as removing the soup spoon just before serving soup. One wonders from what white man they learnt these stern ways. It was great fun, a real Christmas jollification.[125]

For Ennals, this Christmas was fun. For the "annoyed" boys "on their dignity," such fun was not always pleasant.

The topsy-turvy event in 1923 was a tea party. The missionaries served their "boys," who sat like their masters in wicker chairs spread out on the lawn. This Christmas was "sillier than usual," Ennals observed, because he "dressed up as a House boy, with a misfit of a 'jerkin' and acted the clown."[126] Christmas of 1923 is the last year for which there is evidence of a topsy-turvy event at Yakusu. Just as the storm over libeli was raging, just as local Congolese accepted autopsies and hospital births for the first time, just as the mission focus turned from domestic servants to nurses, from dining to surgery, Christmas topsy-turvy meals and teas disappeared. There continued to be pantomimes as well as prize and gift giving for the Congolese, even a special Christmas feast for "our Station people" in 1936, but missionaries concentrated more on their own ceremonies of serenading, eating plum pudding, and prayer.[127]

"Christmas laughter" continued, but like so much else at Yakusu, it took on medical inflections. Carnivalesque elements persisted in missionary reactions to early morning Christmas caroling. In 1921, Chesterman had noted that Congolese carolers arrived at the missionary doors at 2:30 in the morning: "Totally unsolicited and quite unnecessary attempt at imitation of the Herald Angels, on the part of a group of waits from the town. Eventually paid to move on. Conversation unrecorded." Others arrived at 5:30: "Slightly better effort by the mixed station choir. Slightly less severe welcome."[128] By 1936, Dr. Browne was playing pranks on the early morning Congolese carolers seeking small coins. The nurses and nursing students who came to his house at 4:30 A.M., and the boarding school girls who arrived a bit later, received a few centimes. The "various house-boys" followed,

> all in one great band, to disturb the night with their singing which was not quite so harmonious. . . . I'm afraid that Holmes and I were very naughty. In order to convey to them our disapproval of many of their discords, Holmes got a 20 c.c. syringe, and filled it with water, and pointed the nozzle through our curtains, and directed the contents of the syringe into the wide-open mouth of the most unharmonious chorister.[129]

Browne had more fun at a Christmas dinner for the missionary staff: "I had a pirate's mask, and flatter myself that I looked the part as I menaced a table-girl with a carving-knife!"[130] He resumed his caroling capers in 1937, this time with his colleague, Dr. Knights, insisting to his family readers that "if you have any preconceived ideas of how goody-goody missionaries are, you had better skip this paragraph!!" He and Knights

> rigged up an electric light in a skull which we borrowed from the Hospital anatomical collection. This skull was suspended by thin string so that it dangled in my open window. The light was made to come and go by means of a simple switch I could work from my bed, in conjunction with a battery. The result was devastating. . . . [W]hen the first band of carollers had assembled outside my window . . . they noticed a grotesquely illuminated skull beating time! Then, by means of a stick, the skull nodded in conjunction with the music! In the pitch darkness of the early morning, the effect was excellent. . . . In order to heighten the effect, first Knights and then I would appear in the dining room window, some distance away. When they put out their hands for our little gift . . . we felt that they had earned their money.[131]

Two nights later, the missionary nurses had a party for the missionaries, and Browne offered to lend a "couple of boys to help at table." One was "duly decked out as an English doctor, . . . with a complete rig-out of European clothes, and stethoscope and bay, and Trilby hat, and horned-rimmed spectacles." The other came dressed as a surgeon, with cap, mask, and gown. "This had a great reception" among the missionary guests.[132]

Did these Christmas pranks consist of, in Bakhtin's words, "purely negative satire"? Or was there an "ambivalence" and "philosophic content" to this Christmas "recreational drollery"?[133] Africa, in popular European representations, is aligned with the lower half of the human body, associated as it is with darkness, bestiality, and twisted, "amorous bondage."[134] Popular, "folk" laughter, Bakhtin tells us, is "topographical." It is a low culture, sexualized burlesque; it turns on the grotesque, the scatological, and the carnivalesque. It produces jokes through and about the "lower bodily stratum." These combined associations—Africa as bodily and worldly bottom, and the human bottom as absurdly funny—colored, indeed produced, racial, minstrel, imperial laughter. In colonial contexts, unlike on British stages and within European caricatures, these coupled associations produced colonizing—violent, embodied, sexualized—joking relationships. "Topsy-turvy" aspects of daily life made colonial Africa seem alternately mirthful and ridiculous for Dan Crawford's readers. Similarly, Yakusu's missionaries improvised with long-standing, church-tolerated, European practices of "Christmas laughter" in apparently wholesome ways with their carnivalesque Christmas jests. The evidence suggests, however, that colonial laughter was more than double in intent and effect. Affection and wholesomeness concealed terror, sadism, and desire. Colonizing greed and laughter bred parody and anger; they also marked memory, bodies, and routine. Curiously, these colonial joking relationships came to life during spectacles and memories of dining and surgery.[135] Just as Nurse Gee witnessed dining as a spectacle for colonized sight-seeing in 1911, and Colonel Bertrand saw surgery as spectacle in 1930, colonial laughter, like Yakusu boys, moved from dining to surgery, too.

Excess

At Yakusu, domestic arrangements and domesticating ambitions were linked to tropes of Yakusu-style evangelism, such as we "can take savages and make them saints."[136] They were also related to boundary making and social marking, especially as the concrete social realities of who ate and slept where, and who served whom when, were worked out. The domestic as a place (home, mission station, hospital, girl's boarding home) and domestication as a process (making home, clearing the forest, soaping faces, rendering feminine and submissive) signified colonial power relations in gendered and racial terms. Domesticity at Yakusu encompassed more than housekeeping and mothercraft. It embraced girls and boys, men and women. Domesticity also included "intimate evangelism," the creation of a "home within the wilderness," and a missionary lady "training rough forest lads in her house."[137] The "knife-and-fork doctrine" was elaborated as metaphor and practice at Yakusu, while "home," too, worked to represent—and create—the boundaries, hierarchies, and intimacies of mission life. Practically, the "knife-and-fork doctrine" was tied to organizing and dividing household labor, teaching hygiene, and finding workers and converts in a context where girls were much less likely than boys to be released by Congolese households. Boy-to-nurse trajectories also operated, as we will see, to reproduce pockets of mission domesticity within an ever-enlarging rural district, especially as an expanding network of rural health dispensaries joined hospital training at Yakusu beginning in the late 1920s.

Hygienic domesticity narratives about boys who became nurses built on classic imperial civilizing figures as found in Defoe, and echoed the historically specific, local stories that became part of Yakusu mission's oral and literary traditions. My point has not been to reveal Yakusu narratives as one more iteration of the European "invention of Africa" (though they were indeed that), but rather to show how these quotations of imperial idioms, once actualized in local mission memory and practice, became forms of moral imagining and remembering that influenced the routines of everyday life. A complex mixture of the Bible, *Robinson Crusoe*, Livingstone's vision, Stanley's adventures, Crawford's topsy-turviness, Morel's "red rubber" tracts, and perhaps even Dickens's *The Pickwick Papers*, fed into and nurtured the moral imperial imaginings of Yakusu's missionaries. They applied this creolized sensibility to their local colonial situation while attending to making history at—and a history for—Yakusu. Salamo's slave-to-mother story, cannibal-to-saint "boy" allegories, dining and surgery spectacles, and Christmas festivities were critical to this making and remaking of history and memory.

Home and holidays—in colonial communities as in metropolitan society— were a comic realm.[138] Yet laughter unleashes uneasiness, scorn, twisted affection, desire, and fun. The equivalence between dining and surgery at Yakusu did not emanate from forms devised by colonizing earnestness and imperial laughter alone. Congolese subjects—middles and lows—also produced dining and surgery as spectacles, while associating them in metaphor. These local parallels and comparisons, we will see, were related to phantasms of a Congolese moral imagination, accessible in forms of remembering about European bodily and eating habits.

An important question remains about the gender asymmetry of colonial evangelical humor, the sobriety of missionary girl tales and the mirthfulness of those about boys. Why, after all, did humor collect around boys and not girls?

Deep-seated anxieties about racial and sexual boundaries in colonial life underlay the common practice of giving colonized Congolese men ambiguous, emas-
culating, degrading work. These same anxieties made colonizing humor significant as a means of control and respite. The liminal quality of mission "boys"
gave these colonial subjects, symbolically likened to cannibal "monkeys," more
autonomy to joke and "signify" back.[139] This liminality was social and symbolic, vocational and sexed; it was positioned in space and embodied in dress.
Yakusu "boys" wore semi-European dress, but shorts rather than pants. They
took orders from white women, and did what in Europe—and in the Congo—
had usually been defined as feminine work: cooking, cleaning, and caretaking.
These "boys" also worked with the topsy-turvy objects of colonial hygiene
jokes: knives, forks, pots, and soap. Indeed, these elements linked them with
popular caricatures of reformed cannibals and *petits nègres*, colonial Congo's
translations—mediated through blackface rubrics—of urban dandy minstrel
figures in mismatched, transgressive clothes.

Though Yakusu's origin fable for boys may have been based on the story of a
future Congolese pastor, first glimpsed carrying a human limb, it is not clear
that it circulated far beyond the daily missionary social gathering among
flowers at Mrs. Millman's riverfront. Yakusu's origin parable for girls was older
and an earnest staple of mission schooling and sermons. The stories of Salamo
and Lititiyo were told and retold, yet only the cannibal-"boy" narrative circulated in jest. What was available in a popular vocabulary of representation
was not insignificant in this difference. Cannibal imagery was integral to the
nineteenth-century rewriting of Africa as the dark continent. And "Congoland" was Africa's cannibal land par excellence in European imaging.[140] Comic
cannibals were pervasive, from Dan Crawford's *Thinking Black* through Belgian
colonial fiction about "Darkest Africa" to advertising about its associated commodities: soap, chocolate, bicycles, and the like. These liminal, transgressive
figures of cartoons and publicity—a cannibal cook boiling up a European; the
half-soaped, half-whitened African figure of soap ads; the joyous, cycling *petits
nègres* advertising bicycles—were not unlike the black boy children of "Ten
Little Niggers" images and the wild, disreputable, Topsy-like pickaninny figures
of minstrel shows.[141] Yet they were male. The laughing, childlike Bamboula[142]
figures of public cannibal humor did not have female, Topsy-like counterparts.
Except, that is, when Europeans would gather and tell lewd jokes—or sing
Salomi verses—among themselves.

Still, we must insist: *Why?* Because, in missionary categories, African men ate
humans, while women were wild, sexual beings, sometimes likened to slaves,
especially to their own female flesh. Woman—like Africa, slavery, and colonialism—*was* excess.[143] The first flaw, cannibalism, was openly funny. It was pre-

posterous and amendable, particularly if these flesh-desiring African men were, like Man Sunday, neutered as boys. Women's excess was scandalous, arousing hidden, dark, desiring laughter. It was for certain and for always. The laughter was shameful. And the only hope was in dead serious, consistent rescripting of the human female narrative as dutiful, clean mother and wife. Woman was also Africa, of course. The female slave Salamo personified enslaved, colonial Africa, just as she should come to signify redemption. The neutered boys became the Topsy figures in this matrix. It was way too risky to let a Congolese woman become a Topsy Salomi if you were serious about colonial evangelism. There is no neutering woman, no containing excess.

Minstrel humor was alive at Yakusu, as the evidence on lantern slide repertoires and missionary sing-alongs suggests. Yet the wild, sexualized Salomi of "Darkies' Sunday School" was tightly contained within an exclusive missionary party as festive Christmas song, except when Salomi emerged within the hidden, sexualized imaging of Yakusu's single women missionaries. This Salomi was perilous, not mirthful. She was a Salomi who needed taming and beating, so missionary logic went. She once appeared in the form of a Mama-girl named Machuli Bolendela who arrived back at the "fence" after 6 P.M., late for "boy" service at dinner, deserving violent blows, perhaps sanitary bucket duty, too. A colonial evangelism based on a Salamo narrative of pure deliverance from sexual slavery through maternity and motherhood meant that the effeminate jesters could be assigned the wild, Topsy roles, arousing shadowy, yearning laughter and affection as they performed. The girls of the "fence" broke from the script nevertheless, especially when the odious greed and envy grew too indulgent. Signifying and defying they did—sometimes secretly, sometimes not, and so they have done in memory since—to separate themselves from the dark, desiring blows of colonial excess.

4 NURSES AND BICYCLES

Things are speeding up in Congo.—"A Visit to Yakusu," *Yakusu Quarterly Notes,* 1934

So, little by little, in spite of this anger, an admiring terror replaced his scorn.—René Maran, *Batouala,* 1921

By 1932, Gladys Owen had left her work as hospital nurse to marry a fellow missionary, Mr. Parris. They were in Yaongama in the BaMbole forest, when a Congolese evangelist came to them and said that "he felt very ill and wanted to return to his village because the spirit of his dead father had come and told him during the night that in two days he would be very ill and that he must prepare to die." The teacher spoke of a dream: "He has called me! He came to me in the night and hit me in the back and my back is now so painful that I cannot stand upright." Gladys Parris explained:

> We told him to go to the dispensary where he would receive medicine which would relieve the pain. However after a day or two he got into such a nervous state because the spirit came every night. One morning when he was relating this to the Infirmier, the Infirmier in sheer desperation gave him some disinfectant and said "Sprinkle this round the room before you go to bed and spirit will not come again." The poor teacher did this and since then he had excellent nights!![1]

How African colonial subjects comprehended biomedicine is a refractory subject. This chapter considers the "enduring problem of historical interpretation" of colonial medicine noted by Megan Vaughan, "the difficulty of knowing how interventions and ideas were 'read' by those at whom they were directed."[2] Because it is so difficult to get "readings" of anonymous patients positioned at the bottom of colonial hierarchies, glimpses of African nurses mediating within clinical practice are critical. The historical processes that have made biomedicine an ambivalent and distinct therapy system in much of contemporary Africa were mediated by middle figures and the "entangled objects"[3] of their work. This missionary letter exposes two transactions: one between English missionary and Congolese teacher, and another between Congolese teacher and Congolese nurse. The nurse, probably none other than Victor Yenga, translated. He and the teacher were middle figures, and disinfectant, through their exchange, became an entangled thing.

This chapter turns to the readings and mediations of Congolese nurses and subaltern subjects. Oral tradition and oral history are so *basic* in African historical studies that the question "can the subaltern speak?" has been posed rarely or quickly shrugged off as misplaced. The formulation colonizer/colonized has too often been conflated with another, equally deforming one, textuality/orality, as if European colonizers only wrote and colonized Africans neither could nor did. Thus, the significance of one of the sources that I use, printed letters written by an emerging elite, Yakusu-trained male nurses like Victor Yenga. Yet not only Congolese letters are valuable. Nor should we assume that missionary-authored texts cannot reveal African readings and mediations. Gayatri Spivak's point was never that subalterns did not speak, but that historians, blind to their own "representations," did not see how their narratives worked to "*speak for*" rather than "*speak to*" subaltern speech, cries, and laughter.[4] The colonial studies' cliché of *colonial encounter* has not been helpful, especially from the vantage point of African studies, as it works once again to skew historical narratives toward one epic-like meeting among two, and too homogeneous, groups. A history of a colonial situation should not run the risk of "re-presenting" a singular *encounter* among colonizers and colonized, but should imagine and render multiple transactions, mediations, and misreadings.

Hence the importance of Gladys Parris's letter. Her act of inscription was a missionary form of remembering rendered with wry amusement, indeed a mirthful missionary disposition that became a genre of its own. Parris "spoke to" the teacher and the nurse, and if her "scene of writing" (in Spivak's words) is handled carefully, these two middle figures can be heard within historical writing. Yet there is no way to handle Parris's "scene of writing" carefully without revealing my own. Thus the mixture of source material for this study includes transactions from my postcolonial fieldwork. I include these not just to refuse authorial transparency stylistically, but also for substantive reasons.[5] The same analytic process—remembering that I was some version of a Gladys Parris—as I recorded and translated subaltern and middle speech has enabled me to hear *who* the Zairians I was speaking with were *speaking to* (a Mademoiselle, a

Madami, Bibi Nesi ["Woman" Nancy], etc.), and it continues to make me wary of speaking for them here.

I do not imagine that Congolese nurses were just filters of memory whose minds collected residue from an oral, subaltern culture.[6] They were in the process of forming one version of a Congolese middle culture. Nurses and teachers circulated ideas, mediated conflicts, translated things, and created a native colonial "high" style as they assumed a middle social position within colonial life. The chapter also considers a genre of oral stories about medicine, mobility, and terror called tokwakwa that Zairians of Yainyongo shared with me in 1989–90. I interrogate these *forms of remembering* as evidence about how colonial medical practice transpired, and how subalterns and middles in one locality imagined biomedicine and its complements.

Missionary medicine has often been portrayed as an anomaly within colonial medicine, as a benevolent, persuasive, sentimental form, an interpretation that has served to underscore the coercive aspect of colonial medicine as practiced by company and state doctors.[7] It has also been in the benevolent, missionary domain that medical work with women and children has been most often situated. State medicine was frequently not gender sensitive, the story goes, and African women were patients in much smaller numbers than men. The correctives of feminist scholars have tended to elaborate what began as an opposition ripe with gendered meanings (soft/hard, gentle/forced), accepting the underlying supposition that missionary healing was the soft side of colonial medicine.[8] The dichotomy does not work here. Colonial evangelism was not soft, and "the" colonial state was not (always) strong.[9] This chapter attends to the visibility of one "sanitary modality" of colonial state forms, as local actors and practices changed through time.[10] Tracing changing mission-state relations through this prism makes it possible to discern *who* represented and performed state forms, and *how.* This chapter examines this visibility through colonial hygiene routines as performed by state agents, Yakusu missionaries, Congolese nurses and chiefs, and "patients." The arrival of roads, dispensaries, plantations, bricks, bicycles, and other signs of a specific interwar modernity into the Yakusu district prove significant. Colonial medicine came with and signified this new mobility. And Congolese subjects, whether subalterns or middles, letter writers or not, made meaning out of the objects of this new, mobile, and concrete modernity in kindred ways.

Indirect Hygiene and Touring Doctors

Motor cars joined rickshaws in the streets of Kinshasa in the early 1920s, and motorcycles, trolleys, and Ford cars appeared in Stanleyville, too. While old forest paths in Yakusu's district had to be cleared to five meters wide, and more and more church members were being recruited for wage work at plantations and mines, a sense of population and labor crisis began to align colonial hygiene touring with demographic censusing.[11]

When Chesterman arrived in 1920, Governor General Maurice Lippens "professed to be 'all out' for two things": hygiene and transport.[12] Indeed, the professionalization of missionary healing at Yakusu coincided with a newly emerging definition of colonial hygiene in the Congo, emphasizing comprehensiveness, sanitary policing, and mobility. As we saw in chapter 2, sleeping sickness control became medical censusing work as mobile teams began systematic surveys after the war.[13] State agreements with medical missionaries who served as médecins agréés[14] coincided with new labor legislation, first enacted in 1921, which made employers responsible for their workers' health. Private enterprises had to provide an infirmary and nurse in each locality where more than 50 workers lived and worked; companies operating in Province Orientale (where Yakusu was located) with more than 1,000 employees had to create a medical service to examine and vaccinate these workers regularly.[15] These new regulations created immense opportunities for Yakusu's medical mission, expanding with its newly trained "medical evangelists" into an area that was being opened up, so to speak, by plantation companies for the first time.

In 1924, state authorities "accepted and encouraged" Yakusu proposals to establish village dispensaries throughout its district. They would be "built by the [state] administrators in brick, fly the Belgian and Red Cross Flags, but be under the supervision of the Mission and served by Yakusu trained boys."[16] Company contracts followed. By the mid-1920s, there was "a happy gang of hopefuls" at Yakusu, young men between the ages of thirteen and twenty, who were living in a hostel, wearing nurse uniforms, playing on the mission football field, and taking pride in their new name, ba-infirmiers. Yakusu's doctors' work as médecins agréés established "an outlet" for these "trained boys" who, once placed in rural dispensaries as nurses, also served as evangelists, healing as God's newest physicians.[17]

One Yakusu-trained nurse was operating a state agricultural post—and future Institut pour l'Etude Agronomique du Congo Belge (INEAC) station—at Yangambi in 1924, and another was awaiting the completion of the Belgika company's dispensary building. Belgika already had 800 men working on rubber and palm plantations on Ile Bertha, and Yakusu's doctor was their official medical officer. In 1927, several additional "commercial companies" paid BMS Yakusu for operating branch dispensaries. The Yakusu mission also sponsored and operated three dispensaries of its own in different villages. By 1928, there were seven company-affiliated dispensaries run by Yakusu-trained nurses, of-

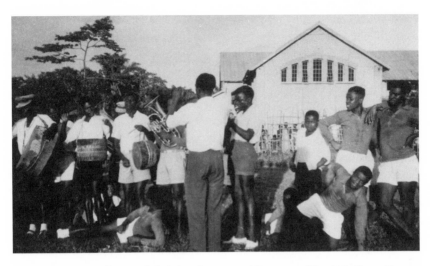

Yakusu nursing students and their band, ca. 1931. (Courtesy of David Lofts, PL Papers, Barton-on-Sea, U.K.)

ficially known as *aides-infirmiers,* for "workmen & families" of five commercial companies.[18] Approving Yakusu as a "benevolent" medical mission represented a way for state authorities to assert control over health care, cut costs, and include missionaries, even Protestant ones, among the bureaucrats whom Congolese subjects met on a daily basis. State power was extended and legitimized, while softening the violent "breaker of rocks" figure, Bula Matari, that dated back to Henry Morton Stanley's embodiment of Belgian colonial power.

New dispensaries meant that outsider nurses went to live among rural peasants and plantation workers. Most Yakusu-trained nurses worked for a year at the hospital and at least two more at a dispensary in Yakusu's district after receiving their diplomas. The father of one nurse was a pioneering BMS Yalemba "boy," Disasi Makulo, a BaTambatamba raid-victim-turned-evangelist who named his son after his personal master, BMS hero George Grenfell. This young Congolese Grenfell began nurse training at Yakusu in 1924, when he was sixteen; three years later, he had completed further training at Stanleyville's nursing school, received a state diploma, and was working at Yalemba's dispensary as a "well paid servant of the Government . . . according to our agreement with the authorities."[19] Three other Yakusu-trained nurses received state diplomas and were appointed to Yakusu, Yalikina, and Ligasa in 1928. By 1931, a dispensary was under construction in Lititiyo's village, Yaokombo.[20]

Yakusu's missionaries were responsible for hygiene touring in a province where rural dispensaries had been encouraged and indirect rule by Congolese chiefs was advanced.[21] By 1933, state authorities had offered Yakusu "complete control, with absolute freedom of organisation, of the medical services for the natives" in about 10,000 square miles of territory, including much of the BaMbole forest.[22] Yakusu signed an agreement with a coffee and rubber planta-tion company expanding in the BaMbole forest a year later. This Antwerp-based company, Bamboli Cultuur Maatschappij, funded three dispensaries, operated by Yakusu's doctors and nurses in the first of a fifteen-year, tripartite agreement among the company, the state, and Yakusu.[23]

State doctors were defining colonial hygiene as a three-pronged program to "conserve human capital" by the early 1930s: curing the sick through hospitals and health centers, protecting health through mobile medicine, and encourag-ing population growth through medical work focused on motherhood and infancy. As the state began to assume responsibility for the health of Congolese "independent natives" (that is, those not protected under labor laws)[24] and emphasize censusing as a part of hygiene work, Yakusu's doctors' responsibil-ities increased. Ennals's first medical tour in 1922 may have been an "adventure," yet he found subsequent rounds "tedious work."[25] Chesterman still called a tour a "joy ride" in 1933, but the "amount of pen pushing to be done in filling in on the immense registers the tediously extorted and deliberately distorted names of fathers, mothers, husbands, wives, and children" proved to be less "amus-ing." His work included a "systematic examination and registration" of about 12,000 people along the river between Yanonge and Isangi. He and his nurses inspected for sleeping sickness and yaws, though the paper pushing had tax implications. Men tried to hide polygynous wives to avoid tax supplements and to produce more than four children by one declared wife to obtain a tax exemption.[26]

In 1935, two doctors examined around 60,000 people during tours. One doctor spent half the year on medical tour; the other toured for eight weeks in addition to making numerous urgent visits to European patients in the district. In 1936, one doctor traveled over 5,000 miles examining some 47,000 people. Dr. Holmes's tour in 1936 consisted of "making each family pass before us and noting their condition" and stamping identity books. Whole villages were "called in for examination," and some "turned up very well." By 1937, Yakusu's doctors were supervising twenty-two church and company dispensaries. They balanced comments about "continual travelling about the district" with dis-claimers about their "closer touch with the natives." Their company and state obligations were hefty, including health care responsibilities for European plan-tation agents and their families resident in the district. Relations became strained when Yakusu, an evangelical medical mission, was asked to make monthly visits to the sixty-one Europeans living at the INEAC station at Yangambi. "Our Baptist supporters in the Homeland would probably object to being called 'I.N.E.A.C. supporters'!!" declared Browne in a letter to Chesterman. These contractual obligations, he added, were "rank slavery." The Belgians at Yangambi, accustomed to Yakusu doctors, also wanted a special sick pavilion built for them at Yakusu where they could pay a missionary nurse for care: "It was a bit difficult to introduce the conception that we were not absolutely enamoured of the prospect of lots of white patients at Yakusu." The INEAC medical contract ceased at the end of 1938.[27]

Yakusu's doctors understood their utility within this local political economy. Chesterman noted in 1933, as their district and authority increased in difficult economic times, "we cost the Government but ten percent of its own organization." Mrs. Millman was skeptical: "Chesterman is cementing his future here. The State finds us useful and uses us. The State will remove us when it suits their purposes." And as Browne snidely remarked, with pleas to his family never to quote him, "my part in the game is to keep the [Congolese] men so fit that they are able to work well, so bringing in pots of money to the shareholders in Belgium!"[28]

In return, Yakusu's doctors were willing to act as sanitary officers—médecins agréés—for Congolese living in their district because it seemed to give them leverage in building "Christ's Kingdom." Medical touring provided occasions for "what is often the only supervised examination of the year to schools in the wayside villages." The subsidies received were significant; without them, Yakusu's missionaries observed, they "could not possibly carry on our extended district work, nor finance the training of our infirmiers, nor properly feed and care for our patients."[29] Some people ran away when a colonial doctor came on tour; others drummed and danced. Hygiene inspections meant that a new form of "weeding" was part of missionary "itinerations" (preaching tours), but touring to evangelize, inspect baptism candidates, and heal remained integral activities. Yakusu's doctors traveled with separate trunks for clothing, food, medicine, and books.

Whether ministering as sanitary police, pronatalist census takers, or pastors, Yakusu's doctors became in many ways colonial agents of a form of indirect rule. The mission became *almost*, yet never completely, its own polity, while its doctors executed the hygiene directives issued by a state-at-various-removes, metropolitan and provincial colonial authorities. Yet Yakusu's medical territory was not constant; as the maps show, the district as well as contracts changed significantly over time.[30] Nor did the capricious agency of another form of indirect rule go away. "We like the B.M.S., and we respect the State, and we welcome the Roman Catholics," said one Congolese chief to a Yakusu doctor during a medical census tour in 1938. If a local chief was "friendly and helpful,"

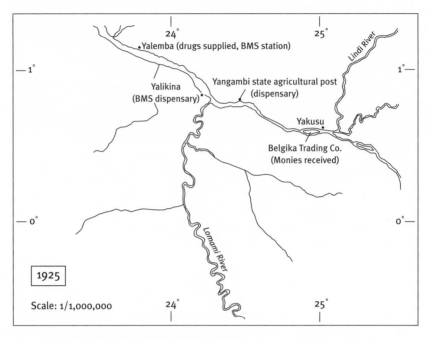

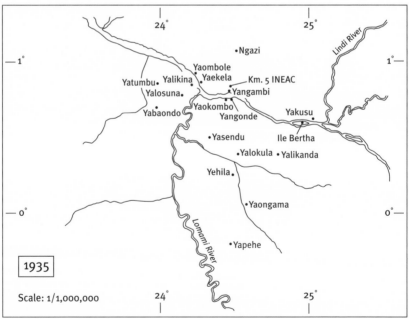

BMS Yakusu-operated health-care sites, 1925, 1935, 1946, 1956.

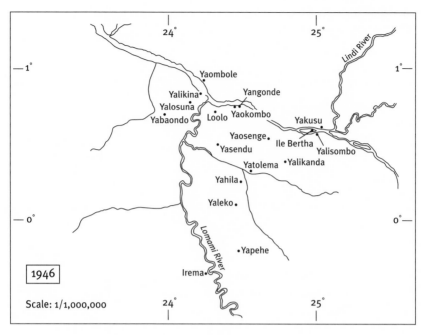

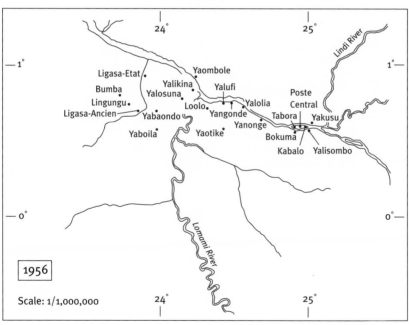

examinations would proceed without "the slightest difficulty."[31] Some chiefs liked bricks and Bibles, yet they could abet or resist a visit of medical passport-stamping doctor evangelists.

Some villages evaded dispensary construction much like they would flee from state agents visiting. Other patients traveled from afar, passing other dispensaries in order to reach a BMS one. Flower beds around the Yaombole dispensary in the 1930s told that mission domesticity had arrived. The Yangonde dispensary functioned as a minihospital with space for inpatients who would journey up to two days for care, staying in the surrounding small huts.[32] Dispensaries began as wattle-and-daub buildings, equipped with drugs, a microscope, a zinc-sheeted table for minor surgery, and sometimes a few huts for lodging patients.[33] By the mid-1930s, dispensaries meant bricks and a new form of obligatory labor in making them, though a new brick-making machine sometimes increased Congolese interest in their construction. Browne would send the machine to villages where state officials had asked for dispensaries. After nailing up the doors and window frames and unpacking all the cases, the doctor would pay his "homages" to the chief, seek his cooperation, and assure him of the "best intentions to cure everybody in his great district." At Lileko, men made bricks in the press, while women carried them in long baskets, a dozen at a time, to the dispensary site. Children assisted, balancing a brick or two on their heads.[34] Yaeme residents were enthusiastic when they learned that they could have a nurse and dispensary. The people of Yaolilemu celebrated when they found out that they would soon have the brick-making machine to construct theirs. Yet Loya's inhabitants struggled to make 20,000 bricks, much to the dissatisfaction of Dr. Holmes, who had expected 10,000 more.[35]

Drugs, tables, window frames, doors, cupboards, an invalid table, drug and patient registers, account books, and a Congolese nurse were among the ingredients of a new dispensary. Bicycles became necessary equipment by the late 1920s. By the 1950s, postwar welfare funding expanded, Yakusu's district included eighteen rural health centers, and nurses received a monthly bicycle allowance in order to travel to the thirty-six satellite treatment centers where they held clinics for infants and pregnant women.[36]

Nurses as Writing Evangelists

It is simply not true that "African medical assistants rarely published, and when they did they wrote about relations with Europeans rather than with Africans."[37] By *Mboli ya Tengai*'s 200th issue in 1929, this "Native Church Magazine" had expanded to eight pages and its circulation was 1,000 copies; the "number of readers" far exceeded this figure. By 1938, 2,600 copies of each monthly issue were printed, and the magazine was being posted to church members—including nurses—working throughout the colony. One missionary estimated that each issue had about 10,000 readers.[38] Christian Congolese in the district were avid readers from the first years in the century; in 1905, the mission sold 10,000 books. Yakusu-trained "teacher-evangelists" or baekesi began to publish letters in *Mboli ya Tengai* in the 1910s; Yakusu-trained nursing men became publishing correspondents some fifteen years later. By the 1920s, mission hygiene lessons advised that Christians should not read or write "at night by the aid of a palm-oil flare." With "the increase in the numbers of [church] readers who were ageing," by the 1950s, one Yakusu nurse toured the district regularly doing refractions so that they could obtain reading glasses.[39]

The words for these two types of colonial translators suggest the colonial "poetics of lexical borrowing":[40] the title "teacher" was expressed in Lokele (*boekesi*), while *infirmier* was borrowed from colonial speech. Yet to reduce the analysis of borrowed lexemes to French terms would misconstrue the complexity of imposition and creativity in the construction of colonial social categories. Where and when and how these writers mediated words and things from colonial milieus provide clues about their social positions, activities, and imaginative labor within larger historical processes of identity formation. Nurses, like teachers, were mobile characters, moving as colonizing strangers, convening, convoking, "itinerating." Yakusu nurses and teachers were usually strangers in the communities in which they worked, and their presence provoked rivalry and strife. Although ba-infirmiers and baekesi possessed important affinities as evangelical "knowledge brokers,"[41] nurses also formed a separate colonial category with distinct work and poetics. Indeed, their letters display the aspirations and whimsy of an emerging colonial social type, mobile rural hygiene workers of the interwar period.

Congolese teachers had long resembled missionaries, and nurses acted as evangelists as well. When teacher Filip Kwaita discussed his travels in the Yafando and Yalinga districts in 1929, he said: "I told them I was only an explorer and bearer of news."[42] Yakusu's "district Infirmiers" were also called "medical evangelists." Their work included preaching and healing, "making a fearless stand against witchcraft, [and] defending their faith before powerful chiefs." Teachers, like nurses, had conflicts with local people over the meaning and use of lisoo (Lokele for medicines and charms).[43] One nursing student wrote in a school composition in 1929: "Many people say that they would never agree to do the unpleasant duties of caring for the sick, but we infirmiers, no, we are willing to help people who are not even of our own tribe, for was it not the work of Jesus?"[44] People thought that nurses had special powers. When Likenyule traveled to Basoko as a nursing student, "doing God's work, helping people," he became sick from "skin rash." This disease "killed many people in Basoko" during his stay: "People were wondering how a nurse could get this disease and came to tell me so. I answered them that no one could live forever. If you are away from home and become sick, trust in God alone." Likenyule concluded: "Wherever we go, Isangi, in Lomani, in schools, in any house of God, people look at us as teachers. For those who work for Jesus, He helps in the name of Jesus."[45]

The term *ba-infirmier* kept Congolese nurses distinct from missionary doctors, who were instead naturalized and proudly so as *ba-nganga,* a Lokele-ized Kingwana expression for healer; thus, one biography of Dr. Browne celebrated him with the title *Bonganga*. The borrowed French term *infirmier* asserted a *kisenji* ("native," "savage," "heathen") antithesis, that is, kanga, the Lokele word for healer or diviner. In English, kanga was glossed pejoratively as "witch doctor." By claiming moral superiority, the new, borrowed term *infirmier* altered the local semantic field. Kanga became not only competitors but foes, the embodiments of basenji at their worst.

A series of essays on forms of sorcery appeared in *Mboli ya Tengai* in the early 1930s. There was one on *lisombo* theft and ailments, another on *likundu* stomach sacks, a third on lightening. Their rich metaphorical detail suggests that they were written by Congolese evangelists, even though they may have been edited by the missionary staff. The lisombo essay began by declaring that this kind of sorcery "is not a true thing," but rather, "a lie which people say to somebody they hate." The author(s) asked readers to learn a new knowledge of the body, its secretions, and the causes of sickness: "Know that what goes on inside of the parts of a person is what makes the body work in a good or a bad way. What comes out of the body has no more use; it is only waste because the things which a person lets out of the body no longer have any usefulness in the body. . . . Sickness is not the result of lisombo." The appeal ended with a concrete one to elders: "Send your children to nursing school so that they can explain very well to you" such matters "one by one." Likewise, after an elaborate description of "a kind of bag which is in the stomach" of a person who "likes to kill people without any goal," the likundu essay stopped short, then shifted to a biological and theological phase, offering an evangelical hygiene lesson:

> The likundu bag of things is not just in some people only. No. It is in all of us because it is a part of us people as well as of animals of the forest. That part called likundu is an organ of the body. . . . Those people who walk during the night, this is not a problem. If they do not go fishing (or hunting), we should only assume that he is a thief, not that he is bewitching people, killing them with likundu.[46]

Some patients were afraid to come to the dispensary for treatment. A man came to see Likenyule one day in Yaokombo after suffering from pneumonia for nine days.

> I asked him again why he did not come sooner. He said that people did not allow him to come to the dispensary saying that nurses do not know anything about diseases caused by bad spirits. "They went with me to one healer who throws people in water to rid them of their bad spirits. Despite their thinking, I came to the dispensary anyway because the disease is not improving at all." I was very sad because he was not breathing well. . . . First of all, I told him to pray. After I gave him the medicines. Every day, the same thing. . . . My patient got strength, he recovered his health. I asked him if he knew God's will. He answered saying: "Truly, God is in heaven because I was sure I had to die soon but God helped me."[47]

Ba-infirmiers had disputes with kanga and their clients over therapies. In 1938, some relatives asked a nurse, Samwele Kamanga, about their pig, which had been lost for three days. When Kamanga said that he had not seen it, they went to a kanga with two francs instead. Kamanga reported that the kanga looked in a mirror and said, "I know who killed your pig." The pig was already dead and cooked, the kanga explained; if they brought him another ten francs, he would track the footprints and tell them who had killed their pig. "(This was a lie)," Kamanga told his readers. He later looked behind "our *Dispensaire,* and I saw a pig that had a bell, and I ran to tell them. . . . They said: 'Truly?'" Kamanga's letter concluded: "Let the cheating stop. Let the cheating stop. Let the cheating stop. Friends, let us not walk in darkness. It is best to walk in light."[48]

One day, Nurse Kamanga and Mama Bandombele (Mrs. Mill) treated a woman "sick in the stomach."

> She was defecating blood, and people were saying that it was the disease of Ikoya. Some of us do not know the cause of sicknesses. When I looked at the excrement in the mirror that has been called Microscope, I saw amoebas, and we gave her oil of emetine. The next morning Mama Bandombele and I went again. Mama saw her wearing an amulet around her hips. Mama took the amulet. It was 2:00. Mama and I, we tore it open and saw nails and parrot feathers and fish inside. This is the cheating of the kanga of us black people. Me, the White Man, Mama Bandombele, and the White Man of the State laughed very hard. The acceptance of the Messiah's death will kill the devil. Romans 6, if you read it through, my friend, you will see the reason for kanga ya basenji.[49]

Dates, hours, and laughter shared with European missionaries marked Kamanga's narrative with authority and prestige. Kamanga condensed basenji life and kanga practice symbolically into one object, an amulet or *likenge*, as he described teaming up with the Mama missionary to investigate bodies.

B. H. Tokwaulu, a student nurse, railed against amulets in 1928: "Let us forget what . . . happened a long time ago about believing in the power of wearing amulets. Those are things done by our ancestors. . . . We have to follow Jesus the Savior. We need to get rid of the habit of wearing amulets because amulets . . . mean you are working for two gods."[50] John Siboko, signing his letter as student infirmier, wrote about seeing a person talking to a likenge at Yanonge, while on a journey in 1932. Siboko asked his traveling companion: "Why is he doing this?" The friend replied: "He is praying to the spirit of the likenge to give his likenge the power to help him." Three days later, at a Belgika company post, Siboko saw "one youngster of the class of the priest putting his knees on the ground" one morning and "muttering" in front of a rosary with prayer. The nursing student thought: "He who is inclined to wear a rosary is also inclined to wear likenge."[51] He asked him:

> "In your church, don't you refuse to wear likenge?" He answered: "It is totally forbidden." I said: "Why is that?" He answered: "Because of God's commandments." I told him: "Kneel only to your God and praise only him" (Matthew 4:10). And he agreed. I asked him again: "Why do you kneel to the rosary?" He replied: "It was given to us to protect and help us during our travels. And also since I am here at Belgika, I do not have a church nearby here, so I have a church which is my rosary and I pray to God."

Siboko showed the Catholic student his Bible and told him to read the words that Jesus spoke to his disciples (John 14:4–7). After reading, the youth told Siboko that when he completed his travels to Stanleyville, he would ask the priest the biblical reason for kneeling to rosaries, "and if he doesn't give me one, I will throw the rosary away and will come to buy the Bible at Yakusu."[52]

Siboko was accounting for other competitors in evangelical nurses' midst, the same Catholic priests who had infuriated Yakusu's missionaries by flooding the region with small medals in 1915.[53] Yet Siboko did not comment on the parallel equation, pervasive in the region, that his interlocutor made: Catholics gave away rosaries, Protestants sold Bibles. Local people spoke of the Baptists' God as the "God of books."[54] They also called BMS missionaries—in drum-signaling messages—spirits from the forest with papers. The Roman Catholic youth would consider switching from one God to the other, but not until he reached his destination. Nurse Likenyule had a similar anxiety about his safety and health during travel. Local Congolese—whether teachers or nurses, Christians or pagans, Catholics or Protestants—sensed the dangers of a journey, and whether carrying along Bibles, likenge, or rosaries, they all used forms of prayer and protection while in transit.

Travel and Style

Nurses wrote about their travels, too. They journeyed with their families to their new posts, and the letters, trucks, and orders of white men determined their itineraries. One nurse, Liita, devoted an entire letter to his first trip to Yaongama, describing how he left Yakusu for Yanonge with a letter from Bosongo Bonganga, the white missionary doctor, for a Mr. Andrades.

> I left Yakusu on January 7, 1930. We took the *camion* [truck] of Mr. Andrades and Mr. Andrades said to me: "This trip will be good and today is the day because the truck is ready for the trip." I accepted the words of the White Man, and this White Man gave me a house for me and Kilima and my wife and my two elder brothers and the youngest of the family.
>
> Very early in the morning, we loaded the camion, and the White Man told me: "It is best that your wife and Kilima and one of your elder brothers go in the camion. And you three take the path not by the river [bokili] because you have your bike." I answered: "Yes, Bwana." And so they began the trip and arrived in Yatolema at noon. We slept at that village. We continued the trip and arrived at Yalifoka, and we left Yalifoka and arrived at Yaongama B.M.S. 78 km. You see, my friends, why did I imagine that that trip was so difficult? I saw very big and long hills and this is true. . . . Me, B. Y. P. Liita Infirmier.[55]

The lexemes for the European truck owner and the Congolese cyclist-nurse— the *Bwana* with his *camion* and the *infirmier* with his *kinga*—impart the domesticating tendencies of colonial lexical borrowing, expressive of the inverted parallels among "going native" and "evolution" in a colonial situation. While the European was domesticated with the Swahili term *Bwana*, the Congolese nurse was worth a French word, *infirmier;* the nurse's means of transportation, a bicycle, was naturalized as *kinga*, whereas the European's truck could not be domesticated. A *camion* remained an inaccessible European object. Nurses may have been privileged characters who sometimes laughed alongside Europeans, yet they also took and followed orders. Their letters tend to report on the confrontations that were their challenge as they went. There was no story of conflict or "itineration" in Liita's letter, however. Rather, a seventy-eight kilometer journey by bicycle in 1930 was sensational; Nurse Liita simply shared this news.

Colonial lexical borrowing may have been poetic, but the poetics were historically concrete. Nurses were educated as evangelists at Yakusu, yet they were also trained to meet state standards for an emerging category of health assistants. The term *infirmier* reflects, therefore, not only local evangelical semantics, but also the seeping in of a state-authored word for a class of colonial workers. Likewise, the seeping into the pages of *Mboli ya Tengai* of two letters about bicycles during the early 1930s corresponds with a period when the extension of commercial cultivation, forced labor (especially in road construction), and police-like, itinerant colonial hygiene converged. These letter-writing nurses were likely the first Congolese cyclists to ride the new roads that opened up the BaMbole forest simultaneously to rubber and coffee plantations, hygienic surveillance, and Yakusu evangelization. As BaMbole hunters and farmers were pressed into road-building gangs and plantation labor, Yakusu's doctors—suddenly forbidden to use porters on medical tours—took to motorbikes.[56] Meanwhile, their ba-infirmiers, assigned to operate newly constructed Yakusu-managed dispensaries, cycled in on bicycles to perform their evangelical nursing labor. All of these developments entered into the BaMbole forest, these middles' letters tell, as if in one wondrous cycling piece. Foremost perhaps among this colonial revolution's panoply of accessory things were dispensaries and bicycles. The 1920s and 1930s were the major decades for the multiplication of bicycles in the colony, and this swell in cycling directly paralleled the addition of roads. These economic and social transformations amounted to the systematic remaking of Congolese rural social space in the name of "modernization,"[57] including that part of the BaMbole forest subject to Yakusu evangelization where the two letters in question were written.

I quote the second letter about bicycles at length. Victor Yenga, the Chestermans' famous "Boy/Man Sunday," wrote this letter about a "big problem" that occurred in his nursing practice on June 16, 1931.

> A young man came to me with a fatty cyst. He told me to do an *Opération* on him. . . . I asked this young man: "Why? Why do you come when your cyst is so big?" I said that I was not able because this is work to be done by a *Bonganga* [a white doctor] himself. And this young man answered that it was not a problem. "Operate on me. I have come to you because my children insult me every single day saying, 'look at the cyst on the leg,' and I get angry saying, 'my mother did not give birth to me with this.' Because of this, I have come to you today to take it away from me." When I heard his words, I felt sorry for him.
>
> I did the work from 8 to 11:30. I was working with the big, loving help of Alonga Samwele. In the middle of the work, when I removed this round fruit of a cyst, I saw this young man tremble because there was a big loss of blood.

Truly, truly, I said to myself I have a problem here. . . . I tried to manage to tie the entire vein because that cyst was on the vein behind the knee, a difficult spot. And I tied. And we put this young man in our house, yes, we watched over him very well. We prayed a lot for this young man. And, I say God helped us with the problem of this young man. I decided I would never do this work of surgery again as long as I live here! . . . Yet how can I refuse to do this work again? I had a dream during the night on my bed. This is what they asked me when I was dreaming. "Why do you refuse this? If you have a talent, if you have something that can heal, don't hide this. If you don't use this, for what good will you be? If you do it, you will gain a good reputation for your talent. How come you are not going to work with your talent?"

The voices in Yenga's dream continued to speak in his letter:

"If you have a bicycle which cost a lot of money, there is no way that you go to Yanonge with your feet. Would you leave your bicycle in your house? If it is so, you are really a fool in this matter. Because there is no reason to hide the bicycle in your house which is the helper of the feet for long trips." So like this these people who were speaking to me placed this idea in my heart. Other people said: "if he knows that it is given to be ridden, then the owner of it should know he should dress up in a wonderful manner."

Then Nurse Yenga ended his letter: "God has helped us by operating on this young man very well; what joy, thank you very much."[58]

This letter reveals the contestation that attended the simultaneous advent of rural health care and forced road construction. When Yenga first arrived to work at Yaongama, he had many patients coming to his dispensaire, yet before long he explained: "we do not see many of them. Truly the reason is their fear of the work that the White Men of the State are doing here." This fearful work was gang labor on the motor roads that BaMbole peasants were forced to construct between the mid-1920s and the mid-1930s, the same period that the new coffee and rubber plantation company, Bamboli Cultuur Maatschappij, expanded operations and recruitment through the forest.[59] When Yenga wrote this letter, Yakusu's missionaries were noting the "increased difficulties and restrictions on native travelling." Most BaMbole villages were "in a state of confusion," some being compelled to move six times during the decade, "for the State and Companies are still not sure that they have chosen the best route for their roads." The rebellious BaMbole so hated the roadwork and their newly sited villages that in "quite a number of villages the people or some of them have gone back into the forest secretly and built a place for themselves and only come out to the main village when they hear that the State man is about!"[60]

Victor Yenga threatened never to perform surgery again after his harrowing experience with a hemorrhaging patient, until he dreamed voices during the night. These voices told him that he could no more hide his medical talent than he could hide his bicycle in his house when he went on long trips to the colonial post of Yanonge, seventy-eight kilometers away. Yenga's dream suggests that his kinga impressed social and vocational identities on him. This contrivance also gave nurses autonomy in movement and fashion, never mind letters and whimsical dreams. Thus, Liita was forced to cycle to Yaongama per the orders of Mr. Andrades, yet his journey over "very big and long hills" inspired his informative letter. The doctor gave Yenga a bicycle for his work, but he dreamed it as a kinga and "helper of the feet for long trips." And the voices in his dream told him that as the owner of a bicycle, he should "dress up in a wonderful manner." Bicycles, perhaps, were as basic to evangelical advancement as such other things as communion cups, Bibles, and likenge- and cyst-removing surgical tools. Yet this colonial thing, which came as an instrument and obligation of nursing work, was also a generic colonial commodity, a symbolic marker of middle status, a marvelous technology, and a manner of dress. Its activity, cycling, released latitude for expressive borrowing and creativity in the historical making of a native colonial "high"—or évolué—style.

Autopsies and Motion

African nurses were necessary workers from the earliest days of the Congo Free State. They were also men.[61] Nursing was not codified as a colonial vocation until the early 1920s, however, at the same time as the state hygiene service was reorganized to focus on the care of Congolese subjects.[62] Medical care had been so selective up until this time that it was still possible to pronounce in 1919 that there was no medical service for "natives."[63] Colonial hygiene was instead aimed at protecting the health of Europeans and Congolese workers and soldiers living in state posts. The need to control epidemic disease, first and foremost sleeping sickness, led to an aggressive, yet still selective system of public health. Lazarets for quarantining patients, forced screening for disease, and medical passports were key.[64] Stanleyville, one of the colony's major cities, did not have a proper native hospital until 1925. "Two dormitories alone cannot constitute a hospital," ran a complaint in 1910 from a Dr. Veroni. He pleaded for a room for autopsies later that year: "I had to do an autopsy on the cadaver of a woman in my courtyard, on a table in the middle of a cloud of flies, a dangerous thing that should never happen."[65]

There was a nursing school in the city but trouble finding students: "It is difficult to find blacks who are intelligent enough. As for the literate [*lettrés*],

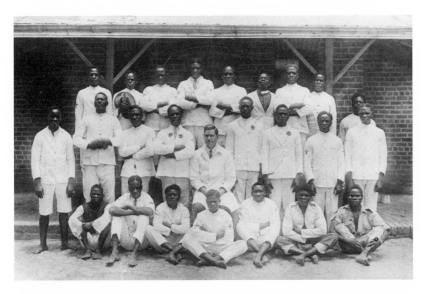

"A group of native nurses," likely working for Union Minière du Haut-Katanga, ca. 1930. (Courtesy of MRAC, Historical Section [61.74.416; gift of R. J. Cornet]. Courtesy of Africa-Museum, Tervuren, Belgium.)

since they find more advantageous positions with private employers, it is impossible to find any who want to follow the courses."[66] When the colonial hygiene bureau decided to increase the number of state nursing schools in the early 1920s, one was opened in Stanleyville.[67] But by 1926, there was a hospital "personnel crisis" in the city, and Minister of the Colonies, Henri Jasper, entertained proposals for increasing student allowances and nurse salaries in order to attract new students to this colonial vocation.[68] Part of the city's "personnel crisis" was the difficulty of finding nurse students who knew French. Another problem was that the province needed nurses not only for Stanleyville but also in its dispensaries in rural and mining areas,[69] where city men could not be persuaded to go work.

The state-run nursing school suffered from competition with nearby Yakusu, which was also turning out trained nurses. Yakusu's fame was not a new worry. As early as 1909, well before Yakusu became an important medical mission in the colony, Stanleyville's state doctor, Veroni, pointed out that this English mission had "a magnificent medication room" and that for reasons of prestige, if none other, he needed one, too.[70] In 1928 Stanleyville officials had misgivings about Yakusu's "indisputable increase in moral authority." Chesterman's *Manuel du dispensaire tropical* had become a nurse-training classic in the colony, and his evangelically trained nurses were being appointed to hospital and dispensary posts throughout the province.[71] Yakusu-trained nurses were known for their intelligent, dedicated work among Europeans in the area. Colonial passengers on mail steamers passing Yakusu in the late 1920s would point to canoes of youth dressed in white and khaki, returning to school at the mission station: " 'Oh yes!' says one 'they are being trained at Yakusu. We shall get some of them for clerks and those hospital boys are going to be very useful to the big companies and plantations.' "[72] In 1937, the director of the botanical research laboratories at the Yangambi station of INEAC requested some Yakusu nurses— "the most reliable native boys he had met"—to work as senior assistants in the chemical laboratory. Four Yakusu-trained nurses were already "running the dispensaries" on INEAC's extensive plantations. By 1943, Yakusu's nursing school was accepting students from as far away as Elisabethville, and its graduates were serving companies between Lisala and the French frontier, near the Anglo-Egyptian Sudan border, and in Uele's mining district.[73]

Stanleyville officials surveyed public opinion among city schoolboys in 1927 as they sought to comprehend—and alter—the image of nursing as inferior, contaminated work. Primary and professional students gave twelve reasons for not enrolling in their city's school for "Native Medical Assistants."

1. One is too easily punished with prison.
2. Certain Sundays one is not free to go out wandering [*se promener*].
3. Certain duties are loathe to us.
4. At night, one is alone at keeping watch, and in case of death, one must transport cadavers.
5. For the least fault, they withhold five, ten, or fifteen francs of salary.
6. We do not like to help with autopsies because of the bad odor given off by the cadavers.
7. One must always go out in the Native Medical Assistant uniform and one is recognized everywhere.
8. In the event of war, nurses are militarized.
9. A nurse works a lot and gains little.
10. We don't like to be night guardian.
11. They take ordinary blacks [*les noirs ordinaires*] for the Native Medical Assistant school; the intelligent blacks go into offices.
12. In leaving primary school, one can gain a lot of money as a clerk with traders [*commerçants*] instead of going to the school for Native Medical Assistants.[74]

Discipline, military associations (including a social memory of hygiene-related conscription during World War I), and loathsome cadaver and night duties were among the reasons that city boys discounted urban nursing work in interwar Stanleyville. Their longing for anonymity reinforces the impression of the second-rate, demeaning station of these nocturnal workers, who were obliged to guard and handle bodies, odors, and corpses. Images of confinement and coercion suggest their desire for freedom of movement and leisure time. Unlike Yakusu's "happy gang of hopefuls," they did not associate nursing with capacities to heal, evangelize, write, or cycle.

A young boy's post–World War II "vision" of an "impressive" rural nurse reveals a substantial alteration in the quality and stature of colonial nursing work by the 1950s. Willy De Craemer and Renée C. Fox collected these memories from a Congolese nurse in the lower Congo in the 1960s:

> I went to school in a little village . . . where there was a hospital in which infirmiers and aides-infirmiers worked. . . . When I was in my fourth year of primary school, I used to see the same infirmier on his way to work every morning on his bicycle. He wore a white helmet on his head, with the Belgian emblem and motto "*L'Union fait la Force*," a sign that distinguished him from ordinary workers. . . . At the end of our fifth year in primary school, when we were asked to write on a small slip of paper what school we would like to enter and what we would like to become . . . I was already influenced by my vision of that nurse I used to see every day. And without any doubts I wrote that I wanted to be a nurse.[75]

Yakusu nurses had this kind of prestige by the 1930s.

Maryinez Lyons's history of sleeping sickness exposes how critical mobility was to the history of Belgian colonial medicine. Struggles over transport and movement, especially barriers to mobility authorized in the name of colonial hygiene, fed the expressions of Congolese contempt for and flight from the strictures of sleeping sickness campaigns. As nurses moved about helping doctors inspect the population, Lyons implies, those who they found to be sick or living in sickly areas were condemned to motionlessness.[76] The evidence above also points to the importance of autonomy, mobility, and leisure time to the experience of nursing work. Yakusu nurses had all three. Travel and nursing went hand in hand in the Belgian Congo, at least in rural areas as hygiene touring intensified from the 1920s on. Indeed, the mobile style of nursing may have been a significant part of what made the vocation attractive.

Remembering Colonial Medicine

Some people ran away when Yakusu doctors and nurses came on tour, but not all did or could. When I queried men and women for memories of colonial

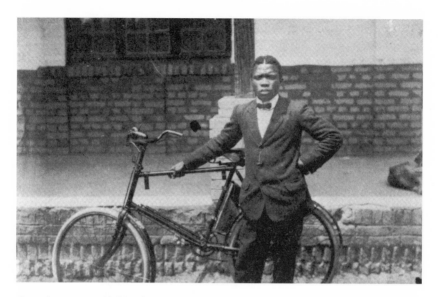

Congolese nurse with bicycle, 1914. First published in Lyons, *Colonial Disease*. (Courtesy of MRAC, Historical Section. Courtesy of Africa-Museum, Tervuren, Belgium.)

medicine and hygiene inspections, many spoke of "the time of Chesterman." Others called it "the time of contracts." Their memories spoke to the ambiguous, overlapping roles of missionary doctors and state doctors, company and mission dispensaries. One old man, Tata Alikuwa, expressed the simultaneity when he explained: "Yakusu, they divided out ba-infirmiers to all the companies. . . . Each month, each month, each year, he would come. So they made *hôpitalo*. . . . They divided out hôpitalo . . . each village with its own hôpitalo. . . ."[77] Yainyongo's chief, known as Pesapesa (Money Money), said that BMS doctors and state doctors had been "the same," but also different from each other during this period when "the State gave doctors who went every place in the forest for *control*." Both types arrived to do census and medical work: "When I was young, I saw the BMS doctor come to do *visites* . . . [and] afterwards the doctors of the State." Missionaries stayed in special, state-constructed houses "for whites to sleep in," and village residents "would make a few houses for the boys and the nurses." Before the completion of roads, the missionaries

would come set up beds, mosquito nets for Madami and the children. They would have guards to take care of them. . . . Sometimes they were carried in *kipoi* [hammocks], four people to carry the child, four people to carry the doctor. . . . It was a lot of work to carry them. . . . People would sing . . . "Where will it stop? This chief or doctor, he will stop where? He will stop at such and such a place." This was the song of carrying whites of the state or the doctor. . . . They were carried very high. It was very nice, huge work . . . [necessary] because of the streams. There were no bridges. The paths were bad, forest paths.

State doctors were more harsh: "When they would say come for census and stuff, some would run. The state people would come with police, do roll call, and send some to prison." These "state people" came "to push work . . . entering the forest, doing medical visits. . . . They were teaching how to make roads so they could pass by foot or by bicycle."[78] Another man, Lofemba, said: "The doctors would come and make inspections . . . *Recensement* [census]. . . . They would put you naked. They would look all places."[79] Tata Alikuwa elaborated: "They would get you here in the neck, saying, 'Come first.' . . . If there was a sickness there, that was it! They would come with a shot. They would prick you."[80] Pesapesa, who had been a child at the time, remembered fear and flight: "They were afraid because of shots, syringes. They would run. Us, children, we would cry. The ba-infirmier would stop us. We were afraid of shots. There were no pills." Yakusu's doctors would call each man to come forward with his wife and children, take their names, and inspect them in a house.

> The father would enter, would take off all his clothes, all his clothes, and [the doctor would] look at the whole body. If he was sick then he [the doctor] would write it on this paper for *recensement médical*. . . . They would call—the doctors, the nurses. You would be naked. If you were sick, they would send you. They would put you in the boat with a motor. You would be hospitalized. . . . Each time, each time, every three–four months, they would come. If they didn't come, the state would send their doctors.[81]

The nurses remain oblique figures in these memories. The doctor would come with "his ba-infirmier." "They would call—doctors, nurses." "The ba-infirmier would stop us." Nurses and their dispensaries were less menacing than the images of doctors touring with syringes to inject people and their tinned food to eat: "They would travel with *ba-boi* . . . also with nurses, satchels, supplies from Yakusu. At eight o'clock, they would finish their *copi*, their cans of food."[82] People were ambivalent and many were afraid: "They had a good *système* . . . coming, having medicines. People were happy, but if they said you were sick, you would start to cry . . . fearing going to the hospital, faraway. If you did not have a strong heart, you could not go. You would say the white man was coming to take people to remove them in order to go and kill them."[83]

This imagery of tinned food and bodily removals is closely aligned to a genre of terrifying stories known as tokwakwa that circulated in the region. Congolese were not systematically refusing medical care. To the contrary, people were traveling long distances to see doctors at Yakusu and thousands were examined every year. Yet—somehow—they understood medicine through these tales of whites devouring black flesh.

Tokwakwa as Tales

Tokwakwa tales are not specific to the Kisangani region, even though the word is. They are part of a larger genre of stories about the terrifying things that Europeans did with black bodies. Tokwakwa were found under various local names—according to the rhythms and events of specific local histories—throughout most of colonial Congo and across its borders as well in the Sudan, Angola, Zambia, Uganda, and Kenya. Rik Ceyssens has called them "collective representations." Luise White labels them "rumors" and "gossip." I find Jan Vansina's definition of a tale useful: "They never have a beginning . . . and they never end, but rather disappear into later tales."[84] Such a definition allows for Ceyssens's *longue durée* analysis, documenting similar constructions of Europeans from the sixteenth century in the lower Congo. Tales also turn attention to historical appearances and disappearances of tokwakwa strands within a local social context. Finally, tales insist on memory as performance.

It seems odd that no one has considered it important to publish a full performance of this storied genre as it unfolded within a local, ethnographic "scene of writing."[85] I first heard a tokwakwa tale by accident, while speaking to the oldest man in the village where I lived. Tata Alikuwa was telling me about the 1893 battle among Belgian officers and BaTambatamba, which had occurred in the very spot where we were speaking. He slipped quickly to colonial taxation, first as a form of extracting Congolese payment for the bullets that the Belgians had used in this battle at Romée, then to taxation as forced road labor, then to the consequence of not paying—imprisonment. Finally, at the urging of his ever-so-keen daughter, Bibi Mari-Jeanne, a young woman for whom colonialism was *only* memory and performance, he arrived at a tokwakwa tale. Tata Alikuwa referred to the BaTambatamba as BaNgwana:

> So the whites came from above saying, "Don't kill, don't kill." . . . The time of killing was no more. . . . We were fighting with the BaNgwana. To get ourselves out of slavery, we paid taxes. Up until today, there is taxation. . . . It started because of their bullets, which ended up inside the BaNgwana. They were fighting with the BaNgwana. The bullets were all gone. . . . The BaNgwana took our grandfathers as slaves. So the whites came: "Don't do

that." The BaNgwana got mad. They fought with the whites. . . . So it was like that, that the State said: "Well, our bullets are lost. We will hold you ransom until you pay a tax." If you didn't pay the tax, they would put you in prison for two months. . . . That was the tax of before. Fields, roads, putting bridges . . . so cars could pass. . . . The tax because of paying for the bullets, the money of the Belgians. If a man couldn't pay tax, you were inside two months . . . in prison. . . . If you killed someone, they sent you to the *parquet* [court of justice]. They spread you out. . . .

When Tata said, "they spread you out," his daughter instantly interrupted: "They had a hook, the kind they use to kill fish, this hook of the white men." Tata Alikuwa explained that if you killed someone, they would put a black cloth over your eyes. You would be confessing, but the hook was right there in front of you: "They would torment you. . . . Doctors would go with you in the motorcar to throw you there in the place where they eat meat."

Father and daughter continued to alternate:

F: They torment you with this thing, this hook. It climbs up. It gets you here. Then it pierces you here, under the head, under the chin, at the neck. Then doctors, doctors again, now they come to get you. . . . White men, doctors of white men.

D: They come to remove you from there. They send you in their truck. They go with you there to the place where there are people. People go to eat you there, like corn beef or another *modèle*. . . .

F: Corn beef. . . . They eat.

D: They eat you. The whites were eating people. . . .

Tata broadened his narrative once again and returned to roads:

So, we black people, we worked off fines up to the millions. . . . Our history of black people, it was like this, the whites came first, going around saying the black people will kill us here. . . . They were going around looking for roads, saying there is nothing. They thought we had a place to hide from fighting with them, so the white man built roads. They saw there was nothing, so they warned us . . . if you do wrong . . . they would send you to the parquet to kill you.

"To make sardines, corn beef," Bibi Mari-Jeanne interjected again, prodding her father on. He continued:

If they saw you on the road, they would kill you. They would take you. They would put you in the motorcar that had a canvas cover. They would take you to the pit down in the earth, that hole in the ground. It would go from here as far as the Romée River concealing people . . . [all the way to] Kisangani. . . . They would build it well with cement and all that stuff. They would take someone and put him there. They would close the lock up above. They would feed you white man's food, cow, meat of pig . . . in this big enclosure.

Bibi Mari-Jeanne explained that there was a special kind of "trap of the whites." Suddenly, it would fall and the hook would get you: "They make a small hole. They put the trap here on the board. . . . A hole. They dig a hole. They put the board up high." Her father added: "But they stay here with a rope. . . . White men, many white men . . . when you do wrong [*kusamba*], many whites are just there. . . . It wasn't at the parquet. They removed you from the parquet to come to this house here of confessing . . . to the house of the trap."[86]

There are multiple versions of tokwakwa stories, alternately called *bakumbata*, "those who grab or enclose you." *Likumbata* is the substantive, "the name of the kind of work for those who were waiting for someone, clasping them in their arms, and killing them. Likumbata is the murder of people."[87] Tata Alikuwa added: "A tokwakwa has no house. He has nothing. He just waits for you, kills you . . . puts you in a sack, waits for their truck." They were equally "those people of the central prison, those who were in jail year after year."[88]

Not all versions of tokwakwa are as medicalized as was the conversation between Tata and his daughter. Some tales move, as did Ceyssens's exegesis, more directly to tinned food: "We just heard; they were sending them to a secret European butcher's shop in order to cut up and eat people. Big white men would eat there in their hotel. Yes. That's what we heard. So us, our fathers and mothers at the *kilomètre* [road marker], they were very afraid." Or: "We heard that there in Kisangani, one bwana, he bought a can of sardines. I don't know his name. . . . A black man . . . opened the can . . . saw the hand of a person . . . [and] showed it to his friends. Well! They returned to the white man. . . . That white man, he gave that bwana many clothes, many francs, many things for the house. He said: 'Go home.' He took many more sardines, many. He gave them to that bwana."[89]

Also important were flashlights, "truncheons with electric current," reminiscent of truck headlights and surgical lights that made one "die in the eyes."

They would divide up flashlights. This torch; it had current. . . . When they would go *kai!* your eyes would not see well again. . . . They would catch you with the rope of the current *tiii*. . . . They would carry batteries. . . . You start to go down. They tie you up. They put you in a sack.[90]

Even Christmastime was imbricated in the dangers: "Everyone knew, saying that the convicts hide during December to kill us."

The sounds of vehicles told of tokwakwa: "At night, that motorcar of the

State, it would be going *vuu,* making the sound of *pepe, pepe* in the island. . . . You stand up. . . . They throw in those sacks." Roads were central to the disappearance of people and to tokwakwa tales.

> Our fathers and our mothers, they were going by the roads of trucks, the Yanonge road or the Kisangani road. Many people were dying; we wouldn't see their corpses. We wouldn't see the dead. Others, especially the roads of trucks or those leaving from Yangambi to go to Kisangani, or leaving Kisangani for Banalia, going to Buta, Ituri, Bafwasende, Ubundu, Opala, Yangambi, Yanonge, Isangi, Bukavu, Bunia, Isiro. . . . They would look for him. They wouldn't know where he died, where he went. It was tribe after tribe. They were saying it was the people of prison who had hidden.[91]

One man called it "their truck opération." People mentioned over and over again that the most dangerous place to be was at the "islands," on the roads in the empty spaces between villages. The risk was being caught from behind, thrown into a sack, into a truck, taken to Stanleyville, and made into tinned food for the fat white men who ate in hotels.

> They enter into the motorcar. They go with you. . . . They put you in that house. They give you shots and bathe you and prepare you very well. . . . *Teee,* you become nice. You don't speak again. Now you grow fat. That time, if they want to eat you, they eat you. . . . Some could do up to a year. They were washing, preparing you, giving shots, so that [you] became well with vitamins. They would eat you. . . . Doctors were doing that thing as well. They would look to see if a person was nice. They would give you shots. They would say, "He is dead." . . . They would say, "Us, ourselves, we will dress him in clothes, we will clean him. We will put him in the village." . . . Now they would go with you, and you were [actually] staying there in the house while they were doing their opérations to remove the flesh. . . . They sew you up. They apply cotton balls. They shave you. They dress you. . . . They dress you in clothes. They put you in a coffin. They say, "This man, we are going to give him to the village. Don't open [the coffin] again." They bury you.[92]

Such flesh removals were also opérations.

Mupendakula and Badjoko

Colonial medical performances were media that communicated ideas, images, and gestures, and remade old metaphors. *Mboli ya Tengai* letters and tokwakwa tales evoked contrary, kindred fantasies about the control and use of these new historical entanglements. Nurses and some of their patients were active users of dispensaries, medicines, and papers. Tokwakwa-tellers actively used the new media, too, often as idioms to remember and perhaps to terrify and control. Vaughan has contended that "in the history of large parts of Africa biomedicine arrived with the state, as part of the state, and perhaps as an embodiment of it."[93] Yakusu's history and tokwakwa tales do not contradict this argument, but they complicate it. Biomedicine arrived with evangelism, a plantation economy, and intensifying commerce and mobility in much of Yakusu's forest district in the interwar years. Its visibility—and sounds and smells—embodied much more than state power. European doctors and Congolese nurses combined and blurred state-, mission-, plantation-, and middle-based forms of colonial biopower. As mobility and commerce increased, medical care came to the "bush," surgery became a part of rural practice, and nurses dreamed about bicycles. Roads and autopsies came in tandem, joined by bicycles, touring doctors, dispensaries, reified villages, and grueling, forced road labor. Imaginations ran wild and concrete.

These contrasting sources correspond somewhat, but never completely, to two different colonial social categories: middle figures, such as nurses, and the "lows" of colonial hierarchies, subaltern peasants. Each source seems to date to the 1920s and 1930s, when, as one missionary expressed it, life in the Congo was "speeding up." Both letters and tokwakwa touched on and were nourished by the new forms of mobility, medicine, labor, space, and speed of this period. The letters tell of a new, middle-authored, mixed and mixed-up lexicon that rejected likenge for diplomas, microscopes, and bicycles. The nurse figure was preeminent, as was his dispensary space. This new style was imposed, in a sense, from above. Likenyule, Yenga, and their counterparts labored and moved as diminutives in relation to European missionaries and plantation agents.[94] Yet such semiotics did not diminish their capacity to make meaning and derive power from their microscopes, surgeries, bicycles, and papers. Their style contained a force and created its own diminutive as they posed Congolese basenji as inferior subjects of trials and laughter. These authoring subjects elaborated a contradictory colonial consciousness. Such was Yenga's move when he gave the teacher disinfectant. This gesture was no less composite and contrary than his letter, accepting the moral metaphor proposed by his dream. This central metaphor of Yenga's letter spoke to surgery and bicycles, cutting and cycling, as simultaneous novelties. Trucks and autopsies were central and simultaneous in tokwakwa. The contrast is significant. The nurse envisioned his vehicle as a cue to dress up and cycle. Tokwakwa tell of style, too; not of an individual capacity to brandish, quote, and consume colonial objects, but rather, of a capacity to be consumed by new colonial styles, as the raw bodies of these tales. Tokwakwa and middles' letters, as historical sources, reveal the contrary metaphors that colonial subjects made in comparing the new circulatory networks of roads and medicine, the mobilities and surgeries through which new social bodies were being created. So aligned with wonder were bicycles for one and all, it seems, that they are absent from tokwakwa. These sinister, sardonic tales were, despite their "admiring terror," too scornful to embrace this marvelous and almost accessible technology that moved as if by wind.[95] Nevertheless, the social power of this public scorn may have made Nurse Yenga—before his "big problem" and dream as hesitant to show off his bicycle as to cut into a BaMbole cyst.

I know such stories not only because reproductive ritual was so central to my research, but also because my own eating and food-sharing habits were a continual source of discussion. I was compared—sometimes favorably, sometimes not—to the generic category of colonial white person who makes one stand and wait while he or she is eating, and eats abundant amounts, but never ever shares his or her supplies or meals. Tokwakwa are also linked along the Upper Congo and in the BaMbole forest to a set of stories about a sometimes generic, sometimes specific colonial agent known for his voracious appetite and taste for whipping people. People remember their nickname for him, Mupendakula or "He-likes-to-eat." Mupendakula emerged as a verb in tokwakwa tales: "They *mupendakula*-ed him." Middle-aged men recalled their fathers saying: "my child, a white man who was here, his name, Mupendakula." He was as old as colonial civilities: "When the white man came, he came . . . to civilize us, you see. Father explained to me the matter of Mupendakula." One man, Baba Manzanza, remembered his father describing how Mupendakula would whip people all over their bodies until blood came, and then if you did not have the strength to walk again, he would tell his men to dig up the earth and bury you, "and you were still speaking."[96]

Many in Yainyongo recalled Mupendakula as the white man who came around, driving the only motorcar that ever appeared there, to make speeches to work hard because the "war of Watsa was raging," named for the northeastern Congolese base where many conscripts were sent. He told parents that the state needed their youth, and that they should meanwhile work extra hard to collect rubber for the war. Benoît Verhaegen's research confirms this association between Mupendakula and the hardships of World War II–forced labor. These "togbaba" or "togwawa" stories, he argues, especially surged in the Stanleyville region during the intense rubber labor demands of the war, not unlike how they must have done during the earlier "red rubber" period. Congolese had nicknamed a Monsieur Declerq, colonial agent at Yanonge, "Mupendakula" before the war. The time of the "war of Watsa" echoed, like Declercq's nickname, memories of the "red rubber" abuses of the Congo Free State period.[97]

People tended to move from Mupendakula stories backward in time to Badjoko stories.[98] Mupendakula was a Belgian state agent during both the interwar and war periods. Badjoko, who we met in chapter 1, was the only Congolese appointed as a state agent. This "chef de poste" at Yanonge from 1900 until 1932 was known in colonial circles for having "saved Stanleyville from an Arab attack in 1892" and having "developed" the Yanonge region. He twice visited Belgium, where he was received by King Leopold II and King Albert.[99] Badjoko is remembered locally as a Bangala stranger from downriver who rose from serving as a "boy" of a Belgian colonial officer to the one who harshly imposed rubber collecting on local people from his post at Yanonge. People spoke vividly about the cruelty of this outsider: Badjoko was a "bad man" who had many police, used a whip, and "did the work of the state." When he married a Yakusu church member in 1906, the church expelled his new wife because Badjoko was already married.[100] Badjoko wanted to join libeli in 1910, but the word was no: "he was not a Lokele." His sons by a Lokele wife, however, entered libeli in 1924. Badjoko was buying church books through an intermediary in 1933.[101] Pesapesa recalled seeing him in 1944 when, he said, Badjoko was ninety-eight years old and Pesapesa ten. A colonial source considered Badjoko "more than seventy" in 1950, at which time he had "obtained an agricultural concession at Lileko and established an important plantation there." Tokwakwa likely circulated around this tax-collector-turned-road-builder; he personally oversaw the hard labor that went into constructing a thirty-kilometer road linking "his plantation" to larger roads.[102] Papers were not absent from this reputation. Nor were BaTambatamba attributes. Mama Tula said Badjoko, the "first sultan from Lileko to Yakoso," received his state post "because he worked first with the whites and knew to write. They took him and put him at Yanonge." She added: "I heard that his family knew many medicines." His medical powers were associated with river streams and the animals that he kept there.[103]

Mupendakula was associated with liking to eat, his big size, and burying people alive. Badjoko was associated with ndimo and whippings. Badjoko's historical and social proximity to the BaTambatamba and their methods—adopting local idioms of power, for example—may explain the difference. Early tokwakwa variants—which circulated around BaTambatamba, Badjoko, and the spaces that they occupied—were marked by rubber, whips, water spirits, crocodiles, and cruel strangers taking local women as wives. Trucks, roads, pits, coffins, live burials, and surgical flesh removal were tokwakwa idioms from the 1920s on. They produced, in conjunction with one Monsieur Declercq's actions, at least one Mupendakula figure as well as a Stanleyville butcher shop and hotel, and in muted form, as we will see, Yakusu's Bonganga, Dr. Stanley G. Browne.

Autopsies and Childbearing

Tokwakwa stories tell of dining and surgery. They suggest that each of these colonial routines entailed a perverse spurning of local notions of good and proper eating. Procreation and gestation are often likened in central Africa to proper cooking, tending a fire, and serving a meal. Indeed, these metaphors comparing procreation with eating, wombs with hearths, and infertility with theft and violence—as well as "summarizing and elaborating understandings of how the world works and what threatens it"—are, I imagine, central to and as old as any regional protolexicon of words, things, and senses. Good and proper sharing of cooked food poses contraries: bad, illicit wealth; selfish and secretive eating; hidden, stolen food and body parts; a boiled-over cooking pot; or too many male cooks tending the same fetal fire.[104] I learned about good eating as generous sharing of food while at Yainyongo and other localities in the region. Good and proper eating is the language of everyday life, and of male and female reproductive ritual. Both men and women regaled me with stories of ritual periods—libeli, likiilo, bowai, and wale—when they had been removed from production and fattened at feasts. Everyday envy, too, is expressed around hunger and selfishness with food. Tokwakwa tales resonate with these feasting periods in inverted fashion. They echo local lisombo idioms of stolen blood, hair, and nails used to harm, kill, and—with stolen menstrual blood and placenta pieces—block a woman's fertility. Tokwakwa are also repeated, in a sense, with contemporary *fonoli* tales of disappeared people who live on as invisible slaves after their corpses are thought buried, and do a live, rich person's work. Fonoli and crocodile-man idioms are closely related.

Selfishness with food remains tied to the dangers of mixing the "waters" (sperm) of multiple lovers with a single pregnancy, and to envious women who enter cabinets to steal menstrual blood and block a neighbor or relative's fertility. Moreover, food sharing and aid in childbearing travel along the same social networks within and among households in Yainyongo. Women who send each other plates of cooked food from time to time also help each other during pregnancy, childbirth, and the postnatal period of fattening known as wale. Cooking is central to these practices, but so is fat as beauty and fattening as wealth, integrated as they are to these periodic ritual expressions of female bounty, seclusion, and protected leisure.

An ungenerous cook or a selfish eater is not just a local category for European diners. It is a fundamental, deeply sedimented one used to shame and abuse selfish neighbors and kin who hide rather than share food. A new wife does not make her own hearth until she comes out of bowai. Her womb being ready and her fire lit, she must show her good heart and share her cooked

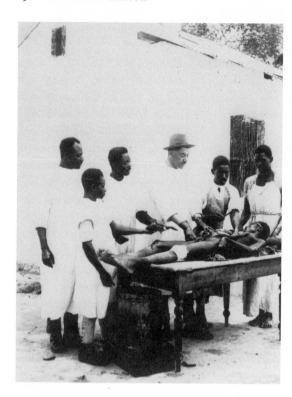

Dr. G. Fronville giving an open-air autopsy lesson to Congolese nurses in Elisabethville, ca. 1925. From G. Fronville, "Six années de pratique chirurgicale chez les noirs du Katanga." (Courtesy of the Institute of Tropical Medicine, Antwerp, Belgium.)

meals. If a new wife is seen as selfish with food, her birth-attending kin of the same household will wait until she has given birth to her first live baby to shame her. They will wait to express their anger until the moment of a successful, accomplished birth, when she can no longer accuse them of tampering with her fertility. They will complain about her greed by refusing to bury her placenta, known as the Mama, saying that they dare not perform this task because if she should have trouble becoming pregnant again, they do not want to be open to accusations that they tampered with this key to her fecundity.

As we saw in chapter 2, when the Yakusu hospital was under construction in 1924 and the foundations and inner rooms exposed, local women became afraid to pass by the site to go to the market for weeks. People told stories about bad doctors and their plans to cut up victims and put them in tins for sale. At play in this Congolese imaging of the hospital was a tokwakwa idiom of bad eating, which posed a threat to women's fertility. Autopsies also nourished tokwakwa. Dr. Veroni, as we saw, was performing autopsies in Stanleyville as early as 1910. They became a routine part of nurse training—and the vocation's reputation and avoidance—during the 1920s. Colonial doctors furtively removed body parts for subsequent study. The kin of a syphilitic patient, who had died in her eighth month of pregnancy in the Ituri forest in the mid-1940s, became disturbed when her corpse was removed from the hospital. They ended up wailing outside the doors of a long-unused autopsy room in a patch of forest. The doctor, a syphilis specialist known among colonials for his multiple concubines, each thoroughly screened by him for venereal disease, surreptitiously removed the dead fetus from the woman's body, keeping it for further study. This was not an isolated incident, even if unused autopsy rooms were rare. Such wailing and suspicion nurtured tokwakwa. The people of Province Orientale—who moved along the roads linking the Kilo-Moto gold mines, Stanleyville, and the BaMbole forest—had no lack of new source material from daily life. Not only did people travel off to mines, plantations, and other work sites and never come back, but a key incentive for colonial medical research in gynecology, obstetrics, and pediatrics was implicitly the ready availability of a dead and dissectible subject population. Dr. P. G. Janssens reported on 1,873 autopsies on infants in the post–World War II period at Kilo-Moto facilities, located out one of the main "truck roads" leading away from Stanleyville.[105]

Both obstetric deliveries and autopsies, Gladys Owen observed in 1929, became acceptable procedures at Yakusu's hospital at precisely the same time.[106] Tokwakwa explain why consent to autopsies and hospital childbearing come together in this historical colonial double. Interventions into wombs and corpses, birth and death—postmortems and obstetrics—were, in local categories, the most intimate forms of colonial penetration possible. Dining and surgery, as tokwakwa imply (and as Ceyssens noted for eastern *mutumbula*, "collective representations" in general), entailed disembowelment, the cutting open of that which is round or swollen, an image pregnant with, in Feldman-Savelsberg's words, "theft and violence," "plundered kitchens, empty wombs, and lonely hearths."[107] Autopsy imagery was central to the infertility anxieties of tokwakwa, where it was paired with cutting into the belly or womb. The same metaphorical double emerged in history, in the tacit social rejection of tokwakwa as a basenji genre, as middle figures accepted and performed these bodily violations.

Those who rejected and accepted were those who had social access to—and wrote—the new vocabulary of evangelical hygiene. They were the letter writers and nurses of *Mboli ya Tengai*, who had been taught to think of the body as composed of mechanical "parts"—not unlike spokes, brakes, and a chain—which, as we saw earlier in this chapter, make "the body work in a good or a bad way." They found it easy to declare "the things which a person lets out of the body" as "only waste," and to pronounce lisombo "not a true thing," but "a lie which people say to somebody they hate."[108] Recall, too, how schoolboys at

Yakusu remembered and wrote about libeli in the early 1930s. Libeli was a lie, they said. The big men who organized libeli sensed that the Yakusu church and schoolboys threatened their capacity to compose power and wealth. Schoolboys condemned libeli in their compositions as theft and selfish eating. Yet youth were keen to compose new wealth and power through cutting, writing, and cycling. Such was Victor Yenga's transformation.

Scenes of Telling

Tokwakwa remained active through the 1950s. Indeed, such stories are still passed along, as I discovered, from old to young today. Tokwakwa, remember, have no beginning and no end, but they *are* historical. They emerge(d) out of and disappear(ed) into other tales, including the recollected tales of daily life. Tokwakwa strands also emerged from and disappeared into local historical experience in Yakusu's district at several junctures—when Yenga saw surgical gloves as black human hands in 1921, when the hospital was under construction in 1924, and, as we will see, when childbearing moved to this new evangelical space of confinement.

Tata Alikuwa slipped rapidly along a chain of linked metaphors, from bullets to taxation to roads to prison to being "spread out" by tokwakwa, and once he got to these scary stories with his daughter's urging, she had a considerable appetite for more. Gyan Prakash has argued that "the staging of science also enacted other performances" within a colonial situation "because the subject of representation (the West, science, 'the native') . . . can never contain and control, the act of its signification." The subaltern may be absent from colonial discourse "as speaking subjects" (though this is mighty debatable), but mutumbula and tokwakwa tales were performances in which the colonized "found a place as knowing subjects."[109] Tokwakwa tales, like bicycles, moved along roads as they carried and remade meaning, and they demonstrate how these new arteries and bodily technologies were intertwined imaginatively, metaphorically, in a word, historically. They are also intermixed with assumptions about tinned food as unshared fare. In comparing autopsies with bad eating, tokwakwa help account for the Congolese fascination with missionary dining and surgery in Yakusu's district, and for the disturbances that could erupt during these spectacles. Local people discussed and remembered these occasions through tokwakwa, likely prodding each other on as Bibi Mari-Jeanne did with her father.

Variants of these stories are very old in the area; we saw tokwakwa strands in the discussion of libeli and BaTambatamba powers in chapters 1 and 2. People told me that when BaTambatamba raided their villages in the late nineteenth century, these first colonial overlords "ate" them, not an uncommon expression in central Africa for control and abuse.[110] This BaTambatamba eating went together with investing their power in crocodiles or ndimo. Fears of prisoners predated roads. In 1917, some teachers in the Eso forest (south of Isangi) who were on their way to Yakusu for classes found themselves the subjects of to-kwakwa accusations in a Komo village near Yafunga: "They said we were prowling round to steal something and some said we were runaways from Stanleyville. . . . They said everybody had heard of our flight and they had been told to kill us like any wild beast if we came their way."[111]

Who "wrote" tokwakwa? Ceyssens defined "modern Mutumbula" by the images of tinned human food found in missionary accounts of Congolese imaging of Europeans from the late nineteenth century. Yet he also noted that the "vocabulary" of mutumbula had since changed.[112] This more recently embedded vocabulary—hotels, doctors, trucks, surgical instruments, and roads and their "islands"—speaks to the fast modernity of tokwakwa and the interwar ruptures that produced them. Ceyssens aligned tokwakwa with his "urban genre" of mutumbula stories. Many tokwakwa variants include particular sites in Stanleyville: a butcher's shop, white hotels, the prison, parquet, and the "Pourquoi Pas" bar.[113] Some men in Yainyongo knew these versions, especially those who had spent periods living in the city. Most, however, knew tokwakwa from the vantage point of road "islands," finding a stranger stealing food in a field, or hearing the sound of trucks going "vuu, vuu, vuu" in the night. The people of Yainyongo-Romée, in a sense, were still writing tokwakwa during my field "scene of writing" while answering my questions about how local Congolese viewed biomedicine and white people. Verhaegen has suggested that tokwakwa were a form of kin-based social control. Hence: "How to keep the children off the streets and in before dark? Scare the living daylights out of them with tokwakwa." I appreciate this line of interpretation and have heard it from Zairian intellectuals, too. But tokwakwa would have also been told to European colonials, not unlike the way they were told to me. Tokwakwa came in a cluster with other stories about kind, generous white people and modern, mermaid-like, Ndiya figures who as ambivalent, white spirits live as seductive temptresses in rivers, lure with watches on their wrists, and steal children who disappear from the river's edge. Ceyssens's evidence as well as recent Africanist scholarship suggest that there is a long, enduring history to white strangers being enraptured by such tales. I certainly experienced them as part of my larger local education in how to behave properly, how to accept food as a special female guest, and when and how to share food as the rich patron I was supposed to be. Stories of Mupendakula and tokwakwa often tumbled out with others about nice and generous white people who are the spirits of a local person who died and returned as a colonial patron. Indeed, this was the reason that the people of Yainyongo gave for why Mupendakula was—like me—unusually kind to them.

Tokwakwa tales and nurses' letters should not be construed as exclusive domains. One source may be oral and the other written, but identifying authorship and the contexts of reception are never obvious tasks. Just as we need to be careful not to approach colonial histories in terms of easy dualisms, we also need to avoid conflating "rumors" with subalterns.[114] As the evidence on Victor Yenga has shown, colonial middles were not only privy to such tales; they would have partially participated in and told tokwakwa as they moved in and out of local geographies of *asili* (natural, customary) and *kizungu* (colonized) space. When Yenga compared surgery to cycling at age twenty-one in Yaongama, he was claiming the honor of his access to these new technologies. Yet as a ten-year-old "table boy" at Yakusu, he saw Chesterman's gloves as cooking, black human hands. The incident was not simply recuperated as Man/Boy Friday for the *Reader's Digest;* more significantly, this tokwakwa thread was domesticated at Yakusu as mission parable, theater, and a middle-told basenji joke.

Baba Manzanza was telling a strand of a tokwakwa story when he said that people had feared touring doctors who told the sick that they had to go to the hospital "faraway." He stressed that those without "strong hearts" would not go, saying that the white doctor wanted to "take people to remove them in order to go and kill them."[115] Baba Manzanza, proud of going to both school and the hospital during his many years spent in kizungu, was declaring his "strong heart" as he defined tokwakwa. A person in kizungu was not cut off from tokwakwa. Likewise, people read *Mboli ya Tengai* letters aloud in villages, and nurses addressed their interlocutors as readers and listeners.[116]

Most, but not all, of the people in Yainyongo-Romée who shared these stories with me were once middles, if rather low and semiliterate middles. They called themselves "children of classes," those who came "out of asili" and "went to school." Research occasions of tokwakwa-telling reenacted complex gestures of colonial translation. There was a facility in contextualizing these stories for me, a stranger to and a subject of tokwakwa: "So like that us, black people, we believed, saying white people during the time of the Belgians, even now we believe it, saying whites eat us in secret. They don't show it. They eat us. So like that we fear whites." Or: "This is just our thoughts of black people. . . . We are just used to thinking like that." Or, more directly, when I asked Pesapesa if people thought that human bodies became white people's food, he said: We were "food for white people because they did not give any to us. . . . Many times, they didn't give any to us . . . that of tokwakwa."[117] The point was, in part, a challenge.

Local people did not systematically reject biomedical care; rather, some traveled far to see Yakusu's doctors and undergo surgeries. Some fled medical tours, but not all could. Reactions were mixed. The new social realities made therapeutic vocabularies and decision making more complex than ever before, while providing rich material for local, collective imaginations. Some ran away or hid wives. Some got caught, whipped, sent to prison. Others rejoiced when a Yakusu missionary gave them their "coveted piece of paper,"[118] some version of a colonial medical passport. Yakusu's doctors had neither time for intimate evangelical healing while on their sanitary census tours nor much power to recuperate and direct local narratives.

Such had been Chesterman's labor—recuperation and domestication—when authoring Boy/Man Sunday. Such, too, was his crocodile-seizing work in the Lokele town along the river where church roots and a Lokele middle consciousness ran as deep as their BaTambatamba marrying and paddling days. Chesterman was working overtime on recovering and diverting this tokwakwa strand, the crocodile's nickname, in his and the church's favor in 1933 and 1934. Yet church roots were not easily laid in the BaMbole forest. Indiscipline and secretive forest homes came as second nature among these trappers and farmers whom the Zanzibari and their middles saw as enslavable basenji. Missionaries met these subaltern subjects as village populations lined up for inspection. History and location made elegant missionary entries by river steamer both of another era and out of reach. Road building and labor extraction for plantation and mining economies within BaMbole terrain were violent processes, not easily rewritten as convincing church parables. But these experiences easily folded into familiar frames for remembering slave raiding, rainbow control, and blood flowing down a trickle of a waterfall.

5 BABIES AND FORCEPS

We had no choice, you see.—Dorothy Daniel, Corse Staunton, 1991

All work is not a matter of saying: "Do this, do that."—Malia Winnie, Kisangani, 1989

In 1956, a pregnant woman making a journey along the Congo River stopped at Yakusu's hospital for antenatal care. Local people called the English midwife who worked there Bokondoko because the name sounds like a moving motorcar if repeated several times, and this Mademoiselle was the first woman ever seen driving a Land Rover. Mary Fagg's nickname also meant that she worked with expertise and authority; she worked like a man. And so it seemed she did as she moved about in the station vehicle from the mid-1950s through the 1970s, energetically supervising a new series of baby clinics along the river. Bokondoko told this Congolese woman expecting her ninth child that she had anemia and should stay for treatment until her delivery. The woman agreed, though her hospital chart indicated that, often absent from her bed, she missed injections. When she went into labor a month later, the anemia had hardly improved. The case proved a difficult one. Bokondoko had to call the missionary doctor away from a Sunday afternoon rest to assist with obstetric forceps.[1]

When Bokondoko told me this story some thirty years later in England, she explained that up until this time, the use of forceps had not been associated with live births at Yakusu. She did not give the woman's name—Boyali—rather, she prefaced her story by saying that the pregnant woman reminded her of a London cockney upstart. Her impression was confirmed when the mother, ecstatic about her live baby, wanted to name the newborn after the doctor's instrument. "Folicepi, Folicepi," the Congolese mother had chanted. Fagg laughed in telling the story, and concluded by saying that she had convinced the woman that Emmanuel was a better name.[2]

What Bokondoko told me in 1990, however, differed from her printed words in the *Yakusu Quarterly Notes*. In 1956, she wrote:

> Progress was slow, but her spirits never flagged and she laughed and joked in true cockney fashion, keeping her old mother in order and taking a lively interest in everything that was said or done. Finally we fetched doctor and he helped her over the final stage. Much excitement accompanied the arrival of a fine son, her ninth baby, and grandma's joy was given vent to in a dance. She trotted and stamped, clapped and sang, with each turn bowing to the baby and announcing his name. During this exhibition Boyali was shouting "Be quiet, mother, oh! be quiet," with annoyance in her tones "that is not his name. He is to be called Emmanuel for surely God has been with us in our trouble."[3]

What was erased in text holds a counterpart effaced from memory. When Mary Fagg wrote, she did not explain the relationship between the doctor's instrument and the joyful, repressed name. A baby named after forceps was too indelicate for her reading public of British mission supporters. Her published article never voiced the word, yet it brought into relief an old grandma as lay birth attendant, condensing a generational conflict that memory omitted or consciousness never grasped. The textual episode reveals the path by which, to use an abiding English category, "the man-midwife"[4] arrived on the scene. It suggests, too, what this summoning and entry with forceps comprehended: Boyali kept "her old mother in order." Whether the rivalry over the baby's name was simultaneous or sequential, Bokondoko seems not to have understood the competing, complicitous dynamics involved. Thus, she easily transposed the generational tensions of "old mother" versus daughter-parturient that she observed in 1956 into their colonial homology thirty years later, missionary versus colonized subject. What enabled this conflation was the one consistency in her two renditions, the mother's identity. Fagg never veered on her use of a British evangelical analogy to classify this colonized woman. Uncouth and jocular, Boyali resembled a cockney woman of London's East End. Indeed, this same association was what made the Folicepi story range from mirthful to too bawdy to write.

Colonized subjects, as Fagg's divergent accounts show, vied over local baby-naming practice and novel biomedical instruments, and they refigured birth ritual within Yakusu's maternity ward. This chapter demonstrates that these historical processes were marked by gender, generation, and race, and mediated by forms of producing and remembering hospitalized childbearing. And they contained debates over particular technologies and surgeries. These refigurations were mediated less by individuals' therapeutic itineraries than by a historical, collective itinerary,[5] the passage of a Congolese locality through colonial birthing space and the course of biomedical maternity care through a subject people's lives.

Missionary-authored accounts are a key resource in this analysis.[6] Yet such textual episodes tend to be truncated, telling little about what happened before a woman arrived at a hospital and after she went home, and often comprising no more than a single scene that transpired within a biomedical social field. The number, patterns, and novelties of such incidents enable an analysis of "paths"[7] to medicalized childbearing; the gestures of old grandmas, midwives, and doctors; and the use and refiguration of obstetric technologies. Many provide glimpses of obstetric transactions among colonizer and colonized. Others give insight into exchanges among Congolese middle and low figures, the social action of kin and friends, and factors that influenced the organization of a parturient's care. I also draw on oral testimony collected in Zaire and England, including from the British and Congolese midwives who worked at Yakusu. Memory does not abridge and dismember social action as does contemporary writing. The value of oral forms of remembering lies in what they conjoin and how they stray from the researcher's intentions and expectations.

Birth in Print

In 1915, a leading Congolese girl teacher at Yakusu gave birth at the station. As Mrs. Millman watched, an angry "old woman" mother and an "accomplice . . . dragged" the young woman "out into the brilliant moonlight" to deliver the baby that the older mother apparently did not want. When her daughter had married a mission-trained teacher and carpenter who had been to England, the mother had been so upset that she had refused to eat. A Stanleyville judge had officiated, and the husband gave the "bridewealth" directly to his wife. The "neat, comfortable little home" with wooden cabinets, doors, and tables that the husband made did not impress. "I'll tire you all out," the mother said of her daily visits to "rave" at her daughter's door. Once her daughter became pregnant, the mother claimed that the baby would not survive, though Mrs. Millman observed from a distance the successful childbirth scene "there under the stars." Mrs. Millman felt triumphant until the day the new mother abandoned her baby in her neatly carpentered house and returned home to her mother. The elder mother tried to kill the baby when her daughter returned to the station again. The experience summarizes the danger of old Congolese "grannies" for Mrs. Millman: "Tribal customs are very, very strong, and we must be brave and patient."[8]

Mrs. Millman did not write publicly about childbirth again until 1929, when she contributed a happy story of the first in Yakusu's hospital. A meteorite had just fallen, and this "bolt from the blue" gave divine authorization for Ana, a young Christian woman, to have a hospital delivery, which pushed aside old clay-caked Congolese women and their powerful charms. Mrs. Millman, Nurse Gladys Owen, and a group of young station women left such "old birds of prey" back at Ana's doorway as they led her away at the onset of labor. A brand-new hospital room, a figurative manger where curtains fluttered and flowers quivered was their destination. The missionary women managed the case, though Dr. Chesterman appeared briefly. A Congolese nursing man, the hospital's "head assistant," remained "just outside the door." His role was messenger once the baby was born. The father arrived after the fact from Stanleyville, completing Mrs. Millman's story: "there were angels who leaned to earth to look at Joseph bending over his wife and child."[9]

These two birth episodes suggest that the "patience" Mrs. Millman had called for in 1915 had paid off by 1929. Thirteen explicit accounts of childbirth cases, including Fagg's, appeared in BMS missionary magazines between 1910 and 1956, most in the *Yakusu Quarterly Notes*.[10] Hospital life, orphan work, and nurse and midwife training were frequent topics in Yakusu's quarterly, and motherhood a recurrent theme. Birth was rare. Missionary magazines were an inappropriate venue for the "'shadow-side' of marriage" or being "in the family way."[11] Procreation, like forceps, reached public discussion only in veiled, euphemistic terms. Nurse Owen felt frustrated as she learned more about local obstetric needs because the subject's indelicacy prevented her from writing to mission supporters: "sometimes such awful things happen in midwifery in the villages that one is almost afraid to write it down. . . . It is something about which we cannot write to ordinary Christian Endeavorers & Sunday schools, but the members of various women meetings could be asked to specially pray for these poor women."[12] The reticence lingered into the 1950s. Chesterman took some thirty years to report on his first "midder" (childbirth) case of the early 1920s.

Because there are so few published birth episodes, their trajectory and fault lines may be easily charted. The Congolese ones constitute a neat mission allegory about the triumph and varieties of colonial evangelical "man-midwifery." A husband "in a state of terror" ran to Nurse Gee to come help his wife, dying in childbirth, in 1914. By 1920, Chesterman was "called in" to handle a "breech with delayed head." A "poor woman" came in by canoe from a village twelve miles away in 1933 "suffering terribly"; her baby nearly died of asphyxia, until the doctor cleared the air passages. Mrs. Millman introduced the voice of a Congolese church woman praising the doctor in saving this infant's life: "God does wonderful things through His servants." Another woman arrived at Yakusu in 1939 by canoe, in which she had just given birth to twins, "one almost

dead" but soon saved. A young woman "was in the Presence of her Maker"—
she died—before an obstetric operation "actually began" in 1936, but "a lovely
boy was saved" by the missionary doctor. A Yakusu-trained Congolese nurse
working in the Topoke forest was summoned to help with a childbirth case in
1948; he handled it with guidance from the nearby Dr. Browne, and the occasion afforded the opportunity for a thanksgiving service. Finally, a doctor
intervened with forceps to save the life of Folicepi (Emmanuel) in 1956. Thus,
the wicked old grannies of 1915, caked in clay in 1929, were progressively kept in
order and at a safe distance, as new kinds of Christian attendants became
ordinary.[13]

Four of the thirteen printed episodes were about European, not Congolese,
childbearing. One involved a Yakusu missionary before the station had its own
physician; when Mrs. Smith went into labor in 1910, her colleagues called for
the nearest state doctor. He came by canoe at night to deliver the baby, staying
"only one day" and insisting that the Smiths "should take the first opportunity
of going to England" before returning to the nearby sleeping sickness camp.[14]
The other white cases clustered in the early 1930s; two were wives of plantation
company agents working in Yakusu's district. Mrs. Mill, a trained nurse, responded to an "urgent call" to help the wife of a Lomami Company agent
working in the Topoke forest in 1930. Chesterman used the mission steamer to
reach a "white lady" in "difficult labor" in 1932; he reported saving her life, with
"the little girl being actually born aboard." In 1933, the BMS nurse in charge of
Yaongama's dispensary—perhaps Victor Yenga—was credited with managing
"a white midwifery case in the bush where no other medical help could be
obtained." This case inverted racial expectations, making the incident news-
worthy. The Yakusu-trained nurse was hardly mere messenger boy here. Nor
was he alone; his wife, "one of the hospital-trained girls," helped him deliver
this baby of a Bamboli company agent.[15]

Like all public transcripts,[16] these contain fractures, omissions, and exag-
gerations, some scrupulously construed, some accidental. The episodes also
reveal that Congolese people were turning to missionary doctors and nurses for
assistance, including during childbirth emergencies. European deliveries were
significant, too. Mrs. Millman's 1929 rendering carefully excluded old Congolese grannies and male medical personnel from the birthing room; these were
important fault lines. Yet old grannies were present in the Yakusu maternity
ward even in the last published case, the Folicepi delivery of 1956. The figure
absent from the published episodes is a hospital-trained Congolese midwife.
The male nurse in the "bush," not his wife with hospital training, was hero in
1933. Rather, the story line reads: mission midwifery spread in space as a beneficent presence, so much so that European male doctors and Yakusu-trained

nursing men were progressively accepted in emergency cases far from the central hospital. Private letters, diaries, and memories confirm *some* of this projected public transcript, as we will see.

Bolau and "Untold Things"

When Protestant women missionaries working in "Congoland" gathered for conferences, they would ask each other: "How can we get the girls?" or "What are we going to give them to take the place of their heathen dances?"[17] In 1911, one woman missionary doctor asserted the "unparalleled opportunity" of childbirth, of approaching a Congolese woman in "her hours of greatest need," of "greatest spiritual accessibility and receptivity."[18] Chesterman spoke similarly, but not until 1940: "No service rendered by a mission to a community is more appreciated and brings more vital contact with the people than does midwifery."[19] Yakusu came relatively late to the realization that childbirth might be a fertile domain for Christian domesticity and evangelization. Concerns about polygyny were part of the turning point. So was a woman named Bolau.

Mrs. Millman had opposed the selection of specially trained nurse-midwives as missionaries in early 1920: "in our villages, there is *rarely* need to interfere as normal is the birth of the child." Maternal mortality was, she thought, exceptional.[20] When Nurse Owen arrived in 1923, "to have a woman patient was almost unheard of & I myself was *never* called out to a midwifery case." By 1929, she noticed, the new hospital was nearly completed, and patients were accepting hospital births and autopsies for the first time. There were usually "at least four women in the general ward & a few midwifery in-patients amongst our Station women to say nothing of the District visits." Owen credited Mrs. Millman: "Our midwifery work seems to be on the upward move at last & we have Mama Mokili to thank for that for it is she who has talked to the women and encouraged them to come."[21]

Phyllis Lofts viewed the early history of midwifery at Yakusu differently. The "breakthrough," according to her, began with "district work" in midwifery at Yakusu, a pattern of missionary nurses—first Owen and then Nurse Lofts herself—assisting with local births in local homes. Soon after Lofts arrived in 1926, an anxious hospital construction worker approached Chesterman for help. His wife was pregnant again, he had watched two babies die, and he was worried. If this third one died, too, his "family would press him to take another wife, and that he could not do—he was a Christian." Chesterman asked Lofts to go, understanding that the presence of a man would not be acceptable to local women.[22] His advice was to "sit in the corner of the hut and observe; only offering to help if an emergency arose." A midwife named Bolau was there.

After some hours the baby arrived—asphyxiated—and the wailing commenced among the older women outside. Here was my opportunity, and I offered to help, and Bolau exclaimed "yes, do!" I took the baby and gave the usual treatment and soon he gave a yap. Bolau looked astonished, and became excited as he repeated his protests. She shouted to the women outside "Stop your noise! Listen!" and the scene turned to joy. We soon had the mother and baby son more comfortable, and shared in a fervent prayer of thanksgiving together. That "Yes" of Bolau's started the "breakthrough."[23]

Birth attendance afforded new forms of social power in mission life. Gladys Owen, too, added prayers to birth gatherings. One day, for instance, Owen feared that a hurricane lamp would be knocked over as the women "danced off some of their excitement." She suggested giving thanks to God before she left: "There was dead silence as I prayed but the minute the Amen was said the noise & rejoicings began again."[24] When Owen visited a hospital carpenter's wife in 1929, she found this "dreadful heathen" of whom she was "very fond" in the middle of hiding a pot of medicines. The woman and her mother had been using monkey tail fur and parrot feathers to treat her feverish baby. Owen "laughed it off & took the little party along to hospital & gave baby some quinine." Scolding was unnecessary, the missionary midwife explained, "since I stayed up all night with her when her baby was born & so she always feels ashamed if I catch her doing anything which she knows is not approved of on the Station."[25]

In her own words, Phyllis Lofts became "initiated into the mysteries of midwifery among these Congolese folk" through her role in attending home births. Bolau was a "medicine woman" who controlled the "realm of native medicine and treatment in midwifery and child welfare."[26] Through Lofts's association with Bolau in "district work," she was able to write a detailed ethnographic account—the only one available—of local birthing practice.

> The patient sat on a log, with a friend sitting behind her, so that when pains came she could clasp the friend's neck to assist in "pushing"; . . . Further encouragement was given by friends around, by beating her head with a broom. Bolau sat on a log facing her—and at times examined her to watch for the appearance of the baby's head, using not only her hands, but her dusty toes, in the process.[27]

Lofts did not explain the purpose of toes, still used by midwives to keep fecal matter from dirtying the final stages of birth. Yet she did elaborate on the ingenuity of the local technique for guarding against tearing. As soon as the

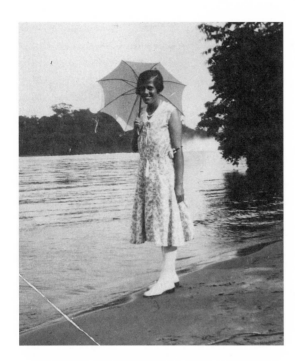

Nurse Phyllis Lofts at
Chopa Falls, a missionary
recreation spot up the
Lindi River, ca. 1927.
(Courtesy of David Lofts,
PL Papers, Barton-on-Sea,
U.K.)

head of the baby became visible, the birth "helpers lifted the patient on to a raffia sling, so that the pressure of it was at the site of the perineum, and gently swung her."[28] Lofts was critical of the tendency to encourage pushing from the early stages of labor: by the time a parturient "reached the second stage she was exhausted." Other local midwifery practices seemed benign. Thus, Lofts accepted instructions to tap the parturient's head with a broom when the placenta seemed delayed.[29]

Lofts's contact with a "medicine woman" was controversial. According to Nurse Owen, Congolese women suffered "untold things at the hands of the old grannies, who are dirty beyond description & steeped in the darkest of superstition."[30] Knowing that Lofts was tapping brooms under Bolau's influence was likely a good part of what moved Mrs. Millman to create a hospital room for Ana's delivery: "What peace is here!" Mrs. Millman exclaimed in 1929. "No beating on the head with a native broom to keep the poor mother-to-be from giving away to fatigue."[31] Nonetheless, the first hospital birth was mediated through the knowledge Lofts gained in working beside Bolau. Lofts's willingness to learn from and help Bolau, who was aligned with the dangerous "old granny" category, is absent from the mission's public story line of events that we saw above.

The crowds and perceived squalor were inconveniences of district work. Owen had little choice but to accede to local Congolese habits as she squatted to deliver babies under what to her were cramped conditions. She slipped in the mud on the way to one birth, began to laugh, and was picked up by a "crowd of women" who led her to a woman in labor lying on a mud floor. About seven women squeezed into the small room awaited her, too: "I could only just fit myself in by squatting on a tiny stool with my knees up to my chin." Owen delivered this baby with her legs caked in mud.[32]

Colonial notions of cleanliness, as much as old granny phobia, inspired the missionary movement of birth to the hospital. Once a doctor had arrived at the station, however, people began to show up at the hospital during obstetric emergencies seeking help. Within months of Ana's hospital delivery, a Congolese woman arrived, four days after giving birth to a stillborn baby, with a retained placenta. The umbilical cord remained uncut, in keeping with local practice. Owen was incredulous: "would you believe it they had never separated the baby from her (which was dead of course). Isn't it just *awful,* just imagine that poor woman, her first baby, born dead & left lying attached to her for four days! in this hot country too! to[o] awful for words."[33] A month later, Lofts and Owen saw "one of those ghastly cases which one hears about in lectures at home but never expects to meet." The baby, dead in utero in a transverse position, "simply could not be got away whole." Chesterman was away on tour, so the two missionary nurses performed the embryotomy without him. The two hours spent dismembering a fetus and extracting it in parts was agonizing for Gladys Owen: "how we prayed silently while we worked."[34] Their surgery saved the mother's life.

Lowering maternal mortality was never the express purpose of colonial midwifery at Yakusu. Evangelization, "getting the girls," and producing a "trained staff of female nurses" were the missionaries' goals. Training girls as hospital workers was fraught with difficulties because people refused to let girls nurse the sick. People were afraid that "when they were menstruating the spirits would 'use' them and cause the death of the sick one." Those girls who "took up the training did so at their peril," as they were "often cruelly criticised by the non-Christian community for breaking taboo."[35] Mrs. and Mr. Millman published *A Mothercraft Manual* for "senior girls" in 1929, and noted that the problem was that "native mothers" refused to accept unmarried girls as assistants during childbirth. Nurse Owen echoed: "the women here will not allow a single girl to see a baby born."[36] While parturients refused the help and hands of single girls, mothers and grandmothers were protecting their daughters from seeing the blood of childbirth that, in local words, "kills eyes."

Again, Bolau helped. When Yakusu's classes for the first four "girl nurses" began in 1929, no "practice work" in midwifery was possible. Six more hospital births followed Ana's that year. Yet the girls in training, all ready with their special nursing caps with tiny red crosses and "white pinafores over their school frocks," were unable to witness any of them. So Owen organized an "ante-natal clinic" in February 1930 to secure promises from pregnant station residents to give birth with missionary assistance. The girls observed their first birth in March.[37] Bolau, according to Lofts, was responsible: she was the one who "tackled the heathen objectors" and diminished "many of the tabus which had forbidden girls to do such work." Eighteen babies were born in the midwifery department of the hospital in 1930, three times as many as in 1929. Bolau also " 'mothered' the girl-trainees." Most came from Mrs. Millman's "house" of girls and the new boarding "fence" at Yakusu. When the chief of Yakoso accused a girl-nurse of making one of his wives ill while in the hospital, for example, Bolau defended her. Bolau and this girl-nurse went together to lead a thanksgiving service in the village after the sick woman recovered.[38]

These struggles over girl-nurses were about local categories for female blood,[39] the difficulties these meanings caused in a hospital situation, and appropriate relations among senior and junior women. The blood of childbirth and the blood of menstruation remain distinct today, as do their significance and potential uses. A woman who is only three to four months pregnant carries a *lisole*, not a *lieme*. A lieme moves within the mother; a lisole emits a dangerous gas. A woman carrying a lisole is as dangerous as a menstruating woman. Neither are supposed to visit someone who is sick or a Mama Wale, that is, a woman in her postnatal or wale period of rest and seclusion. Men, women, and youth alike explained to me that a lisole, made of blood and water, is like menstrual blood; the mixture possesses a gas that can sting and kill someone. "The breast milk of a Mama Wale will dry up," I heard many times about why a newly pregnant woman should not visit the frail or sit on another woman's stool. A lisole's bloody gas is never seen, only touched. Women caution each other to be careful where to sit. The sight of blood from parturition is dangerous to girls and women alike. The midwife and others who tended to a woman in birth performed *lilembu* in 1989 to neutralize the danger of seeing this blinding blood, which also endangers crops and hunting.

More than thirty years after their initial encounter, Lofts wrote of Bolau as Yakusu's heroine of hospital midwifery. Lofts's story, like most missionary narratives, was one of transformation. Yet Bolau was no Salamo, the icon whose cultural production Mrs. Millman oversaw. Bolau's metamorphosis did not fit the simplified, linear, domesticity narratives that Mrs. Millman's reading public was accustomed to hearing. She was neither former slave nor orphan, neither young nor helpless. She was a "heathen" with "great influence in the area" when

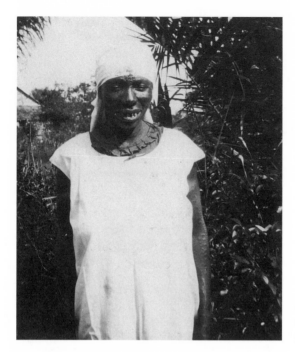

Bolau, ca. 1932. (Courtesy
of David Lofts, PL Papers,
Barton-on-Sea, U.K.)

Lofts first met her: "She was not a witch doctor, but one who did believe . . . that
illness was chiefly because the patient had upset the evil spirits." Bolau "aimed
at seeking some way of appeasing" these spirits: "she concocted 'medicines,' she
said abracadabras over the patient and in her own way did some curious
treatments, some of which increased the suffering and brought terror to all
concerned." Bolau's local reputation as esteemed healer was enhanced, Lofts
implied, because her mother had been banished in about 1893 after a poison
ordeal found her responsible for killing seventeen people when smallpox swept
through their village. An infant at the time, Bolau moved with her mother to
the "'sanctuary' village in the forest, where witches were made to go." She
"never forgot her old mother," still visiting her in the forest when Lofts knew
her as a Christian hospital worker.[40] An abiding European idiom, a "midwife-
witch,"[41] was at play in missionary constructions of "old grannies," as it was in
Lofts's description of Bolau as a "medicine woman" who held local midwifery
"in her own power, and in such secrecy" that she at first seemed unapproach-
able. By 1932, Bolau was a "radiant Christian," church member, and "native
midwife" at Yakusu's hospital.[42] Yet she only appeared in the *Yakusu Quarterly
Notes* once, and then as "first deaconess and Christian mid-wife" when she died
in 1940.[43]

Bolau's exclusion from print underlines the contradictory, perhaps even hotly disputed risks that this old granny figure represented, and the subtle negotiation and exchange that characterized the first years of evangelical midwifery at Yakusu. When Bolau first came to work at the hospital, she had only recently been baptized. Lofts imagined Bolau would continue seeking adultery confessions as she always had when labor was prolonged. Such rubbing of "the abdomen with special pebbles, with incantations etc." was what the "old cronies outside" expected the first time Lofts and Bolau had a case where "there was some delay." Lofts remembered the importance of such confession practices to Bolau's "reputation" as a midwife. The missionary nurse recalled reminding herself: "Be patient; she is young in the Christian faith." Instead, Bolau went to these local women waiting outside and said, "I know just what you're expecting me to do! I shall not do so, for I now know that we should pray to God, and ask His help—so shut your eyes and listen while I pray for this woman!"[44]

This innovation was, as Lofts told it, Bolau's move. Why had this missionary nurse tapped whisks on parturient's heads? She could not see any harm in it, and Bolau had told her to do so. Likewise, when Lofts first saved an asphyxiated child, she had Bolau's permission to intervene. A hospital birth meant there was a firmer spatial boundary keeping "old cronies" outside, but these lay birth attendants were clearly still *inside* both Lofts and Bolau's perceptions of how to administer—and produce—this birth scene. The difference was confidence in and power to change birth ritual. Bolau had both. Lofts, to her credit, knew she had neither. Older female figures with specialized knowledge, such as Bolau, were critical in achieving consent, in recoding ritual. Medicalized childbearing was not simply about persuasion. A figure like Bolau—and my hunch is that there were many Bolaus in evangelical settings in colonial Africa[45]—had the authority to insist, control, and intervene. Bolau substituted prayer for pebbled confessions, but it is unlikely that she went biomedical or evangelical in one fell swoop. When she went to tell the old women outside the delivery room that she was going to pray, there was a door that ostensibly excluded them, but Bolau opened it to declare and defend her refigurations. Indeed, Bolau's local knowledge of social action, and her sense of new obstetric and evangelical duty, extended far beyond a mud room's walls, the borders of hospital confinement, and the borders of the mission station.

Two "Caesars"

One day, Bolau heard that Senga, a woman in nearby Yatumbu, had been sent to the forest to die. Senga had been in labor for four days without giving birth when people decided that "the spirits were angry, and she must go there—

nothing more could be done for her." Bolau asked for a hospital stretcher and two male nurses to help. The story was a key one in Lofts's narrative:

> Off went Bolau, and rescued this woman, and brought her to the hospital, followed by angry men with spears, threatening Bolau that if this woman, Senga, died, they would kill her. Dr. Raymond Holmes performed a Cae- sarean operation, and at the window of the theatre stood these angry men, threatening revenge. Senga was placed in a single room, and Bolau tended her that afternoon. At 4.30 she said she was going home, and I did not blame her—she had certainly had a critical day. But she was back in ¼ hour—with her palette-bed; "Should I leave her here and not help her? If those men came and snatched her away and returned her to the forest, she would suffer and die; no, I shall nurse her day and night." She did so, and accompanied Senga back to Yatumbu in due time; and after that, she would go there on Sunday mornings and bring Senga to our Church for the morning service.[46]

Bolau's act of removing the dying woman from the forest infuriated the men and women of Yatumbu. Some who carried spears threatened to kill Bolau. Even after the doctor had removed the baby that died within her, saving the mother's life, Bolau still feared that some men would try to seize Senga from the hospital and take her back to the forest.[47] The decision making likely began among women in Yatumbu: Senga's midwife or midwives, perhaps her own mother, almost certainly her mother-in-law and other women of her husband's house with whom she shared cooked food and now her childbirth labor. Yet men would have deliberated and argued, too, during those four days with a woman in agony from obstructed labor, a baby jammed in her pelvis. A diag- nosis of social danger from angry spirits was present in the decision to remove Senga from the village. People associated the forest with the dead and their spirits, just as they do today. The spirit of Senga's father had recently threatened her when she went to the forest to collect wood: "Dead leaves blew up in her face, and a log was thrown at her. . . . She . . . heard a voice saying, 'Now you are to be punished, for I have never received my dues in food and payments.' "[48] Senga, terrified, expected to die.

Forest banishments and visits from spirits were not uncommon in Yakusu's district or in records of evangelical medical practice. A BaMbole man was late for church one day because "spirits of the forest had come to his wife in the night and fought with her." He was sure that if he had not "held her down she would most certainly have been taken away."[49] It was also common for a dying person, or one associated with causing death, to be banished to the forest. So it had been with Bolau's mother in 1893; so it remained in the 1930s. Nurses and missionaries tried to rescue people from such local expulsions. In 1932, a dispensary nurse had a pneumonia patient, who had been sent deep into the forest to die, "fixed up in a hut at the end of the Village." In 1937, however, Mr. Parris was unable to persuade men to go into the forest and carry a very sick woman to Yakusu's hospital because they feared, in his words, "her spells." The same men had been obliged "to drag her weary body some four or five miles into the depth of the forest" after village proceedings concluded she was a "witch."[50]

Bolau—as a Christian, hospital midwife, and healing daughter of the forest—had multiple forms of social power at her disposal. She likely drew on them all when she challenged the diagnosis that Senga should be sent away to die. Conflict followed—and preceded—Bolau's bold move. There had been "a good deal of quarreling in her town as to what was to be done" with Senga, before Bolau was even apprised of the situation. Lofts said that old women were responsible for "decreeing that she must go to the forest." Clearly, some of the men were prepared to defend the prescription of the old women. Yet others— Lofts called them "some enlightened people"—sought hospital "help." They set the stage for Lofts's heroine, the brave woman raised in the forest, to enter with a hospital stretcher.[51] A missionary doctor followed with more obvious technology of operative obstetrics, yet Bolau, not Dr. Holmes, was the subject of threats and abuse.

Although still alive in 1936, Bolau was absent from accounts of a cesarean section that took place at Yakusu that year. So were all Congolese midwives and girl-nurses. Dr. Chesterman left Yakusu in 1936, going back to London to work as the head medical officer at the BMS headquarters. Holmes became the senior doctor, and an enthusiastic surgeon who had grown up on stories about Congolese cannibals, Dr. Stanley Browne, arrived.

Three months after Browne's arrival, a young woman of sixteen, the wife of a mission worker, came into the hospital to give birth to her first child. After several hours in labor, Browne became convinced that a vaginal delivery would be impossible given the "extreme smallness" of her pelvic bones. So, he explained, "the only thing to do to save her life and that of the babe was an operation." The husband consented, calling his wife's kin to come "in the darkness." Once their consent had been obtained, a process that involved "some difficulty," Browne proceeded. In a private letter to his family, the doctor reported:

At about a quarter past nine, all was in readiness in the Hospital, and the patient was on the table. We do most of our anaesthetics here by the spinal route; I was just going to give the anaesthetic, the needle was in position, when the girl (who was very nervous) nearly jumped off the table. This must have torn a vein in her spinal canal, for she died of respiratory failure in about two minutes. It was a ghastly experience for us all—for me, for the people in the theatre, and the crow[d]s of friends and relatives, who were gathered round the windows of the operating theatre. However, I realised quickly that something should be done, so while Nurse was busy doing artificial respiration, I operated on the dead woman and extracted a living babe. I then massaged the woman's heart for twenty minutes, and injected a drug into the muscle of the heart wall—but all was unavailing, she could not be brought back to life. The baby was a big one for the Congo, and received all the necessary care and attention.[52]

The incident provoked an uproar. While the husband and the woman's father "received the news in good part," they were not the only ones involved. The sounds of wailing kept Stanley Browne from sleeping. By five o'clock in the morning, "great crowds gathered outside the Hospital" were arguing over who caused this death: the doctor who had performed the surgery or the husband who had consented to it. Browne thought these relatives and "heathen villagers" were "wild-looking folk, armed with knives, and other ugly weapons." As for himself: "I can tell you that I looked much more calm than I actually felt deep down." The doctor believed their anger was misplaced: "they could not see that even although the woman had died, she would certainly have died had nothing been done, and that her death was quite unexpected and due to her own moving during the injection of the anaesthetic." The surgeon assumed that a live baby was as important as a live mother.[53] But in local eyes, to save an infant from a dead mother was ludicrous, even murder. The dead mother's kin did not want the live baby that was removed from her dead body, and this baby was added to the station's orphan list. The baby was named Amos because the mission press where his father worked was printing the book of Amos at the time. But the baby had no mother. Gladys Parris stepped in as caretaker instead.[54]

The two cesarean episodes show how outcomes in maternal life influenced the meaning people made of a cesarean section. When Senga survived after her dead baby was removed, Bolau still feared that the woman's life would not satisfy the angry men and women of Yatumbu. But in the end, the men did not try to seize the convalescent patient from her hospital bed and return her to the forest. Moreover, Senga became a Christian. In the second case, the kin did not want the live baby that Browne had removed from the mother's dead body. A woman had died in childbirth, one of the most dear losses of life possible.

If childbirth proceeds without incident, it is a female affair. "Go ask the women," some men would say to me. "That is not our matter." Yet if the mother dies, the common metaphor about birth—childbearing is dying—is no longer metaphor. Birth has become death. And the death of an adult woman, especially one of childbearing age and in the very act of giving birth, is an affair for men to resolve. After a baby is born, the father should present a chicken to the male elders of the kin group (bokulu, or "house") of the mother. This chicken is symbolic payment. It represents the labor of childbearing and the blood that was lost to produce a child. It compensates the parturient's kin for the danger through which the mother has passed. The childbirth chicken must be paid whether the child survives or not. It does not celebrate a live birth; it compensates for the lost blood of a live mother. If the baby dies, wailing is discouraged. Quite the contrary occurs when a grown person dies; then when not to wail constitutes evidence of foul play. Likewise, a childbirth chicken symbolizes the much larger set of payments that are transferred to maternal kin (*muyomba*) whenever an adult dies. These payments are at their highest if a mother dies in childbirth.[55] This kind of death is so serious that the mother's kin go with lances and spears, as if in war, to demand that this death be paid for dearly. Midwives are also open to accusations of foul play.

We saw that libeli turned on female reproductive idioms, such as the dying of birthing. Childbearing remains associated with warrior idioms: the battle of birth, the winning of a war that a woman who brings a baby into the world achieves. The gesture of men gathering with spears was reduced to caricature in these two missionary-authored episodes. Yet each case was thick with meaning. While a woman is in labor, tension is high. Her male kin, who are not present for the birth, wait with their "hearts up wondering if she will die or not die or if the baby will die." People sing to celebrate if all goes well as if "to say we had a huge matter, hard and dangerous. Now we relax and our hearts cool off." The singing captures the midwife's point of view, too, as if to say "I was a witness," for she, too, would find herself in trouble if the mother dies. A popular Lingala song, encouraged by Mobutu's regime, declared birth as wealth, and development reinforced this equation; it concluded with: "the girl has fought a war."[56]

A Mama Midwife and a Cockney Technicienne

I spoke in 1989 with one of the first Congolese women trained as a midwife at Yakusu's hospital in the 1930s. Malia Winnie was Bolau's junior. She had been raised by Mrs. Millman in her boarding home, and went on to work in Yakusu's labor and delivery ward for over thirty years. When I asked Malia Winnie about cesarean sections, she lowered her voice and spoke more slowly: "They were doing cesareans, but not very many. . . . Doctor Browne, he started the cesarean affair." Dr. Browne liked the "work of the knife" too much. Mothers and babies had died from his surgical kind of childbearing, and local women had become afraid to go to the hospital. "When I came, there were not many cesareans again," Malia Winnie declared. "There were no more baby corpses, there were

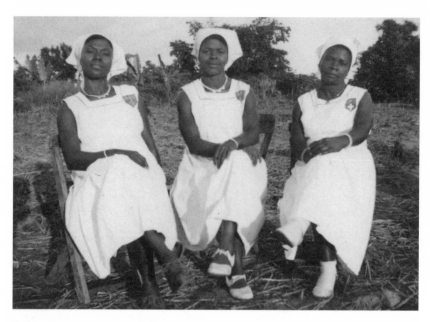

"Malia Winnie, Hana, Miliama," three Yakusu midwives, left to right, ca. 1931. (Courtesy of David Lofts, PL Papers, Barton-on-Sea, U.K.)

no more women to die. Before, with that one who started cesareans, they were dying. I think even three or four." Dr. Browne had not understood, she explained, that "childbearing is dying." Giving birth takes women to the mouth of the grave, said Malia Winnie; this doctor's kind of surgical childbearing was taking women to the mouth of the grave, but they were not coming back.[57]

Malia Winnie (as I will call Wini Kolo Litoi Malia here) had moved into Mrs. Millman's girl's house at the age of eight, when her father, a BMS teacher from Baulo named Paul Litoi, died in 1924. Though her mother was still alive, she was not a Christian.[58] Malia Winnie recalled that it had been Mrs. Millman who decided she should become a girl nurse: "Madame, she didn't want me to go to school again. . . . 'I want you to enter hospital work.' So I entered hospital work."[59] Her heroes were Chesterman and Lofts. They trained Malia Winnie, one of the first girl nurses in the early 1930s.

After receiving her midwife diploma at age fifteen in 1931, Malia Winnie married a teacher evangelist, Tokolokaya. His work took them to Liyeke on the Lomami and then to Yalikina, where by 1933, Malia Winnie was a mother.[60] Tata Tula recalled her "work of delivering women," though he moved immediately to her autonomy and her stormy relationship with her husband: "Malia Winnie stayed here coming from her Tolombo village." A woman refusing polygyny was a rarity in the 1930s. Even more rare was an independent woman with a full-time job at the station. Hence, Tula's unsolicited explanation that "they left each other because Malia didn't like to stay with two wives. She refused it. . . . She left him."[61] Malia Winnie did not mention her marriage. She remembered Holmes and Chesterman calling her to come back and work at Yakusu after Browne did cesarean sections: "The time I went again, the work came out of their hands. Dr. Holmes gave me the work. 'It is no longer our work, it is Malia's work.' Two women died. Right there and then, fear got to people. They started to go backwards. So Chesterman, he looked and said, 'No, we get one woman, one village girl.' "[62]

Malia Winnie was pregnant and living back in Baulo at the time. "Call your Tolombo people!" she recalled being told. Baulo women also spread the news: " 'Heee! A Baulo girl, she got the job. We have ours there. Let's go, that's all.' So women started to come to the hospital, because me, I had started to work—to deliver babies." Soon after she began work, she was busy preparing the linen and clothes for Yakusu's new maternity ward. The provincial governor came and gave her his hand at the official opening in 1939: "Do your work," he said. "I have heard about your work. It makes me happy. Do your work." Malia Winnie took credit for the new ward's success: "They didn't like it in the village again. They said: 'Heee! One of ours is over there!' "[63]

During the early 1940s, Malia Winnie was identifying pregnant women and persuading them to come to the hospital's latest "venture," an antenatal clinic held during market time on Saturday mornings. She would go the few steps away from the hospital, "inviting, persuading, and compelling" women—some formerly station girls, some not—to come. The clinic roll listed thirty-eight women in two months. Malia Winnie also worked on the ward and in the delivery room. Her son, Manwele, came with her as a toddler, trotting around the hospital corridors and carrying patient charts. Being a mother enhanced Malia's social power in and outside the hospital, and perhaps also in relation to the missionary nurses, who were required to be unmarried. Malia Winnie enjoyed "bossing the girls about" and, according to Muriel Lean, another Yakusu missionary nurse, they accepted her authority: "strange as it may seem to us they all take no end of abuse from her without a murmur." In 1942, Lean wrote Chesterman back in London that Malia Winnie was like a "staff-nurse" who could manage any case when the missionary nurse was busy: "She had twins a fortnight ago, the second a breech, and managed them by herself. She loves to get all the girl pupils round her at a time like this and has them waiting on her, but she does make them work properly." When Lean was ill, Malia Winnie delivered her midwifery lectures to the students.[64] Malia Winnie boasted that she could deliver ten babies in a day, while the missionary nurses became, in her words, techniciennes, "just watching me, that's all."[65]

When Dorothy Daniel arrived in 1945, Malia Winnie was still a central actor in Yakusu's maternity ward. Daniel appreciated Malia Winnie's work and accepted her style. Malia Winnie was "temperamental," Daniel told me. Nor did everyone like her. Her knack for writing incriminating letters may have inspired caution. In 1944, she wrote to Bosongo Bonganga (the White Doctor) informing him that another missionary, Dr. P. Austin, had told her several times that if he saw her face again he would vomit.[66] One "had to be in good with Malia," Daniel said, otherwise she would get angry and storm off. The risk, as Daniel saw it, was not only losing Malia Winnie but parturients as well. Acquiescence, especially after the cesarean death of 1936, was the order of the day. When I met Daniel in her home in England, she said that she was shocked when she discovered patients went to bathe in the river the day after a delivery. Another nurse, Stanley Browne's sister Winifred, had found this odd in 1940: "Even the morning after the babe has been born you may see them going down to the river and bathe!! . . . Can you imagine an English woman doing this?" Daniel remembered Dr. Holmes telling her in 1945: "Leave them alone, Dorothy, they'll be all right." How long did patients stay? "It didn't matter to us how long they stayed," Daniel declared. "Most only stayed a few days. They'd decide when they were ready and then they'd pick up and go off. We were just happy to get them at all, you see. It was still early. . . . It was something just to get them."[67]

She and Holmes would never know exactly what Malia Winnie was doing, Daniel explained, especially when Malia would "go off into the forest."

—She'd handle births out there, we knew that.
—For the hospital?
—No, not for the hospital, but she'd go off. Raymond Holmes would say, "Have you seen Malia Winnie?" "She's gone to the village." "Gone to the village, has she?"

Daniel imitated Holmes's amusement as she spoke. She and the missionary doctor knew "gone to the village" meant that Malia Winnie was off being a midwife somewhere else: "We had no choice, you see."

Quick-witted and street-smart, Dorothy Daniel came from the very background that Mary Fagg imagined she saw in the woman who named her baby after obstetric forceps. Daniel would certainly not have told the Congolese woman to choose Emmanuel instead. "I am a cockney and proud of it," Daniel told me; she was born in 1917 and raised in London's East End. Her parents had died when she was twelve. She first became a Christian, she said, because one dark November night after her parents had died, a lady across the way brought her and her elder brothers an apple pie. The following Sunday the lady returned and asked if Dorothy would like to go to Sunday School at the East London Tabernacle. Dorothy asked one of her brothers what to do: " 'Go,' he said, 'We might get another apple pie.' "[68]

Daniel became a devout Baptist who bent to Malia Winnie's ways and joined Dr. Holmes in attitude. The politics of the labor ward were simple in her view. Malia Winnie was "big on enemies," and "we had no choice." But Daniel did want women to come in to give birth, and she wanted to train midwives. In her time, in her way, and under the guiding influence of Holmes, these politics meant letting Malia Winnie and the women patients do pretty much what they wanted. Holmes was a mild-mannered and modest man who everyone—Congolese and British—remembered fondly, if at all. There are no unseemly stories about him. He left no research publication record, and he is also the only male medical missionary who ever appears in the photographic record beaming with a Congolese baby in his arms. A former missionary whispered to me that Dr. Holmes liked to heal while Dr. Browne liked to cut. Holmes was also able to laugh and have good fun. So, we saw, did Browne. Yet their definitions of good fun seem to have differed, even if Holmes assisted Browne with a syringe during his first year of Christmas carol pranks. Holmes was amused by Malia Winnie's double practice, and he would tease the spectators who gathered to watch him operate in Yakusu's theater. When he removed a hernia sac, he would hold it aloft in a teasing way to show that there had been no foul play. One day, the humor turned sour when he threw a bloody piece of hernia sac at his spectators. Someone caught it, and a "row" ensued about how the bodily part would be used.[69] So ended this form of play, though quietly so. Holmes's name appeared in the memories of some Congolese hospital students and workers, but unlike the beloved Chesterman and the feared Browne, former patients did not retain his name.

Nor did they retain Daniel's. Neither did Malia Winnie, even though she was central to Dorothy Daniel's wit. Daniel remembered that she would enter the labor ward to find some old woman demanding that a woman in labor name her lovers. "I would get the baby into the world," she said, while the Congolese women "would do their business."

> Afterward I would take the girls into the sewing room, which was also the lecture room, and talk with them, explain why it had been a delayed delivery—the medical reasons. Malia Winnie would be there with her hands on her hips, watching and glaring. What she told them afterward is anyone's business. They would say "Yes, Mademoiselle, no, Mademoiselle, three bags full, Mademoiselle."

After Daniel's explanations, the midwives in training would go off with Malia Winnie: "She'd put the finishing touches on."[70]

"Could a parturient have other women present at her birth?" I asked. "It was hopeless to keep people out," Daniel replied. "They would just go off." Yet the way the "old mums" wanted the woman to push before it was time was "quite a difficulty." Here, Daniel set limits. "You had to be hard on them," she said, recalling how she would tell them, "Stop! or I'll put you out." Missionary acceptance did not mean an absence of power. There was plenty of power. Congolese midwives described their training at Yakusu as a series of commands: "Do this, do that." They obeyed Malia Winnie. They obeyed Yakusu's missionary nurses and doctors. They likely obeyed older patients, too. Daniel did not completely accede control, though her concerns lay elsewhere: "The wretched pushing down was the greatest bother." She wanted successful vaginal deliveries, untorn parturients, and well-trained midwives. Malia Winnie's "finishing touches" did not interfere with live babies and live mothers, and the girl-nurses passed their exams.[71]

Consider again the image of Malia Winnie in the sewing room with her hands on her hips glaring as this Mademoiselle-nurse taught. Gestures were important to power in this period. Malia Winnie was making herself the commanding Congolese Mama in a situation where the missionary midwife had little capacity to interrogate what she did. Nor was it expected that she should. Lokele exams focused on commands necessary for specific work. Daniel had to translate sentences like:

—Wait near the woman till the placenta has come out. If you do not see it before half-an-hour has passed, come and call me at once.
—Give that woman an enema this evening. When that woman begins to feel birth-pains call me.
—What Lazy Folk! I'm amazed that you dare to sit down while I am staying here to watch you.
—Haven't I told you once and for all that I will not have rudeness from you?[72]

Daniel could read gestures, but never knew Lokele well. "We had no choice, you see," was her refrain. Malia Winnie would go off in the middle of a case and come back with a handful of herbs for the patient to drink. She would say that everything was going to be fine, Daniel said, "whereas I could see it was going to be a forceps delivery." Why stop Malia Winnie from getting some herbs to give the woman a drink? "If we'd refused or tried to stop, they would have just gone off. We had to accept, you see."[73]

Malia Winnie Does Not Go to Jail

Malia Winnie recalled the Sunday she was called away from church to care for a woman relative, Esther Lokangu, who was afraid of the doctor. She had led Lokangu to the labor ward and delivered the baby. Stanley Browne scolded her afterward; he even wanted to send her to jail because she had aided this woman without his permission. She recalled that he came to tell her that she had done the wrong thing when Esther Lokangu had come to her with labor pains. Malia Winnie was able to say to the accusing Browne: "Trouble, what trouble? I do not see any trouble. This baby came into the world just the way all babies do, and I felt a cold wind come into the room, and it was Bwana [God], and He came into the room and showed me what to do." She was also able to say "what trouble?" while pointing to a live mother and a live baby. The mother was alive, the baby was alive, and Malia Winnie did not go to jail. "The child itself is living up to today. 'Winnie,' of course, she got my name," Malia Winnie took pleasure in concluding her story. This baby did not have to be named after a book of the Bible like Amos, Browne's "Caesar" baby, did. It was a happy birth, and the live mother named her live baby after the attending midwife.

Dorothy Daniel recalled that Esther Lokangu had survived an ectopic pregnancy. This prior surgery—likely a salpingectomy with a partial uterine resection, as was common in removing fallopian tube gestations in the 1950s—would have made Browne cautious about the risk of uterine rupture in a subsequent pregnancy. The same logic about prior uterine scarring is, in fact, why cesarean sections are avoided today in contexts like Yakusu, where women may not be biomedically supervised during subsequent deliveries. What Malia Winnie remembered, however, was not Lokangu's medical history, but that she had been told not to go to the hospital after a fight with the doctor. She was just sitting at home when rumors began to circulate that Esther and her baby would die if the doctor delivered the baby.

> I stayed at home, and then people said, "Hey there, if the doctor delivers Esther, Esther and the baby will die." . . . Sunday, it happened like this. They called me. We went to church first, to pray there. "Hee, Mama, come here." Me, I said [to myself], "This matter, if there is a problem with the pregnancy, what will it be like?" Arriving then, the head of the baby was already in the birth canal. Me, I said, "No. They will cut my throat." I carried her there. . . . I carried her by the arm, the child started to come out. I went with her to the Queen Astrid Maternity Ward, put her on the bed like this, and the baby came. The doctor said, "Hey!" Me: "I didn't know you said a black person couldn't deliver her. If you had told me before, then I wouldn't have done it." He wanted to take me up to the State. . . . This hand, [I swear by it], the baby Esther gave birth to was totally a white person, with white fingers. . . .[74]

Malia Winnie posed Browne's prohibition in terms of her race, not her expertise. I once asked Malia Winnie, "Who taught you the work of a midwife?"

Her answer was similar to the way in which local healers explain their knowledge of medicinal plants. They go to collect them and, while in the forest, the wind blows, spirits come to them, and they know which bark or leaves to collect and how to use them.[75] Malia Winnie responded:

> We were working there together, us and Loftsie and Chestermani in that Reine Astrid maternity. The know-how of delivering babies, I got it from *Bwana* [God] himself. I didn't tell anyone. I was just there with this work in my heart. A time when women, even ten, even eight, even six, came at night, it was just me, all alone. If it surpassed me, I called Doctor or Mademoiselle to come there. That time was over. Then I stayed there, me alone. If it was too much for me, the sisters couldn't do a thing either. The work of the doctor it would enter. And so it was that we were there. God blessed us. He Himself taught me to deliver babies, it was Jesus Christ himself, by the word of God.[76]

This conviction probably had nothing to do with Malia Winnie's capacity to stand up to Dr. Browne. Standing up to men who did her wrong was not a problem for this midwife with "enemies." Yet this conviction enabled her to articulate her indignation in medical and theological terms—"It was a normal birth" and "God was guiding me"—that her medical missionary accuser had to understand.

She also spoke to me in local idioms. Malia Winnie spoke about childbearing being a struggle with death. She spoke about a good, healthy baby being born pale white, holding onto a cluster of ideas that link the whiteness of pemba and bodily coverings with health, protection, abundant breast milk, and infant survival. Colonial color categories perhaps reinforced the idea that a reddish, pale baby is an auspicious sign, yet the white chalk of pemba is ancient in local color categories and healing practice. Nurse Gee saw many pemba-smeared patients at Yakusu in the 1910s. Babies are still decorated with pemba marks, as is the house of a Mama Wale. Pemba protects against illness, bad spirits, and menstruating girls and lisole-carrying women emitting the dangerous gas that can dry up breast milk. Malia Winnie would go back to her village when she was a Mama Wale. She did not stay inside by a fire like many women did. She went to be fed and waited on as an honored Mama Wale should be, and possibly also to protect her baby's skin from sunlight so that it would not darken quickly.

Malia Winnie told me about the importance of being tough in childbearing as in life and, when the moment is right, doing the hard work involved. Hitting a parturient into action was sometimes necessary. "It's work, enormous work. Me, I don't like to hit the woman. Unless she is flimsy and hanging there lifeless, *goi goi*, defying all. If she has strength, she'll push out the baby. Those of *goi goi*, dangling there like this . . . the person wants to die. It's bad." Malia Winnie used other local techniques when the need arose. She knew the same animal meta-phors that popular midwives and village women used to perform types of childbearing, their breathing patterns, their rhythms of feeling contractions and chanting, "I am dying, oh."[77] She also thought that having one woman hold a parturient from behind, as is still often done, was helpful in difficult cases. She would ask one midwife to support the woman from behind, empowering her to push.

> We wouldn't do it for nothing, only if problems appeared. . . . Doctor knew, Mademoiselle knew. . . . The one behind, she would be Fear for the woman, thus to give her heart a little happiness, to say "push your baby, so it comes out." . . . Some couldn't do it themselves, only if someone came behind them. . . . "O.K. now, push hard!" . . . Another woman would be here in front. Another there behind. You help her. It's only a matter of helping her strength.[78]

Malia Winnie also privileged the biomedical logic that she had gained in her hospital training about birthing periods and measuring the dilation of the cervix. Did "Loftsie" and "Chestermani" add the Christian dimension to this logic that Malia Winnie so effectively turned against Browne? Perhaps it was Malia Winnie's own mixture of Olombo and Christian healing idioms. Perhaps, too, Bolau had already beat her to it. Malia Winnie attributed her flawless record as a midwife to her understanding what local popular midwives did not: "Childbearing has its own time." Those who think giving birth is just a matter of pushing out the baby as quickly as possible, they "will send her to die."

> Me, I don't like the woman to tear. I don't like her to have hemorrhaging. I don't like her to get tired. If you wait until the time of the child such as God put there, she will give birth well. This one of pushing, pushing—"Do this, do that"—the woman's body will be pressed. So it will be another matter, either exhaustion, or the baby will die, or the mother cannot [push] again.[79]

Pushing was Daniel's battle as it was Lofts's. Bolau likely came to change this old habit; Malia Winnie probably began by accepting new hospital routines in this regard. But they all had to struggle with lay birth attendants who brought their logic of "do this, do that" into the hospital birthing room. In smaller Yalemba, Winifred Browne had "17 people in the small accouchement room" when two women were in labor in 1942: "Now I've insisted on only the nearest relatives." Nora Carrington, who was in Yalemba in the 1950s, said the cries of relatives outside the maternity door telling the woman to push the baby out sounded "like a football match."[80] Their efforts prevailed. Not that local Congolese habit in asili space has changed, but it is common knowledge from Kisangani to Yainyongo-Romée and beyond that what most distinguishes a kizungu birth in a hospital, from an asili one administered by a mbotesa is the timing and duration of pushing.

When I asked Dorothy Daniel about pebbles and adultery confessions, she said: "Yes, they'd rub anything on their stomachs. . . . The intelligence the baby was supposed to have before it was born was enormous. We had to go along, you see, we had no choice. We knew it was a lot of tripe."[81] Malia Winnie never told me that she performed adultery confessions. When I pressed her, she suggested that an old grandmother may have introduced them into hospital space. Malia Winnie located confessions in time. "That matter" was a "before" in her chronology. "Many, many lessons" and new rules came afterward. "That matter, it was forbidden, that matter. . . . Missionary medical people didn't like it. They refused it saying: 'this kisenji matter, don't you come with it here!' "

> It was before. That time when we were taught to deliver women . . . there were no longer these problems . . . of lazy, wasted words. . . . They came, they asked: "You went around with how many men?" . . . "If you were with other men, say it then." Words like that . . . in our time, you washed your hands. That was only talk. . . . You wash your hands, you enter your fingers. If the water hasn't broken yet, you say: "don't push the baby." . . . It's all kisenji, that's all.

What did kisenji mean? "Lack of intelligence, so it gives these thoughts. Lack of intelligence. They don't know the time of birthing. They don't know the time of an infant giving birth pains. Because birth has its time."[82]

Metropolitan conventions about childbirth and sexuality marked missionary birth narratives by omission and erasure. Congolese counterparts to this British evangelical timidity need to be unpacked from what the evidence suggests about the use of rumor and camouflage, critical subaltern tactics of eclipsing some of the stringencies of colonial life. Mama Tula whispered to me one day that she had seen Malia Winnie eliciting confessions. Her whisper was revealing. Forms of secrecy are not static, however. Women whisper about such confessions among each other, and a midwife must never repeat what she has heard confessed.[83]

The evidence reveals several junctures when there was a reconfiguration in maternity power in and near Yakusu. The first came with missionary access to birth; Phyllis Lofts observed rituals with pebbles and confessions, yet she did not intervene. The arena of debate shifted when mission midwifery moved from "district work" to the hospital, when Bolau rejected pebbles for prayer.

The terms of debate were refigured several times, especially as the parties were transposed. Malia Winnie would have had a greater need to prove herself as a midwife in local terms than Bolau; she may have reintroduced pebbles alongside prayer or at least not objected when grandmothers did so. The time of "many, many lessons" and missionary discipline was certainly not Dorothy Daniel's time nor Muriel Lean's. Yet once it came—after the war, after Holmes's and Daniel's departures in 1948 and 1950, likely after Bokondoko's arrival in 1951, too—new forms of colonial camouflage[84] would have been necessary. I suspect that Malia Winnie's altercation with Dr. Browne also dates from this new period in mission midwifery at Yakusu. Once again there was a reconfiguration of power in the maternity ward. Mary Fagg's arrival is part of the story. So, too, are operative obstetrics. Indeed, we must return to Browne's cesarean section of 1936 and the handling of obstetric emergencies in its wake.

"Removing Dead Babies"

Unlike Senga, the name of Amos's mother is nowhere to be found in missionary sources. Her anonymity contrasts with the symbolic weight that her death by a miscarried spinal injection assumed. The case, a cesarean section that saved Amos, had immediate and lasting consequences. Two days later, a woman came to the hospital after being in labor for two days with twins. Dr. Browne declared it a case of obstructed labor and decided "unfortunately it was too late to do anything . . . and we had to send her out to die."[85] Other operations were begun and then abandoned in 1937 because, in Browne's words, "in the interests of the work it is unwise to have a death on the table."[86] While Yakusu's doctors became cautious, Congolese sensed that it was dangerous to give birth at the hospital.

When the new maternity ward opened in 1939, it "met the approval and admiration of all except the old village midwives." So reported Nurse Lean: "These fearing 'the hope of their gains was gone' spread false rumours—the building was for white folk only, the ward was too big and would be very cold at night, mothers confined there would have to pay 150 francs to get out, mothers must stay in the ward till the babies could walk, patients were only admitted if in great difficulties and village help failed."[87] When I spoke with Yakusu's hospital pharmacist, Papa Boshanene, in 1989, he explained that women "before were afraid, saying: 'If you go to the hospital, they will kill you.' . . . There was trouble before."[88]

Tokwakwa tales about the Yakusu hospital were recurrent, yet historically specific. Malia Winnie recalled that intravenous equipment in the labor ward engendered rumors at first: " 'I won't go there. They are going to eat me, cut my arm.' . . . We said: 'Come sit there, so that you might see what we do.' So that ended the mess."[89] We saw that tokwakwa tales were alive in 1924 at the height of the struggle over libeli, when women were afraid to pass the hospital construction site. They surged again around Dr. Browne's blunder of 1936, became encoded with his name at this time, and were still active, although recast, when the new ward opened in 1939. Lean aligned the "false rumours" with old grannies. Yet not only old grannies told—or believed—tokwakwa. Malia Winnie, already a trained "girl-nurse" and mother at some twenty years of age, believed Browne-embedded tokwakwa tales, too. Her tokwakwa variants—in which Browne figures as near enemy-butcher and she as heroic, fashionable, soothing hospital midwife—likely served her reputation and command well. Malia Winnie evoked collective, rational fear of the doctor and his surgery, while claiming a pivotal role for herself:

> They started cesareans because that doctor that we had, Dr. Browne, he only liked to work if it was the work of the knife. When I entered, I forbid it. I forbid the work of the knife. Even if a baby came with one foot, I could get it out. Women wanted to forbid going to the hospital, to give birth there. . . . Me, so, I came with my tough will, because the world isn't good, they will come to imprison me. They didn't like it. The women liked me though. Not one woman was buried. I just worked fine, soothing them.[90]

There were no more cesarean sections at Yakusu after Browne's debacle of 1936 until the 1950s. Indeed, there is only one documented cesarean section between 1936 and 1955; Daniel recorded it in her birth register on March 14, 1950.[91] Yet the "work of the knife"—obstetric surgery—did not end at Yakusu. As Browne noted in 1943: "We have had some difficult midder cases lately—at night, of course, and I have had to operate, removing dead babies, etc."[92] "Removing dead babies" meant performing embryotomies, the "ghastly" operation that Owen and Lofts had used to save a mother's life in 1929. In 1942, Dr. Browne wrote to his family about the "terribly slow work" of teaching "even the rudiments" to the six midwife students.

> After I had spent an extremely arduous and mentally exhausting hour performing an obstetric operation, with all the girls watching, they were asked to describe exactly what I did and why. Two of the girls gave a sort of homily or sermon on the benefits of a Mission Hospital, two others described something entirely out of their imagination, while one girl was so overcome that she could only write: "And we wondered with great astonishment to see what the doctor did."[93]

The girls' responses were not so surprising. When Gladys Owen helped Phyllis Lofts dismember a fetus in order to extract it in 1929, she said it was "too awful to write about." The missionary nurses, too, turned to homily: "how we prayed silently while we worked."[94] Doctors found embryotomies ghastly, too. Laura Briggs has shown that American doctors justified their preference for cesareans in the 1870s, when many still likened this surgery to murder, by the "kind of suffering" that craniotomies "inflicted on *physicians*" who performed them.[95] Seventeenth-century English surgeons also tried to avoid craniotomies. Indeed, forceps are what first enabled eighteenth-century doctors who removed dead, obstructed babies by craniotomy—"the traditional staple of obstetric surgery"—to earn the status of "man-midwives," that is, practitioners associated with live babies.[96] What is remarkable is less the "overcome" Congolese "girls in training" than Browne's expectation that they should help when he did such a "destructive operation,"[97] and that they, in turn, found homilies rather than tokwakwa tales to express their wonder and astonishment. Why was he *not* afraid of more bad press? And did they not tell tokwakwa among each other?

There is no evidence that there was ever an uproar over embryotomies at Yakusu, not even a hint of Congolese moral outrage. Yet many women who underwent these surgeries died in the end. The number of these surgeries increased in the 1950s, just as cesarean sections returned as the method of choice. When I asked the old mission man, Tata Tula, if women ever feared giving birth in the hospital, he said:

> To fear, no. . . . In our villages many women were dying giving birth. But the doctor came. No fearing, just going. Because to give birth to a child, they [mbotesa] will just remove the arm, while the whole body is in the belly of the women; they will make medicines, ah! what is this!! Another child puts a foot first; afterwards our women . . . [are there] just looking at the feet. It is not going to go back. *She dies.* . . . If the doctor sees it like that he will cut. He will remove the infant.[98]

Tula's emphasis in his birth = death equation is significant, especially because this mission man simultaneously expressed a missionarylike, antigranny attitude. "*She dies,*" he said, to chide mbotesa. Doctors, he praised, cut and removed infants to save the lives of mothers. Thus, "no fearing, just going."[99]

Dorothy Daniel could not remember any cesarean sections during her five years at Yakusu. "We only opened one tummy the whole time I was there," she said. The case was Esther Lokangu's ectopic pregnancy: the fallopian tube had burst, the woman was moribund, and the hospital had no blood. No one would give blood, Daniel said, because doing so meant "putting your spirit into another spirit."[100] Dr. Holmes persuaded Esther's husband, the mission printer Samwele Lokangu, that surgery was the only chance. Daniel went to fetch a soup ladle from her kitchen to reintroduce the blood that had collected in the patient's abdominal cavity back into her veins through a gauze-lined funnel. Esther Lokangu survived.[101] An autotransfusion to save the life of a woman dying from a burst tubal pregnancy was not unique at Yakusu or in the Belgian Congo.[102] Such heroism with blood and ladles, however, was not replicable for most obstetric emergencies.

Mary Fagg recalled that when she first arrived in 1951, "*Caesarean Section* was not popular, rarely performed and the mortality rate was high (no blood!)." "No blood!" was a problem everywhere, not just at Yakusu or in Africa. Only after the Second World War did transfusion technology and blood banking become routine in Europe, reducing the mortality associated with C-sections.[103] Transfusions at Yakusu required on-the-spot donors, and donors did not appear without a concerted effort. In 1954, it took four hours—"the suspense was terrible"—to find willing donors with compatible blood for a patient who was admitted eight hours after giving birth to twins and needed blood.[104]

A medical report in 1955 cheered that a cesarean section had been performed at Yakusu, recasting a complicated history of conflict and refusal in facile, evolutionary terms (much as Mrs. Millman had cast the future in 1915): "Until now in this area of the Congo, Caesarean operation has been refused because of prejudice and superstition—it is good to know that this is now breaking down."[105] Fagg reported on two cesarean sections in early 1956; at least four others followed before the close of 1957.[106] The availability of blood for transfusions and of antibiotics to prevent infection had made these surgeries safe, though under other social circumstances, both could have been possible at least a decade earlier.[107] Sulfonamides became available in Europe from about 1937, and were introduced at Yakusu after the Second World War. Before antibiotics, cesarean sections had carried a major risk of infection, and the maternal mortality rate was high. With both antibiotics and blood transfusions, however, the risks of a craniotomy or embryotomy—uterine perforation or unremoved fetal matter leading to sepsis—may have been higher than the risks of a cesarean.[108] Until then, an embryotomy represented a medically appropriate as well as, at Yakusu, a culturally acceptable way of trying to save a mother's life. A telling sign is that missionary women were not exempt from embryotomies at Protestant Yakusu; an Unevangelized Fields Mission missionary underwent a craniotomy at Yakusu in 1946.[109] Caution about exposing Congolese women to uterine scarring—and thus, the risk of uterine rupture during a subsequent, unmonitored pregnancy—was active logic during Fagg's tenure at Yakusu (1951–72), although the celebratory tone of the 1955 report implies otherwise.[110] The same convergence of logics keeps embryotomies part of obstetric practice in some parts of Africa today.[111]

The data suggest that embryotomies declined at Yakusu once cesarean sections became, in Fagg's words, "more acceptable."[112] In 1945–50, 70 percent of the 280 Congolese births that Daniel attended were normal vertex deliveries with no complications.[113] The other 30 percent varied from minor complications, such as a tear needing a few sutures, to much more serious ones: postpartum hemorrhage, spontaneous abortion, placenta previa, stillbirths and retained placentas needing removal, a ruptured uterus, and maternal death. Nine cases were forceps deliveries, three were embryotomies, and one was the 1950 cesarean section that Daniel forgot ever happened.[114] Between mid-1953 and early 1959, of sixty-one cases in an obstetric operations register, there were fifteen forceps cases and thirteen destructive operations. The number of embryotomies—six—was especially high in 1955.[115] This cluster may have encouraged the change in attitude about cesareans. The number of embryotomies decreased once C-sections came into play. There was only one destructive operation in 1956; there were two in 1957.

After Amos's delivery by cesarean section following the death of his mother, both European and Congolese cultural logics and wills constrained Dr. Browne and his colleagues to the "compassion" of craniotomies.[116] Yakusu's doctors were called on to save not babies' lives, but mothers' lives. Calls for instrumental interventions came very late, often after a woman had been in labor for several days and the baby was already dead. Under the circumstances, embryotomy was often the only chance of saving a mother's life.[117] The emergency-oriented character of Yakusu doctors' obstetric practices is a striking feature of these cases—and it, too, had a cultural as well as a medical logic.

Yakusu's hospital had two distinct obstetric patient profiles. By the 1930s, one set of obstetric patients lived close by and could easily walk or be paddled to the hospital; they tended to be church members or the wives of workers living at the mission station, who had regular encouragement to receive antenatal observation.[118] Their numbers were small, and Ana in 1929 was the very first. The other set of patients came from farther away to seek help. Yakusu's medical missionaries began to see these "ghastly" cases in precisely the same year, though Nurse Gee had a glimpse as early as 1914. After the hospital and then its maternity ward opened, missionary doctors were no longer *called in* to village cases; women had to find their way to them, or at least to the riverbank by canoe.

Winifred Browne was exceptional because from her base at the downriver BMS post of Yalemba in 1941 and 1942, she would answer village and canoe calls for "midder" help. Her daily diary reveals how much her practice was dominated by those to whom she had given antenatal care. These women had names and identities: "I'm expecting another midder case soon, Balomboya, Victor Maculo's wife, 1st baby." This "Mama Monganga" knew when they were due, admitted them at the onset of labor pains or well before, scheduled inductions

("Gave Ngbangha medical induction—v. small pelvis, bad posterior lie of babe"), administered morphine when she thought a woman in labor needed it, and visited them afterward in their homes. She also learned about beliefs shunning colostrum and favoring tinned milk. Though fewer proportionally than at Yakusu, most of her emergencies were anonymous women who arrived by canoe long after labor had begun, sometimes with obstructed labor, but often with retained placentas up to six days after a child was born.

The intimate quality of relationships generated by continuous care is absent in the Yakusu evidence. There were early admissions of women from nearby villages diagnosed with toxemia, Daniel noted; some women, at least, were receiving antenatal care. Winifred Browne also kept a diary during the short period that she stayed at Yakusu in 1943. The names she knew at Yakusu were not those of the parturients, but of the Congolese midwives—Folo, Salamu, Malieti, Limengo—whom she helped deliver babies, sometimes their first cases.[119]

From 1945 to 1950, according to Dorothy Daniel's register, less than half of the 280 parturient Congolese women that she attended lived at the mission station or nearby, especially at Yakoso and villages immediately upstream from the station. These women had easy access to the hospital when they went into labor.[120] Scattered evidence from 1929 on suggests that Yakusu was always handling a considerable proportion of emergency cases, with women coming in after days and days of labor with impacted, long-dead fetuses within their exhausted wombs. The number of late admissions and especially unplanned, late-arriving emergencies is the most striking aspect of Daniel's register. In almost 10 percent of all cases, the woman arrived at the hospital late. Twenty-one women had been in labor many hours, sometimes days, before even setting out for the hospital. It was these women who came from afar, often by canoe, who were most likely to undergo craniotomies and forceps deliveries; these women were also most likely to die. Because those who came from faraway arrived in the gravest condition, craniotomy was often the intervention of choice, if not the only one available.

Several factors were shifting as cesarean sections began to be practiced again at Yakusu during the late 1950s. Blood transfusions made C-sections much safer for the mother. Antenatal care had commenced under Mary Fagg. She not only identified Boyali as in need of hospital treatment for anemia until she gave birth, but her district clinic work extended antenatal care over a much wider space. It is likely that Dr. Browne's struggle with Malia Winnie over her intervention in the Esther Lokangu case was, at least in part, his defense of the better antenatal screening for potential emergencies that Yakusu patients were supposed to receive. He knew about Lokangu's previous ectopic pregnancy, appreciated the fact that her uterus had already been cut into during this ladle-marked operation, and feared uterine rupture in the event of an inadequately monitored vaginal delivery. During the 1950s, maternity wards were going up throughout the Belgian Congo, and most Congolese women in Yakusu's district had shorter distances to travel and greater incentives to participate in social obstetrics as new facilities and technologies arrived in their midst.

Mission Midwifery

As a Protestant mission, Yakusu combined its interest in hospitalizing birth with promoting domesticity. Christian women who lived at the station were the express focus of maternity efforts; maternal hygiene would enable monogamous marriage, clean lives and bodies, and spiritual transformation. A woman in childbearing crisis, seen as particularly open to conversion, could make a good parable. But Yakusu's missionaries did not seek out these crises any more than other colonial doctors did. Just as Mrs. Millman invoked biblical symbolism in narrating a story of hospital childbirth, Congolese ascriptions of meaning were encouraged when couched in Christian terms. Mrs. Millman was keen to tell of a station woman who rose in a church meeting to testify about the miracle she witnessed when the mission doctor saved the life of an asphyxiated baby.[121] Some Congolese pregnant women spoke of the "magic of the waters of baptism" and sought to be baptized "before the child came."[122] Mrs. Millman was pleased with such talk, and it went to press.

The impact of high infant mortality on the capacity of Christian converts to remain monogamous became a mission concern. The Yakusu church forbade polygyny in 1908.[123] Consequently, many men did not join the church. Given the rate of infant mortality in the region, which was as high as 50 percent during the late 1920s,[124] the rule interfered with men's capacity to have many living children. Other men were expelled because they took a second wife after their first did not prove fertile or had not produced surviving children. As one man explained in 1913: "If you follow Baptism you will die out; there will be no people because you will only marry one wife."[125] Basuwa of Yatolema, a church evangelist, watched his wife give birth to eight babies, all of whom died. His father's people "heaped abuse" on him: "Remember So-and-so he was a teacher and had no children; but he left the work and now has three healthy children." Others took up the tale, and everybody said, "Why don't you do something? What's the use of saying I am a man of God, when God doesn't help you?" Basuwa took up his hymn book instead, becoming a hero in the *Yakusu Quarterly Notes*.[126] But hymns and church work did not console most Congolese men in similar situations. One old man was known in Yainyongo-Romée as Tata Alikuwa or "Mr. He Was" because he was a BMS church teacher until he was fired for marrying a second wife after his first did not give birth to surviving children. Tata Alikuwa lost his church job, but he became a father; his nickname keeps alive his story. Mrs. Millman understood the power of such stories.[127] And many Congolese mission men, as we saw with Lofts's "breakthrough" case, sought obstetric assistance for their wives.

Mission midwifery first came into play at Yakusu in 1914 as an emergency service where Congolese women with retained placentas or obstructed labor called for help, walked in, or arrived by canoe. Bolau's vision of what midwifery services should be was remarkably different from anything that came before or has come since. She wanted not only to rescue a woman dying in childbirth, but to recast local etiologies—how people interpreted why Senga was afflicted with a blocked birth, a condition called *lokwamisa*. Bolau's move pitted her not against missionaries, but against the men and women who had decided that Senga should be banished to the forest and left to die. Once the men were involved, they were pitted against the surgeon, yet they were also spectators of a surgery that saved the mother's life. Bolau was already a renowned healer, midwife, and grown woman by the time she met Phyllis Lofts and learned new biomedical techniques for handling neonatal asphyxia. She also began to substitute prayer for pebbles and confessions in a case of prolonged labor. Thus, some of her new techniques were biomedical and evangelical, not unlike the mixture of approaches that Yakusu's evangelical missionaries practiced. Critical to the role that Bolau played was Lofts's approach. Critical to Bolau's reputation, and likely to her capacity to cross the boundary into the hospital world, was her special knowledge of forest medicines. Bolau became a Christian, and saving Senga from the forest was part of how she imagined her new work. But Bolau's idea did not easily catch on. Women kept arriving at Yakusu for help in obstetric help in emergencies, as many still did in 1990.

Malia Winnie had long experience with multiple missionaries before she became a midwife. Dr. Chesterman and Nurse Lofts were her teachers, and they remained her heroes.[128] Not so Dr. Browne, who unlike Lofts and Daniel, imagined he could be in control; Malia Winnie soon detested him. Stanley Browne was an expert surgeon, and he became a renowned leprologist as well as the subject of two florid biographies published in 1960 and 1980.[129] But he had no sense in 1936 that a patient brought into as bewildering a space as Yakusu's operating theater should be held still to prevent movement during the administration of a spinal. Malia Winnie's hostility may well have made his reputation as a bad doctor spread. Browne was never the only doctor at Yakusu; he was junior to Holmes until the early 1950s. It was likely the modest Holmes who decided that there must be no more deaths on Yakusu's operating table and asked Malia Winnie to come back to restore confidence just as Yakusu's first maternity ward opened its doors in 1939. He, Muriel Lean, and Dorothy Daniel gave Malia Winnie considerable reign to be boss in the maternity ward.

Malia Winnie did not go out and rescue pregnant women for hospital deliveries as Bolau did. She started a parallel practice, and Holmes and Daniel knew and would joke about this fact. Daniel also did not mind the accoutrements and medicines from local practice that were introduced into Yakusu's delivery room by Malia Winnie and lay birth attendants. She had one goal: to get a parturient not to begin pushing until the right moment in terms of dilation. She let the rest go with a laugh, admitting that her Lokele was weak and "we were lucky just to get anyone."

Colonial birthing rooms were important arenas for secrecy. The historian must weigh how the evidence available—whether contemporary or postcolonial in vintage, whether textual or oral in form—was abridged or edited in answer to competing needs for knowledge, rumor, and camouflage. Victorian prudery worked to erase obstetric detail from written, missionary-authored sources as late as the 1950s. Postcolonial memory, too, remains marked by assertions of secrecy.

Papa Boshanene spoke of "trouble before." Certainly moral outrage over failed cesarean sections was part of this trouble. Yet there were other, earlier troubles as well. A Congolese grandmother feared the baby born to her improperly married mission daughter in 1915, just as local women feared that European clothing would harm their fertility at the time of libeli in 1910. Women were afraid of becoming tinned food when they saw the hospital construction site in the mid-1920s, just as libeli of 1924 raged. People began to accept both autopsies and hospital childbirth in 1929, just as the rebound from libeli peaked and at the same time that Mrs. Millman guided Ana on the path to becoming the hospital's first parturient. Trouble did not end there. The crucial local factor in any birth was for the mother to survive, ensuring that the expression "birthing is dying" remained figurative, that birth blood was symbolized in a chicken and not realized in the death of a mother. The chronology of obstetric interventions reveals that what mattered was not any specific obstetric technology, such as forceps or a craniotomy crotchet, but how Congolese kin and birth attendants interpreted the use and outcome of an instrument.

Reproduction and maternalism, long-standing idioms at Yakusu, were medicalized only from the 1920s. Even then, what the Yakusu mission published about medical work with women and infants tended to be about baby contests and orphans. Mrs. Millman's vignette called "Mothercraft on the Congo" drew on the Salamo story of a mother bringing her daughter to be raised in Millman's boarding school: "Mama, mother her, for she is such a baby."[130] There was rarely a medicalized discourse about infant mortality. Nor were maternal

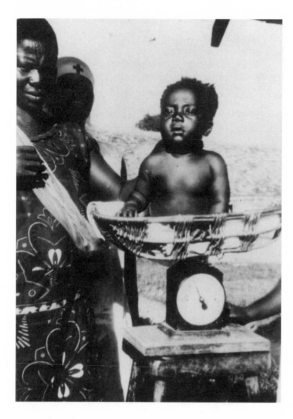

"The prize baby" at a
Yakusu baby contest,
ca. 1929. (Courtesy of
David Lofts, PL Papers,
Barton-on-Sea, U.K.)

hygiene and medicalized childbearing ever the top priorities of Yakusu's doctors.[131] Tragic narratives about the suffering of Congolese mission workers and evangelists who watched their children die were frequent in the *Yakusu Quarterly Notes*. Unlike elsewhere in Africa at the same time, including in the Belgian Congo, Yakusu's missionaries did not represent this death rate as a crisis. Rather, infant mortality was a routine context of the daily reality of ministering to local people, consoling them in their grief. Likewise, the station's first baby clinics represented evangelical opportunity more than preventive health work. Maternal mortality was absent from missionary rhetoric, as it was from most colonial discourse in the Congo. Still, dying mothers were not absent, as we have seen, from how the history of childbirth unfolded at Yakusu.

Trouble Trouble

What shaped Congolese women's responses to obstetrics was not technology per se, I have been arguing, but rather outcomes in maternal life. The 1936 incident made cesarean sections and Dr. Browne unpopular. Samwele Lokangu was not the first mission man to accept a surgical intervention; mission men were leaders in accepting operative obstetrics. When babies kept dying in his wife's belly during the 1930s, Tata Tula agreed when Chesterman told him, "If I see that the *mimba* [pregnancy] is near, I will go to get her. We will do an opération here, to take out the child." This surgery never occurred.[132] But some husbands trusted doctors, and male kin would gather to sanction these operations. Their decisions influenced women's experiences of childbearing, even if surgery was not performed. Biomedical intervention did not necessarily become central to female memory, however, as the following recollection shows.

One day, I spoke with a Yakoso woman who had given birth in the Yakusu maternity ward during the 1950s. The woman began by describing a repeated, routine experience: how labor pains feel, how she could tell that it was time to set out and walk to the hospital, and how during delivery the medical people would come to catch the baby. Then she came to a concrete memory about the disposal of a placenta. The woman had named her baby Tabu Mateso or Trouble Trouble because of the trouble she underwent. Dr. Browne had proposed surgery. Yet her trouble, as she explained it to me, turned on her future fertility, on tensions in her relations with the female kin of her household, and on the disposal of her placenta. The conversation went like this:

> —If you feel labor pains here, sometimes you yourself can figure it out that it is time, you start down the path to the hospital, to the maternité. At the very time that you go to stay there, God helping, you're just feeling the contractions, feeling the pains. When the time comes for the baby to come out, the medical people come to do their work of receiving the baby. You give birth. Those things that remain in the stomach come to fall out as well after the baby. And so there, coming out of there, they come to put you on the bed. They put you on the bed. People come to say-say to you: "You, you didn't give anyone food, these things that fell down, the placenta, we won't go throw it [in the river] for you." They were say-saying trouble there . . . saying to me: "Me, I won't discard it, you yourself go throw it." If you don't give people food, they say she is selfish, let her go herself to throw away her stuff, just like that they will do it. Afterward, they give food and cook water on the fire, I go to lie down. They're there giving food; you eat as if you gave birth well. You're just eating, talking with the people there. When the time comes to leave, you come to stay in the village.
> —Who refused to throw your placenta? Some of your kin?
> —Yeah. If someone isn't nice, she won't throw it for you. They refuse often

because, saying that if you go on to not give birth again afterward, sometimes it will be said: "That's the one who threw it, so she bewitched her."
So like that they tend to refuse, saying: "I won't go to throw it because they
will come to say I bewitched her placenta."

—So when you gave birth, who threw your placenta?

—That time I gave birth, me, I gave birth to my first child with troubles.
Her name, Tabu, Tabu Mateso [Trouble, Trouble Trouble], because I gave
birth with troubles, and Browne he was still here. One white man, he
stayed here, Browne. . . . I had troubles. That time when he stayed here, if
he would operate today, if four people came, three persons would die.
One, then, he would get well. So it was, I was having big troubles. I went
there to the hospital to be looked at. There I was lying for three days
without eating. I was just in labor, that's all. He said, "No, go call her
father." My husband went off traveling the second day; he went to call my
father. Because Browne said not until, because he was . . . a *bokumi* [church
elder]. He said, "I won't do this work unless her father arrives here." So like
that my husband went off to get them, they by the time they came, the
baby didn't wait again at all, just like this the baby came down. I wasn't
made to do any more work. I gave birth to that baby, a small baby. I stayed
with her in the maternité. People to hold her: Mademoiselle didn't like it
because the heart of the baby might go entirely. . . . I had troubles because
of that first child.

—So did he do an operation?

—He didn't do the operation after all; just like that God gave a hand, I gave
birth, and the men relatives ["fathers"] arrived afterward. . . . God helped
me. They did their asili matters.

—What kind of things?

—To spit-spit saliva, to spit saliva, all the people here, they put their spit
together, they put it in a cup early in the morning, they came to have me
drink it. And so I drank it, and I gave birth to the baby. . . . They saw and
said, "These asili things of ours here is what did this for you."

—What kinds of things?

—Hey, there, aren't there witches there? There in your homeland, aren't
there witches there?

—They said it was troubles with witches?

—Yeah.

—They didn't say it was troubles of going around with someone else
[adultery]?

—No, no.

—They didn't see it like that?

—No.

—They didn't do this thing of naming lovers' names?

—No, no, they didn't do that business. I didn't know that business.[133]

Another woman interjected that in "the old days" and "even today," a newly married woman will be given a place to cook food after she leaves bowai. If a woman cooks and does not share with people, when she gives birth "that day even . . . they will say to you, they'll say, 'She herself, she will dispose of her *eulanda* [placenta]. We, the people of her husband's family, we won't carry it for her, because *she*, she is selfish. She didn't give us anything.'" They will wait until that moment when they can no longer be accused of tampering with her fertility to complain and humiliate her: "So, they will say, they will say, it will be saying only. One, she will agree. They will go to throw it . . . [or] to bury it in the earth."[134]

The catalyst for this woman's memories was less surgery than the humiliation when female kin mocked and abused her, a struggle that was ultimately over her future fertility and the proper sharing of food. "Who finally buried it?" I asked the mother of Trouble Trouble. "They did," she said, "they were just 'say-saying.'" They humiliated her, yet eventually they took care of the placenta. This woman's recollections of childbearing at Yakusu began as an account of a routine, yet an altered routine. The reputation of the doctor was well known. He had wanted to perform surgery, perhaps a cesarean section. Browne insisted that her kin give their permission first. Even though surgery was in the end unnecessary, the arrival of the parturient's male kin likely heightened the teasing of her birth attendants. Their threat to refuse to bury the placenta was degrading; it signified a lack of generosity with food. Thus, the catalyst for this woman's autobiographical memory was not the possibility of surgery, but this struggle among female kin over the disposal of a placenta. The dispute transpired unhampered, as did the saliva therapy, within the walls of the maternity ward. Still, the doctor's proposed therapy somehow had worked to alter the context of debate. The baby was alive, and the saliva therapy showed the value of asili ways. The parturient's male kin were also on the scene, however, called there by the now-cautious Dr. Browne. These men would have been hungry, magnifying postnatal cooking responsibilities for the women in the household. The effects can be glimpsed in their anger, in their teasing and abusing their brother's wife, by acting as if to refuse to tend to her subsequent fertility.

"It's about the End" and Christmas Laughter

Mary Fagg was surprised to hear that craniotomy was still performed at Yakusu in 1989, although she was less shocked when she heard that the fetus would already be dead. Her relief suggests that her doctor colleagues may have been removing not only dead but live babies by destructive operations. I have often wondered about what appears to be a peak in embryotomies just as cesarean sections were "becoming more acceptable" at Yakusu. Craniotomies have been associated in other times and places with malnourished, colonized peoples, racialized surgical experimentation, and an indignant sense of the unworthy affliction such surgeries posed for surgeons. In 1870s' Philadelphia, as Laura Briggs has shown, the case of Josephine Scott—a black woman with a rachitic, contracted pelvis who died after her third craniotomy—"marked a turning point in the willingness of physicians to attempt the caesarean."[135] A black, colonized, Congolese people—tokwakwa-tellers who objected to anything that resembled the disembowelment of women's bodies, who remembered or had heard about the fatal 1936 cesarean section at Yakusu, and whom missionary surgeons (at least Stanley Browne) easily conflated with cannibals—long denied such a turning point to Yakusu's surgeons. Is it possible that this denial may have stirred a punitive current in obstetric practice, expressed either in an increase in embryotomies just as "prejudice and superstition" against cesareans broke asunder or in the demeanor of their execution?

Hired by Browne and deeply respectful of him, Fagg knew these extractive, skull-crushing operations performed on babies as "horrible," "a terrible thing," this surgery of "crushing the babies," where a doctor would "put a horrible spike in, open the skull up, and let all the brain out," sometimes cutting off an arm as well if it was a big baby. A craniotomy, Mary Fagg concluded, is "about the end." Her aesthetic and moral revulsion could not have been stronger. She also knew that Yakusu's doctors had not been doing cesareans when she arrived in 1951, although she referred to previous maternal deaths obliquely. It was not necessarily the parturients who refused, she said, but either the doctor or the family who were "not keen." If there was a risk of losing the mother, she continued, "it was not worth getting them cut up because people would say the surgeon had killed them, and that doesn't work."[136] One can hear some retelling of Stanley Browne's experience speaking through her words. The exigency of detestable embryotomies, their loathsome aesthetics, the sacrificing of beautiful brown babies for the descendants of cannibals—such topoi were likely part of a missionary point of view at Yakusu. A craniotomy may have been an act of human compassion in the seventeenth century, as it was in the ancient world. But by the nineteenth century, obstructed labor and its more gruesome sequelae—craniotomies and vesicovaginal fistulas—became aligned with dark, enslaved skin, at least in some parts of the Anglo-Saxon world, before cesarean sections became more routine.[137] By the 1940s and 1950s—indeed up to today— embryotomies have survived only as a "tropical" necessity, hence more than ever aligned with colonized populations and "the developing world."

What happened to compassion in light of these alignments when a woman was dying of obstructed labor in colonial Africa? If craniotomy felt like an imposed, uncivilized activity at Yakusu—aligned with darkness but unthinkable at home, still performed in a colonial situation in order to prevent accusations of murder by C-section, even though the mother often died by craniotomy anyway—what happened to compassion for maternal life? And what were the implications for physicians? The amount of skill required for a successful embryotomy is considerable, and most colonial doctors would have learned on the job. A cesarean section was easier to perform, and doctors had been trained in the procedure in Europe. The maternal mortality rate was not negligible at Yakusu; of the three embryotomy cases that Daniel noted, all of the women died, one two days later from sepsis and two of uterine rupture.[138] Given that the line between compassion and cruelty was already clouded when it came to craniotomies, what kind of ambivalences and abuses could arise when the leverage of local terror tales and the sight of women dying from obstructed labor made outsider doctors feel obliged to act in "horrible," "terrible" ways? Craniotomies were, it seems, a concession to local African moralities, circumstances, and preferences, yet such a concession, as Fagg's testimony hints, strained the modernizing, pro-baby moralities of Yakusu's missionaries.

On Christmas Day in 1936, the line between compassion and cruelty wore pretty thin. No human medium perhaps is able to tread such a line more coyly than laughter. That year, Browne began his Christmas caroling capers with his doctor colleagues. The possibility of good, affectionate fun in his blinking human skulls irrevocably acquires a sinister, punitive edge in light of this doctor's own need for the catharsis of colonial humor after his experience of being haunted, only a few months before, by men approaching him with knives and spears. Yet this was not the only Christmas laughter of 1936. Someone chose the biblical story of Solomon's judgment as the subject for the annual Christmas play performed by station Congolese for a large and festive gathering on a Yakusu lawn. Christmas plays were a time for teaching moralities, but festively so. In 1936, good and bad motherhood was the theme. There is little detail on how this story from the Old Testament was staged. Yet the surviving, contested baby in the mission play was none other than Amos, the unwanted baby whom Dr. Browne had rescued by cesarean section from the dead, anonymous mother who, depending on one's point of view, jumped when she shouldn't have or was sacrificed—cut up, divided—for the sake of a helpless baby. So up stood a Congolese King Solomon at Yakusu and rendered his judgment that the three-month-old, unwanted Amos must be cut in half, dividing the body between the two wrangling mothers. Once the good and rightful mother pleaded that Amos be saved, of course, Solomon completed his judgment in her favor.[139] Who made this casting decision? Was it merely tactless or something else? Who moralized how? And, most important, who laughed and how? I do not know. But this example demonstrates that Stanley Browne's woes were not only being acted out, but recast as well, during Christmas laughter festivities in 1936. If the play's moral was indeed one of maternal sacrifice for a bonny baby, we do know that the message did not succeed for the next twenty years, either with patients or doctors, in the everyday Yakusu world of operative obstetrics.

6 COLONIAL MATERNITIES

Obstetrical assistance is . . . an efficacious instrument for the rational transformation of native life.—V. Cocq and Fr. Mercken, 1935

La colonie est le paradis de la paperasserie.—Marie-Louise Comeliau, 1945

"Bwana, I have a son since this morning." Or perhaps the approach would be: "My daughter was born at the sixth hour of the day." The Belgian coffee planter would interrupt his work to congratulate the Congolese father whose wife had just given birth in the workers' camp. "*Primo mihi,*" the laborer would say in Swahili, asking for his birth bonus (*prime de naissance*) worth five days' pay. Three to four days later, the mother, the husband, and other kin would approach the plantation headquarters to present the newborn. Only mother, father, and child would be permitted on the colonial veranda or *barza,* and a Mademoiselle—Bwana's sister—would inscribe the baby's name into the plantation's book of children. The "cortege" would continue to the dispensary, where a European nun would examine the mother and child. Then, the family would return to Bwana's house for another birth bonus, a cotton cloth for the wife. "The rites thus being accomplished, baby has nothing else to do but grow, as the weighing inscribed in the dispensary book each week will certify."[1]

These scenes come from Marie-Louise Comeliau's historical novel, *Blancs et Noirs* (1942), set on a plantation in the Kivu region during the interwar period. The independent *colon* was playing paternalist, pronatalist Bwana by paying birth bonuses and advancing bridewealth payments to workers who signed three-year contracts: "If the paternal State has not yet concerned itself . . . with imposing social assistance in such circumstances, the Bwana has provided therein, and the birth bonuses are well appreciated by the personnel."[2] The nun's dispensary was a counterpart to the planter's veranda in Comeliau's images. They demonstrate that family policy in the Belgian Congo was about more than "babies and the state."[3] Belgian colonial pronatalism embraced transactions among working fathers, maternalist employers, and baby-weighing nuns. Independent planters, mining companies, and the Force Publique used social Catholic routines to mark Congolese births with bonuses, inscription, and baby scales.[4] Yet Comeliau's nun was *not* a midwife. Nor was there any attempt, according to Comeliau's popular colonial account, to intervene in the birth process itself; Congolese midwives without any colonial training (*matrones*) handled births in the plantation worker camps.[5] Yet at birth bonus payout and inscription time, a colonial vision of family was at play, limiting those allowed on the veranda to father, mother, and baby.

Consider, too, a scene from British Baptist Yakusu. On November 15, 1939, many people gathered at the station for the official ceremony opening the hospital's new maternity ward,[6] a separate building named Maternité Reine Astrid in memory of Belgium's queen who died in a car accident in 1935. As we saw earlier, when Princess Astrid visited Yakusu and its hospital in 1933, this symbolic colonial mother had been pleased that local women were "coming in ever increasing numbers to have their babies born with the help of the Doctor and nurses."[7] Yakusu's use of a queen's name to bless a colonial hygiene enterprise was not a novelty. The Congo's most important health program for Congolese before World War II, FOREAMI, was named after Queen Elisabeth in 1930; and her image still marked hygiene booklets for Congolese mothers in the postwar period.[8] Such commemorative naming at Yakusu proved effective. No Baptist Missionary Society funds were necessary for the Maternité Reine Astrid. Instead, local Belgian colonial "friends," including at least one plantation company, gave thousands of francs beginning in 1936.[9]

The opening ceremony was "a far bigger do" than Dr. Holmes had expected. The date was November 15, the Fête du Roi in the Congo as in Belgium. Yakusu's senior missionary welcomed the crowd that gathered, including local chiefs, Protestant Congolese, and an official Belgian party that came down from Stanleyville. The provincial governor made a speech in French, the district commissioner followed in Kingwana, and Holmes came last in French and Lokele. The ceremony closed with everyone singing the *Brabançonne*—the Belgian national anthem—and joining in prayer. After giving a tour of the hospital, Holmes held a luncheon for the official party at his home. The other fifty Belgians from Stanleyville went off on the steamer to visit the Belgika plantation at Ile Bertha, returning later to collect the official party. As the boat pulled away from Yakusu for a final time, Holmes and the other missionaries heard "cheers from the visitors who started to sing God save the King." The band soon joined in "with all the officials at the salute." Holmes described the gesture as "altogether a very gracious act," though he had been disturbed during the visit by the "discordant voice" of the chief provincial doctor, Kadener, who was "in his most cynical mood."[10]

Yakusu's missionaries had long been aware that not all state doctors and officials were fond of the British Baptist doctors in their midst. Perhaps this explains the careful mixture of symbols utilized to show off the new ward. An embroidered white linen cloth with the words "Maternité Reine Astrid" decorated the center table. The blankets were scarlet, the head steads were black, and "multi-coloured squares of warm knitting" dressed up the baby cots. A Belgian flag draped a bronze plaque. Pictures of "the Nativity, the Arrival at the Inn, Christ and the Children, and a photograph of Her Late Majesty Queen Astrid" hung from the walls.[11]

An evangelical reading of childbearing was not new at Yakusu, of course. Evoking mission midwifery through biblical metaphors had been Yakusu style since Ana's journey to a manger-like hospital in 1929. Nor was this the first time that Belgian colonial pronatalism made an appearance at the mission. Maternal and infant health care as a movement dedicated to saving the lives of mothers and babies was a global phenomenon by the interwar period. Yet the movement came in distinct national, imperial, regional, and evangelical guises, even if some of the associated objects were global forms.[12] In 1939, a British evangelical guise met a Belgian colonial one at Yakusu. The mixture could be amiable; thus, the anthems. And it could yield money; thus, the philanthropic funds given to this British mission adopting a Belgian royal figure as maternity symbol. Moreover, while traveling downstream to Yakusu on November 15, the Belgian officials and guests had joined in making a collection of 800 francs to be dispensed as primes de naissance (birth bonuses) to the first forty mothers who gave birth in the new building. There had never been monetary handouts for bearing babies at Yakusu before. The opening of this maternité marked the entry of Belgian natalist gifts, reminiscent of those of an interwar coffee planter named Bwana in the Congo's Kivu region.[13]

These two natalist scenes from the Congo—the opening of the Maternité Reine Astrid and Comeliau's plantation depiction—together raise questions about the representativeness of Yakusu as a Congolese site of medicalized childbearing, about strands of influence linking the characters in these scenes, and about the historical and political processes of quotation. This chapter turns to mixtures in metropolitan and colonial natalist forms, mixtures of European and Congolese childbearing and of Protestant and Catholic medical cultures in Yakusu's district, and contradictory mixtures of experiences and *things* in memories of medicalized childbearing. *Mixture* suggests combination and convergence, perhaps confrontation and rivalry. It also implies seemingly integrated or submerged—combined or lost—bits of knowledge and practice. When Belgian colonial, British Baptist, and local natalist metaphors and forms met in and near Yakusu, the processes of borrowing, combination, and theft were intended and improvised, visible and concealed. Medicalized maternity was creolized at and near Yakusu, not only because Belgian forms met British and Catholic met Protestant, not only because Congolese nurses and midwives translated diverse forms of practice and knowledge, but because multiple "metropolitanizations" were involved.[14] I especially explore two such metropolitanizations in the post–World War II period: British Baptist Yakusu and the nearby Catholic state maternité of Yanonge, and their respective engagements with Congolese natalist metaphor, memory, and practice.

"Vigorous Races"

In 1910, when Mrs. Smith gave birth to the first white child born at Yakusu, European colonial life in the Congo was largely a world of unmarried men. Colonial agents and Congolese soldiers were the primary patients of state doctors during this period. Venereal disease, concubines, prostitutes, and patient privacy formed a tangle of medical worries.[15] The frequency of syphilis and gonorrhea seemed "regrettable" but "almost inevitable . . . in a country where love relations are so inconstant and fragile," wrote one colonial doctor in 1909.[16] If a European came down with venereal disease or dysentery, medical officers would seek out his house servants in search of a source.[17] Most hygiene officers were eager to extend sanitary, venereal inspections of state workers to their sexual partners.[18] Indeed, colonial doctors encouraged European men to take live-in Congolese concubines, known euphemistically as ménagères or housekeepers. "Gonorrhea," noted one physician in 1909, "constantly threatens the one who, not having a ménagère, is forced to take chances with women who do this trade rather clandestinely."[19]

Colonial calls for maternités did not begin in the Congo until after the First World War. The focus was babies, not mothers. The Commission pour la Protection des Indigènes voted during its 1912–13 session to support a new organization of "generous" Belgian colonial women, the Ligue pour la Protection de l'Enfance Noire. Like its Belgian counterpart (the Ligue Nationale Belge pour la Protection de l'Enfance du Premier Age), this colonial charitable league was dedicated to saving babies' lives; it had just opened its first baby clinic in Kisantu.[20] Milk-dispensing baby clinics, known as Gouttes de Lait or "Drops of Milk," began to open in Belgium at the turn of the century, particularly among working-class populations. Anxieties about good mothercraft and a decline in breast-feeding were sweeping much of Europe at the time; voluntary organizations providing pasteurized breast milk substitutes were a common response.[21] Over fifteen countries sent representatives to the Second International Conference for "Gouttes de Lait" held in Brussels in 1907. By 1913, the Belgian national league had ninety affiliated projects in the country, including twenty gouttes de lait, forty-three infant clinics, six day care centers, and a restaurant for needy mothers.[22] Meanwhile, the colonial Ligue pour la Protection de l'Enfance Noire reported excessive infant mortality rates in the Congo—50, 75, and 90 percent in some regions, according to its 1913 survey—and operated a few baby clinics there.[23]

At that time, doctors, Catholic missionaries, and state agents lamented the low birthrate as well as the high infant death rate in the colony. "We must try to have much more numerous births," pleaded Veroni, a state doctor from Stanleyville, in 1910. A 1903 state circular authorized free rations for pregnant and nursing wives of Congolese state workers, and an extra half-ration for those with more than two children. By 1910, Province Orientale authorities were giving tax exemptions to Congolese fathers with more than four children. Some Catholic missionaries, too, were giving birth bonuses to parents with many children.[24] Yet, as with all colonial hygiene for Congolese prior to the war, natalist measures were unevenly and capriciously applied. Some officials could see no economic benefit in tax exemptions for fathers with numerous children. Others argued that such a measure "would lead blacks to no longer be Malthusians without knowing it."[25]

Venereal disease, dysentery, and sleeping sickness were the primary *public* health concerns before World War I. There were few European women in the colony, and most African patients were men. One doctor, F. Houssiau, for instance, treated only one white woman in Leopoldville in 1910. Another 1,279 Congolese women were a tiny minority of the Congolese patients seen in the city; the other 97 percent were men.[26] The Congo remained a masculine place of adventure and danger—out-of-bounds for ladies, mothers, and wives. If the tropics did not make a wife sterile, she would only be in a man's way, "a chain at her husband's feet."[27] To send out a brand-new official with his wife was an amusing idea for A. Detry, state magistrate at Stanleyville, in 1912. What would happen, he asked, when she discovered that there was no looking glass in her hotel room or when her husband had to announce that she was pregnant? How would the husband travel? A journey was "almost impossible with a white woman at his side," noted Dr. Veroni, "never mind the inconveniences of another nature that it is not up to me to advise you about."[28]

Missionary women were the exceptions to this logic. Some were Catholic nuns. The first congregation arrived in 1891, and another five before 1900, though there were only 288 nuns in the Congo, affiliated with thirteen congregations, in 1923.[29] The first Protestant missionary woman came to the lower Congo in 1879; there were several more, including single women missionaries, by the mid-1880s.[30] If "an isolated white family" welcomed a Belgian traveler to their home in 1910, it was usually an Anglo-Saxon housewife who was responsible for the cozy scene. The "initiative and courage" of these missionary wives, explained one author, came from the "secular hiving off [*essaimage*] of their nation and a virile and free education." Belgian women, instead, were "much less well prepared for colonial life" because they, "our young girls," in keeping with their "homebound [*casanière*] race" were "overprotected by their families." An image of a Belgian woman giving birth in the Congo clinched this eugenic argument. Without her mother and other relatives present, and with a doctor rarely close by, no one would be there to help her except a "black chambermaid, very often incompetent, negligent and unclean." Moreover, "what a long convalescence awaits her under this debilitating climate." Belgian women would have to go home to give birth, therefore, which would make pregnancy such a "calamity" that the "perfidious advice of neo-Malthusianism"—(that is, "use birth control")—would be observed. Finally, a white child born and raised in the Congo was at risk of "degeneracy." A Belgian woman's "primordial marital duty" was to create "a sound and large family, to continue a vigorous race," and "this duty of course must keep a wife in her natal country."[31]

A "vigorous race" with large and sound families versus a "degenerate," unhealthy one of Malthusians: these were the same eugenic polarities that Émile Zola popularized for his francophone reading public with his 1899 novel, *Fécondité*. The book promoted "patriotic procreation," though with fierce anticlerical sentiments and an imperial twist. Faith lay not in the Church, but in the Nation and Empire, in Zola's novel. So the enterprising French colon returning from French colonial Niger—part of "the other France," "the future France"—made clear with his visionary words in the novel's concluding scene: "We shall swarm and swarm and fill the world."[32] My point is not to liken Belgian imperial pronatalisms with Zola's representations of such preoccupations in France and its empire. Rather, Zola's *Fécondité* as counterpoint shows how distinct both Belgian and French imaginaries *and* Catholic and anticlerical orientations were, and thus how extraordinarily versatile a eugenic lexicon could be. In 1910, Belgian colonial visionaries (some Catholic, some not) used this same popular vocabulary of opposites—vigorous, fecund races versus degenerate birth control practitioners—to articulate two objectives. The first was to foster large, monogamous Congolese families among soldiers and other state workers in "semi-civilized" colonial posts. Second, Belgian women should be protected from the dangers of the Congo's degenerate, tropical climate, so they could fulfill their duty as mothers for their Belgian national "race." A decade later, this malleable vocabulary was still viable, but for different purposes and with radically different effects.

Colony as Mother

After the First World War, Belgian colonial eugenic logic shifted. Concubinage, long justified as a prophylactic against venereal disease, was pronounced a source of corruption and shameful maladies instead. Respectable Belgian housewives were to accompany their husbands to the Congo as a patriotic duty, safeguarding them from the moral dangers of living alone in a tropical climate. Efforts to nationalize the European population of the Congo as Belgian were also involved, as were attempts to build popular pride in the empire among Belgian citizens. "Colonial Days" were first celebrated in Belgium in 1921. Not unlike Empire Days in Britain, they were intended to raise money for colonial charities and instill imperial patriotism. At last, so it was said, "the Congo begins to identify with the mother-country" and "all citizens finally realize the grand colonial idea."[33]

Population loss, infertility, and low birthrates were central worries, therefore, in the metropole and colony alike. Demographic concerns were not unfounded in the Congo. Most colonial commentators assumed that there had been a drastic population decline since conquest, and reports of villages with no children were frequent for some regions.[34] The low fertility reported for the forest region may well have been linked with the atrocities of the "red rubber" period of violent, coerced labor and women hostages, which led to one of the major international human rights scandals in world history, as well as to King Leopold II's loss of his private colony to Belgium in 1908.[35]

Yet the new sense of demographic emergency that emerged during the 1920s expressed more than guilt for a colonial regime gone wrong. Depopulation in Belgium became a pressing issue in this strongly Catholic country after the First World War, when a decline in the birthrate and the devastating tally of war casualties fueled widespread anxiety. Pronatalist propaganda and proposals proliferated, ranging from the scientific activities of the Société Belge d'Eugénique to the popular pro-family tracts of the Ligue des Familles Nombreuses de Belgique. Major family allocation legislation, explicitly aimed at "encouraging births and large families," followed in 1930, along with such measures as birth bonuses and progressive tax reductions for large families. The Oeuvre Nationale de l'Enfance, which became an official state body after the war, was funding antenatal and baby clinics in Belgium and the Congo by the mid-1930s.[36]

Interwar metropolitan hysteria about depopulation spilled over into Belgium's colonial field when the colony was, for the first time, squarely under Catholic domination, much more so indeed than Belgium itself. The transposition to the colonies of the ideas emanating from social Catholic pronatalist movements in Belgium was an easy passage in political terms; the Ministry of the Colonies was controlled by the Catholic Party with few exceptions from the mid-1920s to the mid-1950s, as close missionary ties and ministerial appointments testified.[37]

Colonial demographic panic was not only a Catholic phenomenon, however; industrial labor anxieties reinforced concerns about population as the colony underwent the greatest mineral development in Africa during the interwar period. The largest copper mining company, Union Minière du Haut-Katanga, took a lead; its policies shaped how the colonial state attempted to manage the impact of growing industry and associated (male) labor migration on the capacities of urban and rural (increasingly, predominantly female) populations to reproduce themselves. Union Minière decided to train Congolese as skilled and stabilized workers in the 1920s; it ended an exclusively male migrant labor system, began to pay family wages to skilled African workers, and encouraged their wives and children to live in mining compounds, where they received housing, education, and health care. The company also initiated a pioneering maternal and infant health care program. These measures were anomalous in interwar colonial Africa. Elaborate investments in socially reproducing a labor force and protecting the health and natality of workers' families were unknown elsewhere before the close of the Second World War. Understanding this Belgian colonial exceptionalism requires noticing how integral maternal metaphors and procreative logic were to the convergence of interests among capital, church, and state on Congo's Copperbelt. "Social reproduction" does not do justice to the increasing birthrate that Union Minière attempted—and achieved!—in Katanga. Indeed, increasing natality and lowering infant mortality rates in the mining labor force were at the core of the matter.[38]

Catholic missionaries had long been preoccupied by Congolese "prejudices that separate spouses," that is, birth spacing practices. Congolese mothers tended to breast-feed their babies for two or three years, abstaining from sexual relations until they had weaned their toddlers to avoid, so Congolese widely believed, the pernicious effects of sperm on breast milk and infant survival. Postpartum abstinence and sustained breast-feeding seemed to buttress polygyny in the Congo. During the 1920s and 1930s, Catholic missionaries welcomed the technocratic discourse of new colonial experts, especially doctors and demographers, which highlighted the consequences of these postnatal practices on the birthrate. Union Minière worked hard to institute monogamy, breast-feeding schedules, and early weaning, and it achieved shorter birth intervals and a higher birthrate among mining families.[39]

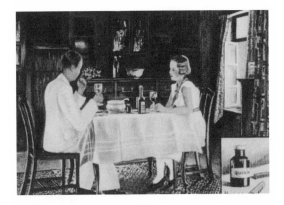

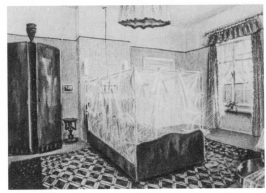

"In the Congo, Europeans take quinine every day to prevent fever [malaria]. . . . At night, they sleep under a mosquito net to avoid mosquito bites." A set of "do-do" hygiene messages directed at Belgians wondering about living conditions in the Congo, 1948. From Francis Lambin, *Congo Belge, publié sous les auspices du Ministère des Colonies et du Fonds Colonial de Propagande Economique et Sociale*, 180.

Colonial anxieties about the sexual, procreative, and maternal practices of Africans *and* Europeans in the colony were implicit in these solutions of the 1920s. Dr. Houssiau still argued against white women accompanying their husbands to the Congo; a tropical climate could kill, this honorary colonial medical inspector and former colonial doctor said in a Cercle d'Etudes Coloniales speech at the University of Brussels in 1928. Houssiau thought the idea of establishing Belgian families in the Congo to stop promiscuity between white men and "négresses" was a naive notion propagated by Catholic missionaries. Doctors systematically underreported venereal disease in order to protect patient privacy, he explained, usually declaring it as malaria instead. Moreover, some Belgian colonial mothers were negligent because they did not give quinine to their children and would go out dancing, leaving them alone with a "boy." "Haven't cases of gonorrheal vulvitis been seen among young white girls of 2–5 years?" Houssiau asked.[40] On the other hand, the same fears of racial mixture inspired the industrial pronatalism and the dreams of new family forms emerging in the Copperbelt. Belgian women were encouraged to come to the Congo to make families, establish bedrooms and dining rooms, and take quinine alongside their husbands just as African wives were encouraged to reside in mining compounds. Indeed, notions of stabilizing Congolese families coincided remarkably with the first calls to transform the colony from a male place of conquest and adventure to a family place of charity and honor.

Pierre Daye, a Belgian nationalist journalist, was among those who publicized the need for white women to go to the Congo in order to "diminish the degrading custom of the black ménagère." The tone and class content of arguments also shifted. The representative story had changed from Detry's of 1910—about a well-to-do woman who broke down in tears because her hotel room had no mirror—to Daye's image of a weeping working-class girl from Liège traveling to meet her fiancé, a worker in an important Equateur company; she was crying because she would have to live without movies and bistros.[41] Most commentators agreed that Belgian women must go to the Congo because ménagères sullied colonial honor and respectability; European wives would protect and watch over white male morality, while also preventing the spread of venereal disease.[42] Moreover, with a new colonial interest in protecting Congolese fertility and maternity, there would be something for European women to do. They would be the symbols and models of good motherhood, and they would help do the work. They would show colonialism at its best—as an upstanding, helpful enterprise—as they weighed infants and distributed clothes, milk, and quinine at baby clinics.

A medical infrastructure, which would allow white women to give birth and safely raise and feed babies in the Congo, became regarded as necessary to induce larger numbers of Belgian women to come to the colony.[43] Calls for maternity hospitals began in the early 1920s. A 1921 plan included maternities for white women in all provincial capitals and district headquarters as well as "maternity dispensaries" in more remote posts.[44] Money was budgeted for twelve European district maternities to be constructed in 1926.[45] By 1931, state regulations required the wives of European state workers to give birth in the state-operated maternities.[46] The numbers of white women giving birth in state medical facilities in the Congo increased from 40 in 1915, to 137 in 1925, to 232 in 1935.[47] In 1914, there were less than 30 women per 100 white men in the colony. Between 1928 and 1935, the sex ratio rose from 35 women for every 100 men to 50 per 100; in the 1950s, there were more than 80 women per 100 men.[48]

Margaret Sally Eulick, an American, was already pregnant when she went with her husband from Missouri to a small and remote diamond mining camp at Luaco. She traveled over 100 miles to Tshikapa, the headquarters of the mining company, Forminière, whose white community had a "make-believe golf course" and cocktail gatherings, a month before she gave birth in 1923. Her Forminière doctor was more interested in tropical disease than in her pregnancy, she noted.[49] Not all private enterprises had comparable facilities for European workers' wives. Houssiau contended in 1928 that no nursing mother or woman in the final months of pregnancy should go to the Congo until after weaning her child, yet he observed that many private companies did not heed this advice.[50] The wives of company agents working in rural areas were often isolated, and when they gave birth, they had to turn at the last minute to whatever help could be found nearby. Yakusu's missionaries, we saw, assisted some white women in their region. Mrs. Mill received an "urgent call" to help a Lomami Company agent's wife in 1930. Chesterman went off by mission steamer to reach a "white lady" in "difficult labor" in 1932. And a BMS nursing man and his wife assisted the wife of a Bamboli company agent in 1933.[51]

The mission station at Yakusu became an important medical center for parturient missionary wives. During the 1930s, English-speaking Protestant missionaries came from as far as Tanganyika for confinements. "We were expecting a Mrs Jones of the Seventh Day Adventist Mission to arrive here next month," wrote Nurse Owen in 1931.[52] Letters arrived months in advance: "Now we have letters from a trader's wife, and an American doctor and his bride and also from an American and his wife coming here for her confinement." Yakusu's missionary nurses reorganized where they slept to accommodate these visitors requiring maternity nursing: "Phyllis went to Mrs Ennals drawing room & I gave Mrs Jones my room & took to Phyllis's as I am to nurse Mrs Jones." By 1937, Gladys Parris thought the hospital "could easily do with three full time white nurses especially when there are white patients & there nearly always are!"[53] Managing missionary pregnancies determined the schedules of the missionary doctors and nurses. A rushed Holmes noted in 1939 that "Mrs. Knights babe is due any time now and the sooner the better for I have still another journey to do before the end of the year." Pending deliveries of white women "immobilized" Yakusu's doctors well into the 1940s.[54]

Helping the wives of private plantation agents and colonial functionaries remained part of Yakusu's district medical obligations as well. Browne received an urgent message in 1943 to cross the river and tend to an INEAC doctor's wife in labor at Yangambi.[55] A Madame Wafflereut journeyed to Yakusu from a Belgika company post on Ile Bertha to give birth in 1947.[56] In 1948, the INEAC doctor, Barlovatz, asked Browne to attend his wife and suggested an inducing agent that Browne could use to coordinate the birth with his busy traveling schedule.[57] Yakusu's missionary nurses continued to provide private nursing services to white women, and it was hoped that their help would lead to donations to Yakusu's medical work.[58]

As the population of Belgian women grew during the interwar period, childbearing in the Congo became more medicalized and hospital based than it was in the metropole. By the late 1940s, a colonial women's journal carried advice columns on raising white babies in the "bush."[59] Lectures for future colonials in Brussels continued to emphasize the "danger of the black mistress" and insist that it was "necessary to leave as a family, whatever the risks." Jean-Marie Habig, who did much of this teaching on the "Psychopathology of the European and the Black," specialized in this racialized, sexualized discourse. "It is antinatural to force a man to live single in a hot climate . . . where the sexuality of the native, his immoderate need of women and the variety of them, forms an atmosphere which permeates bit by bit the white man."[60] Colonial women were still advised to go to a maternity three or four weeks before their due dates, although they were also told what to do if they did not reach a hospital in time.[61] The colonial women's union and Catholic nuns organized baby clinics and day care centers for European women, especially in Katanga. By the 1950s, infant mortality was lower among Belgian infants in the colony than in the metropole, indicating how well developed this infrastructure had become.[62] Most women living in Belgium continued to have home births, attended by professional midwives or doctors, until after World War II. Indeed, maternities, long associated with indigent and unwed mothers, did not become the norm in Belgium until the

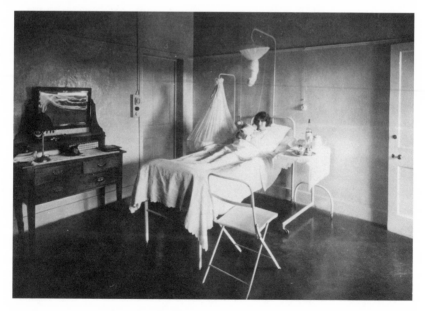

"Patient rooms are cheerful and furnished with the greatest comfort," 23 February 1931. European woman in a maternity room at a hospital for whites in Katanga. Perhaps a publicity photo; location indicated as "Panda?" by curator. (Courtesy of MRAC, Historical Section [59.61.303; gift of C. Héla]. Courtesy of Africa-Museum, Tervuren, Belgium.)

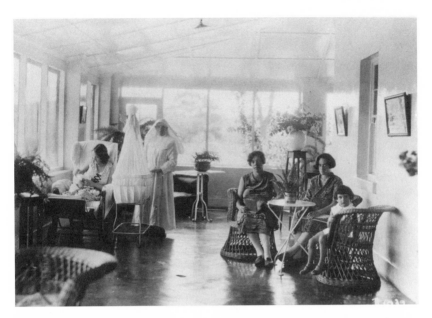

The room in a maternity for European women in Katanga "where the convalescents rest," 23 February 1931. Again location indicated as "Panda?" Perhaps another publicity photograph, though the intention of showing the scene of poor white—perhaps Greek or Portuguese—visitors at the side is unclear. (Courtesy of MRAC, Historical Section [59.61.305; gift of C. Héla]. Courtesy of Africa-Museum, Tervuren, Belgium.)

bureaucratic requirements of postwar health insurance legislation effected a sudden and rapid hospitalization of childbearing.[63]

Social Obstetrics and Nuns

"Social obstetrics," one manifestation of interwar social hygiene activity, was not directed only at European women in the Congo. Indeed, Houssiau complained that medical improvements for white women lagged behind those for Congolese women in Leopoldville.[64] In the 1920s, midwife schools opened and official maternity dictates appeared. The first school training Congolese women as midwives opened in 1924 at Baudouinville; several more followed before the end of the decade (including state schools at Boma, Leopoldville, and Stanleyville; a Red Cross school at Pawa; and the BMS school at Yakusu). One circular insisted that breast milk substitutes or wet nurses be found for the orphans of Congolese mothers who died in childbirth. Another specified that in all Congolese hospital facilities, special areas were required not only for "civilized natives" but for women "in confinement" as well.[65]

In addition, as the assumption that relocating childbirth to clinical settings would inspire better social hygiene took hold, pressing for—and evasion of—hospital deliveries began. Catholic missionaries were among those who urged Congolese women to give birth in town hospitals and rural clinics. In 1926, village women ran away at the sight of beckoning nuns from Boma. Others fled at the last moment from the more rural Red Cross maternité in Pawa, in the gold-mining district in Province Orientale.[66]

Soldiers' wives could not easily run away. Rather, most state-provided reproductive health care for Congolese was a branch of military medicine in the interwar period.[67] In 1921, Dr. Fronville and his nurse, Mademoiselle Sirtaine, studied fertility and gynecological disease by examining soldiers' wives in Katanga. The corpse of one wife, who died in Elisabethville's military camp from a ruptured ectopic pregnancy on a Sunday afternoon, was carried to the hospital for an autopsy the next day.[68] Dr. Rebuffat studied venereal disease and miscarriage as well as pelvic disproportion and ethnicity by examining soldiers' wives living in Coquilhatville's military camps.[69] The wives of soldiers may have been more important as a subject population for state doctors than their husbands were. A European officer regularly took roll to be sure that wives attended the biweekly antenatal clinics in Irebu's and Elisabethville's military camps.[70] Soldiers' wives were also the principal parturients in most state-operated maternities through the 1930s. Fronville was not alone in taking special interest in gynecological surgery—an emerging field of colonial medicine that he called "a true mine to exploit."[71] Venereal disease surveillance, reproductive surgery, and autopsies were commonplace in tightly controlled milieus like mining compounds and military camps, where Congolese monogamy, family health care, and medical research were seen as vital to worker health and productivity.

Yet colonial gynecological and obstetric care did not begin because private companies and the Force Publique forced miners' and soldiers' wives to receive it. Operative obstetrics began early in the century with Congolese parturients and their kin, who showed up seeking help from colonial surgeons when a woman suffered from obstructed labor or the sequelae of a difficult delivery. A Congolese woman with labor obstructed by a transverse lie was an unusual surgery case for a Dr. Grossule at Basoko in 1907.[72] Houssiau operated on a woman with a vesicovaginal fistula who came to him after giving birth in Leopoldville in 1910.[73] A Dr. Pulieri's Coquilhatville caseload in 1912 included three operations to remove placenta pieces.[74] These were uncommon cases before the First World War. Yet they suggest an important theme, which also appears in the history of obstetrics at Yakusu. Doctors were able to save the lives of women dying in childbirth. And Congolese, unsolicited, actively sought out this kind of biomedical care during emergencies. Indeed, the beginnings of health care for women and mothers in the Congo lay, in great part, with these same Congolese women.

When a Belgian obstetrician and a leader in the Catholic organization, Aide Médicale aux Missions, prepared a major report on social obstetrics in the Congo in 1935, they argued that assistance to pregnant women and mothers remained "embryonic." V. Cocq and Fr. Mercken's bibliography included documentation on forms of maternity care in Australia, Soviet Russia, the United States, France, Britain, India, French Equatorial Africa, Morocco, Algeria, Malaysia, South Africa, Cameroon, and fascist Italy. This gamut reveals the global scale of population, social hygiene, and maternalist movements during the 1930s. These eugenics-oriented movements were exceedingly diverse, embracing fascists, socialists, liberal democrats, and social Catholics, and ranging from early "negative" visions of state-organized racialized sterilization (as eventually promoted in Nazi Germany) to the more benign "positive eugenics" of state-legislated family allocations favoring natality and large families that flourished in Belgium. An idealization of motherhood was common, if differently weighted, across this spectrum. So, too, was a reliance on the technocratic expertise of social professionals, especially doctors, social workers, and demographers.[75]

Social obstetrics on the scale practiced in Union Minière compounds was, in Cocq and Mercken's words, in keeping with the "eugenic tranquillity necessary for the flowering of the race." They contended that it should be extended to all Congolese contexts. Belgium remained an important reference point, and Belgian Catholic social hygiene movements a significant influence, especially after the war. Yet the Congo also offered opportunities for Catholic social policy and authoritarian-inspired technocratic planning that were not available at home.[76] Union Minière's family health program represented one such convergence, though within the tight confines of an enclosed and semi-carceral industrial environment. Descriptions of the progressive sanitation and socialization of new workers and their wives through a series of spatial and hygienic transformations point to the minute, regimented kind of control of Union Minière's family health and maternity care programs.[77]

Union Minière began its family health program in conjunction with the Catholic church in Katanga in 1925. Unlike Comeliau's portrayal of an interwar private enterprise scheme, it included maternity wards, antenatal care, maternal care, special rations for pregnant women and nursing mothers, and mess halls for feeding—and thus weaning—children between the ages of two and four. Because there was strict company control over participation, Union Minière was able to track the demographic results achieved: a decline in worker and infant mortality along with an increasing birthrate, which was associated with limiting the duration of breast-feeding.[78]

The first director of the Fonds Reine Elisabeth pour l'Assistance Médicale aux Indigènes (FOREAMI), Dr. Dupuy, expressed his admiration for the kind of selectivity and honing of superior, monogamous, fertile families that industrial conditions offered. Indeed, the centrality of maternal care to social hygiene came to the fore in the Congo with the founding of FOREAMI by royal decree in 1930. The Congo's most significant "native medical assistance" organization, FOREAMI was funded by the Belgian state and the Ministry of the Colonies. It made "growth of human capital" the cornerstone of its objectives. Organized on an intensive scale, first in the Lower Congo and later extended to Kwango, FOREAMI aimed at an extraordinarily minute and authoritarian demographic and medical censusing of local populations. Staff were to work by teams, "hut by hut," with a European doctor, according to Dupuy, personally touching every patient.[79]

As FOREAMI took shape, the emphasis in maternity care, as in all colonial health care for Congolese subjects, began to shift markedly toward social medicine and demographic control.[80] A language of positive eugenics, closely aligned with interwar Belgian Catholic medical thought, permeated FOREAMI plans, just as it did Cocq and Mercken's 1935 call for colonywide social obstetrics. What was novel about FOREAMI in 1930 was its orientation toward those left behind in rural areas, while labor recruiters picked off youthful men for wage labor at mines and plantations.

When FOREAMI's director first declared its objectives, he argued that missionary nurses would be inadequate to meet them. Dupuy wanted nuns not only to be nurses, but to serve as midwives as well. The coding of infant care as nuns' work was widespread by the 1930s. Yet as Comeliau's anecdote suggested, midwifery tended to be left to Congolese women, the so-called matrones of her semifictional account. The colonial state, however, increasingly found it convenient and cost-effective to turn over nursing care to the Catholic church. A group of lay nurses had accompanied the first large group of state doctors sent to the colony in 1919, and references to these women—such as Elisabethville's Mademoiselle Sirtaine—were common into the mid-1920s. Still, these unmarried lay nurses proved unsatisfactory, expensive, and inclined to "appeal to a higher rank" without passing through "the doctors on whom they depend directly." One doctor complained in 1922, "A little modesty would not hurt some of these young ladies."[81] Many of the lay nurses, it was said, had "abandoned their posts" to marry. The solution became: "It is necessary to have nuns come."[82]

The governor general never hid "his intention of reducing as much as possible the number of lay nurses" since, for each lay nurse replaced, two new nursing nuns could be hired to meet the labor requirements of the colony's expanding medical infrastructure. Yet there were few nuns in the Belgian Congo at the

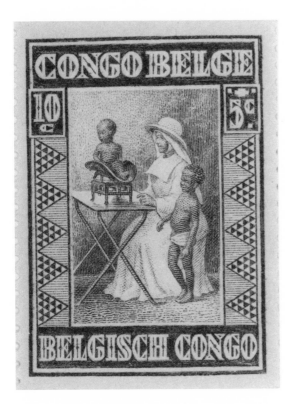

Belgian Congo semi-charity postage stamp of "Nurse Weighing Child." Issued on January 16, 1930, as part of a nine-part series intended "to aid welfare work among the natives, especially the children." Others in the series included first aid station, missionary and child, Congo hospital, dispensary service, convalescent area, instruction on bathing infant, operating room, and nursing students.

time, and even fewer who were able and willing to work as midwives.[83] Locating religious orders whose nuns would act as midwives in the Congo was not always easy or straightforward.

Although Christian charity as practiced by female religious orders had embraced medical work and hospital nursing for centuries, midwifery had rarely been in the hands of these Catholic congregations. In seventeenth- and eighteenth-century France, for example, older, married women served as parish midwives and worked in association with parish priests. These lay women handled the indelicate work of delivering babies and seeking bastardy or paternity confessions from childbearing women. In Europe and North America, as in Africa, the practice of soliciting sexual confessions was not uncommon, and it seems to have been undertaken primarily when a woman was in labor. Abiding associations of childbirth with pollution and midwifery with sexual confessions made midwifery unlikely—even unthinkable and prohibited—work for nuns in the medieval and early modern periods.[84] In some congregations, such as the Soeurs Franciscaines de Marie, these rules endured into the twentieth century.

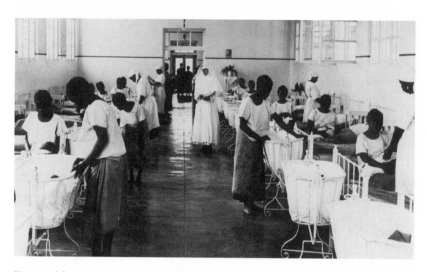

"Hospital for natives at Elisabethville. The maternity," 1945. Congopresse photograph by E. Lebied. (Courtesy of MRAC, Historical Section [no. 72.25/2]. Courtesy of Africa-Museum, Tervuren, Belgium.)

No one seems to have noticed this prohibition in Stanleyville, where the Soeurs Franciscaines had served as nurses from at least 1911, until state authorities requested more Franciscaine nuns for the city in 1925. The request included seven nurses and a midwife because the state needed some qualified European women to oversee the city's new midwife school. There was some discussion of terminating all contracts with the congregation, based in Stanleyville since the 1900s, because of the Franciscaines' "quite severe regulation: they do not handle births. They must work in twos for certain duties, etc." The issue was only resolved when the Franciscaines agreed that nun-midwives from another religious order would join them in an associated capacity (as *agrégée accoucheuse diplômée*). The evidence suggests that other religious orders made similar agreements, and that special solicitations went out to hospital congregations so as to locate nuns who could touch the blood of childbirth.[85]

Although an additional twenty-two female religious orders arrived to work in the Congo during the first half of the 1930s, only forty nuns, working in thirty locations and representing only fifteen of the Congo's fifty orders, were working as midwives in 1935. By this time, the state was no longer recruiting lay nurses; the major Catholic medical missionary organization pleaded with congregations that they begin to do their share in the field of social obstetrics, pointing out that midwifery services were too often provided by Protestant missions instead.[86] The pleas were effective. Many Catholic orders were operating maternities by the late 1940s, and they included nuns with midwife diplomas among their members. There were 184 maternity wards or hospitals directed by religious missions in 1948, and the numbers of congregations, midwife nuns, and supervised births continued to rise through the 1950s. There were 1,057 nuns in the colony by 1935, 1,456 in 1940, and 2,890 (2,356 Belgian, 534 foreign) in 1957. This swell in colonial nuns and nun-midwives coincided with the expanding, state-funded medical infrastructure for Congolese women and children. Colonial authors began to speak of "black maternities and white nuns" in the Congo in the 1950s. Indeed, by this time, most European nurse and midwife positions in the colony's state—and many company—hospitals were held by nuns.[87]

Baptist Meets Catholic, British Meets Belgian

This chapter began with mixtures. Small, intimate gatherings among British Baptists and Belgians—Catholic or not—did not survive after the war. Yet mixtures among Belgian and British, Catholic and Protestant, mission and state programs did. Catholic nuns arrived as specialists in midwifery and social obstetrics in Yakusu's district, and those at Yanonge were officially operating under BMS Yakusu supervision in the 1950s. Some British still met Belgians privately, but Yakusu's doctors were no longer needed as the doctors of Belgians in their region. Indeed, Yakusu became engulfed in a much larger colonial, at times global, set of processes after the Second World War.

By the time Malia Winnie shook the provincial governor's hand at the opening of the Maternité Reine Astrid in 1939, medicalized childbearing was a significant *Catholic* endeavor for colonial subjects in the Congo. It was not the first time that pronatalist agendas of Belgian private interests and state authorities had punctuated a key transition in maternal and infant health care at Yakusu. Madame Dardenne, who went on to found the Union des Femmes Coloniales, visited Yakusu "on behalf of the Queen and women of Belgium" in 1921. When Yakusu's first baby clinic opened in 1924, the scales and medicines came from a Belgian charitable organization; further donations to the BMS stations of Yakusu and Yalemba came from the Ligue pour la Protection de l'Enfance Noire au Congo Belge two years later.[88] Soon after Nurse Owen began baby clinics in two nearby villages in 1931, Dr. Chesterman sought state subsidies for her work. An evangelical service preceded each clinic, though classic objects of colonial maternities—scales, quinine, soap—were also there. There was nothing *specially* Belgian about these elements, even if they were in this local instance *specifically* so. Rather, baby scales, quinine, and soap were, by the 1930s, part of global cultural flows.[89]

The number of births at Yakusu was never large. There were 6 births in 1929,

18 in 1930, and 36 in 1938. A marked increase followed the opening of the Maternité Reine Astrid; there were 64 births at Yakusu in 1939, 109 in 1941, and 180 in 1949. Yet even in Yakusu's peak year before independence—1959—only 249 women gave birth at the Maternité Reine Astrid.[90] The significance of hospital childbearing at Yakusu never lay in numbers, but in the fuss: evangelical fuss about churchmen's wives as parturients, safe deliveries of babies of local Baptist parents, and midwife training, imagined as sound domestic education for the future wives of Yakusu-trained male nurses and evangelists. Mama Tula was about sixty or sixty-five years old when I met her. Her mother had given birth to all her children in Yakoso during the 1920s and 1930s; Mama Tula had given birth to all of hers in Yakusu's maternity ward during the 1940s and 1950s. This was a consistent pattern for the women of Yakoso, especially for a woman trained in mission schools. Yet Yakusu never tried to take over childbirth in a wide area. Moreover, this Baptist mission did not baptize infants as Catholic-operated state maternities did. Nor did this Protestant hospital intervene forcefully into intimate matters surrounding childbearing practice.

Nonetheless, Yakusu was operating in a changed world after World War II. State hygiene imperatives were felt more strongly and directly than ever before, particularly in maternal and infant health care. Thus in 1946, when the state began to pay a bonus of 150 francs for each baby born to a nonsalaried "independent native" (*indigène libre*), "provided the accouchement was attended by a State-recognized white person," Yakusu's missionary committee decided to pay the same amount for each child born at Yakusu to a mission worker.[91] Maternity wards began to be built almost everywhere. The Fonds du Bien-Etre Indigènes (FBEI), a colonial native welfare fund inaugurated in 1947, provided capital grants for building the maternity facilities first called for during the 1920s.[92] In 1948, the Isangi territory of which Yakusu was a part became the site of an FBEI project to reduce infant mortality.[93] Yakusu's doctors, as médecins agréés, helped in executing the plans, which included constructing separate maternity and baby clinic units adjacent to ten existing rural dispensaries. Yakusu-trained Congolese nurses handled a midwifery case in a rural dispensary occasionally. But now, for the first time, Yakusu began to place newly trained midwives in company (especially Belgika), state, and church dispensary posts in its district.

New Midwives

Yakusu's missionaries followed the guidelines of Belgian maternalist efforts more than ever before as they professionalized their midwifery training program, hired a district training midwife, and awarded state-recognized diplo-

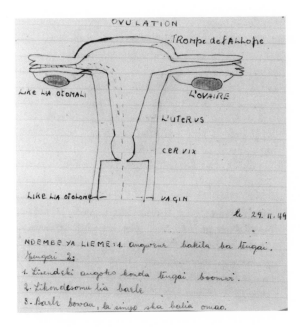

Ovulation lesson drawing from midwife student's notebook. From Madame Daniël Christophe Beimo Isengi, "Cours d'Obstétrique—Njaso ya Mbotesa," Yakusu, 24 November 1949. (Courtesy of Madame Isengi, Kisangani.)

mas. Their Baptist Congolese midwives, in huge demand, began to act independently from the mission as they went off to work in Catholic state hospitals and manage their own rural maternities.

The postwar changes in colonial maternity policy certainly encouraged Stanley Browne to hire Yakusu's first professional district and training midwife in the early 1950s. Mary Fagg recalled her interview with the missionary-surgeon-turned-leprologist. Her professional and theological credentials could not have been better; he examined her driving skills and made sure she was not going to the Congo in hopes of finding a husband. And Fagg's background as a district midwife in Britain served her well at Yakusu. Malia Winnie said that she "taught with her readings" and changed midwifery training at Yakusu with "the words of teaching." Fagg achieved a good command of Lokele, and she gave detailed lessons. She also "took the work beyond Yakusu, teee, organizing women faraway in villages."[94] She organized antenatal and baby clinics along the Congo River in Yakusu's district, eventually adding clinics for two to five year olds as well. Fagg would travel for up to ten days, often with midwife students, visiting two to four villages a day, holding evangelical services, selling books, participating in "palavers," seeing patients, delivering hygiene talks, and offering sewing classes.

The number of pupils increased after Fagg came, and for the first time, Yakusu's hospital school was issuing state-recognized midwife assistant diplomas. Four of the eight students who began in February 1952 had close mission ties, including the daughters of Malia Winnie, Pastor Lititiyo, and Liaocho, a former hospital evangelist, as well as an orphan raised at Yakusu.[95] Nine students were enrolled for *aide-accoucheuse* training in 1956, and five received state-recognized diplomas the same year.[96]

Yet the new generation of students in the officially recognized aide-accoucheuse school seemed sassy and out of line when they began to get pregnant and demand better food. Several midwife students joined, or even initiated, the forest strike of 1953.[97] The strike survives in memory, as we saw in chapter 3, in terms of food and the greed of single missionary women. Disciplinary measures were also involved in these "times of temptation" and "muddy waters" (as Fagg described them). Stealing, promiscuity, premarital pregnancy, and "run-away marriages" were among the "grounds of immorality" that led to dismissals.[98] In 1958, four out of ten new students were expelled for "moral palavers," and since being "out after dark unchaperoned" was against "hospital discipline," no students received diplomas.[99] Two more, "one already pregnant, the other for disobedience," were dismissed in 1959.[100]

Malia Winnie was the "night service midwife" in the hospital during this period, and having divorced, she also lived in Yakusu's "fence" as a senior Mama of the midwife students: "she rules with no uncertain sway in her own world, and the girls of today, naughty, wayward, disobedient, will 'take it' from Iya Malia Winnie and are not anxious to be [in] her bad books."[101] Malia Winnie recalled giving orders to midwife students who came after her: "When a woman came, I was just sitting there, watching how they would work. So: 'Do this, do that.' . . . Me, I was there only showing all the ways."[102] Others focused on Mary Fagg as teacher instead: "Mademoiselle came to teach you: 'Do this, do that.' . . . Thus, a class. I wasn't afraid."[103] Many postwar midwives remembered Malia Winnie as teacher "because she had finished long before."[104]

Generational conflict and difference are clear. Malia Winnie was their Mama, most remembered; they had to obey her. Yet ambivalence was strong among some: "Our Mama that one, she gave some of us bad trouble . . . because when we finished class . . . Malia went with our names to Doctor saying: 'They are bad children.' . . . So Doctor said . . . 'we won't give them their certificates. They will just die for nothing.'" Indeed, many midwife students in this postwar cohort ultimately rejected her. They resented her seeming alliance with missionary women against them. Moreover, they were less drawn to local birth customs than was Malia Winnie; while manipulating with greater ease a French obstetric vocabulary, they considered adultery confessions and local birthing positions kisenji. One student, Machuli Georgine, explained: "Us, we forbid asili matters, saying: 'Don't bring that into the maternity. If you like it, do it in the village.'

Because there in the village, they like, when a woman gives birth, for someone to stay behind her back. In the maternity, the woman lies on the bed. We don't like someone to climb up to sit behind her back." Others swore that Malia Winnie had an uncanny ability to know if an unborn baby would be a boy or a girl. Anger about Malia Winnie's role in hospital discipline lingered in memory: "When we came to the hospital then she was our Mama showing us the work, 'do this.' She was showing us the work with force is all. Showing us nicely didn't exist."[105]

Mary Fagg standardized and professionalized midwife training at Yakusu during this period. Yakusu's long-standing rule that only one family member could accompany a parturient into the birthing room was also enforced during Fagg's term, considerably diminishing the power of lay birth attendants from the years when Dorothy Daniel and Malia Winnie shared power in Yakusu's maternity. The "times of temptation" were, however, also about struggles over the status of aides-accoucheuses in postwar Congo.

There were troubles dating from the late 1920s, as we saw, in finding young Congolese women willing to accept midwifery training. Although Malia Winnie used her position as midwife to enhance her reputation and that of the maternity ward, the hospital continued to struggle to find midwife students who would not "have to be made to come" during the early 1940s. Too many still had "the idea that they were doing us a favour by working in hospital."[106] Bodily troubles and cultural discord over midwifery practice continued at Yakusu. Yet the legitimacy and prestige of the work changed when the larger body politic—a pronatalist colonial state—began so decisively to shape childbearing practices and midwifery work. Congolese midwife became a recognized, semiprofessional category as maternities expanded throughout the colony, including through Yakusu's rural plantation district. By the 1950s, the official aide-accoucheuse training and diplomas that Yakusu's school offered led to paid professional jobs, and gave these Congolese women authority and negotiating power over their working conditions and salaries.

At Yakusu, the new state-recognized category led to debates about pay.[107] Mission salaries for Congolese medical workers were lower than the state's, prompting Yakusu's "medical boys"—nurses—to go on strike in early 1944.[108] In 1947, Yakusu's missionaries agreed that aide-accoucheuse salaries should be progressively increased over five years until they reached the state maximum of 250 francs per month.[109] There was a shortage of trained Congolese midwives as FBEI-funded maternity annexes went up and most private enterprises added maternities to their health services. Yakusu-trained midwives were in hot demand, and they must have known it. Letters seeking Yakusu-trained girls came to the mission's medical director from companies and state medical facilities within the province. An agricultural and industrial company, BIARO, wrote asking if a Yakusu-trained midwife was available for work in 1956, as did the state doctor in the Yahuma *territoire*.[110] Several worked at Isangi's state hospital, under the supervision of Catholic nuns.

Yakusu-trained midwives wrote letters, too. They wrote to Yakusu's medical director in Lokele, demanding evidence of their diplomas for state and company jobs as well as asking for salary increases. Josephine Koto wrote to a Dr. Wyatt in 1957 for her midwife diploma; she could not be paid at the Isangi state hospital without it. Machuli Georgine remembered refusing work at Yalemba because she had been asked by a missionary to work at this BMS post without pay. She recalled that John Carrington did not understand the local risks involved when he said, "Here at the mission [at Yalemba], there isn't any money to pay you. If you like, just do the work of delivering women free." She did so for a while, but recollected telling herself that midwifery "is the work of going to defend yourself against accusations. If it is bad and a woman dies . . . no one will be with me. I will go stay in a bad place, and I won't be paid a thing." So she stopped working without pay.[111]

Yakusu's efforts to medicalize childbearing had always been directed at helping the parturient wives of churchmen and providing midwife training, imagined as sound domestic preparation for future spouses of Yakusu nurses and evangelists. A husband-and-wife team, Kialia and Luta, took charge of the Yaombole dispensary in 1935.[112] Although two out of six midwife students in 1943 were unlikely to receive diplomas because they found "French medical terms almost impossible to master," Muriel Lean assumed that they would be "really useful in helping sick folk, wherever they may be after marriage, and can certainly take an accouchement quite well." When Yakusu's midwife diplomas were not yet recognized by the state during the 1940s, several nurses' wives were helping out in dispensaries and "company folk are finding them useful." Lean concluded that "the next best thing" to state recognition would be a "matrimonial agency, to see that our girls are paired off with our boys."[113] The missionaries continued to set up husband-wife, nurse-midwife teams in rural dispensaries after the war.[114]

Madeleine Lititiyo was an important exception. After her graduation in 1956, she returned to the village of her father, Pastor Lititiyo: "only the fact that this girl can live in her own home makes such a piece of work possible for an unmarried girl."[115] She became responsible for the state-funded dispensary in Yangonde. The brick dispensary annex had never before been used, but over fifty mothers came to Madeleine Lititiyo's clinic on the first day. Within ten days, she had managed five deliveries, and over seventy mothers were soon coming regularly to her baby clinic.[116] She observed 353 pregnancies and delivered 213 babies in 1957, almost as many as at Yakusu's well-staffed maternity in the same year. Excluding the 200-some births that took place at Yakusu each year, the number of births at maternities under Yakusu's jurisdiction grew from 321 in 1951 to 1,003 in 1957. This increase was not evenly distributed. Forty percent of the increase came from births at the Yanonge maternity; another 20 percent was due to Madeleine Lititiyo's work at Yangonde.[117] In 1956, Lititiyo's nurse colleague at Yangonde, Janson Baofa, wrote to Yakusu's medical director reporting that the state administrator from Isangi had been "astonished" during a recent visit to see women giving birth under the care of "Mandeleni" and "he would like to know . . . about her salary." Baofa cautioned: "since I did not have anything to tell him, I inform you only."[118] Madeleine Lititiyo herself wrote a year later demanding a raise, much to the shock of Dr. Browne. She also requested mosquito netting for the maternity beds.[119] This midwife knew that she had power by the time she wrote. She was working in a period when Yakusu doctors were having to account for the number of maternity births taking place in their jurisdiction, and state administrators were impressed by a Congolese woman managing a maternity on her own with evident ease and numerical results.

Yanonge, which was also located in Yakusu's district, became representative of a new, postwar Belgian colonial vision of maternity care. Funds from local companies and the FBEI led to the construction of a hospital with a maternity building, dispensary, and small orphanage. The foundation for the Yanonge hospital and adjacent maternity was laid in 1952 and construction ended in 1957. Pregnant women awaited the onset of labor in a special hostel built for this purpose at the maternity site. This infrastructure enabled Yanonge to bring two-thirds of the pregnancies it observed into its ward for deliveries—and baptisms. The Soeurs Hospitalières de Sainte-Elisabeth of Luxembourg operated the facility until the rebellion in 1964, registering close to 500 births a year. They had an ambulance at their disposal, another common feature of FBEI-related funding. The nuns conducted antenatal and baby clinics in the plantation region and gave pregnant women who were close to term free rides to the special waiting hostel.[120] Yanonge's new maternity quickly surpassed Yakusu's numbers. There were 232 registered hospital births at Yakusu in 1956, whereas there were 456 at Yanonge. Yanonge's capacity to transport and provide housing to pregnant women permitted it to administer the deliveries of 66 percent of the pregnancies observed (406 births for 614 pregnancies in 1957), while Yakusu delivered 51 percent (219 out of 426).[121]

The Catholic nuns at Yanonge utilized the services of Congolese women in midwifery cases. While Shangazi Angelani was living in Yanonge with her husband, who worked at the Catholic mission, she was accosted by a nun one day when she was visiting a sick child at the dispensary. The nun said that she wanted to teach Angelani midwifery work: "We will work in one place together." Angelani also recalled her lessons: "First look, then receive the child. If

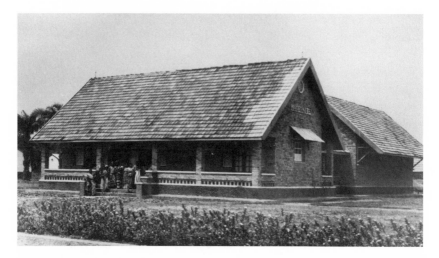

"The Sainte Elisabeth Maternity at Yanonge, constructed with the aid of the Fonds du Bien-Etre Indigène," ca. 1955. Congopresse photograph by C. Lamote. (Courtesy of MRAC, Historical Section [CID 72.43/23; 55.96.1270]. Courtesy of Africa-Museum, Tervuren, Belgium.)

there is a problem, ring this bell and I will come." This woman, who lived in Yainyongo-Romée in 1989, remembered being the only Congolese to work at Yanonge at the time. She would hear knocking at her door at night, and would call Soeur Alois only if she had trouble. The nun would come, give a shot, and say to Angelani, "Stay at work." In this early period, Yanonge's nuns found it useful, according to Angelani's recollections, to encourage her to ask for adultery confessions from the women who gave birth; perhaps they added their own words about sin. Angelani said that she would take a white leaf, *kalilanga*, with her to the hospital to give to the parturient to chew and swallow. If the patient had been with other men, the child would come out. The nuns knew, and said, "Ask her. . . . When she names. . . . If she does not give birth easily, ask her! . . . 'did you mess around with someone else?' " Angelani exclaimed, "They knew, eh? The baby is there making trouble in the tummy. The baby is there making trouble in the tummy. You would ask her. The baby would come out. She messed around with someone."[122]

Papers and Presents

The postwar extension of maternity services to Congolese women entailed new, colonial objects as well as new, Congolese personnel. Birth certificates and confinement statistics became routine. At Yakusu, from the opening of Maternité Reine Astrid in 1937, gender-coded, pink and blue birth certificates were "not the least of the many attractions of the Ward," especially since this was "where Father comes into his own." As the mother would gather "pots and pans and baby on discharge-day," according to Nurse Lean, "Father takes the Birth Certificate to be put amongst the treasured papers in his box."[123]

The Belgian colonial effort to medicalize childbirth attests to what Crawford Young has called a "diluted form of indirect rule." "Assimilationist currents," the impulse to use maternities as part of new évolué roles and representations, were balanced by a "premium upon immediate efficiency."[124] "Evolution" was stronger before postwar funds permitted efficiency on a wide scale, opening up maternity doors to a majority of Congolese women. The medicalization of childbirth was tied to the increasing bureaucratization of colonial life, and high attendance statistics in maternity wards were a by-product of a pronatalist colonial welfare state. As in Belgium itself, the medicalizing impulse was fed by the postwar paper requirements of managing daily life.[125] Medicalizing birth was not only about giving birth in the Congo, but about counting—privileging and enumerating—birth. The bureaucratic imperatives of *colonial inscription,* the demographic arm of the sanitary modality of colonial rule, effected this intense pressure on getting numbers. This squeeze was also where significant amounts of Congolese clamor lay.

The legal obligation to register births and deaths, first introduced in 1940,

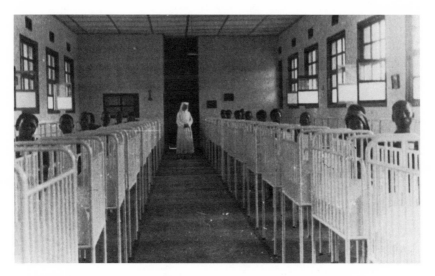

Maternity at Fataki, ca. 1955. (Courtesy of KADOC, Leuven, Belgium.)

had been extended to 92 percent of the Congolese population by 1955. Registered births rose by 44 percent from 1953 to 1958, unlike death registration,
which only increased by 3 percent. Almost all deliveries in cities as well as "an
important fraction of those in rural areas" were occurring in maternity settings,
where hospital staff prepared the birth certificates that were later presented in
colonial offices for official birth registration. The "high proportion of hospital
deliveries" stimulated more complete registration and increased the accuracy of
the recorded data, especially as regards the date of birth. Additionally, according to colonial demographer Anatole Romaniuk, the increase in registered
births was due to the family allowance benefits provided to "all employed
persons, both in private enterprise and in governmental service, provided legal
proof of a birth was given."[126] What began as isolated programs for select
groups of workers' wives became, after the war, part of a massive set of "policies
pursued in rural areas [that] . . . imposed modernity on the countryside." As
independence approached, the atmosphere was "no more taxes, no more cotton, no more census-takers, no more vaccinaters, no more identity cards, no
more army recruiters."[127] Yet the call was for more and better maternities.

These requirements yielded confusion at the time. In 1955, the Leopoldville
native advisory council took up the African population's complaints about the
Hôpital des Congolais. District Commissioner Tordeur began the discussion by
declaring that the Congolese perception that women who did not give birth at
the hospital were subject to fines was "inexact." "What is true," he said, "is that
the registration of births requires that after a birth, the doctor should seriously
examine the parturient and present a birth certificate." Tordeur explained that
it was the examination and the certificate that were charged to the Congolese,
and that "this billing had been interpreted as constituting a fine." He asked
those present to "rectify the error by spreading in the township the true interpretation of facts."[128] Indeed, "living in translation" began to permeate all of
colonial life in a situation where birth translated into an object of inscription—
a birth certificate—and where this inscription, in turn, virtually imposed the
routines and "entangled objects" of maternity births.[129]

Memories of how birthing was socially organized by the FBEI-funded maternity at Yanonge suggest rigidity and excessive emphasis on maintaining an
antiseptic environment. Women had to remove all their clothing when they
arrived and don sterilized hospital clothing. Kin could be present—indeed, they
were relied on for cooking parturients' food—but they were never allowed in
the ultraclean ward. Mama Mosa, a hospital midwife, showed me the interior of
the former maternity, a building nearly as large as the adjacent hospital, though
empty—except for squatters living there—since the rebellion hit Yanonge hard
in the mid-1960s. The former patient ward was a long narrow room that used to

contain twenty-four beds, twelve along each side. Each was for a mother and her newborn, except for two places at the end: "they put one bed for those who lost a baby. Those women, they had their own bed in those days; no one else could sleep there. Others, if the pregnancy was looking for a way to fall down [in a miscarriage or preterm delivery]—they could calm the matter, saying, 'don't come out'—they too had their special bed." The complex of vacated buildings included one where two Congolese midwives had lived, a baby clinic or kilo room, a cooking place for sterilizing the clothes given to each woman as she entered the ward, and a storeroom that held the baby clothes that were given to each mother as she left. Each woman was given a shot of penicillin and vitamins to "get the dirty blood out of the body," Mama Mosa explained.[130] She also said that there had been a huge pit behind the maternity. The Congolese midwives would take the placentas there, wrapped in a cloth provided by the kin, and throw them into the pit, returning the cloth to the family afterward. At Isangi, another nun-operated state hospital nearby, the hospital staff disposed of placentas in a latrine. Placenta disposal became a hospital affair in these Catholic colonial institutions of the 1950s. Yakusu's staff never dreamed of attempting this; maternity staff instead gave the placenta to the parturient's kin, and they threw it in the river or buried it. At Yanonge, too, hospital disposals are no more: "It is over now. The ba-soeurs are gone."[131]

Sometimes, when expecting mothers arrived at night, they had to wait until morning to get a bed. Many came to Yanonge. On arrival, they were given maternity clothes. They could not take anything else into the maternity ward with them, Mama Mosa explained, except a lamp and matches so that they could look at their babies at night. No relatives were allowed inside. Only the midwives could enter, except for two men. One was the man who swept. The other had the job of writing the names of the newborns in a huge book and counting the number of births each month. When the mothers left, the mid-wives would cook the maternity clothes in a big pot "with a medicine given to them by the ba-soeurs," and then fold and put them away. The mothers would leave with a "gift for the child," clothes and a blanket. When they returned to attend kilo, when their babies were weighed, they would receive another gift, soap and medicines for the baby. Mama Mosa called this period "the time of bathing babies" because the "nun put each baby in its own towel" and the Congolese midwives bathed the newborns. It was also a time of gifts: "after giving birth, the nun came to her office. When a woman gave birth, she could give salt, rice, oil, bananas. When a woman gave birth, she received her ration."[132]

The Bamboli Company likely paid for the rations and blankets for its work-ers' wives; the state had begun paying 150 francs, in two 75-franc allotments, as birth bonuses for nonsalaried Congolese (indigènes libres). People at Yanonge talked about "the time of the nuns," "the time of before," when there was a small truck, "this ambulance," to "transport our women from fifteen kilometers, twenty kilometers away, bringing them to give birth here. . . . After a day, two days, she gave birth." Once the ambulance arrived in 1957, the nuns—one always remembered as Soeur Alois—would go forty-two kilometers away to the Bamboli work centers of Yasendo and Yatolema. "From these small houses there, they were getting women with pregnancies," and after their hospital stay, Sister Alois "would put them in the van again and return them to their villages."[133]

Almost all of the thirty-five women from whom I collected reproductive histories in Yainyongo-Romée had some experience of childbearing in a colonial maternity, most at Yanonge. Why did they go? Nuns roaming with ambulances played a key role. How did they remember this colonial experience? Mama Somboli, a mbotesa at the village of Ikongo, told me that she had given birth to several of her children in a Kisangani maternity in the 1950s. She liked going, she remarked, because of the shots. Another woman, Mama Lifoti, recalled that *bazungu* (white people) said they would arrest her husband if she did not go to Yanonge's maternity ward to give birth. That was why she went, she asserted, though she added that she had never given birth before and wanted to be sure that everything went well. She slept in a bed with a mattress for the first time.

Thus the postcolonial female voices that I collected in the field—primarily in Yainyongo-Romée, and also in Yakoso, Yakusu, and Kisangani—alternated between two kinds of statements, sometimes in the same narrative. One went like this: "There were beds with mattresses, and they gave me baby clothes and soap" or "I had the comfort of a bed and morning coffee, and I left with baby clothes." The other ran: "The time of maternity wards had come" or "I went to give birth at the hospital because otherwise they would have fined my husband or thrown him in jail." The first kind of statement is not easily unpacked from postcolonial nostalgia about the time when state and mission provided health care, often free, and gave away clothes, food, and soap—a nostalgia that my presence, as a white Mademoiselle, likely elicited. The second, when elaborated, includes a cluster of ideas about the coercive power of the state and the need to give birth in a hospital in order to have the newborn inscribed in the identity book of his father. Indeed, two concrete elements fueled participation in colonial pronatalist schemes. One was birth certificates. Concerns with the birthrate went hand in hand with censusing procedures, and as these were systematized in the postwar period, the number of maternity births soared. Both men and women desired these certificates, which were most easily obtained as part of a maternity ward birth. The second was the gifts or birth bonuses that women received for attending clinics and giving birth in maternities.

Boshanene, a Foma man in his sixties who was the hospital pharmacist when I was at Yakusu, said that the popularity of the mission station's maternity followed the arrival of Bokondoko (Mary Fagg) in 1951:

> If she arrived here today, then they would call "Bokondoko, Bokondoko, come with all babies." Mademoiselle would come. She liked to say "give children quinine and clothes." Each month a baby would come to kilo. Each month a baby would come to kilo. If six months passed, they would look to see who got a prize. . . . Once they knew, they would let them do kilos in village after village, village after village. So then people came along to come to give birth in the maternité.[134]

He condensed the changes that accompanied Fagg's arrival into baby clothes. Boshanene was not alone. Others, too, said Fagg was a "good Mademoiselle" because at the end of each year, she would give clothes: "The clothes came from as far as Europe waiting until women gave birth only."[135] Soap for each kilo attendance and brightly colored vests at Christmas and childbirth were Yakusu habits in the 1950s: "The one who came with her baby from the first, and there was no absence—she hadn't missed kilo—she would give her one thing, her matabish." Boshanene also mentioned money: "The prize . . . a piece of clothing and 75 francs . . . 75 francs and a blanket."[136] While these monetary birth bonuses at Yakusu were consequences of state forms and subsidies, the mission continued to associate gifts as much as possible with Christmas.

Christmas gifts were an old custom at Yakusu, and in the postwar period, they became conflated with baby clinic gifts. Yakusu had received donations for "specially-supported children" and gifts of garments and schoolbags since early in the twentieth century. Dorothy James had worked in her English parish church, training girls to make garments and bandages for BMS stations in the Congo, before she went to Yakusu as a teacher in 1911; they had sung a song— "the bandage, the net, the cake of soap"—as they worked.[137] Yakusu's missionary nurses lent mothers with sick babies "splendid little vests sent out to us from working parties at home" from 1923 on.[138] Birth gifts at Yakusu dated back to at least the first hospital birth in 1929; Ana received a baby cot. By the early 1930s, "want boxes" of "little garments and the other gifts"—such as clothing, books, and toys—were arriving at Yakusu from England at Christmastime.[139] Parturients paid for a maternity "confinement" in 1940 at Yakusu. But these small sums were compensated for by the rewards given for a maternity birth: "when they go home they have a hand-knitted blanket given to them (only if their baby has been born in the hospital and not in the village or in the canoe coming up to Yakusu!)." Mothers could keep the woolen vest put on the newborn and, if they liked, buy another baby vest or a woolen sling for carrying the baby.[140] During the war, the supply of baby vests from "want boxes" almost ran out. The maternity ward was becoming popular: "They nearly all stay in ten days and some don't want to go out then."[141] By the early 1950s, baby vests were no longer an automatic gesture within Yakusu clinics, even if they remained a maternity birth gift. Rather, mothers received a piece of soap at each baby clinic attendance, while vests were held out as a gift awarded at Christmastime: "all the mothers know that if they attend regularly they will receive one of the brightly coloured vests sent out from our lady workers in our home churches." Baby vests still arrived from England in bms-organized "want boxes" in 1953.[142] By the mid-1950s, 500 baby vests a year were needed for hospital baby clinics and an additional 1,000 cotton garments for two-to-five-year-old children attending Fagg's district toddler clinics. Children's clothes began to be made at Yakusu by the hospital tailor, midwife students, and other station women and girls.[143]

Projected Images and Doctors' Criticisms

Medicalized childbearing was central to a historical movement that began in the 1920s to regender the colony: to reorganize reproductive hygiene, encourage the presence of European women, and promote natality and stable family life. A focus on childbirth and infant care supplanted earlier concerns about venereal disease as a threat contaminating European and select African men. Some European women came as wives and parturients, and some came as nuns and midwives, yet together their arrival permitted the hospitalization of childbearing. Simultaneously, the colony became encoded as mother.

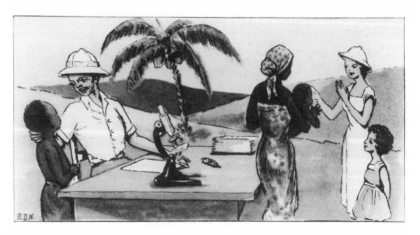

Idealized image in didactic hygiene booklet for Congolese mothers, published by FBEI and FOREAMI, ca. 1953. From Dony, *Mashauri kwa Mama wa Kongo*, 57.

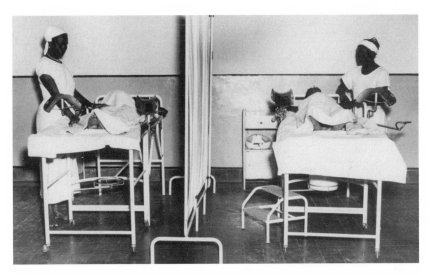

The labor and delivery room at the FBEI-constructed hospital at Tongoni, Kasongo territory, Maniema district, Kivu. Congopresse photograph by H. Goldstein, ca. 1955. (Courtesy of MRAC, Historical Section [IC 72.24.18; 56.22.695]. Courtesy of Africa-Museum, Tervuren, Belgium.)

A standard representation of the goodness of Belgian colonial rule was an idyllic image of colonial motherhood. All the elements of caring benevolence and medical power in tropical society were there: the white man as doctor, at his examining table, with a palm tree in the background, tending to the health of a mother with child. The microscope held center stage. The European woman— more likely the doctor's wife than a nurse—was at the doctor's side. This was a family affair, and there was no mistaking that the European woman was a mother, standing with her healthy daughter. White hands touched black bodies in this scene of colonial mothering of African children. This image was printed as the closing image of a booklet published in about 1953 for Congolese women in the colony's four major lingua franca.[144]

Photographs and postage stamps from the 1950s, especially those intended for European audiences, echoed the didactic images intended for Congolese. Yet these did not represent colonial society as helpful family to the same degree. The white doctor was usually absent from these baby clinic and maternity ward scenes, as was the European woman's child. Rather, promotional photographs from this period increasingly had a technological face, issuing images of the arrival of First World public health care in Africa.[145] Typical scenes included Congolese mothers collectively bathing their infants, lines of parturients in delivery ward beds, orderly hospitals, sophisticated surgery, ambulances and mobile hygiene vehicles, and technology to save the lives of premature babies.[146]

In Elisabethville's hospital for Congolese during the mid-1930s, women came to have their newborns inspected by Catholic nuns: "Behind each young mother walked the husband carrying in a bowl the placenta, which was also shown to the nursing sister, who could tell at a glance if all the afterbirth had been expelled." The maternity sister explained that many "still feel safer delivering in the bush," though by asking the fathers to make "the first fearful steps towards civilization with flyblown placentas in their outstretched hands," they prevented puerperal fever among many mothers.[147] These passages from *The Nun's Story* speak to paternal participation in interwar maternity care in one of the Congo's largest cities and to the centrality of maternity care to popular representations of Belgian colonialism. First published in 1956, this best-selling biography suggested that maternity births and inspected placentas became signs of paternal prestige and "evolution."

The formation of new paternal identities was integral to the colonial projections surrounding new maternities in the Congo. Images of colonial maternity wards became routine in didactic material directed at Congolese: films, hygiene books, newspapers, and comics. Yet Congolese fathers were absent from promotional baby-weighing and baby-washing scenes. They were active critics, however, as the pages of *La Voix du Congolais* show. As maternity births became part of the signs of colonial évolué culture, perhaps no subject was more

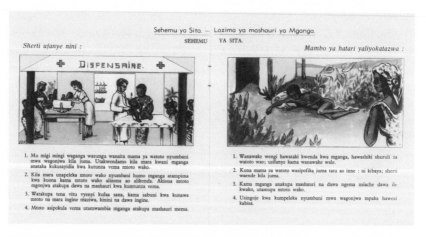

A set of "do-don't" messages about the importance of regular clinic attendance for mothers and infants. From a didactic hygiene booklet for Congolese mothers, published by FBEI and FOREAMI, ca. 1953. From Dony, *Mashauri kwa Mama wa Kongo*, 42–43.

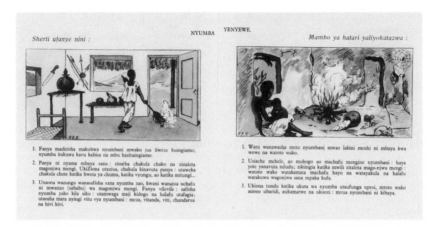

A set of "do-don't" messages about good housekeeping as opposed to the dangers of *wale* fires and smoke for infants. From a didactic hygiene booklet for Congolese mothers, published by FBEI and FOREAMI, ca. 1953. From Dony, *Mashauri kwa Mama wa Kongo*, 24–25.

actively debated than maternity care. One Congolese father wrote from Bau-douinville to complain that women were giving birth at home and four had died after childbearing because the existing maternity was closed; women also were giving birth en route to maternities or in villages because of the long distances and lack of ambulances. From Matadi came complaints that there were no cribs for newborns at the Kinkanda maternity. Many Léopoldville fathers debated conditions in the city's maternities.[148]

New notions of family life were projected at Congolese; images focused on évolué circles, living and dining rooms, baby clinics and maternity wards, and joint spousal preparations for a new baby. Catholic nuns were often present as teachers and midwives. Despite some late-colonial projections of parity among Belgian and Congolese worlds, most representations reveal how medicine was imbricated in the formation of colonial racial hierarchies. The semiotics were less about parallel worlds, less about the colony as mirror image of the metro-pole, than about racial control and diminution as native, achieved in part through a—sometimes sexualized, sometimes satiric—colonial gaze.

In the classic Belgian cartoon about the colonial experience, *Tintin au Congo*, it was not a microscope that was central, but momentarily a gramophone and especially a camera. A camera alone could function as metonym for a Euro-pean, positioning the viewer as dominant: hence, a colonial gaze. Spectator positioning shifted, however, when cartoons were remade as didactic messages for colonial subjects. The semiotics changed from cameras, airplanes, and auto-

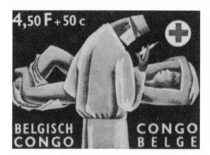 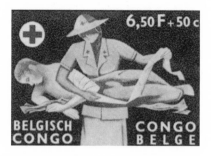

The sexualized and racialized entanglements implicit in this pair of Belgian Congo semi-charity postage stamps celebrating medicalization are eerie today. One can only imagine how these official images were read by those sending and receiving them in the Congo and Belgium at the time. The health care practitioners in each are more ambiguously white; the patients are unambiguously black. These of a patient receiving an injection and a patient being bandaged were issued as part of a three-part series on December 10, 1957; the third was of a female nurse embracing but also holding apart two children. The surtax was for the Red Cross.

mobiles to mirrors and bicycles. Mbumbulu cartoons, a postwar comic strip designed for Congolese readers, depicted men cycling off to visit their female kin in maternity wards. The spectator was no longer positioned as if from an assumed outside, peering in through a camera. The didactic cartoon positions the colonial middle in a self-questioning mode—a "who am I?"—through no less than a mirror with an image of the middle grandfather gazing at his reflection with puzzlement and wonder, just after his son's wife has given birth in a maternité.[149] Mbumbulu cartoons also project a bicycle—the diminutive of a European's automobile, a critical element to the mobility of colonial medicine, and a not insignificant complement to soap—as counterpart to a maternity ward. Nor were these semiotics unrelated to the historical—and gynecological—specificities of the Congo's interwar modernity.

By 1934, some colonial doctors began to notice "the huge progress accomplished over the last few years in obstetrics and gynecology in our hospitals for blacks."[150] Maternity services and buildings were multiplying, and doctors were publishing the records of their gynecological caseloads.[151] Dr. Vander Elst, after six months of gynecological practice in Leopoldville's Hôpital des Noirs, doubted that any hospital in Belgium had a gynecological clinic as "well-equipped and varied." "Orchestra" doctors must "cede place to specialists," he argued. Given the high number of venereal-related, salpingo-ovarian infections, for example, gynecologists were "indispensable in the present period of colonial organization."[152] The postwar period brought greater medical special-

LES AVENTURES DE LA FAMILLE MBUMBULU

(suite)

MBUMBULU EST GRAND-PERE

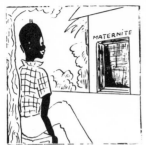

Pierre attend devant la porte de la maternité de la ville. Il est nerveux et impatient... Que se passe-t-il donc?...

Pierre anangoja mbele ya mbango ya nyumba ya wazazi ya mji. Iko wahasira na asiyemuvumilivu... Inapita nini basi?...

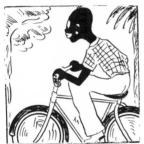

Mais il faut avertir la famille... Pierre se rend en hâte chez ses parents pour leur annoncer la bonne nouvelle...

Lakini inafaa kuarifu jamaa... Pierre akajirudi kwa haraka kwa wuzza wake kwa kuwapasha habari ngema...

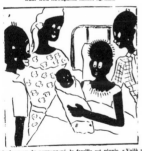

Autour du berceau du nouveau-né, la famille est réunie. « Voilà un solide gaillard, s'écrie Mbumbulu, il me ressemble étonnamment ». Tous rient aux éclats.

Kandokando ya kitanda ya mzaliwa-sasa, jamaa imekusanyika. « Ona kule mfurahivu wa nguvu, analalamika Mbumbulu, inanionekania msangao ». Wote wanacheka kwa makelele.

MBUMBULU NI BABA-MKUBWA

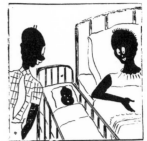

... Agnès vient de mettre au monde un gros garçon! « Quel bel enfant! », s'exclame Pierre. Agnès est souriante et Pierre ne sait comment manifester sa joie.

... Agnès anatoka mukuzala mwanaume kabambi! « Mtoto mzuri gani! », kalalamika Pierre. Agnès iko meheko na Pierre hajue namna ya kuonyesha furaha yake.

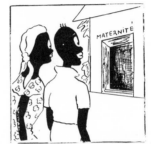

Mbumbulu et Marie sont tout joyeux. « Allons vite à la maternité, dit Mbumbulu, pour féliciter Agnès et faire connaissance avec notre petit-fils ».

Mbumbulu na Marie wako wote wafurahivu. « Tuende mbio ku nyumba ya wazazi, akasema Mbumbulu, kwa kusifu Agnès na kufanya ufahamisho pamojana mwana wetu mdogo ».

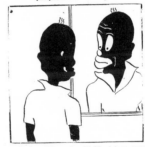

« En un peu plus jeune évidemment, rectifie Mbumbulu, car me voilà maintenant grand-père. Comme le temps passe vite! J'ai peine à croire que j'ai vieilli, mais un coup d'œil à ce miroir suffit, hélas! pour m'en convaincre ».

- Kwa kijana mdogo zaidi, kweli, anamutengeneza Mbumbulu, kwani munione sasa baba-mkubwa. Sawa wakati inapita mbio! Nina tabu kwa kusadiki kama nimezeheka, lakini kadicho ku hiyo kiyo inatosha, hélas! kwa kujiwesapo! »

Bicycles and maternity wards were central to the semiotics of Congolese "evolution," as can be seen in this mimetic moment of self-recognition when the Congolese comic strip star of ten years, Mbumbulu, becomes a grandfather; his son cycles to deliver the news. From the Belgian missionary-authored didactic comic strip that appeared in the equivalent of *Life* magazine for Congolese from 1946 to 1955, *Nos Images,* an official publication. From "Les aventures de la famille Mbumbulu," *Nos Images,* Sw. ed., 8, no. 124, 20 November 1955, 19. (Courtesy of the Bibliothèque Royale, Brussels, Belgium.)

ization. While Stanley Browne's medical career became increasingly focused on leprology, gynecology and obstetrics was for the first time becoming almost a branch of tropical medicine.[153] Belgium's tropical medical literature increasingly featured obstetric topics. Colonial gynecologists and obstetricians in the Congo wrote about anemia and pregnancy; uterine ruptures, fistulas, and tubal pregnancies; eclampsia in urban women; dystocia and pelvic size in particular districts and ethnic areas; and in the late 1950s, *ventouse* (vacuum) extractions and symphysiotomies.[154]

During the late 1920s, doctors spoke of colonial gynecology and obstetrics in terms of depopulation and ensuring the economic future of the colony. While the assumption was that maternities would lower the infant mortality rate, statistics were never kept in such a way as to prove this one way or the other. Maternal mortality was hardly mentioned, though operative obstetrics certainly saved a good many women's lives. In 1929, a Dr. Duboccage suggested that in order to have a "prosperous country" with a high birthrate, the puerperal infection rate must be lowered by relocating the childbirth to maternity wards.[155] Not until 1939 did two colonial doctors publish a critique of maternal and infant health care in the Congo.

Drs. G. Platel and Yv. Vandergoten, a husband-and-wife team, had spent six years in charge of a Mayombe infant clinic subsidized by the Oeuvre Nationale. They argued that such clinics were amateurish baby-weighing ventures that did little more than give advice to Congolese mothers, which given material conditions, these women could not possibly follow. They also questioned colonial statistical methods and claims. The impact of baby clinics on infant mortality had been exaggerated because of the conflation of different kinds of mortality within single analyses. Baby clinics were unable to affect the rate of stillbirths and infant deaths in the first days, they contended; these could only be reduced through better obstetrical assistance and antenatal care. Yet Platel and Vandergoten were opposed to an expansion of maternities: "Except for difficult births, we do not see the benefit that a native can receive from the multiplication of these costly organizations." Most Congolese deliveries did not require biomedical assistance, they asserted. Maternities in the Congo should be reserved for difficult births, as was largely the case in Belgium at the time: "The concentration of pregnant women in maternities determines a movement of population without justification."[156] Institutionalizing childbirth also posed public health dangers, this husband- and-wife doctor team argued: "in concentrating parturients in conditions of promiscuity which are not found in the village, in unclean conditions due to the lack of adequate facilities, in conditions of obstetric assistance which are *not made up for by good will or devotion,* we risk seeing dramatic epidemics of puerperal fever replace some few obstetric deaths."[157]

Such criticism was exceptional, especially before the Second World War. With the inauguration of the FBEI in 1947 and the Oeuvre de la Maternité et de l'Enfance Indigènes (OREAMI) in 1955, money became available for maternity construction as well as research and evaluation. By 1949, Governor General Jungers commented that even if existing baby clinics had "had a happy influence on the black child," they had not lowered infant mortality in the proportions expected, especially given the mass of subsidies provided each year.[158] OREAMI was founded, under the auspices of FOREAMI, to inventory, oversee, and coordinate the colony's diverse maternal and infant health care programs. In 1957, when Marc Vincent, a prominent colonial pediatrician, made a journey throughout Belgian Africa studying maternal and infant health installations for OREAMI, he too criticized the poorly trained workers of baby clinics, notably Catholic nuns, and the lack of systematic antenatal care.[159]

Some doctors thought that Congolese women no longer had to be encouraged to go to maternities. New ones were hardly opened, the colony's leading obstetrician, J. Lambillon, noted, before they were overwhelmed with patients.[160] Lambillon spoke in 1957 from the vantage point of Leopoldville's teeming maternity services and state-of-the-art technologies. He had headed a Fondation Médicale de l'Université de Louvain au Congo clinic in Katana beginning in the late 1930s, before becoming, in 1947, the director of Leopoldville's native maternity, "an incomparable field," in his words, for gynecological practice. He was opposed to satellite maternities that operated without doctors in 1957. He also thought that embryotomies were no longer worthy of any discussion. Forceps deliveries were obsolete, he claimed: and so they tended to be in Leopoldville, where in 1956 there were only 95 forceps deliveries but 602 cesarean sections. Indeed, cesarean sections were undertaken in 5 to 7 percent of Congolese births, but in only 2 percent of those among European women.[161] By 1949, spinal anesthetics had been abandoned for cesareans by Bukavu's doctors because of cases of maternal death during spinal operations. Chloroform was used from 1940 to 1951, though some women were still dying from the anesthesia. The number of cesareans increased dramatically in Bukavu with the introduction of ether in 1952. Almost 6 percent of medically supervised births in Bukavu's native hospital were handled by C-section that year, making Bukavu's rate higher than that in the United States in 1970 and in Britain in 1975.[162] Lambillon's approach assumed it was possible to perfect the technocratic vision of eugenicists of the 1930s. Specialists had arrived, the funds were ample, the most sophisticated biomedical technologies could be easily imported into this colonial situation, and there was a readily available research subject population.

Marc Vincent, on the other hand, was a planner with a vision of primary maternity health care reaching into the most remote parts of the Belgian Congo. As he traveled on his study tour, he witnessed firsthand the unevenness of services and practitioners. His recommendations for OREAMI were largely solid and prescient. He saw the need to professionalize and systematize practice. He especially wanted antenatal referral schemes and favored waiting homes near maternities for pregnant women.[163] No comparable, grand visions came to the Congo again until primary health care arrived with World Health Organization (WHO), United Nations Educational, Scientific and Cultural Organization (UNESCO), and SANRU plans in the late 1970s and 1980s. "Safe motherhood," a new WHO slogan, found its way to Zaire as it did to most of the world around 1985; though most planners thought that they were inventing something unprecedented, many Zairians did not even notice.

Husbands, Honors, and Wale

While doctors debated operative procedures, satellite maternities, and antenatal care, colonial policy led to a medicalization of childbearing. Although Yakusu followed Belgian colonial patterns from 1939, Yakusu's evangelical hospital culture remained distinct from that of Catholic state hospitals. Both kinds of institutions loaned parturients clothes; when Yakusu's maternity opened in 1939, each mother received "a linen bag containing towel, soap, blanket, and six napkins," which she was supposed to return when discharged.[164] Yet birth and baby gifts were broached as much as possible through idioms of Christ's birth and Christmas gifts; there were never rations at Yakusu, and monetary rewards may not have lasted long. The slight increase in hospital births at Yakusu was not representative of maternity birthrates in the colony. The mission station never had a waiting home or an ambulance for transporting pregnant women. When Belgian colonial pronatalism met British Baptist evangelical metaphors and maternity practices at Yakusu, there were explicit and implicit processes of borrowing, translation, and mixture, in keeping with this foreign mission's pragmatic posture on using medicine simultaneously to evangelize and to raise money and survive in a slightly hostile and alien colonial context. The processes of quotation and translation across these fields became ever more complex, as Yakusu trained Congolese midwives to supervise deliveries.

Congolese women who gave birth at maternities continued such practices as postnatal bathing and, at Yakusu, placenta burial because these habits took place outside the time of obstetrical intervention. The importance of these baths may have grown over time, as we will see in chapter 7, as they became equated with shots. Postnatal seclusion practice, too, remained a source of honor for women. Both men and women assert—and regret—that the duration of wale has declined historically. This change may be difficult to quantify and date, but it represents a significant alteration in the role of fathers in natalist practice. Its decline is a source of shame for men, perhaps even more so than for women.

Mixtures in imaging of colonial maternities and childbearing experiences in autobiographical as well as social memory illustrate these points. Mama Komba Lituka gave birth to babies at both Yakusu's and Yanonge's maternities. She recalled food from her stay at Yanonge: "When I gave birth there, I ate well. They were handing out rations, rice, dried fish, oil." Like others, she remembered a nun, Soeur Alois, who gave her a baby blanket when it was time to go home: "She would give a blanket. She would give you, the mother, clothes to wear. She would give those for babies, too. So we left the maternité there. We came back to Yalokombe." Yanonge was an easy canoe ride downstream from Yalokombe, where Komba Lituka lived at the time. Her husband died after she gave birth to their second child. She remarried in Yakoso and went at the last minute to give birth to her third child at Yakusu's maternity: "Me, I was with that pregnancy tiiii, I was just here going around with that pregnancy. And the time itself of giving birth, me, I said: 'Me alone, not that kind of birth pains.' I just stood up like that. Me, I went just me alone up to the maternité." On arriving at the maternity door, she remembered voices calling the Congolese midwife: "Yes, Likenja, come. Likenja come, Likenja come." Komba Lituka stayed for ten days after her delivery, and when she left, "they gave me a baby's vest, saying: 'This is a baby's vest.' We came to the village."[165]

Mama Komba's memories reveal differences in the gifts that she received: food rations and a baby blanket at Yanonge, a baby vest at Yakusu. She also remembered midwives' names: Sister Alois at Yanonge and Likenja at Yakusu. British met Belgian and Protestant met Catholic in Komba Lituka's memories, but most striking is the symmetry by which she concluded each account with a "we" returning home and then a happy, proud period of wale. Komba recalled returning from Yanonge's maternity to Yalokombe: "There, me, I entered the house again, entered wale. That wale there, I was cooking well, I was eating well. And me and my in-laws, when I came out of there, my friends were dancing. There was no trouble at all. No fighting, no anger. We were just all fine." On her return home from Yakusu's maternity to Yakoso, she remembered:

My mother-in-law, that one, she celebrated incredibly, doing good. She gave out palm wine here, just giving it to people. Here again, I entered wale once again. They put me again in the house. My husband went to the river, killing fish, giving them to me. I was cooking, eating. Then I came out of wale. I stayed in two months. I came out. I was going about once again. There was no trouble, not at all.[166]

Unlike the mother of Trouble Trouble, whose kin humiliated her by refusing to bury her placenta, Komba Lituka recalled no fighting, anger, or trouble associated with either of her deliveries or wale periods. Instead, there was feasting, celebration, and her Lokele husband netting fish for her to eat.

Colonized childbearing at Yanonge and Yakusu had an immense impact on delivery, and the ten days or so following a birth, but very little effect on much of local natalist practice. Wale—except through baby clothes—remained relatively untouched. Not that baby clothes were insignificant; keeping babies close to smoky fires soiled baby vests and blankets, and the new clothing kept babies covered and warm. When I asked Tata Bafoya about baby clothes, he said, "whites came and changed the world." The honor and prestige of a long and abundant wale did not die easily, however, even as baby clothes, birth certificates, blankets, and quinine became desirable.

Yakusu's missionaries did not write about wale seclusion until the mid-1940s.[167] By the 1950s, they denounced wale practices as problematic, though some doctors were encountering related burn injuries in the Congo from the 1920s on. E. D. M. White reported in 1954, after she visited the Yalisombo clinic: "We were trying again to think of some way of discouraging the women from keeping up their native custom of sitting in a small mudhut at the back of the house, and being smoke-dried by a huge log fire for at least one month after the birth of a child."[168] The missionaries never understood the cultural reasons underlying the practice, even though wale seclusion in a dark room was less strictly maintained over time.

When I asked why wale became less strictly observed, the most common explanation was that the fire's smoke would sully the baby's clothes. The color-coding of colonial power ironically would have reinforced the desire for light-shaded babies, while the material representation of an auspicious, lavish, fitting birth was increasingly encoded in the prized clothing of kilo Christmas gifts. Malia Winnie went home for her wale periods. "Good plants don't grow here" at the mission, she explained. Yet she also fancied baby vests, and she would snitch a few when the Mademoiselle at the hospital was not looking.[169]

The celebration that comes at the end of a wale parallels the one that begins it: first, the husband gives his wife's father a chicken for the blood of childbirth that she has lost; when the mother of the baby is sent home to her father after her wale, the husband sends her back with another chicken. Usually a husband would decide when a wale period should end, though there could be fights about it. People insisted that wale and bowai were asili practices that predated the BaTambatamba. Wale was a period of rest, staying near a fire, growing fat, lightening skin, smearing oil on one's body, and sitting. During this period, a Mama Wale's house had to be protected from the entry of a woman pregnant with a young fetus or also the baby would not nurse well, or the mother's heart would close up and she would not feel hungry.[170] Wale was also a time of washing with hot water and being helped by female kin.

Some spoke of wale periods of three months. During pregnancy, especially at the end of the lisole period, the family of the husband would, if they liked you, give you food. Indeed, if your in-laws liked you, they would not only give you a lot of food, but also cut a lot of wood and call your family to show the food of wale that they have prepared. "People do not do it anymore. People eat cassava greens only. To give birth is to die. Meaning: you give good food." In her day, Mama Kumbula Wayinoko Rosa told me, her in-laws gave her a lot of food at wale. Her own mother would refuse to eat this food given by the in-laws for her daughter, a Mama Wale, instead cooking her own cassava greens during the three-month period. Wayinoko's first wale was three months, her second two months, and her others lasted three months, yet she was walking about and going to the market, though keeping her baby in the house.[171] Mama Lifoti also remembered wale periods of three months. Her mother came to help her, although her mother-in-law was also there helping to cook and getting wood and water. Lifoti's husband got the food.[172]

Tata Bafoya said a wale lasted three to four months during his time (in the 1920s, 1930s, and even 1940s): "You don't want your wife to go about with your child. She should eat first, grow fat, so the child becomes very big. The person who looks will say, 'Ah! she ate good in the house!' " But times have changed:

> Now, these days, will they put a woman there one month? Even two weeks, three weeks, and she comes out to buy clothes and *mapapa* [cloth wrappers] . . . like the shoes of babies. Me, me, your father, I cannot wear these mapapa of theirs. I come out of the cabinet from bathing. So, me, I get my wife, "give me a hand towel, give me soap, give me my mapapa." Our mapapa of before, they weren't like that. No. Our mapapa of before, they were of good *bahindi* [Indian cloth] and the skins of animals. They would give it [to us] when we came out from bathing. These mapapa a woman wears! You see it: she is nodding, she is going about, she looks here, she looks there. What state of mind has she entered? . . . [T]hey are parading themselves as if they are intoxicated. Me, your old man, I will not look for clothes. It is what sort of thing? It is kind of the children to give them a good mattress, a good bed.

He explained that when a wife was giving birth, the husband would leave her with his mother: "Your mother will care for her. You, the bwana, you go fishing and give fish, buy banana, cassava, and give them." A man also did not "sleep in this house where the woman is sleeping with the child" until it was three months, his mother staying there instead to care for his wife "because they don't want to hurt the baby." This was no longer so: "You, don't you see small babies each time they come to the hospital? Because for the mother and the father to have sex is very bad for the child." When did this change? I asked. "It changed because . . . you white people. *Wazungu,* you changed the world. . . . The time of our fathers, *wababa,* it wasn't like that. All words were clear. All words were clear, my child. Before, no, no, no, no. The child is at the breast and you, the father, go to make love to your wife. Ahhhhh! . . . A woman gives birth today to sleep in the bed today, ahhh!"[173]

I tapped an ambivalent mixture within social memory about maternity births among women in Yainyongo-Romée, too. Many men, especially those who had gone to school and had worked in kizungu during their lives, were proud to speak about the maternity births of their wives. Nonetheless, the rigidity of hospital culture in Catholic-operated, state-financed institutions imposed changes on social forms of organizing maternity care, whether in a plantation district surrounding Yanonge or in a large city, where class distinctions were well advanced. The duration of wale periods declined. Husbands' roles finding food in the immediate postnatal period vanished in maternity contexts, such as Yanonge, where employers were providing rations. And maternity births and the associated baby garments carried prestige for fathers as much as mothers. The contradictions in postcolonial testimony need to be seen in terms of how Congolese moved among mixed social realities of coercive and tempting messages. They also may have ascribed meaning to name-inscribing papers, birth certificates, and identity books, as human-made objects with special capacities to create identities, enhance paternal distinction, and promote infant survival.

7 DEBRIS

The township had not yet completely lost all recollection of the customs of the colonial regime which, if nothing else, had been a great provider of medical care. . . . The time had not yet come when, as soon as someone said that they were going to the hospital . . . they would find scorn and derision poured upon them. . . . As soon as the labour pains started she was to get on a bus that would take her to the clinic at Ntermelen. There the baby would be delivered by a midwife who would provide her when she left with the certificate which was absolutely necessary to benefit by the various social advantages which all officials, even temporary ones, had a right to.—Mongo Beti, *Perpetua and the Habit of Unhappiness,* 1978

When Malia Winnie told me about her conflicts with Dr. Browne at Yakusu's hospital, she swiftly moved without a pause to more recent problems working with young Catholic midwives in Kisangani. Explaining the danger of cesarean sections, she said: "Childbearing is dying, hence I forbid it, saying I don't like it because he himself, our chief, he was one bad man. So, me, I spoke like this, because we do not like each other, us and the Catholics." My questions about colonial cesarean sections took Malia Winnie to Stanley Browne, to conflict with a Protestant evangelical "bad man," and these memories led her instantly, through her subjective, symbolic coding of events, to young Catholic midwives among whom she has worked at Kisangani's state hospital since moving to this city after the rebellion. She told me that she could no longer work with these young Catholic midwives because they did not have a proper sense of professional ethics and abused parturients. She was practicing at home instead, often at night and never with disputes. If a parturient or her kin gives her an argument, she tells them to go find a hospital. She emerged from this intricate tangent wondering if I knew Esther Lokangu, and proceeded to tell me about the day Dr. Browne wanted to send her to jail.

The risk of jail may have brought these seemingly disparate memories together side by side. When Malia Winnie elaborated on her private, quiet practice helping with home deliveries, she emphasized the importance of avoiding shame, steering clear of any dispute over the handling of a case that could lead to threats of jail. The fear was not fanciful. All of the midwives I met who had been trained at Yakusu in the 1950s knew that a few years earlier, about 1985, a conflict between a hospital doctor and the kin of a parturient who had died while giving birth had led to one of their cohorts doing time in a Kisangani jail.

Malia Winnie's postcolonial conflicts with city midwives have been generational and religious. Most midwives trained at Yakusu carried a sense of professional superiority and bitter indignation about working among these younger women who, they held, had inferior training in a hospital school inherited from a Catholic-dominated colonial state. They all believed that their Protestant training at colonial Yakusu was superior. Malia Winnie said that she had refused to work with these young city midwives who don't work when they are eating, demand payments from patients before delivering them, and hit parturients in labor. Protestant-trained midwives and recently trained Catholic ones have different kinds of hearts, she said, reminding me how she coaxes and soothes women in labor, and will not sit down until her work is finished.[1]

The memories and reflections of other Yakusu-trained midwives reveal how much their postrebellion experiences in Kisangani are also mediated through their memories of the 1950s. They recalled that there used to be "drugs of all kinds . . . drugs for deliveries, drugs for treating the baby at the time of being born. . . . We were delivering with gloves, and everything was there on the table. . . . Afterward there was no tetanus, because there were pouches for the babies, infant clothes, bandages and everything." Each day, a mother would take off her clothes and be given fresh ones to wear, until the umbilical cord "was left one week drying. Only then did the mother leave." The midwives would wash the babies and clothe them in hospital-provided vests. By 1989, everything had changed. "The means for a mother to buy clothes, to cover these huge costs today: no way. . . . But now: trouble. Clothes: only if the mother might buy them. Many don't have money, especially in this time after the war." Another interjected: "One woman, she will come without bandages." The first continued:

> There aren't even bandages. Only dirty cloths, here and there. Now it's become what? You give birth, today. Today, today! you go to the village. There in the village, they don't know how to care for a baby. The baby goes and gets tetanus. These days and the ways of before, they aren't the same. We are seeing many troubles of the people because many, they don't have the money to buy clothes and bandages and other things. The time of

before, there was a huge cabinet of these things and medicines that weren't for sale. Now, when everything has to be bought, where will you get it?

Before, if a woman was sick or felt labor pains, she could go to the doctor to explain how she was feeling: "Now it has become, until you pay first. . . . Now, as soon as you arrive, you are asked: 'Do you have money?' So those without money, they go back home." Doctors will no longer do operations, another woman added, "if they haven't seen your money. . . . He will turn you away, saying, 'go to another hospital.' The 15,000 zaires? . . . Nothing, they will not cut until you pay money." A third exclaimed: "Some women have just died right there." Instead, many women give birth at home: "Many! Many! Many! Many!" one said.[2] Statistics from a 1982 study indicate that the number of women giving birth at home in Kisangani, rather than at hospitals and clinics, was substantially higher than in other cities. In major Zairian cities in 1982, 16.4 percent of Zairian women had home births; in Kinshasa, this percentage was only 3.6, whereas in Kisangani, it was 34.3 percent.[3]

I asked who helped if a woman gave birth at home: "Sometimes *ba-accoucheuses*. Sometimes a village person who knows . . . a relative . . . or her mother will deliver her daughter." Another said: "Sometimes she knows an accoucheuse; this midwife, she can help her." A third added: "Other midwives live close by, so they know each other. So someone says, so-and-so, she is a midwife. Let's call her. Even at night, she will go." One woman admitted that she goes to help women and deliver them. Yet another insisted: "But if there is a difficult birth, you can't help. . . . You just say: 'Go to the hospital.' If she doesn't like the hospital, she will just die with it in her."[4]

Many midwives trained at Yakusu during the colonial period worked in Kisangani hospitals during the late 1980s, while also maintaining semiclandestine, informally compensated practices in their neighborhoods. Kisangani's state hospital is located on the outskirts of the city, and urban transportation and hospital conditions deteriorated drastically during the Mobutu years. When their neighbors, Kisangani residents, ask for help with a delivery, these Protestant midwives carefully apprise the likelihood of a normal presentation and delivery before agreeing to attend to a birth in a parturient's home. Yakusu-trained midwives do not risk assisting with a difficult case because if a parturient dies or ends up in medical trouble, the midwife is at risk. They also protect themselves from potential legal reprisals by being sure to have the necessary biomedical equipment at hand: cord clamps, scissors, syringes, needles, and ergometrine. They send the high-risk cases to the hospital. Women who do not give birth in one of Kisangani's hospitals or private clinics, I heard, go later to purchase a birth certificate under-the-table from a member of the hospital staff.

Several studies on the impact of structural adjustment on maternal health in

Africa during the 1980s note the declining numbers of women who give birth in biomedical settings. The assumption tends to be that a hospital birth is not only safer but an indicator of better health conditions.[5] Little is known about the microeconomics of these decisions as well as the quality of care received in various settings. My evidence on Kisangani during the final years of Mobutu's Zaire is incomplete, coming almost exclusively from midwives trained at Yakusu in the colonial period. Yet it suggests that these Protestant-trained midwives were providing a quality of care during home deliveries (and home-based ante- and postnatal care) that was superior to the care possible in an overburdened and underequipped state hospital reeling from the diminished resources and austerity conditions of a corrupt regime, reduced and extorted public expenditures, and structural adjustment exigencies. Most women in a city like Kisangani in 1989 could only consider a clinic delivery if they went to the dilapidated state hospital for the mass population, the former native colonial hospital completed in the mid-1920s. A delivery at a private clinic or the university-affiliated (former European colonial) hospital serving an urban middle class would be perhaps eight times more expensive.[6]

SANRU *among Ruins*

We arrived by canoe at Yalemba at dusk on the third day of our journey. There were images of Yakusu within Yalemba, the neighboring BMS mission post located downriver before the Aruwimi confluence at Basoko. Yalemba was higher up a riverbank, more spread out, less organized in linear, quadrangular form, and rickety. Missionary houses were never converted to brick at Yalemba, as they were at Yakusu. The path by the riverfront with its line of former missionary houses in wood with large verandas was reminiscent of Yakusu. Brick, however, is less destructible. Yalemba was BMS domesticity in slow ruins. BMS missionaries never returned to Yalemba after those from both stations fled in 1964.

At Yalemba, like everywhere in the region, the rebellion of the mid-1960s was the defining chronological marker for everyone who was at least twenty-five in 1989. Nostalgia for life "before the war" at Yalemba meant that Yakusu's missionary nurse and I were escorted to the former home of single women missionaries; there, we were to spend the night, even though it resembled a condemned building. We walked carefully over broken slats, quite literally, so as not to fall through the floor. The bathroom and toilet were inaccessible, hanging from mere floorboards. We bathed with a bucket in our bedroom. There were enough gaping holes to throw the used bathwater down through one of them. The wood floor was caving in just before our bedroom door. The bed frame was there, but the mattress long gone. They set the table for all of us with china from a glass-doored buffet, turning the soup bowls facedown. Dinner arrived in large plastic washbasins, placed in the center of the table. Yakusu's nurses saw the humor. The church elder and Yalemba nurse joined us. The elder said grace.

The going energy at Yalemba was regret. The church elder measured historical time in missionaries' periods of service and mission buildings. He, a mission man born and bred at Yalemba, gave me a tour of station sites the next day. He was eager to tell me the history of each missionary house, showing me the Carrington house, the former boarding home for girls, the present church and former church building, and the spot where George Grenfell pitched his tent when he came to found the station in 1905. The dispensary had built-in cement benches set in an open breezeway in the middle of the structure. These benches, at once functioning as waiting room and sanctuary for religious services and hygiene lessons, expressed the interchangeability of evangelism and hygiene. Way in the back of the station there was a small brick house, off by itself, built with FBEI money, where a state-sponsored nurse used to work. A married nurse-and-midwife team conducted the present dispensary, still a church operation, but since the mid-1980s, also run as a "self-financing" SANRU health center with Yakusu as its central reference hospital.

Our arrival—a BMS missionary nurse, two Yakusu-trained nurses, and me—as part of a Yakusu-organized tour of old church dispensaries within its relatively new SANRU health zone was a big event, at least for the church elder who measured history by the comings and goings of BMS missionaries. I had a chance to witness forms of domesticity, hospitality, and prayer on this journey. I also witnessed, as I did throughout this trip, structural adjustment–imposed, primary health care at work.

The SANRU project, billed as "a self-sustaining, community-supported, primary health care system," was founded to prevent and treat the "ten most prevalent public health problems" in rural health zones in Zaire. Franklin C. Baer, an American Mennonite missionary working as project manager in SANRU's headquarters in Kinshasa in 1989, told me that the project's objective was to decentralize the management and financing of primary health care through a health zone concept. The idea of zones was accepted at the national level in 1974–75, he said, and SANRU began, as a USAID-funded project, in 1982. USAID officers in Kinshasa boasted that SANRU, a forty-million-dollar project, was "the biggest bilateral health project in Africa" in 1989. The lack of knowledge about Belgian colonial health care was plain at USAID and SANRU headquarters. USAID-affiliated staff defined, for example, "user fees" and "self-financing" as major colonial legacies, giving legitimacy to their own austerity policies.[7] They were surprised to learn that in Yakusu's zone, SANRU was a new bureaucracy and funding source for primary health care that was being imposed on top of a mission-organized, state- and company-backed, primary health care network that had been in place since the 1930s.[8]

SANRU began with fifty zones in 1982; by early 1989, there were ninety. The USAID subsidized training, vehicles, and the first six months' worth of drugs to get a zone operational. The Eglise du Christ au Zaire (ECZ), a consortium of Protestant churches that included the BMS, implemented the project with technical assistance from USAID in Zaire and the Peace Corps. Funding to train popular midwives as TBAS, traditional birth attendants with some biomedical training, was an important component of SANRU plans. Baer was especially proud of SANRU's training programs for TBAS, particularly those at Karawa, where there were 100 to 125 TBAS working in the zone, and Nyankunde.[9] Yakusu was a SANRU zone from the beginning. When I arrived seven years later, in 1989, technical assistance had shifted from money for antenatal and TBA training to better bicycles and water sanitation (spring capping and latrine construction). The agenda had also been adjusted from "the ten most prevalent public health problems" to an "emphasis on fee-for-service and self-sufficiency" as a tenet of primary health care in Zaire. A 1987 report declared: "User fees to finance the health care delivery system are well accepted at all levels in Zaire."[10] Yet an audit that same year found that assessments of the "financial sustainability of the projects' health care system" had never been required. There were problems with cash management and self-financing procedures from 1984. By late 1986, a SANRU evaluation report indicated that the legal status of rural health zones had not been established. "Community involvement" was excellent in some zones, while in others, there were problems of "changing zone tactics" and "community organizing." "Supervision, financial and logistic management, and monitoring" needed "strengthening" at all rural health zone levels. U.S.-made bicycles "proved ill-adapted for rural use." There were ultimately two types of SANRU zones, according to a 1992 final report written after USAID personnel in Zaire were evacuated due to widespread looting in Kinshasa in September 1991 and after the April 1992 USAID decision to terminate assistance to Zaire. (The project continued "in a much diminished form, with funding from UNICEF" as as well as remaining USAID-Zaire funds, "despite anarchy, hyper-inflation, and limited external support.") Some zones received only government subsidies, and SANRU was effectively acting "as a shadow Ministry of Health." Other zones—such as Karawa, Nyankunde, and Yakusu—were served by (mainly Protestant) religious missions; in these zones, SANRU mostly provided "complementary assistance, especially in the areas of training and supervision."[11] Both types experienced the imperatives of self-financing and cost recovery, however.

By 1989, pharmaceutical cost recovery as a method of financing primary health care was a growing agenda within structural adjustment–oriented USAID planning. These imperatives were new in Yakusu's zone then, and I observed Yakusu's nurses struggling to implement them. Evangelization had almost dropped out of this former BMS and then SANRU-era dispensary network. The bureaucratic imperatives of self-financing—pharmaceutical and salary cost recovery through patient fees—were paramount. Yet self-financing was multiple in meaning, and state forms were blurred in their visibility. Every meal began with grace, the eye nurse especially saw patients wherever we stopped, but there were neither evangelical services nor hygiene inspections. Records were tallied and inspected, some local disputes adjudicated, and drugs and supplies sold. Meanwhile, the Yakusu nurses and driver engaged in their own parallel activities: their gracious courier service and the purchasing of forest products for resale from Yakusu.

War, Memory, and Soap

Throughout my stay in Zaire, the conversations I had revealed a duality to social memory. On the one hand, there were horror stories of being whipped, taxed, buried alive, and carried away in sacks to become white people's wealth and food. On the other hand, people expressed regret that the times of many bicycles and bandages were no more. The ideas of some former soldiers and Mouvement Populaire de la Révolution (MPR) party members seemed refracted, mechanically and cautiously, through Mobutu speeches then current on radio and television: we were the slaves of the Belgians, and now we have freedom. Others complained when soldiers and party men arrived in their villages demanding fines. Some spoke about the meaning of the pregnant woman image on Mobutu's walking stick. But the breaking point in local historical imaginations was neither independence nor Mobutu; the dividing line in history was, simply, "the war" of the mid-1960s.

Everyone's memories were marked by the rebellion: Mama Sila with her bullet scars; the BaTula and Papa Lokangu who guarded the mission station keys and all missionary property; the elder at Yalemba who missed missionaries; all kinds of people who had been continually in flight in the forest for two or three years; and Yakusu nurses and hospital administrators who had lost fathers and uncles, having been seen, as were all Lokele intellectuals who lost their lives, as the enemy. At the Yanonge hospital, memories of Soeur Alois, her ambulance, and all the women giving birth at the hospital were alive. Nevertheless: "We were like that until the time the war arrived. We were afraid, we ran away. Even me, I spent three years in the forest. I didn't come out quickly. Slowly I came out and arrived here." A new hospital administrator took charge, and midwifery services began again. I asked who handled births during the time of the war, while in flight in the forest. "There out in the middle of the forest, you couldn't deliver a woman in the middle of the forest. . . . We scattered, that's how we were. That time, women weren't giving birth anymore. During that time God helped a lot of people; they weren't giving birth anymore. . . . There, there wasn't anything like a maternity ward because in the middle of the forest, we scattered here and there, running." Someone added: "Unless a pregnancy itself entered the forest, people were startled with fear. They weren't having babies anymore."[12]

Although the Yakusu mission was under partial occupation by Simba rebels from early August 1964, the missionaries were not evacuated until late November, the day after the Belgian-American paratrooper operation began in Stanleyville. During and after the evacuation, some mission buildings were ransacked and burned to the ground, though hospital and church archives went unscathed. Congolese nurses were among those who were vulnerable in this period, and many fled to live in the forest.[13] Lombale was a soft-spoken, slow-speaking man, a well-educated believer and foreign-traveled and -trained nurse, who began his career in nursing school at Yakusu in the 1950s and remembered the rebellion years well. More recently, SANRU funds had allowed him to attend a two-month public health course at Johns Hopkins University. For twenty months during the rebellion, he, his wife, and his children had lived among and worked for the BaSimba, deep in the forest north of Kisangani. They carefully hid all signs of class, education, difference, and contact with the outside. He learned to hunt and trap animals in the forest, and was considered a good and polite worker for the BaSimba. Surreptitiously, he continued his nursing. He acted as midwife for his wife and other women. He camouflaged salt-based medicinal concoctions with blue so it would not be recognized.[14] And he made an infant food from local palm wine and other forest products, distributing it quietly to mothers, many of whom came to live close by his house. These women continue to worship him today in Kisangani, fueling his popularity among women in the city. Ever present during the rebellion was the threat of being killed if you acted more comfortable or of a higher class than anyone else, or if you possessed any item with outside, urban origins.[15] Lombale finally escaped by canoe, paddling for two nights with his wife and children, hiding up small streams during the day. This flight was possible only after he met the secretive, camouflaged people who helped him. They plied a trade between the worlds of the Simba forest and Kisangani, with their double sets of forest and city clothing, always hiding the wrong set for each within a special kind of dugout log. "They were clever," he said, as he knew he was in hiding salt-based medicine for his children and escaping by night.

After the rebellion, Lombale came back to Yakusu and, as he told it, almost single-handedly refounded the dispensary network. He traveled from one village to the next, finding boys to be nurses, training them at Yakusu, and sending them back to work in rural dispensaries. He also told me of the little bundles of salt and soap that he would wrap up and give to the poor during his dispensary tours. The first BMS missionaries returned to the region in 1968. Mary Fagg was among them. There was no doctor again until 1975. Fagg focused on preventing anemia among pregnant women, and persuading multiparous women and their husbands to accept birth control, distributing all the iron pills and contraceptives she could get to prevent childbirth emergencies that she could not handle without a doctor—hemorrhaging, uterine ruptures, and transverse lies. She had a harrowing experience trying to take one woman who was dying of obstructed labor up to Kisangani for a C-section, only to discover that the doctors did not work weekends; the woman did not survive until Monday. Occasionally, a mission doctor passing through Kisangani could be persuaded to come to Yakusu for a day of surgery, and the early morning enthusiastic preparations and daylong, window-gathering spectacle resembled, in her words, "a garden party."[16]

Yanonge's nuns were not as fortunate as Yakusu's missionaries. Yanonge was hit very hard during the rebellion. A Zairian priest and primary schoolteacher in the town's Catholic mission told me that they, like all intellectuals and traders, had been vulnerable. Most fled into the forest. Three nuns of the Soeurs de Sainte-Elisabeth of Luxembourg were among the Europeans assassinated by the BaSimba in Kisangani. No nuns ever returned to Yanonge. Maternity services continued next door in the main hospital in 1989, but Yanonge's maternity building never reopened. It was a sorry site in 1989, surrounded with overgrown weeds and inhabited by some squatters who entered and left from behind. The hospital director and midwife spoke with me at length; there were no archives. Many women were still coming to the hospital's kilo, "but birth, many are giving birth at home." Village women especially, even if they were in difficulty, "can't come again to the hospital." No ambulance was part of the story: "Many people. . . . give birth there, somewhere at the side, in a corner, because there is no automobile now like there was during the time of the *ba-soeurs*." Yet it was also "a matter of the State; it issued the matter of paying. It wasn't us."[17]

Women used to pay before the war, but "little, little money. During that time money wasn't dear." Another said: "Those money prices of before, would I still know them? It was three francs, two francs, ten francs, as you wished. In 1970, my daughter became a mother; I paid thirty zaires to the maternity hospital. I paid the midwife-assistant three bottles of beer. . . . I gave her *longonya* [celebratory gift of thanks, usually of alcohol] because she did my daughter well." Were midwife gifts common? I asked. "We do it like that. It's just a matter of the wishes of the husband of the woman. But we have started to ask for soap to

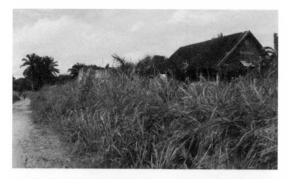

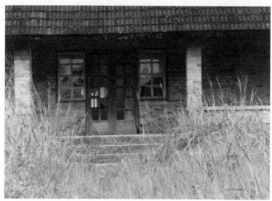

(*Top*) Yanonge maternity hospital building, 1989. (*Bottom*) Front door of old Yanonge maternity hospital building, 1989. Photographs by author.

wash our hands. Before a woman arrives, we ask for soap. When you finish your work, if that husband has a good heart, he can make you happy saying you took the dirtiness of my wife like that. In the way he wants to thank you, he can thank you." Not that many came anymore, and those who did knew to come with soap. "Now we have become just black people," Yanonge's hospital midwife explained, effectively recalling a period of hospital soap aplenty and a distinct, middle category of hospital workers who used it. "So we ask for soap so we can wash our hands before work." What about asili practices at Yanonge? I inquired. "They follow asili, black people. . . . They do medicines ya asili. . . . If the time is ready, it will come out, that's all. Us of the hospital. . . . We look, that's all."[18]

Yakusu Deliveries

I was just crawling into bed when I heard pounding at the door: "We have a case, a ventouse." I walked in the dark through Yakusu's hospital courtyard, noticing the stars in the sky. Women were snoring in the maternity ward as I passed through to the delivery room. Minishe, the head Zairian midwife at Yakusu, was there, apologizing for waking me in the night. The parturient looked at me. The older woman there—wearing a headband around her cropped, almost shaved gray hair—was her mother, I thought. She seemed to say hello, even with friendliness. The parturient, naked, was perhaps less pleased, though in pain. I stood against the wall. A blue tube was inserted up the woman's vagina. Her feet were wrapped within bands of cloth hanging from metal circular rings at the end of stirruplike structures. It looked mighty uncomfortable. Minishe occasionally told an assistant to pump the metal tubular vacuum extractor, known in French as a ventouse, to which the blue hose was attached. When the woman began to complain of a cramp in her leg, her mother reached for a crumpled-up cloth and put it under her upper thigh. Minishe became angry. She yelled at the soon-to-be grandmother about the clean hospital cloth that her daughter was lying on. The mother removed the crumpled one she brought from home. Minishe also threatened, saying she would throw the mother out if she misbehaved again.

Within five to ten minutes, Minishe began pulling. Before long, the metal cup of the extractor emerged slowly out of the woman's vulva. Soon, I could see a hairy scalp attached to it. The woman held on with a tough, cringing face. The tension in the room was enormous. During the last moments, her mother held her forehead and hand, touching her for the first time. The assistant held one foot in place, another woman the other. Minishe kept pulling. Finally, the baby was out, swung over onto a table and crying for the first time. Throughout the delivery, the woman had moaned, almost singing, in pain. Minishe had remained clinical, calm, in control.

The assistant struggled with putting on some gloves, then aspirated the child. As the infant lay on the table, I noticed the pieces of newspaper in which the gloves had been sterilized lying next to the baby's body: "HIV and Children" was the headline. The assistant then moved the baby, blood and all, to an uncovered scale in a small alcove. Minishe was waiting on the placenta, still performing calmly and carefully, without words or emotion. The mother sat off to the side on the bed. The parturient and the mother watched the baby, whom neither had yet touched, until the assistant brought the newborn wrapped in a hospital cloth back to the mother's bed. The mother began speaking to her child. Another relative also came close to watch the baby. When Minishe pulled on the cord, the placenta emerged. She moved it around in her hands as she meticulously examined it, and then let it drop into the plastic tray below the delivery table that had been catching all the blood. She pulled the bands loose and released the woman's legs. The woman gasped in pain and relief. Minishe squeezed more blood out from the woman and cleaned her up. She removed the hospital cloth beneath her, so she was lying on the yellow plastic alone.

The nurse took the baby and bathed it over a sink in cold water. She was angry that there was no towel when she turned to bring the baby back. The other relative returned with a bag of things, including a brand-new towel. Just after the placenta had been delivered, Minishe said to me, "It is over." I was still lingering. Another younger woman, well-dressed in a full Zairian woman's *kikwembe* suit, came in with a smiling face, eager to see the child. Minishe said to me: "You are going to leave now, aren't you?" I left.

Minishe, a young woman trained at the mission school during the 1980s, did not remember the time of many bandages and bicycles or the war. Yet she had plenty of respect. Susan Chalmers, the missionary midwife, told me that there was no procedure that Minishe could not perform as well as she did. And the one day we spoke at length, Minishe was quick to point out that she could understand everything that was said among the women present at a birth. She only lets one family member enter at a time, she explained, and if the relative tells the parturient to push too soon, she calls in another family member instead. She thought that too many visitors were allowed in Yakusu's maternity at once, and envied the tidier, more regimented conditions at private clinics in Kisangani, where there is a visiting hour every afternoon and only one visitor can enter at a time. Women were still being washed with very hot water in Yakusu's maternity; mothers and grandmothers were helping with these baths, and there was little, Susan said, that maternity staff could do about it other than being sure that the water was not scalding. Though rarely, some women who came in with prolonged labor, came in with leaves on their abdomen or a compound of medicines in their vagina. The maternity's maternal mortality rate had been high in 1988: five deaths for only about 500 deliveries. Both midwives noted that many women came in very late to deliver, often waiting until they were fully dilated, fearing that if they went too soon the contractions might stop. Others came in trauma.

When SANRU began to influence Yakusu in 1982, the mission's medical agenda began to focus on antenatal care for the first time. Sterilized birth packets—comprised of razor blade, cotton ball, bandage, gauze swabs, and ties for the umbilical cord—began to be sold at kilo, now antenatal clinics, in the Yakusu zone. The BMS mission was able to add Sue Evans as a second nurse-midwife to the missionary staff. She trained district nurses in antenatal care and referral criteria, and undertook a small TBA training program of some five popular midwives in Yalengi, a village near Yakusu.[19] By the time I arrived, Evans was long gone. I met the Yalengi TBAS. They were still handling cases in the local dispensary and referring problematic ones up the road to the hospital. The birth packets were also still for sale. And the hospital had hired its first trained male nurse-midwife ever, a point of considerable local consternation. But mobility was needed, and bicycles were gendered objects: He, Wenda, was cycling to do his clinics along the river, at sites where church contacts were strong.

There was, then, theoretically an operating SANRU system in Yakusu's enlarged zone for referring patients from small dispensaries to larger rural health centers (primarily Lotokila and Yatolema) and to Yakusu as the central reference hospital. Since Evans had left, however, many of the nurses whom she had trained had moved on. No one had taken over antenatal and obstetric training of the male nurses operating rural posts, especially those beyond Wenda's bicycle's reach. Thus, women dying in childbirth still arrived from afar. For example, a fifteen-year-old, small (1 m, 43 cm) girl who had received antenatal care at Yatolema had arrived at Yakusu undelivered the year before. She went into labor on a Monday and not until the Wednesday, in response to her mother's pleading, did the nurse agree that she should be referred to Yakusu. Difficulties of transport meant that she did not arrive until the Friday with a baby, by then dead for forty-eight to sixty hours, "jammed into her pelvis." If the nurse had understood SANRU's antenatal referral sheets properly, said Susan Chalmers, the missionary nurse-midwife then at Yakusu, he would have known months earlier that a young woman of fifteen who was under a meter and a half in height was an obvious high-risk case. He should have sent the girl to Yakusu to wait for her delivery when she became seven and a half months pregnant. Instead, the girl underwent a "traumatic delivery" that ended in a "very nasty" craniotomy at Yakusu. She was lucky, Chalmers added, that she did not die or leave with a fistula; she did have severe difficulties walking and was incontinent for a while afterward.[20]

The church elder in Yalemba wore a winter wool hat pulled to his ears, a brightly flowered shirt in pastels, and patterned ladies' sunglasses. Fancy gear, I understood more profoundly a few weeks later when I stayed in the homes of two church pastors. The house of one was an anomaly in a poor, riverain Olombo village. It was well constructed, with an enclosure and separate kitchen out back, and bananas growing on the path to the separated latrine and bath. Most people had small homes and cooked right out in front of them. When I asked Yakusu's Pastor Botondo why, he said, "the people are weak," though he was pained by my question and by what he avoided calling poverty. Church youth sang songs about temptation and death: no one can escape death, were the words of one church song, even if you board a boat for Kinshasa or an airplane for America. On Sundays, these youth would go to a metal-roofed chapel in a white building with large windows, whose wooden bars alternated in color from red to Zairian lime green. It became so full that children sat under the altar table. Bunches of fresh flowers were tied to pillars and hung from bushes outside. Women wore scarves; most were white. There was one large red star on the back church wall with a red cross with lime green stars on each side. One green star was effaced; the other had a heart inside it and a chalice beneath it.

People in these villages possessed little: their houses, dishes, pots, pans, fire stand, table stands for drying dishes, and a few clothes. One village pastor wore a ragged straw hat. Another wore a dirty, tattered lady's hat made of pink cloth. He carried an old frayed briefcase tied up with a rope. His Lokele Bible was crumbling, and his stepson went off to school in a T-shirt so torn that the front hardly held together anymore. Most of the women in the village where I lived wore used chiffon nightgowns as daily work clothes. The youth in this village did not go to church, except one young Protestant adherent who was in charge of organizing services and collecting offerings for what people called the women's church (the men went to the Catholic chapel because offerings were not required).[21] They spoke a special youth language called *Kimbile,* which only they could understand and through which they fabricated unofficial names, different than those on their identity cards. They would also run off downstream by canoe to join up with the periodic moving city—the mail boat with a string of barges, markets, discos, and brothels—as it plied its last stretch upstream to Kisangani. They might not reappear for a couple of days, after dancing, drinking, buying used clothes, visiting in the city, and making the easy downstream journey back. One *mungwana* [sing. of BaNgwana, "Arabisé"] alone still lived in the vicinity of this village, which was located near the old BaTambatamba swimming hole. He passed through from time to time by foot on his way to the state offices at Yanonge, always wearing the same bright lime polyester abacost with an image of Mobutu imprinted on it.

A Placenta Delivery

I heard that Mama Mateso was pregnant one day when I was visiting her neighbor. We overheard Mama Mateso's husband fighting with his wife. The neighbor feared that his hitting would hurt her pregnancy. Some children nearby were playing with a small turtle that they had found in the forest as we spoke. The subject returned to pregnancy. Some women will not eat turtles when pregnant for fear that the baby will act like a turtle during labor, coming close to being born and then withdrawing its head again up the birth canal.

One day, I went to see Mama Sila, the young midwife with bullet scars from the rebellion who had moved from the BaMbole forest to the riverain village after the war. She was eating a soup of turtle, mushrooms, and crab when two older women—the "mothers" of the pregnant girl—passed by. They said that Mama Mateso might be entering labor. Mama Sila and I followed them to her house. Mama Mateso was on a bed in pain. Her stomach had been smeared with green leaves. Mama Sila sent for another mixture called *ndembu,* the same name she used for the mixture she had smeared on my swollen foot that morning. She said it would keep "bad spirits" away. As Mama Sila worked to help this woman, she talked defensively to me: "I am not paid, not at all. I am just helping women, those who cannot get to the hospital." She told Mama Mateso to perform an enema with water, red pepper, and other medicine. She refused to name the medicine for me: "My knowledge is worth money." Later in the day, Mama Sila and I returned. The woman was in an adjacent room on her back, lying on some dried leaves, close to the fire, with a homemade lamp made with a wick of burning cloth placed in palm oil by her side.

Another day, Bibi Mari-Jeanne told me that Mama Lisongomi would deliver the pregnant woman, even though Mama Sila had tended her that one day. Finally, one morning at about seven o'clock, Mari-Jeanne called me to say that Mama Mateso was giving birth. We went quickly to Mama Sila's. Mama Mateso was crouched on the ground in the corner of this midwife's house, sitting on a small piece of wood on top of a piece of burlap spread before her. The baby was already born, lying at her feet peacefully. The umbilical cord was still attached to the child and to the placenta yet inside. One woman said, "Let's get palm kernels, so the placenta will come out."

Soon, Mama Sila entered with a *mbuu,* the kind of conical container that women use to bale water when they go to gather fish in low-lying water. She placed palm kernels and some water inside this mud-fishing tool and held it over the woman's head, shaking the mbuu so that the water dripped out of its funnel-like hole. She spoke to the placenta: "Come down, drop down now, Placenta." She also moved the mbuu so that the mother could drop her head back and drink a bit of the same water. As she did so, Mama Sila again addressed the placenta: "Come down, Placenta, if this woman messed around with a man, come down. If her husband messed around with a woman, come down." Then Mama Sila grasped the cord with a *liatato* leaf and pulled, repeating as she did, "Come down, Placenta." Out it came onto the burlap piece beneath the woman, and Mama Sila covered it under a portion of the burlap right away. There is no other use for this cord-pulling leaf, Mama Sila told me. Usually it is avoided because it makes skin scratch and swell.

Mama Sila went to get a commercial razor blade as others searched for string. Then, she tied the string tightly around the cord about six inches away from the infant and cut the cord. Gauze pads, cotton, and one long piece of gauze appeared out of a small bag. Mama Sila used them to cover and wrap the cord, and to keep it snug against the baby's body. Another bag with infant clothes and a towel appeared. Mama Sila sorted through the clothes, choosing some large underwear and a shirt. She dressed the baby, covered it in the towel, and handed the wrapped infant to a woman who took the baby away to the mother's house. A single palm oil flame provided the only light in the dark room. The mother remained behind until women found an old cloth and made her a belt to catch the blood of childbirth. She wrapped another complete piece of cloth around her waist "to keep her stomach from dancing" because there was still blood inside.

By the time the new mother stood to leave, many women had arrived to see. A few sang the lines of a birth song called "Kelekele" or "Thank You." A few took seats inside the room. About ten others passed through to look. No men were there. The mother told me afterward that she had prepared the gauze, cotton, and brand-new clothes and towel for the birth. She went to kilo the first time during the fifth month and continued until the eighth, when she bought this SANRU home birth kit. She said she would begin to go to kilo again with the baby every week after a month had passed.

At one point, someone appeared with about two-thirds of a bar of soap, the kind manufactured from palm oil by the Kisangani-based company, Sorgeri. Mama Sila complained that it was not a full bar. Someone added that even if a woman goes to a hospital, she must give a full bar of soap to the woman who has delivered her. The discussion continued: how would Mama Sila be compensated for her work? The new mother said that her husband had been to the forest to look for food, but he hadn't found anything. Mama Sila said that the woman would smear her with oil mixed with pounded medicine, and she (Sila) would reap much cassava. Someone else told me that Sila would receive 500 zaires, food, and palm wine. If you go to Yalokombe, you have to pay 1,500 zaires, they said; it costs too much, and there is no reason. One can give birth safely here in the village. One woman said that she once accompanied a relative to a rural health center, wincing as she described how her relative had to lie down with her legs pulled apart and back. When the woman was in labor, the *munganga* (nurse), a woman, demanded money before she would help: "Give money. Give money." They paid 500 zaires. After the baby was born, they also gave her food and soap.

The mother, suddenly a Mama Wale, returned home. When I asked about the placenta, Mama Sila said that she would not touch it. It was hidden there under the burlap. If she did and anything went wrong, she would be blamed. As Mama Kumbula Wayinoko Rosa cleaned up the area, she told me that Mama Mateso's mother had died when she was an infant, so she, Mama Rosa, had breast-fed and raised her. As effective mother, then, she went and got a small, child-size *bofala* (a basketlike construction for transporting cassava to the market) and a knife. She wrapped up the burlap with the placenta inside and used the knife to scrape away any remaining blood that had oozed onto the floor. This bloody dirt she added to the bofala with some paper she had used to gather it. After tidying it up, she crossed the road the small distance back to the woman's house. She lay the bofala down outside and went to touch the baby, who was lying next to the mother on the bed and even closer to the fire. They commented to each other that the mother's "big sister" had missed the birth because she had gone to sell tangerines in Kisangani. Mama Mateso's husband was behind the house, moving about with hesitant gestures, a shovel in his hand. I had heard that he would bury the placenta, as the shovel seemed to confirm. Yet he took the shortest route to the river, climbed down the hill, paused to roll up his pant legs, and waded a few feet into the water. He let the bofala float down the river as he unwrapped the burlap, allowing the placenta to drift away. He saved the piece of burlap, shaking and turning it within the water to clean it out. As I left, he was reaching for some stones to rub the piece of burlap cleaner.[22]

One morning a couple of days later, after a night of heavy rain and cool winds, the village began to move more slowly than usual. Tata Alikuwa sat in his chair observing while people passed across the compound. Soon, moral practice was under review. An old man who stayed at the school village nearby came to see Alikuwa. Their fathers were big and small brothers to each other. The man was also related to Mama Mateso's matrikin, and he explained that he had come to urge Mama Rosa to go with him to Mama Mateso's husband and demand his chicken. "Birthing is dying," Alikuwa explained to me. A father must pay for the mother's loss of blood. "Come on, come on," the other man urged Mama Rosa. She left with him and came back shortly alone. "Had she gone there? Had they agreed?" "No," she had refused: "this was not a good man." He would take chickens without reciprocating as he should. The father's kin should give a chicken to the mother's, but her kin should also give a chicken to the father's kin afterward.

Mama Sila emerged from her house one morning with some ndembu paste on a shard of pottery. We went together and woke up Mama Mateso and her husband for lilembu. The husband went off to call his "little brother," Jimi, who would go hunting with him in the forest that day. Mama Sila and Mama Mateso began, spitting on their hands first, then taking the paste in each other's hands and rubbing it over their bare breasts with a bit on their arms and backs, too. Then Mama Sila did Bibi Mari-Jeanne as Bibi Mari-Jeanne did her. The other women present at the birth who had seen the placenta were also there. Mama Sila put a bit on me, and Mama Mateso smeared me. Then the two men came, and both Mama Sila and Mama Mateso smeared them. They spoke during this lilembu of the good luck that would come to them in their fields, in hunting, and in commerce. Papa Jimi was the only one present who had not seen the placenta. The rest of us, they explained, were protecting ourselves from the danger to crops and life that this sight entailed. Papa Jimi was there for the good luck needed for a day of hunting for food for the midwife and Mama Wale. Mama Sila reminded Mama Mateso's husband this morning that he must cross to Yalokombe that day and explain to the nurse that they had tried to make it to his rural health center, but his wife had given birth while en route. He was to pay for the birth certificate—at some 1000 zaires—so as to prevent the *groupement* chief from writing a letter to the *collectivité* chief about Mama Sila's role in this birth.

When I later went to talk with Mama Mateso, she detailed her pregnancies: one was a miscarriage, and her first birth was a hospital delivery. When pregnant, she performed enemas from the fifth month so the baby would slip out easily. Her husband took care of the placenta, so if she had trouble getting pregnant again, it would be only his fault. The umbilical cord would be buried with a new plantain tree to promote many more births. She and her husband would have separate beds for two years, until the child began walking. The only compensation for Mama Sila would be money. They had not yet agreed on a price. Nor had her husband gone to fetch a birth certificate yet. There was no money. She said her wale would last one month. She called Mama Rosa her older sister. Her older sister was coming to squeeze the blood out of her during three daily baths. Her sister was also coming from the opposite end of the village to cook for her each day.

I wandered over in the evening to see this Mama Wale bathed. Mama Rosa carried a tub of very hot water into the cabinet. Mama Mateso lay on the kind of palm leaves used to roof a house. Her sister took a cloth, dipped it in the water, and pressed down with force on her abdomen as Mama Mateso cried out and writhed in pain. After about four or five such pressings, she turned over to have her back bathed. More great cries. Then, she sat with her knees bent while her sister bathed and pressed her arms. Next, moving in front of her as Mama Mateso spread her legs open, the sister splashed piping hot water at her vulva. "There are wounds there," her sister said, "and many more in her womb. It is necessary to remove all the dirt and sores." "Had she torn?" I asked. "Yes, and there are many cuts inside." She would continue to "squeeze her with force" like this until the day the umbilical cord fell off. Then, she would give her an enema of medicine and very hot water, and these trials would be over: "She will get her strength again. She will work again."

A Trip to Yalokombe

Bibi Viviane's house was just across from the one where I lived. She came by to chat, complaining that her baby was moving and causing her pain. Two women took a bit of sand from the ground and put it on top of her bare stomach as she sat on the bed out in the midday shade. Once the sand had been shaken off, they confirmed that her baby was indeed moving inside. About a week later, Bibi Viviane stopped by to have another woman cut her breasts with a razor and spread *bosau* into the cuts. Small scars from former cutting sessions were plain. She said that she had been doing this every day for a week and would continue until she gave birth because she had *baketcha,* a malady of hurtful breasts before giving birth. Mama Lisongomi had been advising her, telling her that if she did not cicatrize with bosau, she would have problems with her breast milk. Viviane bought her bosau from a very old woman who lives up the hill. A black powder resembling charcoal, it came from the wood of a tree that had been burned and pounded. Viviane did not know the name of the tree, so I asked Mama Lisongomi. She said she did not know what Mama Meli uses for her bosau, but she knows her own. Mama Lisongomi will deliver her, Bibi Viviane told me that day. Mama Lisongomi had also advised her to eat every morning to prevent an ear sickness in the baby.

About two weeks later, Bibi Viviane came by with another black powder to promote easy labor that her mother had sent her from Kisangani. A woman friend cut small gashes on her breasts, just above her pubic hair, and on her back as the mother said to do. She was planning to go to kilo a few days later at Yalokombe. A few days earlier, I went with her to see her visiting "mother-in-law," Mama Collette, the daughter of Mama Yamba. Everyone agreed that this woman was a specialist in "medicines for the pathway of birth." Bibi Viviane explained that she would pay her, otherwise she would not give her any. Mama Yamba, too, had sold her the powder for her breasts. Viviane thought that Mama Yamba's daughter would sell her an enema medicine, but she gave her lokwamisa medicine instead. She told her to pound *basatubasatu* leaves with *lososo* fruit and then to drink this tea. She also told her to take a root and pound it with local, unrefined salt, cicatrizing it on her back and lower stomach. If she did not take this medicine, she was told, she would not give birth quickly. The medicine would also protect her from getting the illness of anyone who has been cicatrized in the same chair. We went there on Monday. Rain prevented Bibi Viviane from looking for the lososo fruit on Tuesday, and on Wednesday, she could not find any in the forest. The other medicine had arrived from her mother in the meantime, so she used it instead.

One day, she came into my room alone to talk. She spoke of her anticipated period as a Mama Wale. Her wale would last for three months, she boasted: "I will not go outside. I will not cook or work. I will bathe, eat, and care for the baby." She recalled her bowai period of seclusion after she was married. She did not go outside for two years. She did not work, did not cook. All she did was bathe—three times a day—and eat. Her skin got light like mine, "peee!"[23] Others, especially her mother-in-law and sister-in-law, did the cooking and drew water for her baths. No one saw her except some small children and her husband. If she went out at all, she wore a cloth over her head, so most of her face and head were covered. She only saw the inside of her house and the cabinet, or toilet and bathing area. She had first arrived in the village at night. For two years, she said, she did not know what it looked like. Nor did people know who she was. When she emerged from her bowai, she came out peee! wearing new clothes. There was a big celebration with drumming, dancing, food, and palm wine.

As Bibi Viviane's labor drew closer, I went with her to her house to drink some palm wine. Her young husband and Baba Manzanza were there. Her husband announced that his wife would not give birth in the village. He would take her to the "hospital" across the river instead. "Why?" "Because it costs less money. Here in the village, there are many words, many matters. You have to generously thank the midwife and still go to the Yalokombe nurse to get a birth certificate as well." Baba Manzanza insisted the problem was the lover-naming that would be involved in a village birth. He said that the husband did not want to have to be questioned. The husband did not deny this argument. Bibi Viviane countered that it was precisely why she wanted a village birth. Someone told me later that they were all joking. The next day, Bibi Viviane explained that because it was her first birth and no one knew if she would give birth easily, her husband wanted to take her to a health center. Her husband also preferred the "hospital" because there would be shots.

A few factors were significant in this reasoning: the economics of midwife compensation and state paper requirements; a value judgment that a maternity birth is safer because of shots; and the village, conjugal, and kin politics of the "many words" surrounding a village birth, including the risk of fines and the apparent male fear of and female desire for adultery confessions. They may have been joking, yet no small amount of gender tension resided in Baba Manzanza's voice as he disparaged confession practices as devious and charlatan. This derision was distinct from his other views about local practices surrounding childbirth. He knew from experience, for example, that if a woman with a young pregnancy enters the house of a Mama Wale, the Mama Wale will not eat well again, her heart will close up, and the child will become dark and die. He also told me that adultery confessions differ by gender: if it is the woman who confesses, the husband will not hear. If it is the man who confesses, however, the wife will hear. Bibi Viviane never expressed her preference for a village birth in terms of support. She seemed to defer to her husband. Other women kept telling me that she had the power to decide for herself and would prevail.

Finally, one day at 5:30 in the morning, Bibi Viviane called me. They were waiting for me in a canoe by the time that I had dressed. Her husband, her mother-in-law, Mama Afeno, and also two "sisters" from her husband's house were there. One sister had been up all night with her the night before. Bibi sat flat in the pirogue, her legs stretched out in front of her as the women gave her last-minute advice. Do not push until the nurse tells you to or you will exhaust yourself, they said, thus incorporating kizungu advice. When we arrived, the health center was empty. It was Sunday and the nurse was at church. Bibi Viviane's husband went to call him; it was at least a half hour, if not an hour, before he came. He examined her stomach, inserted his hand in her vagina, prepared a few instruments (cord ligatures, scissors) in a metal dish with disinfectant, and said it would be about one and a half hours. He went to his office to see other patients.

As Bibi Viviane's pains became more intense, she sat in the hallway with her back to the wall for a while. Mama Afeno went to get a small tray of *matembele* leaves and cut them up in water. She spread the water over Viviane's stomach, saying, "Come out, come out, your kin are out here." The coldness of the water would make the infant want to come out. Otherwise, no one touched her. She reached to grab the leg of a nearby table during contractions, complaining that she was feeling cold. "Ninakufa, Mama," came an early cry of pain that continued with greater intensity: "I am dying, Mama. I am dying, my mother. Where are you?" The women wanted her to walk around to help the baby move inside. "Leave me alone, leave me," Bibi Viviane objected. "Stop, stop," they insisted. They walked her down the steep riverbank once again, then had her undress and enter the river. They wanted her to get wet so the baby would feel cold and come out. Many times after going to the river, a woman will give birth, they said.

They took Bibi Viviane back to the delivery table in the far room of the health center, a flat, metal-covered table with not even a pail at the end to catch the blood. The nurse came in again, said he could see the head, and told her to start to push. It was nearing ten o'clock. Bibi began to insist that the nurse stay with her and no longer retreat to his office, grabbing his hand at one point so he would not leave. He did begin to stay more, and when she pushed, he would move his fingers, inserting them into her vagina to open the birth canal at the bottom more and more.

By eleven o'clock, panic was in the air. Things were not moving as quickly as the women thought that they should. One woman had retreated into an adjacent room, while the other two stayed by Bibi Viviane's side, guiding her when it came time to push. Worries of adultery set in. They went outside and questioned her husband about whether he had slept with other women. I remained with Bibi and the nurse. He was not surprised that the husband was being questioned, and probably would not have been as amused as he was if I had not been there. About fifteen minutes later, one of the women came in with a bowl of water. The four women took turns taking a mouthful of water and spitting it over her stomach, speaking to the baby and to ancestors: "Come out, come out. There is no hate or problems here, come out." They were asking three deceased relatives to release the infant. The three ancestors called were all *bayomba* or womb relatives of the father, the husband's mother, his brother's mother, and the Tata (grandfather) of his mother's matriclan.

The nurse continued to spread water over the woman's stomach periodically. I asked him about it. He, too, believes that the sensation of coldness can give the infant the longing to come out. I sought to classify: "Was this a hospital or an asili practice?" "It is both," he said, as in this case it clearly was. The energy in the room became taut when the nurse began insisting, as the women did, that she push very intensely during each contraction. One woman placed one hand behind her head and the other over her mouth: the first hand was so that her body did not slip back on the table, the second so that her mouth was covered and could not cry. After two contractions like this, the nurse told her to stop and let Bibi Viviane push herself.

Finally, the nurse began to tell Bibi to try to not let the baby retreat again, but to push very, very hard. He began pushing from above on her stomach. Hard. He tried to show one of the women how to do it: "Don't be afraid," he said, "you can push very hard." He told a woman to do this as he rubbed his hand around the bottom of the baby's head. Then he took over again. A big pushing scene followed. The nurse essentially took the pushing over from Bibi and forced the baby out by exerting tremendous pressure on the top of her uterus with his hands. He told me later that he realized that she no longer had the energy to push the infant out, and so he did it for her. It was a terrifying thing to watch, this pushing out of a baby's body from a woman's birth canal through applying force on the fundus, the upper end of the uterus. After the baby was out and wrapped in a cloth, the nurse simply pulled out the placenta. He did not examine it, leaving it on the end of the table under a cloth. It later fell to the ground into the pool of blood. The new mother nearly fainted as she got up from the table minutes later. The women caught her, and the nurse came in with an injection of ergometrine, saying she had lost a lot of blood.[24]

Before we left, we went to the nurse's house. Bibi Viviane's husband went to purchase some local whiskey as a longonya, a gift of drink made by someone who has had good luck. The nurse talked about having worked with Mademoiselle Fagg and Sue Evans. He was, I learned, a *garçon de salle* only, never a trained nurse, though he had assisted Evans with antenatal care.[25] Some village women told me later that he was known for encouraging women to give birth in an asili way, even assisting parturients who sat on the floor of the health center as if they were at home. He complained to me that he was tired and there was no one to replace him. His elaborate house, with a whole row of lanterns hanging ready to light each room in the evening, suggested that he was not doing so badly. Bibi Viviane's husband accompanied the nurse to his office afterward, paid at the reduced price for a woman who has attended antenatal kilos, and came back with a birth certificate.[26] We left.

A City Mother Arrives

About a month later, Bibi Viviane's mother came to visit her from Kisangani. The three of us talked together about her birth. Bibi recalled when she nearly fainted: she did not know where she was. She was happy that she did not die because she knew she had lost a lot of blood. The way the nurse pushed the baby out of her is an asili way of handling a *cas grave* (serious case), they explained. She was worried because she still felt pain near the top of her stomach when pounding bananas. Her mother was angry: "My child was treated like an animal." She had paid for her daughter to go to a kilo with some nuns in Kisangani, and Viviane had told her she would return to give birth in the city. The mother was upset that she had gone to Yalokombe for this "modèle ya asili," this local method of pressing and forcing down on the womb: "If she gave birth the first time in this rough way, what will happen again when she gives birth? She will be exhausted." She wanted her to give birth *ku kuzungu*—with white nuns, a "place of white skin," she emphasized—so that she would not "die like an animal." Viviane's mother had given birth to all her children in maternity wards, except Bibi Viviane, her first. She gave birth to her at home, but with a gentle woman who used modèle ya hôpitalo (the hospital style). She lay on a bed; it was modèle ya kizungu.

Bibi Viviane was less taken by arguments about delivery styles. Hers was a cas grave, she said, because bad people wanted to kill her or her baby. The nurse first saw the baby's head at nine o'clock, she reminded me, but she did not give birth until noon. When the baby became blocked, she explained, the women got water and matembela leaves, and put three stones in the mixture. There were three stones because, they said, her husband had gone around with three women. All those women were now mothers. Adultery is forbidden; it leads to *sanga*.[27] A baby only likes the "water" of its own father. If a mother or father goes around with someone else, the baby will meet the "water" of another man or the smell of another woman. Hence, they had called on the three deceased kin to send good wishes and spit their blessings, so if there was any anger there, the baby would still come out. The fact that the baby still did not come out at this point was proof that it was not a problem of adultery, but a problem of bad people. She also thought it was good that we had crossed to Yalokombe since it was early morning and people—bad people—did not know she was in labor. They hated me because you—the white lady researcher—wanted to help me, because you were interested in me due to my pregnancy. "No," her mother interrupted: "No, follow God. Put your eyes there."

When she first arrived back in Yainyongo, Mama Machozi gave Viviane a medicine to drink so that her heart would open up, her breasts would fill, and she would nurse well and eat plenty. She spread another medicine around the house so that a menstruating woman or a woman bearing a young, lisole pregnancy would not be able to come near and close her heart, killing her appetite and making her child turn black. A sister came to bathe her, heating water until it was boiling vigorously. Then she put a cloth in the water and squeezed it on Viviane's stomach until big clots of blood emerged. Bibi Viviane cried. Her sister tossed more piping hot water at her vulva. Bibi Viviane cried out so loudly that the old man across the way got out of his chair to find out what was going on. This sister came three times a day to bathe her. Bibi Viviane also avoided drinking water. If she did, she said, it would mix in her stomach with the blood and *busaa* ("a white blood") would come out. She does not want the bad smell in this place where her baby was born. They had just recently given her an enema with *wenge* to remove the blood of childbirth. Wenge bark is a very strong drug. She felt faint. There were wounds inside, she explained. Her back was sore, thus she had cuts inside there by her back. They will give her another wenge enema with red pepper the following week to remove the blood that has turned to busaa.

Once her mother had come, the sister had gone home. Her mother was bathing her, but not with boiling water. She told Viviane to sit in the water afterward. Her mother said she refused "the way of boiling water." She is used to the way of the hospital: "I changed. This modèle will kill my child. This dose is too strong." Still, she did press on her stomach and throw water at her vulva. "Why do the women like such hot water?" I asked. They explained that it was because shots and medicines of white people were not there: "This boiling water is like a shot, and one will heal and get strong. If you don't use this hot water, you will not pound banana paste again."

Viviane's mother said that "in the time of our mothers," after being bathed like this, the Mama Wale went back to her bed with her back close to a fire, so these wounds would dry up and heal. This was no longer done, she continued, because the smoke ruined things and burned the baby's skin. The baby will lose weight. In her mother's time, there were no clothes. The baby was naked. "Yet God has changed the world. We have changed the world including this smoke. Before there were no clothes, even when I was a girl." She was no more than fifty, so she was a girl during the 1940s. Some women still do stay close to a fire after giving birth, others said, even though the baby will lose weight: "We have started to have wale ya kizungu, keeping the hot baths but no longer staying close to the fire after birth." A major reason for staying away from the fire was the cost of baby clothes. Smoke ruins them. To prepare well for a new baby costs 10,000 zaires, they calculated, then around twenty dollars or about one-tenth of the average annual income in the country. If a woman had a small budget, and could only buy a towel, shirt, and underwear for her newborn, it would cost 500 to 800 zaires, then a dollar or two, still a considerable percent of the annual cash available to a household.

Another day I met with the other female kin who had been present at this delivery. If Bibi Viviane's baby had been a boy, it would have died. It was only because it was a girl that it did not die. Women have strong hearts. The real problem at the health center, however, was the way Bibi Viviane pushed, the women explained. They echoed Malia Winnie's voice as they accused her of not having been a "person." Viviane did not push the baby hard enough. Perhaps if it had been in the village, there might have been a problem of bad people. But the problem in this case was that Bibi Viviane did not push well. That was why they tried to hold a hand over her mouth when they wanted her to push. They covered her head and mouth so that all her breath would go through her body, pushing the baby out.[28] They also loosened her hair threads to help her get the strength to push.

Lokwamisa, or a Blocked Birth

Her discomfort grew as her birth approached. So Mama Sila, herself a midwife and healer, indeed the one who had helped Mama Mateso, told me one morning when I passed by and found her preparing an enema. Bark from the *litumbe* tree and *kengembululu* rope were brewing on the fire so she could clean her stomach and provide slipperiness (*buthelezi*) for the baby. She showed what buthelezi meant as she took a bit out with a spoon and it slipped back into the pot in the slimy way okra might. She had had a dream the night before. Her mother, who had died, appeared. Mama Sila told her to come to help her because she was tired and about to give birth. She also broke out in a big sweat during the night. She said that the spirits of dead relatives had come to spit good blessings on her birth with this sweat. The dream and her heavy sweating were auspicious. Mama Sila was happy. That evening before sleeping, I came to see Mama Sila again. She had spread the palm oil–based salve called ndembu on her stomach and was very uncomfortable.

Days passed and Mama Sila still did not give birth, despite continued discomfort, many enemas, and much fetal movement inside. She told me one day that she would have a lilembu ceremony, calling together women from both her mother and father's clans to smear her with ndembu and bless her with saliva. She needed palm wine to call them. The enemas she had been doing morning and night over the last few days were supposed to bring her baby out. The medicine she had been using was also the name of her affliction of delayed birth: lokwamisa. Mama Machozi was selling one kind, but Bibi Marcelline gave her another. Mama Sila mixed her own into this. *Liesu* was one kind of leaf that women would pound and cook with pepper to make an enema for lok-wamisa. The word *lokwamisa* comes from the verb "to block." Mama Sila explained: "You don't give birth. You just sit there like this. It's a sickness. You will not give birth quickly. Your day of labor will not come quickly." Lokwamisa is an illness caused by the medicine of a bad person who, for example, puts it in your chair. As Mama Sila described: "They did Ma Liyaoto like that. They are bewitching me because Madami will do me well."[29]

Again, I was implicated. And my name had changed to Madami. People did not call me Mademoiselle while I was in Yainyongo as they did at Yakusu, where the Mademoiselle category was strong and I was living in the house of a series of Mademoiselle midwives, including Bokondoko and Sue Evans. I was instantly domesticated at Yainyongo as a young, local woman, affectionately called Bibi Nesi. Assumptions about celibacy disappeared in this shift from Mademoiselle. Indeed, women were keen to ask me personal, sexual questions that no one would dare ask a Mademoiselle at Yakusu. No one who knew me well had ever called me Madami before; it was more of an anonymous appellation used coyly, perhaps snidely, in Kisangani's market. Mama Sila reminded me in this mo-ment of code switching to Madami that when it came to discussions of envy and fears of sorcery, I had the ambivalent qualities of a white colonial lady.[29]

I accompanied Mama Sila when she went to her "little mother" to have her birthing blessed and receive good wishes from her *BaTata,* deceased "fathers," so "she would give birth well." She was also going to get some of her little mother's lokwamisa medicines. One was for an enema. Another required the bones of a male chicken, and it was rubbed into cuts made on the stomach and back. As we walked through the forest together to Yanonge, she explained again: "Lokwamisa is when bad people stop you from giving birth when your time is due. It is happening to me because Madami is paying so much attention to me." She had also had more dreams. Bad people had thrown a big rock into her house to block her birth with lokwamisa. In another, her mother was sitting on her bed laughing at her as she was giving birth. She was there to help, but she just sat laughing. Mama Sila removed the baby herself. Again, she woke up in big sweat. Again, she interpreted the sweat as a blessing, as her mother's saliva.[30] When I asked another woman about lokwamisa, her first response was: "A medicine. A bad person puts a medicine in your stool, and when a pregnant woman sits there, then she can't give birth." She also said lokwamisa can only be cured with a medicine smeared into cuts on the lower abdomen and lower back, and to be effective, the medicine must be bought and applied by the same person who put the bad medicine in your stool.

Finally one afternoon, Shangazi Angelani came to tell me that Mama Sila was in labor and I should come. I arrived as rain began to fall. Her husband came into the house to smear ndembu on her stomach and to spit his blessings on her. Mama Sila does not like cold water and matembele leaves, someone remarked. She just smears ndembu to encourage the baby to come out. Mama Sila left the room a couple of times, saying she would check how many fingers away she was. She tried various positions, walking about, squatting, lying down. Mostly, she stood upright with her hands on her waist. There were some men around when I arrived, though they soon dispersed, and Mama Sila moved outside by the fire for a while. Only women were left: Shangazi Angelani, myself, and Mama Sila's eleven-year-old daughter, who was taking care of her two younger siblings. The men and the noise had made her afraid, Mama Sila told me.

We moved back inside the small, two-room house. Mama Lisongomi had gone to look for one of her medicines for Mama Sila to drink. When a crowd of women entered, Mama Sila asked me to send them away. She wanted me to bring a burning log from one room into the other. She put the bone of a turtle that I had helped her eat months ago on the burning log, smelled the smoke, then placed it close to her vulva. The child is not yet coming and going back in, she observed, but this medicine is just to be sure that it does not. Meanwhile, Shangazi Angelani was telling me her own stories of working for Yanonge's nuns once again. The next thing I knew, Mama Sila was sitting on the edge of the bed with her hands behind her back, and then she abruptly stood up. That was her last stand in pain. In seconds, Angelani had her lying down on the bed, said she saw the child's head, and told her to start pushing. She assisted with some fundal pressure and wanted me to help, too. I pretended to obey. By evening, women had smeared white kaolin with *lomboyomboyo* leaves on the baby's forehead as well as Mama Sila's forehead, breasts, midchest, and the backs of her neck and upper arms. This was to protect them from *kisila*, the dangerous gas of a woman bearing a young, not-yet-moving lisole pregnancy. Her visiting "sister" was newly pregnant, so the risk of kisila was high.

"Let Them Go Find a Pirogue and Go to the Hospital"

When I spoke with Mama Lisongomi, she told me that the first time she delivered a baby it was because she was needed. "*Kema, kema, kema!*" she recalled telling the woman: "Push! Push! Push!" There was no one else to help, and afterward she never stopped. "How many has she delivered?" I asked. "Even two hundred," she replied, noting that the first baby she ever delivered is the mother of a child who herself was recently married. So she learned and helped women.

Mama Lisongomi quickly moved on to how *basongo* ("white people") had come and said it was bad to give birth in the village: "The women who delivered babies before, no more delivering except at the hôpitalo only. If a woman has labor pains, you will come with her to a hôpitalo. She will give birth there." These basongo came after the rebellion, after the nuns had gone. Still, women come to her and say that hôpitalo are far away or "run from the hospital saying the hospital is bad, men deliver women there. We who gave birth long before, we did not give birth with men." Nor was it so in the time of the nuns. "Women refuse saying, 'The man of someone might come look at me? What kind of thing is this?' So they see problems, and they come and wake me up." Knowing that the hospital is far and they will not go ku bazungu (that is, to "white"-influenced space), she goes and delivers them: "Bibi Nesi, can you imagine a woman who goes into labor at night crossing the river!!?" Women do not pay her. She may receive a bit of palm wine, but never money. At Yalokombe, women must pay, while if she helps them, she takes a risk with l'Etat. Remembering this, she said angrily, "Let them go to the hospital," even claiming at one point that she had left the work. The next time we spoke, she told me that she had taught her daughter about her midwifery medicines. Together, they have maintained lilembu and *ikwakona* rituals, that is, the mutual smearing of palm oil on each other's bodies to neutralize the sight of childbirth blood and the giving of food as gratitude afterward. In general, however, these customs have been reduced into giving *molofu* (alcohol) or nothing at all. Again, Mama Lisongomi's resentment surfaced: "Let them go find a pirogue and go to the hospital."

The State of "Right Now"

Most agreed that before the rebellion, no one paid for a maternity birth, unless perhaps if drugs were needed. No one paid for a birth certificate either. Since the rebellion, you must pay a nurse for this document. One man said there were not fines per se for giving birth in a village, but if you went years later to try to get this document, authorities would know that you had been hiding a village birth and fine you. The village chief, however, insisted:

If *l'Etat* knows that you didn't go with your wife to the maternité over there to give birth, they make that man pay a fine. . . . Before it was the Ba-

Mademoiselle and ba-soeur who were coming to visit the villages in a small truck looking for those who were pregnant. . . . That's what the State-of-before used to be like. Afterward, the State-of-these-days, it's up to you yourself. You will search for a pirogue. You will search for a bicycle to carry a woman who is going to have a baby. So, there are many who give birth in the village. So, like these women sitting right here, they help. They tend to births very well. If the State-of-right-now hears about it, it issues a fine because you gave birth in the village. . . . Before, people were giving birth in the village without fines. Not too long ago, fines appeared. . . . It's not soldiers, it's the *service territorial.* . . . Sometimes, the medical service of nurses makes you pay a fine of 500 zaires. . . . This woman gave birth, and her husband, they paid . . .[31]

The people of "the State-of-right-now" were those that Lisongomi called basongo. One day, I went to attend a meeting with state representatives who came to inform the village people about taxes and hygiene requirements. They said that basongo would be coming to make a hygiene inspection of village cabinets. "So who are these white people?" I asked.

Basongo are people with power who come from the outside, people asserted: "When these people of l'Etat come, we have to cook for them and feed them and take care of them, and it is a lot of trouble." Who is called *bosongo* (sing. of basongo), muzungu, *mundele,* or "white" is not about skin color in postcolonial Zaire; rather, it is about domesticity, wealth, style. Tata Tula acquired the designation bosongo, as he did the title Monsieur, during the late-colonial period, long after leaving his job as mission clerk. He was chef de poste for Belgika, managing one of its plantation posts and driving a company car. "Basongo will eat and tell you just to sit and wait. We could never do that," people told me both at and outside of the Yakusu station. This kizungu habit remained a missionary practice at Yakusu when I was there, and Zairians living at the mission station resented what they read as racial arrogance and a continued coloniality in their midst. Yet eating and telling others to sit and wait were also class-based practices, I learned, performed by big men, soldiers, state agents, and perhaps some nurses in the postrebellion period. This kind of eating defined them as basongo. The fact that the same social category also ate the wealth they appropriated through fines and birth certificates only confirmed the sinister nature of their meals. So I thought, too, when I met a commissaire's assistant from Kinshasa, posted in the remote state post of Opala on the middle Lomami, boasting that he had been working hard—fining people—to stamp out home births and encourage their location in the still active, colonial-built hospital instead.

How are we to explain this relish for birth fines in an era when the World Health Organization's Safe Motherhood Initiative was encouraging even more TBA training programs and sterile birth packet sales? Structural adjustment is too vague. The principle of self-financing through user fees is more precise, especially in the twisted context of Zaire where Mobutu's self-financing had multiple, sinister, indeed anthropophagic meanings for years. User fees are keeping women all over Africa from going to hospitals and health centers for biomedical assistance during childbirth. Why should we be surprised to find the same economic constraints in Zaire? Yet user fees are still too vague for a location where there used to be nuns who picked a pregnant woman up in a vehicle and showered her with gifts of food as a Mama Wale, and where in 1990 the closest alternative was a male nurse who had little more to offer than what would be available in a village except ergometrine injections and birth certificates? The chief's words were telling. He distinguished three states: the State of "before," the State of "these days," and the State of "right now." "Not too long ago, fines appeared," he said. "It's not soldiers, it's the service territorial. . . . Sometimes, the medical service of nurses makes you pay a fine of 500 zaires." He expressed it as a "need": "The state is frightening people so that they don't just give birth in the village. They need to make a little threat so that the person is afraid to give birth in the village and goes to give birth in the maternité."[32] "Not too long ago" was certainly since SANRU began in 1982, and perhaps more recently with cost-recovery imperatives.

The principle of self-financing through user fees had intensified as a SANRU agenda in the mid-1980s. USAID-affiliated SANRU personnel in Kinshasa expressed concern to me that the Zairian government was not paying the salaries of those in zone offices as it should, and that these, too, were coming from user fees instead.[33] A 1986 cost-recovery study concluded that "on an average, health zones were able to finance approximately 79 percent of their operating costs."[34] A subsequent "health care demand" study, however, conducted over two weeks in two Zairian zones, found that only 44 to 55 percent of persons were using biomedical clinics, while 25 to 33 percent were relying solely on pharmacies for their health care. These figures imply that people could not afford SANRU fees, though only 1 percent were using "traditional care"—results that the author admitted were "suspicious."[35]

No specific studies on the use of SANRU obstetric and midwifery services exist, as far as I know. SANRU statistics from 1987 indicated enormous variability in the proportion of health areas (zone sections) that had maternities (8 to 100 percent), the proportion of babies born at maternities (1 to 99 percent), and the proportion of zone localities with TBAs who had undergone biomedical training (0 to 83 percent). Yakusu was not included in these apparently unpublished reports, which Baer kindly had printed out of a computer for me.[36] Still, such data would not have helped much to understand the kinds of processes that I was observing.

The breach between USAID generalities and the kind of ethnographic data that I collected, whereby mbotesa felt afraid to help women in childbirth and husbands scrambled to obtain birth certificates for babies born under a mbotesa's care, was wide. The reason one mbotesa in a village with a SANRU health center was afraid to practice anymore was because the SANRU nurse who needed user and drug fees, perhaps to prove "financial sustainability" but more likely for personal "self-financing," had threatened to call in the State of "right now." And this State, in light of Baer's fears about user fees going to pay for zone managers' salaries and USAID questions about the legal status of a rural health zone, was as the chief suggested, some amalgamation not of soldiers, but of a district or territoire-level of authority and "the medical service of nurses." In areas where mbotesa were not being converted into acronym-bearing, fee-collecting, patient-referring, SANRU-associated TBAS (as was the case in all but one village of Yakusu's zone, where Sue Evans trained a group of five mbotesa as TBAS), they were being threatened with fines and jail.

"Jealousy Is Hunger"

"Jealousy is hunger," Evans-Pritchard's "witch doctor" said in one of his chants.[37] People were struggling with hunger in Yainyongo every day in 1989, while considerable informal sharing and a strong ethic against the "shame of greediness" prevailed. Nevertheless, jealousy was everywhere, as was bickering over debts and unfair treatment. I imagined a fair amount of hiding of wealth was going on; I know that food was hidden. One day, I entered the old colonial house of a much-better-off man a few miles upriver from Yainyongo. Papa Lofemba was a proud hunter who managed to have guns and ammunition. There was an established interior: a *salon* (living room) area, a dining table. A kitchen out back. Several wives. A radio. Decorations—Mobutu pictures and authenticité objects—on the walls. Lofemba's house reminded me, in a toned-down, less barricaded way, of the large brick pastor's house where we had stayed in ex-Elisabetha, an old Unilever (HCB) company town, which in 1989 suggested urban sprawl. We had a separate bedroom entrance with padlock and key during this hygiene tour stop. Everything possible in the living room also bore padlocks, the large blue Frigidaire included. There were mermaid and animal-forest scene paintings by a local man who lives in Kinshasa and returned to create "agriculture is it"–type, MPR-colored assemblages displaying farming tools and national fidelity. This pastor had such a picture hanging on a wall.

There was also an old, non-leopard-capped photo of a young Mobutu in military uniform perched atop the blue Frigidaire. Chairs in a circle around a table made this room a salon, and there were even a few doilies for domesticated and pastoral authenticity.

There were neither urban sprawl, Frigidaires, Mobutu photos, nor doilied salons at Yainyongo. No room was fixed. Rather, there was a continual movement as people came and went. Chairs and fires went inside and outside as the weather changed, and as the sun rose and set. There seemed to be a fluidity in domesticity, motion in the location of homes and farms, occasional retreats of several weeks into forest shelters for gathering caterpillars and trapping. This fluidity in homes went with continual building. A house was always falling apart; perhaps it was partially rebuilt; perhaps another was under construction. Bodies moved, too, as men shifted among wives, and as houses went up and down.

Domesticity extended beyond shelter. People seemed to domesticate the land with a similar fluidity. New land was brought under cultivation, and other fields returned to forest. Whole villages could move, as Yainyongo itself has done. Older people in Yainyongo-Romée knew that their village had moved several times in the last hundred years before settling again in the BaTambatamba battle site, which according to social memory was home.[38]

Domesticity was also about eating. With the reification of domesticity and hygiene based on colonial evangelical models came individualized eating, each man with his own plate, spoon, and cup. A man would be served separately and, among those men served, equally. Diners sat at a table, often praying first. At Yainyongo, a more fluid domesticity was still alive. Sharing of food was routine, effected according to subtle hierarchies of gender and age. Men ate more, though they would often gather in kin groups to share from the same bowl. Sisters ate together with their children. There were prohibitions about who could eat with whom (especially surrounding in-laws) and habits about who was served how much. These habits encompassed sharing among households, the passing of plates to another fire, the joining of "brothers" daily over plates, and informal sharing with friends passing by. A guest was a special category, receiving his (or her) own plate. Often a male guest was served in private; he was left to be alone with his food.

Colonial interference in Congolese women's procreative lives at Yakusu intruded in only labor, delivery, and sometimes the first days of the postpartum period, thus in a narrow slice of what is locally construed as a longer span of protective practice. Many beliefs and routines persisted in local space, according to local time, outside colonial purview. Women carried other beliefs and practices to biomedical settings. Practices like postnatal bathing and placenta disposal endured because they were subject neither to obstetric intervention nor usually to colonial forms of knowledge. Labor and delivery, I learned, although pivotal, are but small moments within an extended duration of reproductive decision making. The lives of Lokele, Foma, and BaMbole women are marked by a sequence of seclusion periods. During each of these periods—during adolescence (likiilo), on marriage (bowai), and with each postnatal period (wale)—the women are not supposed to work and should be copiously fed.

These "shoulds" are significant. The abundance of food, the scope of prohibited work, and the length of seclusion are variable. Women call them matters of luck, though it is clear from the boasting that some women can muster that wale is also a matter of wealth and prestige. The luck of a good wale in 1989 was, in part, luck in a husband who would provide: a husband who would go hunting or fishing and provide food; the man who also would decide when his wife should begin to cook, fetch wood and water, and farm again. Yet a man cannot make a good wale. It is the women who step in to help a woman with child care, personal bathing, cooking, water fetching, and the like, which enable her to rest. Everyone, men and women alike, said that wale periods had declined. Some older women remembered staying inside and not working for four or five months. Women of childbearing age in 1989 were rarely receiving a wale of two months. Most women said their wale periods had ended because there was no one else to take care of them and do their work. A decline in interkin resource sharing was key here, I suspect. Cooked food was not only shared among men of the same house who came together to eat from the same plate, as if the old special eating and palaver huts called *ngbaka* still existed. Women also passed cooked food among women of different fires and households. While this passing was usually among relatives in the same bokulu, some was among neighbors and friends as well. Those involved in such passing of cooked food corresponded precisely with wale helpers and birth attendants. And this circle was smaller and more overstretched than ever before.[39] The decline in wale periods also points to an erosion in the necessary kin support to keep husbands from demanding that wives return to food preparation and production. Greater control over decision making by husbands is evident elsewhere, as is a decline in their food-providing roles during a wale. The very fact that there is now a choice about where to give birth means that there is a possibility that husbands will make this decision.

Women of Yainyongo recalled a time when a woman gave birth in an *eelo*, a special clearing in the forest designated for this purpose. Women used to give birth on a large banana leaf placed on the ground, with one woman supporting the parturient from behind while the midwife received the baby from the front. There are no more eelo clearings. Nor did I witness the use of banana leaves. At

Yakusu, one station woman gave birth under the moonlight in 1915; by the late 1920s, women were crowding into an enclosed room of a station house. There was the same kind of crowding in Yainyongo-Romée in 1989. Yet if I asked about where a village birth tended to be located, most women told me the "cabinet," an enclosed bathing and latrine structure that had first been imposed by hygiene authorities during the late 1930s.

People were consuming and reworking their tangled histories, during the 1980s, as they remembered and used local and colonial elements, from eelo to cabinets, wale to maternities. Birth certificates, soap, lokwamisa medicines, enemas, and baby clothes were key elements in local practice surrounding fertility, childbearing, and bodily digestion and flow in 1989. Most of these objects were colonial "remains and debris." My questions and observations exposed complicated childbirth itineraries quite unlike SANRU projections of primary health care circuits linking village-based health committees and re-tooled "traditional birth attendants" to reference hospitals. They also revealed refiguring of this debris in new forms and uses, especially through memories of colonialism and a postcolonial period of "war" and flight.

Some greed could be rebuked and defied as immoral. A greedy man should not receive an undeserved chicken. Yet there was also a new, second economy of greed and morality. Village people were jockeying a complicated economy of compensatory gift giving, underground payoffs, and story fabrication as they enacted new birth rituals during the late 1980s. These rituals involved new price schemes, new forms of state visibility, new threats and fears, and new uses for colonial debris.

Those opting for village births were choosing what was financially the most viable. Convenience was also an important factor; the health center was across the river from this village of farmers with few canoes. The village mbotesa were the ones who were being squeezed. One man spoke of a problem of "double payment." Village midwives demanded a lot of money, he said, and a man still had to go pay dearly for a birth certificate at a health center afterward. Hence, the indignation of someone like the older fisherwoman, Mama Lisongomi, who went up the Romée to collect birth medicines near her rice fields, wading in the water with her daughter Lutia on the way home as they trapped fish in the gigantic, six-foot-long, *ikunduku* basket that she made with her own hands. Hence, perhaps, the style of someone like Mama Sila, the younger mbotesa who came from the BaMbole forest to live bayomba after the war with her husband, a young man who smoked marijuana and knew about BaSimba medicines. Mama Sila's fishing was only the mud fishing of a forest woman using a small, hand-size ikunduku in low-lying water. She had an uncommon, if invidious, magnetism in the village. Mama Sila's house was perched on a hill away from, yet between, the two main arteries. It was neither along the riverfront, as was Mama Lisongomi's house, nor along the other row of houses, running at a right angle to the river. Her house was set almost in a little return to the forest of its own. She came to the women's *mutualité* meetings with bottles of medicine to sell, and likely played on people's fears of misfortune with her rich knowledge of forest medicines.

People divided social space into kizungu (white- or colonial-influenced) and asili (natural, traditional, customary) domains. People would say: "I was living in kizungu then" or "Here in asili, we . . ." People moved between these two realms within their lives and within a single day. Loading a canoe with forest rope or avocados and taking them to sell in Kisangani was a trip to kizungu. So was a journey to Yakusu's hospital. The polarity, then, was spatial, not temporal. Tata Alikuwa explained one night that if a man had at least one child "ku bazungu, in an office there, you will not die" because this child will take care of you. People have long made the best of their differences and advantages, just as earlier generations would have attempted to turn a trip to a BaTamba-tamba stronghold or a colonial plantation work camp or school to their best advantage.

No one thought that asili space was one of continuous, unchanging tradition. They knew that there used to be eelo and special libeli groves. They remembered when each village section (or house) had a ngbaka, where all the men of these related households would gather to talk and eat together the food that women would bring to them there. And they knew that cabinets, roads, and salons were colonial creations that changed the organization of space in their villages. Even though ngbaka were no more, when a wife or daughter handed a senior man of one household a plate of cooked food, the senior men of the other households of the same village "clan" gathered with him to share it together.[40]

This local conceptual geography allowed many people to take birth out of a village to a hospital or health center—ku kizungu—for delivery and shots. Nevertheless, before they left and when they returned home to their asili village, practice went on in many ways uninterrupted, including preparing the lieme for slipping out with a clean body; nourishing it with semen, a substance full of "proteins" that made the baby grow big; cleaning out the blood of childbirth; paying for the loss of a woman's blood with a chicken; burying the cord with a plantain tree to ensure future fertility; and properly disposing of the placenta, a "Mama" being with teeth and a mouth that lives next to the baby during pregnancy and might eat its food, but does not like greens, and whose substance, if tampered with, can be used to block a woman's future fertility.

Some colonial remains had entered local practice. Powdered milk became a lactogene, resembling the white clay that women were accustomed to digesting to prevent milk insufficiency, though this desired commodity was largely out of economic reach in 1989. Baby clothes, those maternity and Christmas gifts of colonial times, were eagerly sought. Mothers obtained them, although they were expensive and likely came with nutritional costs. A newborn was rarely dressed in used clothing, even in a poor village where most people wore castoffs. Indeed, new baby clothing was one of the largest single expenses in giving birth in 1989, especially since feasting and toasting at the close of wale had become so rare.[41] Some colonial absences have consequences; postnatal scalding baths may have intensified in heat and duration once injections became rare.

Birth Is Death

In Mobutu's Zaire, people generally remembered—usually correctly, contrary to USAID assumptions above—that medical and maternity care were free in colonial times. This perception prefaced the explanations people gave me for why there were conflicts over birth choices and midwifery compensation. The complicated subterranean economy of birth payments and fines surrounding village births that I witnessed in 1989 and 1990 was based on the belief that village births were illegal. Yet since transport to a medical center from a remote site was often difficult to find, village midwives were relied on much of the time anyway, particularly when a parturient had already had a successful birth. Since husbands also had to pay off state agents and nurses to be sure that they had the right papers and were not fined for an illicit birth, they saw the need to thank a village midwife as double payment. Village midwives' services, therefore, were diminished by men and ultimately by women. These mbotesa were angry.

Older women recalled the days when there were special lilembu rituals, where all women who touched the blood of childbirth would gather to spread palm oil on each other's bodies to neutralize this blood whose sight "can kill eyes." They remembered that the lilembu was followed by ikwakona: the parturient's female kin would prepare a copious meal, including palm wine and chicken, for the midwife.[42] A crucial turning point in the history of childbirth at Yakusu was convincing mothers and parturients to let young women students witness the blood of birth. Ascriptions of meaning to soap, a condensed, efficacious cleaning agent assisted in this process. Soap, injections, and medicinal enemas condensed meaning in hospital birth ritual, cleansing the dangerous blood, replacing the need for lilembu to remove the danger of the blood that "can kill eyes," and reducing the need for scalding hot, postnatal, blood-removing baths. In 1989, whether in hospitals, health centers, or local homes, lilembu and ikwakona were rare, condensed as they were by the insistence on soap giving from parturient to midwife.

Mbotesa spoke of demanding and deserving compensation in kizungu and asili terms. They expected cash and soap (kizungu), palm wine and chickens (asili). In practice, however, they rarely saw any of it. Except soap. Whether a woman gave birth in her village or the city, at home or in a local hospital or health center, it was her responsibility to provide a bar of soap to her birth attendant. Usually, one bar was given for her use during the delivery and another afterward as a gift, as compensation. Soap, therefore, condensed in late Zairian birth ritual what was once a blood-neutralizing ritual enacted by the parturient, midwife, and all the lay attendants who saw the blood of childbirth, and was followed by a copious cooked meal. The economics of purchasing birth certificates had effectively eliminated the wherewithal for cooked food. Midwives felt robbed by these substitutions and by the depreciation in meaning.

Bernard Hours has argued that "the principal leaven" of negative popular representations of the postcolonial Cameroonian state as l'Etat sorcier (a witchcraft state) is a dysfunctional public health care system lacking drugs joined by the expectation of free medical care inherited from the colonial period.[43] Drugs have not been at the center of my problematic, nor is my subject as vast as all of public health. Postcolonial birth routines demonstrate how childbearing continues to be mediated, even performed, through colonial debris. Thus, I turned less to clinics and drugs than to birth certificates and soap. Yet I also turned to the rhythms of the life cycle, the fluidity of reproduction and pregnancy, and the use of enemas and other medicinal techniques to prevent affliction, neutralize the mixed-up, obstructive bodily fluids of adultery, and unbind blocked fetuses, stuck placentas, and the rotting blood of childbirth.

If we liken the local etiologies and therapies permeating postcolonial birth routines in this small village in Yakusu's district to representations of the fertility-mediated power of Mobutu's postrebellion, "authenticity"-influenced state, we find this now-dead "king for the Congo" and his walking stick. V. S. Naipaul commented that no Zairian he knew during the mid-1970s could explain to him the meaning of the carving on Mobutu's walking stick: "One teacher pretended to not know what was carved, and said 'We would all like to have sticks like that.' "[44]

When I made my dispensary trip with Yakusu's nurses in 1989, two of them began discussing eyeglasses over a breakfast of cassava greens, fish, bread, and papaya. They were saying that many Zairians who wore glasses did not need them. "Isn't it a question of prestige?" I interjected. "Isn't this the Mobutu image, after all?" They laughed. I teased the nurse wearing glasses that all he needed was a leopard hat. "Do you believe there is a force in the world, in things?" they wanted to know. Did I know about Mobutu's walking stick and how he stays in power? Mobutu has a force, a special force invested in his walking stick. There is a pregnant woman sculpted on this staff, they explained.

Everyone knows she is there. People say that until this pregnant woman gives birth, Mobutu is protected and will remain in power. One nurse said that he knew many, many incidents of Mobutu's disappearing, vanishing, in moments of danger. Some people have such powers, he insisted, drawing on local Olombo examples. Mobutu has carried his staff since he came to power, they observed, and he has survived, despite numerous coups and wars. And he fights, they added. When there is a battle, he comes personally and fights. Only God can take his life, these Baptist nurses declared: "God will decide." Until then, "until God fixes things [arrange les choses]," Mobutu "is protected, he hides himself within her," this sculpted pregnant woman, "and cannot die."[45]

In the early 1990s, Zairian television broadcast the same speech by Mobutu, every evening just before the news. "How many fathers?" Mobutu would cry out in Lingala, while raising his hand with authority. The audience would answer in one voice: "One!" The president, encouraged, would continue. "How many mothers?" "One!" "How many tribes?" "How many parties?" "One!" "How many masters?" "One!" The clip would close with thunderous applause, Mobutu lowering his hand, and "a faint smile stealing over his stern countenance."[46] Press photographs confirm an image of Mobutu clutching his sculpted staff with his hand around the pregnant woman's womb. To understand local meanings of this clasp around a pregnant woman who stays pregnant, we need only recall the therapeutic itineraries and life stories of Yainyongo's women. Nothing is more dangerous than bodily, digestive, and fertility-related obstruction. Whether caused by hiding a woman's menstrual blood to block her fertility, stealing placenta pieces to prevent future pregnancies, emitting the dangerous kisila gas that dries up breast milk and closes a nursing mother's heart, or blocking a birth with lokwamisa, an obstructed body embraces infertility in agriculture, in hunting, in all of life.

Remember, the most common expression for childbearing is: giving birth is dying, or birth is death. With these words, Bibi Viviane called out to her mother to come assist her in labor. With these words, Mama Lisongomi declared her refusal of more men and more births: "Giving birth is dying. I have given birth to many. Of my sons, five died. I have seven kids left, two sons, five girls. My children are giving birth. Me, give birth again? No way! I don't want it." The expression also explains the blood debts (chickens) that compensate maternal kin for the loss of the blood of childbirth. One day, I asked the old man, Tata Alikuwa: "Kuzala iko kufa? (Birth is death). What is the meaning of this, Tata?" "The meaning is: give your wife lots of food. She has just been through death. You do not want her to die." In 1989 and 1990, people interacted with the state, imagined or concrete, whenever they organized a birth ritual, sought a birth certificate, or avoided a birth fine, and whenever basongo came and demanded

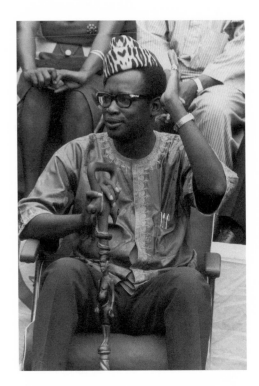

Mobutu Sese Seko posing with his walking stick some four years before he renamed the Congo Zaire. Photograph by Eliot Elisofon in Kinshasa, 1967. (Courtesy of Eliot Elisofon Photographic Archives ["Leadership—General; Congo (Democratic Republic); image no. C 3 ZAI 15.14], National Museum of African Art, Washington, D.C.)

food and fines, or threatened mbotesa in the name of colonial vestiges and postcolonial public health slogans, imposing conditions that were making it more and more difficult for a man to give his wife a proper wale. The popular representation that turned the MPR party motto "One Father" into an image of Mobutu hiding his power inside the pregnant woman carved on his staff of "authentic" authority—his source of power and also his weapon—was none other than a representation of an Etat sorcier, mediated through a pregnant woman's body. It was a representation of a cunning sorcerer blocking birth, of a nation with lokwamisa, of a citizenry who knew as he did that birth is death.

DEPARTURES

When I began this study, historians were debating whether experiences or representations should be privileged as subjects of inquiry and sources of evidence. One path orients analysis toward agency, the other toward knowledge and discourse. This study sought stories and the concrete objects embedded in them. Thus, what mattered was less the force of historical subjects or the representations of cultures than what people did and undid, as they performed ordinary routines and extraordinary tales of daily life. Colonialism was, as its history must be, a storied process.[1] Routines turn analysis to social and symbolic action. Narrative was one such realm of practice. Missionary stories, evidence of an inscribed oral culture, revealed routines of chatting it up and jotting it down in a colonial culture of missionary evangelists. Yakusu's British Baptists, for all their earnestness and antipapal sentiments, laughed and worried about some of the same things as the Belgian planters, officials, and missionaries among whom they lived. They greeted, entertained, dined with, and showed off their mission station to Belgian queens and princes, colonial governors, and provincial doctors. Yakusu's missionaries did not balk at singing the *Brabançonne*, wearing colonial helmets, issuing state medical passports, or invoking "white men's quiet laws" to get a good night's sleep. They displayed pictures of the Belgian king and queen alongside Bible pictures in the hospital, and incorporated other state-issued colonial ingredients into their hierarchies and iconographies of power. Yakusu's *bricoleurs,* whether British or Congolese evangelists, revised and improvised as they reworked biblical verses, colonial hygiene jokes, and local metaphors into new parables and arguments. Both groups translated, but they began with access to different words and things. Congolese evangelists achieved entry to the missionary lexicon, in part, through reading and writing. What makes their letters and the translating activity that they expose so special, compared to oral tales and autobiographical memory, is nothing innate to literacy and texts; rather, it is our privileged access to this lexicon at use, in translation. I have argued that objects assist in dating tokwakwa, but in a markedly different way than letters assist in dating metaphors containing communion cups and bicycles or debates between a kanga and a nurse.

The church was a new judicial body, arbitrating a new moral vision, within as well as outside of medical settings. Yakusu's missionaries also sought state and private company monies to further their evangelical work. Whether acting as sanitary police, pronatalist census takers, or pastors, Yakusu's missionaries became agents of a form of colonial indirect rule. The mission became at times almost its own polity, executing hygiene directives issued by a state-at-various-removes, metropolitan and colonial-based authorities. Colonial medicine in Yakusu's 10,000-square-mile district entailed a merging of the secular and clerical, the official and charitable. The result was a species of hygienic evangelism,[2] personified in British and Congolese evangelical teachers and healers. Maternal and infant health care at Yakusu developed, in this political context, as a priority within missionary medicine. Medicalized childbearing was never the preoccupation among Yakusu's British Baptists that it was among Belgian colonials. For Belgians in the Congo, maternity hospitals were part of a procreative fixation with increasing the birthrate and reforming Congolese sexual, birth control, and marital practices. Yakusu's history includes a polygamy strand of church prohibition and lost church members. Its medical missionaries tried to make it easier for Congolese Baptists to remain monogamous. But this strand may have been less accentuated from the British side than demanded by Congolese Protestants. In addition to generating state subsidies, midwifery at Yakusu was a way to promote a new generation of Congolese Christians and reproduce model monogamous, midwife-nurse spouse teams. Funding missionary medicine involved bending to state prerogatives and incorporating pronatalist agendas, idioms, and objects into what had been a largely fee-paying form of medical care. Yakusu's missionaries and Congolese evangelists added domestic, evangelical mantles to these objects. Birth certificates were color coded by gender at Yakusu, and kilo matabish became knitted Christmas gifts.

Observing postcolonial childbirth routines was integral to this study. Embedded in these routines were colonial elements. Soap, papers, and other signs of colonial debris in contemporary "procedures of consumption" guided many historical questions. Creativity in practices of quotation and appropriation tends to thrive, de Certeau tells us, "where practice ceases to have its own language," thus speech its *own* lexicon or exclusive system of signs.[3] The shifting, variable meanings of things such as soap and papers steered this historical ethnography. I could not look at giving birth alone to understand its medicalization. Counting births—that is, the bureaucracy of colonial demographic imperatives—also had to be considered as a powerful force. A hospital birth did not necessarily mean compliance with colonial desires and rules. Congolese insinuated their own fertility strategies into this seeming obedience. Colonial obstetrics began, after all, because Congolese sought help in childbirth emergencies.

Homemade soap was an early element in domesticity training for Yakusu mission girls. And soap became a vital accoutrement to the work lives of Congolese nursing men who began their evangelical careers cleaning knives and forks for an occupation. Papers, too, were key to the language of practice in colonial evangelical life. A favorite sermon written by a Yakusu missionary tells of a boy who came to work at the station early in the century, was sent on an errand with a leaf (letter) to deliver, and still possessed the same leaf, evidence of the white missionary's power, several years later. Yakusu's missionaries were embedded in a local Congolese moral imagination as spirits from the forest with papers. Their practices as doctors and sanitary agents made them purveyors of letters and medical passports as well as Bibles.

Yakusu's Congolese evangelists were among the first letter writers and publishing authors in the region. They wrote papers, read papers, and collected and distributed papers. Yakusu's British Baptist missionaries were among the first to issue birth certificates in a colonial maternity in their district. They also distributed soap, readers, baby vests, and hygiene documents, but they believed patients should pay for medical care. Birth certificates, a new kind of missionary paper given to fathers, assisted in hospitalizing birth. Similarly, soap and baby clothes attracted mothers to maternity and baby clinic routines. Soap was Malia Winnie's "disinfectant." She linked her knowledge and authority to it. Over and over again, in speaking with me, she interjected the words: "and I washed my hands." Soap and injections worked to condense and displace adultery confessions, while soap and baby vests extended the authority and prestige of hospital childbearing and colonial midwifery.

Soap and papers have positional meaning, and history was materialized in their situational dominance.[4] As debris from colonial experiences, from colonial cultures of domination, soap and papers did not dominate colonial subjects. Congolese appropriated these objects from colonial life, and continue to incorporate this debris into their routines of consumption and practice. Since soap and papers emerged from a culture of domination, their positional meanings remain magnified, especially in birth ritual, giving them their capacity to condense meaning and crystallize history. Surgery had a subversive power at Yakusu, simplifying the meaning of libeli into death and rebirth formulas, and extending the cutting and dividing powers of local evangelists. Enemas and injections also condensed meaning, and they continue to do so in the postcolonial period.

This study has attempted to unmake conventional historical narratives about colonialism, in which symmetry of structure—European imposition and indigenous response—discloses and circumscribes the argument. It was partly for this reason that I alternately interjected revelatory tales from the historical record and my field interviews and observations. Although the emergence and use, misuse and reuse, of a colonial lexicon was the subject of study, asymmetries in social power and gender meanings were my starting points. A foreign mission within a colonial state. Congolese mothers within colonial maternities. A male birth ritual within a colonial evangelical situation. Each of these situations of asymmetry and debate engendered struggle and compromise, misrecognition and redefinition. Each situation led to bargaining over political and cultural ground, especially within the arenas of a medical mission, hygiene surveillance, surgery, and obstetrics. Another more navigational sense of negotiation yielded transitions and crossings in practice, the passage and condensation of objects and meanings. People debated ideas about the relative value of adult and infant life, the meanings and implications of death, illness, and misfortune, fertility and blood, maternal sacrifice, selfishness, and food. Childbirth proved to be a thickly layered and sensitive domain of transactions, exchange, and argument from the mid-1920s on. The terrain of struggle shifted to women's bodies, therefore, just as the visibility of libeli performances ended, surgery performances began, and autopsies became possible.

Tinned food marked tokwakwa dating back to at least the late nineteenth century along the Congo. This tale-telling form garnered surgery within its repertoire of terror and scorn during the 1920s. Roads and trucks arrived in tokwakwa during the 1920s and 1930s as quickly as they arrived in forest life. This swift mobility in ideas and things characterized a new and specific, local colonial modernity of the interwar period. The speed and conjunctures of the 1920s—which coincided with new, technocratic ways of counting lives, measuring populations, and calculating reproductive values—meant that these supposedly Western ways arrived instantly, simultaneously, in the Congo. Medicine and maternity from the 1920s coincided with an unprecedented form of historical consciousness, as life sped up across a new global ecumene, as jazz and rumba rhythms, scheduled airplane flights (the first in the world was Leopoldville to Stanleyville!), and automobiles moved as swiftly between Kinshasa and the Upper Lomami as they did among Havana, Brussels, London, New York, and Accra. This startling fast modernity of the 1920s and 1930s, the period in colonial Belgian Africa when strange medleys produced such wry mirth and enraged terror, explains why the lexicon of debate accreted bicycles and airplanes as signs. Medicalized maternity coincided with this new mobility of ideas, styles, and things. The analysis of childbirth demonstrated continuing eddies of struggle around risks and claims in wealth in persons and things, in fertility and social reproduction. Indeed, this history of childbirth confirms that fertility and reproduction were and remain a key vortex of social action, and thus help explain why bodily markings, clothing, monies, papers, food, and balimo were central terms of debate within earlier clashes over controlling youth and contrary birth rituals for making them men.

The notion of colonial encounter, in the singular, orients historical interpretation, the narrative process itself, toward the epic. This study sought a new vocabulary—in routines, transactions, and exchange—to restore the multiplicity of engagements that can be glimpsed in a historically specific, colonial lexicon. Treating historical episodes—embedded in letters, tokwakwa, and autobiographical memories—as tales and routines enabled the integration of narrative and time with social and cultural analysis. It also illuminated complex asymmetries. Nothing in and near Yakusu was as simple as white pith helmets versus black skins. Gradations and combinations of highs, lows, and middles were constantly shifting, recomposing and decomposing. Each transaction or tale was also a variant, a newly improvised, reworked routine. Some were extraordinary, even if never completely composed, historical stories. These incomplete retellings imparted fancy and ruses, laughter and scorn to white helmets, black skins, and colonial middles. They also demonstrated and confirmed the sometimes global, but always local, lexicon that these historical figures kept at play: crocodiles and bicycles, salt and soap, placentas and baby vests, libeli scars and gramophones. With my presence, the lexicon open for active translation expanded, for a time, to include eelo, animal metaphors for birth pains, and cassette recorders.

I want to return one more time to the central moral metaphor of this study, the 1934 account that compared crocodiles to airplanes. It was not until I was combing data in Brussels, just after my fieldwork in Zaire had ended, that I first paid attention to Chesterman's anecdote. I knew that when I had asked to go to Romée, the historic battle site of 1893 where some Tippu Tib–associated Zanzibari had slave-worked rice plantations by the 1880s, my guides led me first to the place where these ivory and slave traders were known to swim and bathe. Only the BaTambatamba could bathe in this former swimming hole without being eaten, I was told, because only they had special powers over the mermaidlike crocodiles that lived in this pool of water at the time. This spatial form of remembering proved important in this writing of history. But that was all I could remember about crocodiles while sitting in Brussels. With one exception. One day, someone told me that there were no more crocodiles on the Lokele stretch of the river. "Why?" I had asked. "Because they were all killed to make purses for white people." Mamiwata, too, emerged spontaneously in conversation, but I also made this mermaid figure associated with infant death an explicit part of my inquiries. I had never pursued crocodiles as a field subject, so far did they seem then from a history of colonial medicine and childbearing.

I asked myself what I knew about crocodiles and airplanes as I mulled over Chesterman's anecdote. I remembered how the people in the village, near the old BaTambatamba swimming hole where I lived for five months, would tease me that I, their white lady researcher, should see to it that an airplane descended onto village soil one day. All the 300-some people who lived in the village would then board this avion with me, along with everything that we needed to carry on living as *they* were accustomed, meanwhile preserving *my* research into their birthing practices. I would join them in elaborating this droll collective daydream with such baggage as cassava, palm oil, bananas, and palm wine *and* pregnant women, village midwives, forest medicines for retained placentas, and enema stuff galore. We would howl as we rehearsed this game about our farcical gear, the airplane landing on the riverfront, and our taking off together for Ulaya, for Europe. Eventually, we would leave this slapstick fantasy until a next time, when we would repeat with new detail, but always with hilarity and inestimable irony, this burlesque about the white Madami, her airplane, and the premium on midwifery engendered by her work.

I also did not pose questions about airplanes either. But these colonial signs drew my attention more than crocodiles. They also emerged more spontaneously in daily life and in my notes. I spent many evenings trying to record local storytelling around Tata Alikuwa's fire. I requested—and my tape recorder produced—these evening story-recording sessions. People would perform, but they also liked to press rewind and play. Soon, they demanded evenings of listening to their recorded voices telling stories as part of our exchange. Meanwhile, I learned that airplanes figured alongside motorcars and walkie-talkies in moral riddles old men would pose about avenues to wealth and success. I also knew Avion, a fifty-some-year-old Yainyongo man. His was neither an unusual nor inauspicious name. (There were many called Avion, though I never met a young person or a woman with this name.) Someone told me, when I asked, that his mother had named Avion after an airplane because one had flown overhead when she was giving birth to him.

If crocodiles, therefore, were about the terror of certain memories and their spaces, airplanes had something to do with local forms of naming, remembering, jesting, and birthing. Airplanes figured in colonial joking relationships; the moral doublet of 1934 was, in part, a tease. I may not have been aligned with the terror of crocodiles, but I certainly was with the humor of airplanes. And so our burlesque performed it: the postcolonial Madami had the power to land a plane wherever and for whomever she wanted. I also aligned myself with airplanes when I stopped on my bicycle one day as I entered Kisangani because I noticed a boy of no more than fifteen walking along with a huge model DC-10 in his arms. He was on his way to sell this Air Zaïre plane at the city market, before I became its consumer instead. I had seen plenty of model riverboats since I had arrived in Zaire. Those that simulated Mobutu's private riverboat with his helicopter mounted on the back were all the rage at major stops as I traveled downriver. Who bought these? Rural pastors with doilied salons, I discovered, were among those who liked to put *Inakwame* paintings[5]—scenes of a man hanging in peril from a tree branch extending over a river, caught between a ferocious crocodile in the water, a lion on the ground, and a large snake above him in the tree—on their kizungu walls. The boy's Air Zaïre plane was as elaborately detailed as a Mobutu riverboat and also made entirely of found materials—mostly plantain stems and bamboo cores, though with ingenious debris, too. The boy had decked out his DC-10 *ndege* (bird) with scraps of clothing and paper in the MPR colors, a party torch, ten moving wheels, two moving doors, all standing on one sixteen-inch-high, bright blue, four-pronged bird's leg. Not unlike the way the children in my village gathered my used batteries and cassette wrappers and made moving toys with them, the boy had glued the printed Swahili word *Instantenene* on one of the plane's wings. He, of course, had no idea how much this clipped bit of advertising from powdered milk packaging would delight me, a historian of maternity. Much later, when traveling in England, I would learn from missionary memories and photograph albums that during Dr. Browne's era, missionaries tried to direct these forms of artifice. They encouraged local pram building for pushing live infants after a missionary lady showed up with one for her child, though the simulacra never caught on. And they organized station contests where Yakusu had to build miniature rural health dispensaries. Yet playful artifice did not arrive with Europeans and their things, even if imposed gestures of mimicry did. Boys were making model canoes with coverings over the chief or white man's chair and fifty to sixty camwood-colored clay figures crowding the sides from early in the century; there is no reason to think that they did not begin much earlier, even if they added river steamers to their repertoire and showed them to marveling missionaries.[6]

Ever since I began to mull over the terms crocodile and airplane and the moral metaphor that joined them, I let my research lexicon expand to include other signifying objects like bicycles, forks, gramophones, steamers, and prams. I also let my "field" enlarge to include England, Belgium, and the United States, as I wandered in search of memories, photographs, persons, and things. Once I let go of childbirth per se, I was struck over and over again by how much the *chronology* of my research discoveries and travels affected what came into my fold, influencing my capacity to recognize things as evidence for history. As this process continued, I became aware of how much I had not asked about when I was in the "field." To think I never explicitly asked about bicycles, crocodiles, airplanes, Christmas. Yet this evidence accumulated without any prompting on my part until I came to recognize its importance.

Eventually, too, I recognized how linear—indeed, colonial—my research itineraries remained, however postmodern and transnational my literary and analytic aspirations might have become. I only began to catch myself when my friend Jo loaned me her car to tour England, visiting former Yakusu missionaries and their forms of remembering Yakusu. We had an enormous amount in common, I learned, and for the most part I won, if not their hearts, access to their stories, photographs, letters, and jokes. These British Baptists were, after all, the colleagues of those English and Scottish missionaries at Yakusu who had invited me for endless teas, nursed me when I cycled back from my village delirious with malaria, loaned me a camp bed, gave me Christmas gifts, invited me to watch a cesarean section, offered me Bokondoko's former abode as a flat, and let me take the hospital archives to the room I made my study for as long as I wanted. I would joke (with others) that these missionaries thought God had sent me to Yakusu; why else would they have welcomed me so generously and unwarily? Alternately, I would tease (also to others) that these missionaries needed me as an outside interlocutor-therapist. Not all told me their joys and woes, but those who did appreciated my capacity to listen and delve. I became friends with most of them, just as I did with most of my key Zairian "informants" and research assistants. Some missionaries, however, were less aware than Zairians of how they, too, became subjects and objects of my scrutiny. Still, their movements and codes, as much as those of Zairian wives and midwives, were material for my nighttime routine of composing snatches of prose.

A few of Yakusu's missionaries came to visit me one afternoon when I was staying in Yainyongo. They were curious to see. I can still hear and feel the howls of Mama Lisongomi's elegant, round daughter, Mama Lutia, as she reconstructed the scene that these strangers made with the visiting pastor's video camera and a dancing umbrella. I had opened my own movie theater–like existence in this village months before. Women were used to stopping to see what the "historian of enemas," as village youth called me, was asking about over the morning fire, before going on their way to farm and gather in the forest. But an umbrella-holding-missionary Madami dancing to a video camera and time far surpassed any of my own theatrics.

I spent only five of my fourteen months in the field in this village. What gets me still is not how brief it was, nor how complicated were these movements among complexity and caricature. What gets me is how my stay was so strongly marked by love and hate. I have never had neighbors so noisy in their quarrelsomeness. Nor did I ever stop marveling, as I would most mornings in my mosquito-netted camp bed after being wakened by screams of bloody murder over unpaid debts and selfish deeds, how the mood could so quickly shift from ravenous anger to the uproarious cackle of a Mama Lisongomi–like jester figure at work.

Yes, this history is incomplete.[7] My students have helped me appreciate, more than I ever did before, how appreciable and troubling the role of conjecture in African history can be. I have tried to make *when* I guessed and *how* I guessed transparent at every bound, and otherwise to draw attention to positionings and displacements of selves, exposing my manifestations and impositions as observer, tourist, researcher patron, and Mamiwata-like, Peace Corps–esque figure, alternately called Bibi Nesi, Madami, and Mademoiselle.

The worst was how I deliberately said thank you. I always promised myself this would be the limit on transparence, that I need not put in print my mangled attempts to express appreciation, to foster trust and good relations, and—once I had asked for advice—to do what I was told to do. They told me to go to Kisangani's market and meet Mama Lutia there. She would help me buy salted fish, salt, and soap, and arrange for their loading in her canoe. And so she and I did, and later we all awaited her return back "home." I watched what next ensued as if I were in an unnerving nightmare version of a filmic colonial spoof: me, then almost a white colonial Lady Bountiful, trying to extend love and thanks through lame gestures of handing out the soap, salt, and fish to every woman in every household. I was horrified to watch this effort transformed before my eyes into something reminiscent of a colonial baby-weighing scene. I did not personally do the handing out; I left this to the women in the household where I lived. Some women were immediately convinced that these women were cheating them, hoarding goods, taking more than their fair share. Thus, my charitable retreads provoked an awkward, painful, noisy pandemonium and more ravenous anger than multiple breakfast brawls combined.

Only worse was Christmas. I dreaded the possibilities of missionary observances and holiday invitations at Yakusu, so I decided to stay at Yainyongo. Not that I did not get drawn into a station Christmas anyway, but I organized my gifts for Yakusu's missionaries quietly and well in advance. Back at Yainyongo, many went to church in the morning. Others drank instead. I went to the Protestant chapel with others in my household. As we walked back home, we witnessed the worst episode of the effect of ethyl alcohol on empty stomachs that I had seen since I had arrived. This beverage was a by-product of a nearby development disaster, a Chinese-funded agricultural development project of the early 1980s. I once biked through the monotonous, flattened landscape of Lotokila with a man named Yenga, the church's lifaefi collector, as he told me about the horrendous working conditions and loss of peasants' farms. On Christmas, I watched a young woman who had been drinking this alcohol, produced and sold at Lotokila, in the latter stages of a major altercation over the ownership of a drum. Angry men were dragging her across the village. They, too, were drunk, and she was screaming at them, furious, naked, her body tied in ropes.

Within a fortnight, her elder sister, Mama Lutia, was dead. I was incredulous. How had this robust woman, the daughter who had inherited Mama Lisongomi's cackle and had helped me buy and transport the salt, soap, and fish picked up and died so suddenly? The Christmas vision of a bound and gagged female body had been much easier to grasp as postcolonial detritus of a Chinese-funded, Mobutu-promoted development project gone terribly awry. At Christmas, no one had died. I felt alone as interpreter then. But after Ma Lutia died, everyone was busy and fairly unanimous about this latest fonoli tale about a dead daughter, an elegant woman, a clever trader: bad people, bad medicine, jealousy, hate. "If you have luck and wear nice clothes, bad people will kill you. Life is getting worse and worse in Zaire because bad people— balosi—are increasing." They retraced the rapid set of events and decisions for me. Their trips to the dancing healer upriver a village or two. Their attempts to organize a canoe to the same health center across the river where Bibi Viviane had given birth. There were other strands, too: anemia, her blood count, malaria, the difficulties in getting a canoe, and the debates over where to go— across the river to the nurse, or up the river to the kanga with his makeshift hospital and riverfront dancing site.

I only arrived after the fact. I was at Yakusu packing my bags to leave when someone brought me the news. I went downriver the following day, in time to hold Mama Lisongomi as she grieved by her daughter's grave in front of her son's house. She only wanted one thing. To hear her daughter's voice. "Would I please go get my tape recorder and the right tapes," she asked, "so they could all hear Mama Lutia speak and laugh again?" And so our nighttime ritual of recording stories for my research only to play them back for all to hear, the nocturnal movie theater–like spectacle around Tata Alikuwa's fire, became transformed into a final funereal visitation from the dead. This last exchange produced more used batteries as toys for the children, and yet more uses for my tapes and their metaphor, birth is death.

NOTES

Introduction

1. Albert Cook, "Note on Dr. Mitchell's Paper on the Causes of Obstructed Labour in Uganda," *East African Medical Journal* 15 (October 1938): 215–19, esp. 216; J. P. Mitchell, "On the Causes of Obstructed Labour in Uganda," *East African Medical Journal* 15 (October 1938): 205–14; and R. Y. Stones, "On the Causes of Obstructed Labour in Uganda," *East African Medical Journal* 15 (October 1938): 219–20.
2. Cook, "Note on Dr. Mitchell's Paper," 216.
3. Michael Crowder, *The Flogging of Phineas McIntosh: A Tale of Colonial Folly and Injustice, Bechuanaland 1933* (New Haven, Conn.: Yale University Press, 1988). I also retain a notion of the improvisational character of tales: "[T]here is no moment at which a tale is composed. . . . They never have a beginning, a composition, and they never end, but rather disappear into later tales" (Jan Vansina, *Oral Tradition as History* [Madison: University of Wisconsin Press, 1985], 12, 26).
4. Natalie Zemon Davis, "The Shapes of Social History," *Storia della Storiographia* 17 (1990): 28–34.
5. Ruanda-Urundi also came under Belgian administration after the First World War.
6. I prefer the French term *hygiène* to its more circumscribed English cognate *hygiene,* as *hygiène* is more open to multiple meanings, including personal bodily hygiene, domesticity, and social hygiene.
7. See the excellent new edition edited by D. C. R. A. Goonetilleke: Joseph Conrad, *Heart of Darkness* (Peterborough, Ont.: Broadview Literary Texts, 1995).
8. For an excellent historiographical critique of the use and misuse of this term derived from Michel Foucault, see Colin Jones, "Montpellier Medical Students and the Medicalisation of Eighteenth-Century France," in *Problems and Methods in the History of Medicine,* ed. Roy Porter and Andrew Wear (London: Croom, 1987), 57–80. I follow Jones in regarding medicalization as "a dynamic and dialectical process" involving "changing patterns of demand as well as the provision of medical services," new forms of prestige for medical practitioners, and "the development of all kinds of medical syndromes . . . as both individual and societal developments came to be seen through medical spectacles" (ibid., 57–58). Yet I maintain a Foucauldian

sense of biopower and the disciplining of "docile bodies" through the "carceral," tropical "laboratory" of the colony. See especially Michel Foucault, *Discipline and Punish: The Birth of the Prison* (New York: Vintage, 1979). See also Michel Foucault, *History of Sexuality* (New York: Vintage Books, 1985).

9. I borrow this expression from Inderpal Grewal and Caren Kaplan, eds., *Scattered Hegemonies: Postmodernity and Transnational Feminist Practices* (Minneapolis: University of Minnesota Press, 1994) to suggest the complexity of transnational hierarchies and global flows and mediations, especially in a post-1989 world. My fieldwork ended in February 1990, just before the period that Congolese tend to call "the transition," which began, they agree, with Mobutu's announcement of democratization in March 1990.

10. On maternity work in Uganda, see W. D. Foster, *The Church Missionary Society and Modern Medicine in Uganda: The Life of Sir Albert Cook, K.C.M.G., 1870–1951* (Newhaven, East Sussex: Newhaven Press, 1978); Carol Summers, "Intimate Colonialism: The Imperial Production of Reproduction in Uganda, 1907–1925," *Signs* 16 (1991): 787–807; and Megan Vaughan, *Curing Their Ills: Colonial Power and African Illness* (Stanford, Calif.: Stanford University Press, 1991).

11. Raymond Leslie Buell, *The Native Problem in Africa,* 2 vols. (1928; reprint, London: Frank Cass, 1965), 1:390, 607; 2:39–40, 578.

12. Laure Trolli, "Les femmes coloniales et l'enfance noire," *Bulletin de l'Union Coloniale* 17, no. 112 (February 1940): 33–34. Maternal health services were much more advanced in the Belgian Congo than in neighboring French Equatorial Africa; see Rita Headrick, *Colonialism, Health, and Illness in French Equatorial Africa, 1885–1935* (Atlanta, Ga.: African Studies Association, 1994).

13. V. Cocq and Fr. Mercken, "L'assistance obstétricale au Congo belge (y compris le Ruanda-Urundi)," *Gynécologie et Obstétrique* 31, no. 4 (1935): 401–513.

14. FOREAMI, *Rapport annuel,* 1955, 60.

15. Belgium, Office de l'Information et des Relations Publiques pour le Congo Belge et le Ruanda-Urundi, *Health in Belgian Africa* (Brussels: Inforcongo, 1958), 55.

16. For 1947 and 1956, see ibid.; for 1952, see FOREAMI, *Rapport annuel,* 1955, 60.

17. Georges Brausch, *Belgian Administration in the Congo* (London: Oxford University Press, 1961), 8.

18. I draw my vocabulary here from a pioneering analysis of state power in relation to families and reproduction; see Jane Jenson, "Gender and Reproduction: Or, Babies and the State," *Studies in Political Economy* 20 (1986): 9–45.

19. As can be seen in Marie-Louise Comeliau, *Demain, coloniale!* (Antwerp: Editions Zaïre, 1945), 89, 166–72.

20. "Circulaire réglementant la situation des femmes des travailleurs de l'Etat," Intérieur no. 43/a, 21 July 1930, Etat Indépendant du Congo, *Recueil Mensuel des arrêtés, circulaires, instructions et ordres de service* (1903): 98–99. Dr. Veroni, Rapport sanitaire sur le 2ème semestre de l'année 1910, H (841), "Rapports sanitaires des Stanley Falls," Archives Africaines, Brussels [hereafter AA].

21. Cocq and Mercken, "L'assistance obstétricale," 486.

22. For a seminal treatment on the census as a colonial subject, see Bernard S. Cohn, "The Census, Social Structure, and Objectification in South Asia," in *An Anthropologist among the*

Historians and Other Essays (Delhi: Oxford University Press, 1987), 224–54. Maternity, though less commonly used in English than in French, denotes a built structure—a maternity ward or hospital—where childbearing and "confinement" take place; I follow many Congolese men and women in borrowing the French word (*maternité*) for this novel kind of space that became an everyday word and thing in the lexicons of all who were present in the Belgian Congo in the 1950s. Maternity also means motherhood, mothering, indeed natalist practice, and thus I insist on the word's plural senses even more. I often use the word maternity rather than the more common English-language use of maternity ward in keeping with the French, to emphasize that these were freestanding buildings and to suggest not just a built structure but its other senses as well.

23. Nancy Rose Hunt, "'Le bébé en brousse': European Women, African Birth Spacing, and Colonial Intervention in Breast Feeding in the Belgian Congo," *International Journal of African Historical Studies* 21 (1988): 401–32 (hereafter *IJAMS*).

24. The best overview for Belgium remains D. V. Glass, *Population: Policies and Movements in Europe* (Oxford: Oxford University Press, 1940); see also W. De Raes, "Eugenetika in de Belgische medische wereld tijdens het interbellum," *Revue belge d'Histoire contemporaine* 20 (1989): 399–464. Belgium has rarely been included in a growing historiography on social hygiene, pronatalist eugenics, and maternalism in Europe. See, for example, Michael S. Teitelbaum and Jay M. Winter, eds., *Population and Resources in Western Intellectual Traditions* (Cambridge: Cambridge University Press, 1989); Paul Weindling, *Health, Race, and German Politics between National Unification and Nazism, 1870–1945* (Cambridge: Cambridge University Press, 1989); Richard Soloway, *Demography and Degeneration: Eugenics and the Declining Birthrate in Twentieth-Century Britain* (Chapel Hill: University of North Carolina Press, 1990); Mark B. Adams, *The Wellborn Science: Eugenics in Germany, France, Brazil, and Russia* (Oxford: Oxford University Press, 1990); William H. Schneider, *Quality and Quantity: The Quest for Biological Regeneration in Twentieth-Century France* (Cambridge: Cambridge University Press, 1990); Seth Koven and Sonya Michel, eds., *Mothers of a New World: Maternalist Politics and the Origins of Welfare States* (New York: Routledge, 1993); and David G. Horn, *Social Bodies: Science, Reproduction, and Italian Modernity* (Princeton, N.J.: Princeton University Press, 1994).

25. The latter remains quite undeveloped. Studies by John M. Janzen, Kivilu Sabakinu, Maryinez Lyons, and Jean-Luc Vellut are important reading for medical history; studies by Wyatt MacGaffey, Vellut (on E. Cambier), and Allan Roberts ("'Like a Roaring Lion': Tabwa Terrorism in the Late Nineteenth Century," in *Banditry, Rebellion, and Social Protest in Africa*, ed. Donald Crummey [London: James Currey, 1986], 65–86) are among the most innovative mission-related social histories (as opposed to the immensely rich literature on religious movements). For these references, see bibliography; and Jean-Luc Vellut, Florence Loriaux, and Françoise Morimont, *Bibliographie historique du Zaïre à l'époque coloniale (1880–1960): Travaux publiés en 1960–1996* (Louvain-la-Neuve and Tervuren: Centre d'Histoire de l'Afrique and MRAC, 1996). (Note: Contrary to Congolese practice, the surnames of Congolese scholars are not capitalized, and they follow their first names.)

26. "Macrohistory must accept the disclosures of microhistory" (Davis, "Shapes of Social History," 33).

27. J. Clyde Mitchell, *The Kalela Dance: Aspects of Relationships among Urban Africans in Northern Rhodesia,* Rhodes-Livingstone Paper 27 (Manchester: Manchester University Press, 1959), 11–12; and Terence Ranger, *Dance and Society in Eastern Africa, 1890–1970: The Beni Ngoma* (Berkeley: University of California Press, 1975).

28. John M. Janzen, *The Quest for Therapy in Lower Zaire* (Berkeley: University of California Press, 1978), 215. The historical literature on medicine, disease, and healing in Africa is now voluminous. See Steven Feierman's pathbreaking essay, "Struggles for Control: The Social Roots of Health and Healing in Modern Africa," *African Studies Review* 28 (1985): 73–147; and the now dated, but important critical review of the literature by Gwyn Prins, "But What Was the Disease? The Present State of Health and Healing in African Studies," *Past and Present,* no. 124 (August 1989): 159–79. Diverse approaches are represented by the essays (many first published in 1979 and 1981) in Steven Feierman and John M. Janzen, eds., *The Social Basis of Health and Healing in Africa* (Berkeley: University of California Press, 1992); Steven Feierman, "Popular Control over the Institutions of Health: A Historical Study," in *The Professionalisation of Medicine,* ed. Murray Last and G. L. Chavanduka (Manchester: Manchester University Press, 1986), 205–20; Vaughan, *Curing Their Ills;* Shula Marks, *Divided Sisterhood: Race, Class, and Gender in the South African Nursing Profession* (New York: St. Martin's Press, 1994); and Luise White, "Tsetse Visions: Narratives of Blood and Bugs in Colonial Northern Rhodesia, 1931–1939," *Journal of African History* 36 (1995): 219–45.

29. An expression borrowed from Nicholas Thomas's *Entangled Objects: Exchange, Material Culture, and Colonialism in the Pacific* (Cambridge: Harvard University Press, 1991).

30. Terence Ranger, "Godly Medicine: The Ambiguities of Medical Mission in Southeast Tanzania, 1900–1945," *Social Science and Medicine* 15B (1981): 264. On African interpretations of other diseases, see, for example, Charles Van Onselen, "Reactions to Rinderpest in Southern Africa, 1896–1897," *Journal of African History* 8 (1972): 474–88; John Ford, *The Role of Trypanosomiases in African Ecology: A Study of the Tsetse Fly Problem* (Oxford: Clarendon Press, 1971), 192; Victor Turner, *The Drums of Affliction* (Oxford: Clarendon Press and International African Institute, 1968), 654; and White, "Tsetse Visions."

31. The classic source regarding such rumors is Rik Ceyssens, "Mutumbula, mythe de l'opprimé," *Cultures et développement* 7 (1975): 483–536. See also Jean-François Bayart, "Les terroirs et des hommes," in *L'Etat en Afrique: La politique du ventre* (Paris: Fayard, 1989), 317–30; Monica Wilson, *Communal Rituals of the Nyakyusa* (London: Oxford University Press, 1959), 150–51; and essays by Luise White, including "Vampire Priests of Central Africa: African Debates about Labor and Religion in Colonial Northern Uganda," *Comparative Studies in Society and History* 35 (1993): 746–72.

32. Feierman, "Struggles for Control," 123.

33. For the quotation and the consequences for postcolonial Africa, see Alanagh Raikes, "Women's Health in East Africa," *Social Science and Medicine* 28 (1989): 448.

34. *L'Etat sorcier* is the title of his book, though "Childbearing with Dignity" is an exceptional chapter in the argument. Hours draws attention to possible reasons for the exception himself; his research had shifted to anglophone Cameroon, where there was a different—Anglo-Saxon—sense of duty and "the symbolic power of the state figure appeared weaker than in francophone areas." See "Accoucher dans la dignité: un centre de santé rural," in Bernard Hours, *L'Etat sorcier: Santé publique et société au Cameroun* (Paris: Editions l'Harmattan,

1985), 92–108, esp. 97, 108. Also of note is Deborah Gaitskell, "'Getting Close to the Hearts of Mothers': Medical Missionaries among African Women and Children in Johannesburg between the Wars," in *Women and Children First: International Maternal and Infant Welfare, 1870–1945,* ed. Valerie Fildes, Lara Marks, and Hilary Marland (London: Routledge, 1992), 178–202.

35. See, for example, Prins, "But What Was the Disease?" 166; and Vaughan, *Curing Their Ills,* 69–70.

36. Summers, "Intimate Colonialism," 806–7. Thus, colonial medicine for women in this instance remains indistinct from "social engineering" characterizations of colonial medicine. See, for example, Vaughan, *Curing Their Ills,* 73–74; and Maryinez Lyons, *The Colonial Disease: A Social History of Sleeping Sickness in Northern Zaire, 1900–1940* (Cambridge: Cambridge University Press, 1992).

37. Violet Jhala, "The Development of Maternal and Child Welfare Work in Colonial Malawi" (paper presented at the Women in Africa Seminar Series, Department of Extra-Mural Studies, London University, 3 June 1985).

38. Summers, "Intimate Colonialism," 807 n. 66.

39. The caution entailed their attempts to reduce rather than eliminate infibulation and reinfibulation practices. By 1933, there were nearly 200 trained Sudanese midwives working in northern and central Sudan (Mabel Wolff to the British Social Hygiene Council, Inc., February 1933, document 582/10/4–15, Misses Wolff Papers, Sudan Archives, University of Durham). Many thanks to Jennifer (Beinart) Stanton for bringing this collection to my attention. See also Hassan Bella, "Sudanese Village Midwives: Six Decades of Experience with Part-Time Health Workers," in *Advances in International Maternal and Child Health,* ed. D. B. Jelliffe and E. F. P. Jelliffe (Oxford: Clarendon Press, 1984), 4:124–48; Heather Bell, "Midwifery Training and Female Circumcision in the Inter-War Anglo-Egyptian Sudan," *Journal of African History* 39 (1998): 298–312; and Janice Boddy, "Remembering Amal: On Birth and the British in Northern Sudan," in *Pragmatic Women and Body Politics,* ed. Margaret Lock and Patricia A. Kaufert (Cambridge: Cambridge University Press, 1998), 28–57.

40. Wyatt MacGaffey, *Modern Kongo Prophets: Religion in a Plural Society* (Bloomington: Indiana University Press, 1983), 91.

41. Feierman, "Popular Control," 214.

42. T. O. Beidelman, "Witchcraft in Ukaguru," in *Witchcraft and Sorcery in East Africa,* ed. John Middleton and E. H. Winter (London: Routledge and Kegan Paul, 1963), 57–98, esp. 80.

43. Lloyd W. Swantz, "The Role of the Medicine Man among the Zaramo of Dar es Salaam" (Ph.D. diss., University of Dar es Salaam, 1972). Placentas have implications for fertility, and thus it matters who handles them and how; see P. Erny, "Placenta et cordon ombilical dans la tradition africaine," *Psychopathologie africaine* 5 (1969): 139–48.

44. Carolyn Fishel Sargent's work is ethnographic; see *Maternity, Medicine, and Power: Reproductive Decisions in Urban Benin* (Berkeley: University of California Press, 1989). Exceptions include Théophile Obenga, "Naissance et puberté en pays Kongo au XVIIe siècle," *Cahiers congolais d'anthropologie et d'histoire* 9 (1984): 19–30; Catherine Eileen Burns, "Reproductive Labors: The Politics of Women's Health in South Africa, 1900 to 1960" (Ph.D. diss., Northwestern University, 1994); and Boddy, "Remembering Amal."

45. See, for example, Bell, "Midwifery Training and Female Circumcision"; Guilia Berrera, *Dan-*

gerous Liaisons: Colonial Concubinage in Eritrea, 1890–1941, PAS Working Paper no. 1 (Evanston, Ill.: Program of African Studies, Northwestern University, 1996); Boddy, "Remembering Amal"; A. Stacie C. Colwell, "Morphing the Body Collective: Subtexts and Sequelae of Colonial Population Studies," paper presented to Fortieth Annual Meeting of the African Studies Association, Columbus, Ohio, 13–16 November 1997; and Lynn M. Thomas, " '*Ngaitana* (I will circumcise myself)': The Gender and Generational Politics of the 1956 Ban on Clitoridectomy in Meru, Kenya," *Gender and History* 8 (1966): 338–63.

46. A word I borrow with inspiration from Bernard S. Cohn, who identifies several "investigative modalities" of colonial power and knowledge, some of which became sciences with their own professionals. There were certainly hygienic, enumerative, census, and obstetric/gynecological modalities in the Congo; I use "eugenic modality" to argue how closely linked these modalities became in this context. See Bernard S. Cohn, *Colonialism and Its Forms of Knowledge: The British in India* (Princeton, N.J.: Princeton University Press, 1996), 5–11.

47. I borrow the term "meaning-making" from a lecture Philip Corrigan gave at the University of Arizona in January 1993. On "transcoding," see Peter Stallybrass and Allon White, *The Politics and Poetics of Transgression* (Ithaca, N.Y.: Cornell University Press, 1986), 6. On "creolization," see, among others, Ulf Hannerz, *Cultural Complexity: Studies in the Social Organization of Meaning* (New York: Columbia University Press, 1992). On processes of colonial and postcolonial translation, see notably Vicente L. Rafael, *Contracting Colonialism: Translation and Christian Conversion in Tagalog Society under Early Spanish Rule* (Durham, N.C.: Duke University Press, 1993); Johannes Fabian, *Language and Colonial Power: The Appropriation of Swahili in the Former Belgian Congo, 1880–1938* (Berkeley: University of California Press, 1986); Tejaswini Niranjana, *Siting Translation: History, Post-Structuralism, and the Colonial Context* (Berkeley: University of California Press, 1992); and Paul Stuart Landau, *The Realm of the Word: Language, Gender, and Christianity in a Southern African Kingdom* (Portsmouth, N.H.: Heinemann, 1995). On translation, performance, memory, and re-presentation in and of colonial situations, I have drawn inspiration from Greg Dening, *Mr. Bligh's Bad Language: Passion, Power, and the Theatre on the Bounty* (Cambridge: Cambridge University Press, 1992), and its equally extraordinary fictional counterpart, Juan José Saer, *The Witness,* trans. Margaret Jull Costa (London: Serpent's Tail, 1990).

48. Georges Dupré, *Un ordre et sa destruction* (Paris: ORSTOM, 1982); Kwame Anthony Appiah, *In My Father's House: Africa in the Philosophy of Culture* (New York: Oxford University Press, 1992), 56, 8. See also David William Cohen, "Doing Social History from Pim's Doorway," in *Reliving the Past: The Worlds of Social History,* ed. Oliver Zunz (Chapel Hill: University of North Carolina Press, 1985); and John Lonsdale and Bruce Berman, *Unhappy Valley: Conflict in Kenya and Africa* (London: James Curry, 1992), 330. On colonialism and biopower, see Ann Laura Stoler, *Race and the Education of Desire: Foucault's "History of Sexuality" and the Colonial Order of Things* (Durham, N.C.: Duke University Press, 1995).

49. T. O. Beidelman, *Moral Imagination in Kaguru Modes of Thought* (Bloomington: Indiana University Press, 1986); and Claude Lévi-Strauss, *The Savage Mind* (Chicago: University of Chicago Press, 1970).

50. Lévi-Strauss, *The Savage Mind,* 16–22, 35, 214, 219–20, 231–32, 263.

51. Michel de Certeau, *The Practice of Everyday Life,* trans. Steven Rendall (Berkeley: University of California Press, 1984), 34–35.

52. Jean-François Bayart, *L'Etat en Afrique: La politique du ventre* (Paris: Fayard, 1989), 143–44.

53. I take inspiration here from Jan Vansina's precolonial linguistic, material turn without forgetting that the phrase "*les mots et les choses*" is, and for colonial Africa must also be, Foucault's (Jan Vansina, *Paths in the Rainforests: Toward a History of Political Tradition in Equatorial Africa* [Madison: University of Wisconsin Press, 1990]).

54. The same is true for the term "modernity," which I insist on locating in time—for the purposes of this study, generally the interwar period—and as a form of historical consciousness, in this case of new mobilities characteristic of this period. On "hybridity" as a term of postcolonial cultural affirmation, see, for example, Annie E. Coombes, *Reinventing Africa: Museums, Material Culture, and Popular Imagination* (New Haven, Conn.: Yale University Press, 1994). For a theoretical genealogy of the term, including its origins in colonial vocabularies, see Robert Young, *Colonial Desire* (London: Routledge, 1995).

55. I owe this term to Timothy Burke, who used it during his comments as a discussant at a 1994 African Studies Association panel on the middle class.

56. Johannes Fabian, "Scratching the Surface: Observations on the Poetics of Lexical Borrowing in Shaba Swahili," *Anthropological Linguistics* 24 (1982): 14–50.

57. On "living in translation," see Niranjana, *Siting Translation,* 46. I extend Niranjana's formulation in that I include not only Congolese subalterns and Congolese évolués, but also categories of colonizers, especially missionaries, as performers in translation.

58. Paul Bolya, "Etude ethnographique des coutumes des Mongo, La naissance, Chapitre III," *La Voix du Congolais* 140 (November 1950), 864.

59. An abacost—a word derived from the expression "*à bas costume*" or "down with suits"—was an integral part of male authenticité dress, worn by party officials, state functionaries, and businessmen until the early 1990s.

60. See, too, Nancy Rose Hunt, "Noise over Camouflaged Polygamy, Colonial Mortality Taxation, and a Woman-Naming Crisis in Belgian Africa," *Journal of African History* 32 (1991): 494.

61. Mary Douglas states that the year of conspicuous change among rural Lele was 1953: "Now bicycles, sewing machines, clothing, paraffin lamps were seen everywhere" (Mary Douglas, *The Lele of the Kasai* [London: Oxford University Press, 1963], 62).

62. Ethnographers might call them Foma, an ethnic designation that local people often translate as "Lokele-BaMbole" or "BaMbole who live along the river." For one of the very few ethnographic considerations, see B. Crine, "La structure sociale des Foma (Haut-Zaïre)," *Cahiers du CEDAF* 4 (1972).

63. Italics added. A kilo is an infant health clinic; the name, widely used in the colonial period, derives from the major activity of these sessions, weighing babies.

64. Thus, in 1977, only 4 percent of SANRU zones had integrated "traditional birth attendants" (TBAS), whereas by the close of 1987, 40 percent had TBAS (Franklin C. Baer, "The Role of the Church in Managing Primary Health Care in Zaire" [SANRU Project USAID/DSP/ECZ 660–107, Office of Project Santé Rurale (SANRU), Kinshasa, ca. 1988, unpublished paper]).

65. SANRU brochures; Glenn Rogers, "Child Survival Strategy," (USAID, Kinshasa May 1987, unpublished manuscript); and Franklin C. Baer, "The Primary Health Care Strategy in Zaire" (Office of Project Santé Rurale [SANRU], Kinshasa, ca. 1985, unpublished manuscript).

66. See, for example, Catherine Coquery-Vidrovitch, Alain Forest, and Herbert Weiss, eds., *Rébellions-révolutions au Zaïre, 1963–1965,* 2 vols. (Paris: l'Harmattan, 1987).

67. The literature on the "second economy" in Zaire is immense; see, for example, Janet Mac-Gaffey with Vwakyanakazi Mukohya et al., *The Real Economy of Zaire* (Philadelphia: University of Pennsylvania, 1991). In urban Benin, hospital certification makes it easier to obtain a birth certificate, encouraging hospital deliveries and postdelivery arrivals (Sargent, *Maternity, Medicine, and Power,* 54, 73, 110).

68. de Certeau, *Practice,* viii, xvi–xvii.

69. Christopher C. Taylor's work has been influential here, though my evidence suggests that enemas are key to local conceptions of flow in the Yakusu region. See Christopher C. Taylor, *Milk, Honey, and Money: Changing Concepts in Rwandan Healing* (Washington, D.C.: Smithsonian Institution Press, 1992); and Nancy Rose Hunt, review of *Milk, Honey, and Money,* by Christopher C. Taylor, *International Journal of African Historical Studies* 28 (1995): 458–61.

70. There is a chapter bearing this name in a post-Leopoldian British view of the Congo (E. Alexander Powell, *The Map That Is Half Unrolled: Equatorial Africa from the Indian Ocean to the Atlantic* [London: John Long, 1925], 186–205).

71. The evidence available does not permit rendering all parties within what was an extremely complex social field equally visible here. Belgian and Catholic social actors are more absent than I would have liked, though the sources were mined as much as possible for signs and representations of Belgian subjects and colonial state forms. The riverain fishing people are Lokele, whereas the forest hunters and agriculturists tend to self-identify as BaMbole. BaMbole who have settled close to the river, such as those I lived among in Yainyongo-Romée, a village on the upriver border of the Romée confluence, often call themselves Foma. Their languages are closely related western Bantu languages, although Swahili (Kingwana) is widely spoken, especially in a former Zanzibari plantation site like Yainyongo-Romée. Other forest peoples included in this study are the Topoke (Eso) and Olombo (Turumbu). See Vansina, *Paths;* and Colonel A. Bertrand, "Quelques notes sur la vie politique, le développement, la décadence des petites sociétés bantou du bassin central du Congo," *Revue de l'Institut de Sociologie de Bruxelles* 1 (1920): 75–91.

72. Arjun Appadurai, "Disjuncture and Difference in the Global Cultural Economy," *Public Culture* 2 (1990): 1–24. See also Hannertz, *Cultural Complexity;* Grewal and Kaplan, *Scattered Hegemonies;* and Carol Breckenridge, ed., *Consuming Modernity: Public Culture in a South Asian World* (Minneapolis: University of Minnesota Press, 1995).

73. Jan Vansina's influential methodological endorsement of the validity of oral materials, first published in 1961, ushered in an oral turn in African historical studies. Most historians continued to draw on written sources in significant ways, though the oral is still often privileged methodologically as more African, more "authentic," more important. The publication of Megan Vaughan's *Curing Their Ills* (1991) was the first strikingly Foucauldian discursive analysis of European-authored texts in African historical studies. A linguistic turn is also evident in important recent histories dealing with various kinds of "texts," including songs, legal documents, dreams, and religious writings. I consider the linguistic turn and Africanist restraint with " 'post-' moves" in my "Introduction," *Gender and History* 8 (1996): 323–37. At the height of the oral turn, Africanists tended to neglect African-authored texts even when they were readily available, as Johannes Fabian notes in his epistemological accounting for the lack of scholarly interest in the African-authored Elisabethville history that

Bruce Fetter located and shared with scholars in Lubumbashi in the early 1970s (Johannes Fabian, with Kalundi Mango and with linguistic notes by W. Schicho, *History from Below: The 'Vocabulary of Elisabethville' by André Yav; Texts, Translations, and Interpretive Essay* [Amsterdam: John Benjamins Publishing Company, 1990]). I note some exceptions to this generalization in Nancy Rose Hunt, "Letter-Writing, Nursing Men, and Bicycles in the Belgian Congo: Notes towards the Social Identity of a Colonial Category," in *Paths toward the Past: African Historical Essays in Honor of Jan Vansina*, ed. Robert W. Harms et al. (Atlanta, Ga.: African Studies Association Press, 1994), 187–210.

1   Crocodiles and Wealth

1.   C. C. Chesterman, "A Month's Joy-Ride," *YQN* 95 (October 1933): 13; and Chesterman, "Can You Pull a Crocodile out with a Hook?" *YQN* 99 (October 1934): 13–17.

2.   Edith Millman to Miss Bowser, 30 October 1933, Mrs. Millman file, Baptist Missionary Society Archives, Regent's Park College, Oxford [hereafter BMSA].

3.   Chesterman, "Can You Pull a Crocodile."

4.   The book's only commentary about this vignette was to index it as "crocodile superstition" (H. Sutton Smith, *Yakusu, the Very Heart of Africa: Being Some Account of the Protestant Mission at Stanley Falls, Upper Congo* [London: Carey Press, (1911?)], 51). The event was likely during Smith's tenure, which began in 1899.

5.   John F. Carrington, "The Initiation Language: Lokele Tribe," *African Studies* 6, no. 4 (1947): 196–207, esp. 197.

6.   Libeli resembled the scarification and flagellation in Bali boys' initiations (Bernard, "Une société chez les Babali," *Congo* 2 [1922]: 349–53). Vansina distinguishes between *lilwa* (the titled, ranked associations of the BaMbole) and libeli (a boys' initiation among the Lokele) (Vansina, *Paths in the Rainforests: Toward a History of Political Tradition in Equatorial Africa* [Madison: University of Wisconsin Press, 1990]). My sources permit seeing parallels between BaMbole and Lokele forms of lilwa while focusing on the history of libeli as a form of recomposing wealth and authority among the Yaokanja Lokele. (See also n. 112 in chap. 2.) Bambole lilwa sculptures included crocodile and hanged human figures. On lilwa, see Kalala Nkudi, "Le lilwaakoy des Mbole du Lomami: Essai d'analyse de son symbolisme," *Cahiers du CEDAF* 4 (1979); NKUDI Kalala, "Identité et société: les fondements d'une marginalité. Le cas des Mbole" (Ph.D. diss., UNAZA, Campus de Kisangani, 1977); V. Rouvroy, "Le 'Lilwa' (District de l'Aruwimi. Territoire des Bambole)," *Congo* 1 (1929): 783–98; John F. Carrington, "Lilwaakoi—a Congo Secret Society," *Baptist Quarterly* 12, no. 8 (1947): 237–44; Daniel P. Biebuyck, "Sculpture from the Eastern Zaire Forest Regions: Mbole, Yele, and Pere," *African Arts* 10 (1976): 54–61, 99–100; and Bernadette Van Haute-De Kimpe, "The Mbole and Their Lilwa Sculptures," *Africa Insight* 15, no. 4 (1985): 288–97.

7.   Daniel P. Biebuyck has called such feasting "lavish dinner parties" in his *Lega Culture: Art, Initiation, and Moral Philosophy among a Central African People* (Berkeley: University of California Press, 1973), 107.

8.   Smith, *Yakusu*, 61. The use of the word *lilwa* was so terrifying, and the prohibition on its improper use so strong, that Lokele used an alternative word (*iseke*) for the number nine

because the Lokele word *libwa* was too close in sound to *lilwa* (John F. Carrington, "Sketch of Lokele Grammar (Missionaries of Yakusu)" [Salisbury, U.K., 1984, unpublished manuscript], 20 [copy in my possession]). Mama Tula told me that Yakoso men once tied a woman to a tree for saying the word *lilwa*. People insisted to me in 1989, as they had to Carrington in the 1940s, that the words *lilwa* and *libeli* signified the same thing (Carrington, "Initiation Language").

9. Michael Taussig, *Mimesis and Alterity: A Particular History of the Senses* (New York: Routledge, 1993), 59. For Likenyule's account, see H. Roboam Likenyule, "Ende baina la Masiya. Kola losamo lofi loa Yesu," *Mboli ya Tengai* 324 (May 1934).

10. See, especially, Kambale Munzombo and Shanga Minga, "Une société secrète au Zaïre: les hommes-crocodiles de la zone d'Ubundu," *Africa* (Rome) XLII (1987): 226–38.

11. Taussig, *Mimesis*, 66; and Roger Casement, diary entry for 27 June 1903, HO 161/2, Public Records Office, London, quoted in S. J. S. Cookey, *Britain and the Congo Question, 1885–1913* (London: Longmans, Green, and Co., 1968), 92.

12. Gladys Owen to Miss Bowser, 18 November 1929, Owen file BMSA. The expression "docile bodies" is Michel Foucault's.

13. I draw on Jane I. Guyer's use of Georg Simmel to distinguish composition from accumulation; see Jane I. Guyer, "Wealth in People and Self-Realization in Equatorial Africa," *Man* 28 (1993): 246; and Jane I. Guyer and Samuel M. Eno Belinga, "Wealth in People as Wealth in Knowledge: Accumulation and Composition in Equatorial Africa," *Journal of African History* 36 (1995): 91–120.

14. Taussig, *Mimesis*, 35.

15. Song recorded at a church meeting in Yanonge, 1989.

16. Tata Bafoya Bamanga, with Mama Tula, Yakusu, 25 November 1989. Bafoya Bamanga of Yakoso was the only man that I could locate in this village adjacent to the mission who would speak to me about having entered libeli.

17. This local grammar is, in part, a form of social memory or historical consciousness. I intend *historicity*—that is, local forms of marking, recording, and remembering the past and the passage of time—throughout this discussion, while avoiding the lofty word. The following works have been influential: Gillian Feeley-Harnik, "Finding Memories in Madagascar," in *Images of Memory: On Remembering and Representation,* ed. Susanne Küchler and Walter Melion (Washington, D.C.: Smithsonian Institution Press, 1991), 121–40; Marshall Sahlins, *Islands of History* (Chicago: University of Chicago Press, 1985); Georges Dupré, *Les naissances d'une société: Espace et historicité chez les Beembé du Congo* (Paris: ORSTOM, 1985); and Renato Rosaldo, *Ilongnot Head-Hunting, 1883–1974: A Study in Society and History* (Stanford, Calif.: Stanford University Press, 1980).

18. Carrington, "The Initiation Language," 198.

19. Italics added. *Nyama* signifies animal, and was closely associated with *ndiya* and *ndimo,* types of water spirits, even in the missionaries' lexicon (William Millman, *Vocabulary of Ekele: The Language Spoken by the Lokele Tribe Living between Yanjali and Stanleyville* [Yakusu: Baptist Missionary Society, 1926], 9). See John F. Carrington's reconstruction of Stanley's passage by Yakoso, including these cries of "nyama! lilwa!" (*Ya Mariwa*), in "L'Explorateur Stanley dans la région du Haut Congo," Carrington Papers, typed manuscript, 3, BMSA. See also Henry

Morton Stanley, *Through the Dark Continent: Or, the Sources of the Nile, around the Great Lakes of Equatorial Africa, and down the Livingstone River to the Atlantic Ocean,* vol. 2 (1878; reprint, New York: Dover Publications, 1988), 204. On ndiya, see also T. K. Biaya, "L'Impasse de crise zaïroise dans la peinture populaire urbaine, 1970–1985," in *Art et politiques en Afrique noire/Art and Politics in Black Africa* (Ottawa: Canadian Association of African Studies and Safi Press, 1989), 95–120.

20. C. C. Chesterman, "The Swan Song of the Libeli," *YQN* 65 (January 1926): 19.

21. See Vansina, *Paths,* 110–12, 183.

22. Carrington, "Initiation Language," 196. According to Jan Vansina, such groves were found as far downriver as Basoko (personal communication, 1992).

23. Carrington, "Initiation Language," 196; and Dipo Kesobe, with Baba Manzanza, Yainyongo-Romée, 13 December 1989.

24. Lofanjola-Lisele (Pesapesa), Yainyongo-Romée, 29 December 1989. He added that Topoke "also had their lilwa; even today they have their own [lilwa] language." Not all Lokele were included; the Yawembe, a large and ancient Lokele district further downriver than the Yaokanja district, "refus[ed] to participate in the libeli ceremonies" (Carrington, "Initiation Language," 198). I have been careful to retain informants' lexical borrowing from French, as in grammaire, which I italicized here, in my translations of their Kingwana.

25. Wawima Tshosomo Saile, "Les Lokele et le grand commerce sur le fleuve de la fin du XIXe siècle au début du XXe siècle," Mémoire en Histoire, Université Nationale du Zaïre, Campus de Lubumbashi, 1974, 32. Ndiya is no more exclusive to the Lokele than are water and celestial spirits. Some BaMbole call a rainbow "Ndia," associating, much like the Lokele and Komo, a snakelike animal of the water with the celestial presence of rainbows. Rainbows are as dangerous as the turbulent water creatures: to see the rainbow's aquatic counterpart would cause one to die instantly. People also claim that ochre clay is the excrement of this water animal (Administrateur Territorial Lauwers, "Notes ethnographiques sur la peuplade des Bambole," Yanonghe, 20 March 1932, in Archivalia De Cleene Natal-De Jonghe Edouard, file no. 60, Katholiek Documentatie Onderzoek centrum [hereafter KADOC], Leuven).

26. Saile, "Les Lokele," 33–35.

27. This is Vansina's term; see *Paths.* The local Lokele term is *bokulu,* and people often used the French term *clan* instead.

28. Claude Meillassoux, "Essai d'interprétation du phénomène économique dans les sociétés traditionelles," *Cahiers d'études africaines* 4 (1960): 38–67. For Jane Guyer's many contributions, see chapter 1, note 13 and the bibliography.

29. He drew on Alfred Mahieu's study and saw the collection assembled at the Musée Royal de l'Afrique Centrale (now often called the Africa-Museum) in Tervuren; A. Hingston Quiggin, *A Survey of Primitive Money: The Beginnings of Currency* (1949; reprint, London: Metheun, 1979), 66–67; see also Alfred Mahieu, *Numismatique du Congo, 1485–1924: instruments d'échange, valeurs monétaires, méreaux, médailles* (Brussels: Imprimerie Médicale et Scientifique, [1925?]), 21–22, 116, 120–21. Ngbele or linganda are still an important feature in this museum's public money display.

30. Quiggin, *Survey,* 64 (Quiggin's source here is E. Torday and T. A. Joyce, *Notes ethnographiques sur les populations habitant les bassins du Kasai et du Kwango oriental,* 1922, II, 202).

31. Lokele considered Mba, Komo, and Bali as strangers, "non-Lokele," that is, batshuaka (whereas Wagenia, Olombo, and Foma were considered Lokele in origin). Those batshuaka women acquired without bridewealth were disdained as *bekoa* (slaves). Many of these were Mba women either offered to Lokele as gifts or pawns, or acquired by Lokele who could not afford bridewealth for a Lokele bride. Lokele would have capitalized on the economic complementarity of the region as various houses, villages, and districts expanded the economic space for trade. The Yakoso Lokele especially pushed up the Lindi and controlled access to trade in this direction, meanwhile giving *likenja* brides to Mba chiefs in return for the right to buy canoes and paddles. When this expansion occurred and the scope of likenja-type marriages are unclear. See the important study by Saile, "Les Lokele," esp. 84, 100–105. Colonel A. Bertrand noted two types of Lokele wives: wives "of knives" (of bridewealth goods) and wives "of shields" (war captives) (Bertrand, "Quelques notes sur la vie politique, le développement, la décadence des petites sociétés bantou du bassin central du Congo," *Revue de l'Institut de Sociologie de Bruxelles* 1 [1920]: 84). According to Baruti Lokomba, Yawembe Lokele would go up the Lomami long ago to procure slaves, but he does not date this (Baruti Lokomba, "Structure et fonctionnement des institutions politiques traditionnelles chez les Lokele [Haut-Zaïre]," *Cahiers du CEDAF* 8 [1972]: 16–17). They might have been Lokele clients of Rachid, the Tippu Tib–associated Zanzibari who assumed power at Isangi. See, too, Baruti Lokomba, "Kisangani centre urbain et les Lokele," in *Kisangani, 1876–1976: Histoire d'une ville,* ed. Benoît Verhaegen (Kinshasa: Presses Universitaires du Zaïre, 1975), 64; Vansina, *Paths,* 104, 180.

32. Bernard, "Une société," 353 n. 1; Vansina, *Paths,* 175; and Carrington, "Initiation Language." On the absence of drum signaling in libeli, see John F. Carrington, *A Comparative Study of Some Central African Gong-Languages* (Brussels: IRCB, 1949), 75.

33. Curtis A. Keim, "The Mangbetu Worldview under Colonial Stress: *Nebeli,*" in *African Reflections: Art from Northeastern Zaire,* ed. Enid Schildkrout and Curtis A. Keim (Seattle: University of Washington Press, 1990), 190–93, 261 n. 21.

34. I follow Jan Vansina's stress on fashion (Vansina, *Paths*), and E. E. Evans-Pritchard's on the mobility of new medicines; E. E. Evans-Pritchard, *Witchcraft, Oracles, and Magic among the Azande* (1937; reprint, Oxford: Oxford University Press, 1985). On ritual change associated with colonial turbulence among the Komo, see Wauthier De Mahieu, *Qui a obstrué la cascade: Analyse sémantique du rituel de la circoncision chez les Komo du Zaïre* (Cambridge: Cambridge University Press, 1985).

35. I follow David Northrup's synthesis closely here; see David Northrup, *Beyond the Bend in the River: African Labor in Eastern Zaire, 1865–1940* (Athens: Ohio University Center for International Studies, 1988), 23–29, esp. 29. See, too, Jonathon Glassman, *Feasts and Riot: Revelry, Rebellion, and Popular Consciousness on the Swahili Coast, 1856–1888* (Portsmouth, N.H.: Heinemann, 1995), 58. On brides as gifts, and the story of a marital treaty between the Zanzibari and the chief of Yainyongo, see Lofanjola-Lisele (Pesapesa), Yainyongo-Romée, 29 December 1989. Abdul Sheriff notes that Zanzibari had expanded north to the Lindi and the confluence of the Lomami and the Lualaba by the early 1870s (Sheriff, *Slaves, Spices, and Ivory in Zanzibar: Integration of an East African Commercial Empire into the World Economy, 1770–1873* [Athens: Ohio University Press, 1987], 200 n82).

36. See the extended passage in Henry Morton Stanley, *The Congo and the Founding of Its Free State: A Story of Work and Exploration* (New York: Harper and Brothers, 1885), 138–53. Giles Bibeau describes these "depredations" in more benign terms (Giles Bibeau, "La communauté musulmane de Kisangani," in *Kisangani, 1876–1976: Histoire d'une ville*, ed. Benoît Verhaegen [Kinshasa: Presses Universitaires du Zaïre, 1975], 190 [incl. n. 15], 223).

37. A. Delcommune, *Vingt années de vie africaine: Récits de voyages, d'aventures et d'exploration au Congo belge (1874–1893)*, vol. 1 (Brussels: Larcier, 1922), 297–300, 302–3. P. Ceulemans's 1958 study has received minimal reconsideration for this region. Much more work like that of Ramazani Solo on BaTambatamba-Topoke interactions at Yanonge and Romée is needed. See P. Ceulemans, *La question arabe et le Congo (1883–1892)* (Brussels: ARSC, 1958); Bibeau, "La communauté musulmane de Kisangani"; Ramazani Solo, "Implantation des Topoke à Yanonge," *Cahiers du CRIDE* 65–66 (July–August 1982), 195–224; and Benoît Verhaegen, ed., *La vie de Disasi Makulo recueillie par son fils Makulo Akambu*, in *Notes, travaux, documents du CRIDE* 4 (Kisangani: Université de Kisangani, 1982).

38. The word *lokele* was also associated with a special spoon with a wooden handle that women used in order to take food from a pot (Lokomba, "Structure et fonctionnement," 11–13).

39. Mama Tula Sophie, Yakusu, 8 August 1989.

40. And so I call them here. A. Delcommune called them the " 'Matam-Matambas,' c'est-à-dire des Arabes" (Delcommune, *Vingt années*, 302). On the "Atama-Atama" among the BaMbole, see Osumaka Likaka, "Rural Protest: The Mbole against Belgian Rule, 1897–1959," *IJAHS* 27 (1994): 589–617. Jan Vansina claims that the "Matambatamba" came from "Matampa country" (Vansina, *Paths*, 240–41). My informants sometimes called them BaKusu, but regardless, insisted how mixed in origin BaTambatamba were, an argument also found elsewhere; for example, Bibeau, "La communauté musulmane de Kisangani," 195.

41. Lofanjola-Lisele (Pesapesa), Yainyongo-Romée, 29 December 1989; Tata Bafoya Bamanga, with Mama Tula, Yakusu, 25 November 1989.

42. René Cambier, "Note de la carte des campagnes antiesclavagistes," in *Atlas général du Congo et du Ruanda-Urundi*, vol. 14 (Brussels: ARSOM, 1948–60), 3; and Adolphe Lejeune-Choquet, *Histoire militaire du Congo* (Brussels: Alfred Castaigne, 1906), 104–5.

43. George Grenfell to A. H. Baynes, 2 May 1898, Box A/20, BMSA.

44. George Grenfell to E. G. Sargent, 21 May 1898, Box A/20, BMSA; and George Grenfell to A. H. Baynes, 9 September 1902, Box A/20, BMSA.

45. Vansina, *Paths*, 91–92; J. P. Gosse, "Les méthodes et engins de pêche des Lokele," *Bulletin Agricole du Congo Belge* 2 (1961): 335–85.

46. W. H. White to A. H. Baynes in *Missionary Herald*, 1 May 1896, 377. Some raid victims became local chiefs and soldiers; one found his way to Boma for a few years ("Letters from Rev. H. Sutton Smith of Yakusu," *Missionary Herald*, September 1901, 437–39).

47. Smith, *Yakusu*, 27, 24.

48. J. Butterworth, "Mokili in Congo," typescript, n.d. [ca. 1955], 52–54, BMSA.

49. Mr. Kempton, ca. 1901, quoted in Smith, *Yakusu*, 212.

50. "Litoi" sermon notes [by W. H. Ford?] in Carrington Private Papers, Salisbury. See, too, Mrs. Mill, "First Impressions," *YQN* 44 (October 1919); and A. G. Mills, "A Dying Leper," *YQN* 99 (October 1934): 3.

51. Sulila's passage may have involved a ransom fee, such as was paid for Salamo: "she was passed over to Salamo's husband by an Arab for whom he had made some furniture" (E. R. Millman, "Our Girls: Sulila of the Lomami River," *YQN* 36 [September 1917]: 5–7). The only other evidence on nursemaids is that Mrs. Millman had a Congolese *nourrice* for her own baby in 1909 (Prince Albert, "Voyage au Congo belge par Cape Town," ca. 1909, dossier 75, 94, Archives du Palais Royal, Brussels).

52. A. M. Delathuy, *Jezuiten in Kongo met zwaard en kruis* (Berchem: EPO, 1986). See, too, "ransoming" in Fanny E. Guinness, *The New World of Central Africa, with a History of the First Christian Mission on the Congo* (London: Hodder and Stoughton, 1890).

53. Smith, *Yakusu*, 105.

54. E. J. Glave, "Cruelty in the Congo Free State," *Century Magazine* 54, no. 32 (May–October 1897): 699–715, esp. 705.

55. E. D. Morel, *Red Rubber: The Story of the Rubber Slave Trade Flourishing on the Congo in the Year of Grace, 1906* (1906; reprint, New York: Haskell House, 1970), 87–88.

56. George Grenfell to A. H. Baynes, 10 September 1904, Box A/20, BMSA.

57. Smith, *Yakusu*, 96, 145.

58. Lofanjola-Lisele (Pesapesa), Yainyongo-Romée, 29 December 1989. Italics added.

59. Lofemba, Yainyongo-Romée, 7 January 1990. On spatial and visceral memories, see Feeley-Harnik, "Finding Memories."

60. Lofanjola-Lisele (Pesapesa), Yainyongo-Romée, 7 April 1989. Italics added. Ancient color categories were at the very least being reinforced during this first period of Zanzibari colonialism; see chapter 7, esp. note 23.

61. Regardless, crocodiles, ndimo, and Mamiwata are distinct phenomena (Lofemba, Yainyongo-Romée, 7 January 1990). On Mamiwata, among other accounts, see Lofanjola-Lisele (Pesapesa), Yainyongo-Romée, 7 April 1989. See chapter 3, esp. note 111.

62. Such amphibious creatures aptly symbolize persons in ritual transition between two age grades, according to Wauthier De Mahieu, who also explains the symbolism of crocodiles and rainbows in Komo circumcision ritual; see De Mahieu, *Qui a obstrué la cascade*, 63–65, 191–92, 198, 208, 222, 257–60, 282, 365 (rainbow). On Bonama, consider this Lokele text: "When the village people see the water spirit, Bonama, during the day, they will clutch their children quickly. They will take coals from the fire to smear their children on the forehead. Since they have seen that Bonama is standing in the river, they will say: 'Don't bathe the children in the river because Bonama is deep in the river.' . . . People say that when a kid sees Bonama with his eyes, he is truly going to die. They say that the rain will fall down. Bonama blocks the rain from falling so that he does not move down the river. We say that when the rainbow threatens war, its shadow goes up in the sky. . . . If someone has something to do with Bonama, he will cling to it and die. . . . If Bonama blocks the river, people don't want to drink the water because Bonama is going to block your stomach, except those who drink a little with charcoal and herbs. We say that Bonama is in the water during the day. For ourselves we know even when bathing during the day, let's keep water in our mouths and throw it down and we will see what we just said. Even when Bonama comes, he does not release the rain . . . because the mother who has a child understands so that seeing Bonama she takes *shele* putting some on the forehead of the child" (Lokele

manuscripts and student essays [likely from W. H. Ford Papers] in Carrington Private Papers, Salisbury).

63. Mama Tula, Yakusu, 25 November 1989. Kayumba, the BaTambatamba chief of the chefferie arabisée at Romée, put the water hole and the crocodiles/mermaids in the place at the Longbondo stream; when his son took over as chief, he acquired power over these water spirits (Lofanjola-Lisele (Pesapesa), Yainyongo-Romée, 7 April 1989). Kayumba was invested as chief of this chefferie arabisée in 1913 and remained in power until 1944 (with a couple years of revocation from 1939) (Solo, "Implantation," 9). On the autonomy of BaTambatamba from Romée after resettling on Kisangani's left bank at Lubunga, see Bibeau, "La communauté musulmane de Kisangani," 230–31. On Badjoko, see also chapter 4, esp. page 188.

64. Smith, *Yakusu*, 62, 199. By 1901, there were 180 students at Yakusu from sixteen different "towns" and eight "tribes," and many by this time were Lokele (ibid., 212).

65. All previous quotations here are from ibid., 62, 205.

66. Ibid., 62–64.

67. William Millman, "The Tribal Initiation Ceremony of the Lokele," *International Review of Missions* 16 (1927): 365–66.

68. Walter Henry Stapleton, "Yakusu Station, Upper Congo River," *Missionary Herald*, January 1903, 36.

69. Smith, *Yakusu*, 64, 216.

70. Stapleton, "Yakusu Station," 37.

71. Ibid.

72. Ibid., 36. They compared its "obviously farcical character" to a Masonic Brotherhood (Smith, *Yakusu*, 64–65).

73. On "laughable," see S. Osborne Kempton to A. H. Baynes, in "The Beginning of the Gospel of Jesus Christ in Yakusu," *Missionary Herald*, September 1902, 412.

74. Northrup, *Beyond the Bend*, 60, 74; and Jules Marchal, *E. D. Morel contre Léopold II: L'Histoire du Congo, 1900–1910*, 2 vols. (Paris: l'Harmattan, 1996), 50–52.

75. Carrington, "Initiation Language." On local and European-manufactured shoka, as well as other local lances and iron monies, see also Sir Harry Johnston, *George Grenfell and the Congo*, 2 vols. (London: Hutchinson and Co., 1908), 789–97; *Geldformen und Zierperlen der Naturvölker. Führer durch das Museum für Völkerkunde und Schweizerische* (Basel: Museum für Volkskunde, 1961), 30; J. D. E. Schmeltz and J. P. B. de J. de Jong, *Ethnographisch Album van het Stroomgebied van den Congo* (Haarlem: H. Kleinmann and Co., 1904–1916), plate 63; and W. Holman Bentley, *Pioneering on the Congo* (London: Religious Tract Society, 1900), 293–95. The history of local iron, salt, and net monies, *shoka d'Europe*, and their relative values in and near Romée and Yanonge warrants separate treatment. Useful in understanding the severe reduction in quality, weight, craftmanship, and aesthetics of a "shoka d'Europe" were the following: Octave Elskens, "Liste des objets de collections envoyé à M. le Chef de Zone, Stanleyville. Monnaies indigènes," 3 November 1909, Romée, Dossier Ethnographique no. 78; Fiches muséographiques nos. 786–805 [envoi Badjoko], 917–52 [envoi Elskens]; and collection of Congolese monies and *linganda* lances, esp. museum objects nos. 946–50 (all in the Ethnographic Section, Musée Royal de l'Afrique Centrale [hereafter MRAC] [Africa-Museum], Tervuren).

76. George Grenfell, 1903, quoted in Johnston, *George Grenfell,* 797.

77. Smith, *Yakusu,* 5.

78. Emphasis on "tribute" added; H. Sutton Smith to A. H. Baynes, in "Tidings from Our Remotest Congo Station," *Missionary Herald,* March 1902, 97–98. In 1909, those who failed to pay on time were forced to "work it out by forty hours of labour on a plantation" ("Baptisms," *YQN* 12 [December 1909]: 5).

79. Smith, *Yakusu,* 222.

80. Smith, *Yakusu,* 224, 237. In 1899, the mission published its first Lokele title, and Lokele was chosen to replace Swahili as the medium of church communication and evangelical instruction within the district (ibid., 198–99).

81. See Carrington, *Comparative Study,* 84, 91, 92, 94, 97, 98, 99, 101. Carrington learned and appreciated the nuances of local slit drum–signaling poetry, and wrote up his fascinating data for both scholarly and popular audiences; see also his *Talking Drums of Africa* (London: Carey Kingsgate Press, 1949), 48–52, esp. 49. Thanks go to Eugenia Herbert for giving me a copy of a related, apparently radio-broadcast recording of Carrington on Lokele drum signaling. See also P. Austin, "Some African Beliefs," *YQN* 135 (January 1944): 6–8; and John F. Carrington, "Puff! Puff! Puff!," *YQN* 145 (1950): 19–23.

82. "Njaso—Ikumbe" (Yakusu church minutes logbook), District Pastor's Office, Yakusu, 31 July and 7 August 1904.

83. On hemp (basili) smoking, see 3 November 1905, 2 February 1906, 5 October 1907, in "Njaso—Ikumbe," 1904–33.

84. "Njaso—Ikumbe," 1904–33, esp. 5 October 1907. By 1921, camwood body painting was "being given up" and "the wooden troughs used for the preparation of this powder are being turned over in large quantities to Mr. Millman who is having them burnt. It is the nearest approach to 'idol burning'" (letter by A. G. Mill, 9 November 1921, quoted in John N. Sinclair, "Our Storied Past: A Saga of Six Lives Molded into Three Families and Lived out on Four Continents" [Roseville, Minn., 1992, unpublished manuscript]).

85. Jean Baluti excepted those from Yakusu from his proposition, suggesting that those of the station, as wage laborers, had easy access to this money form. "Njaso—Ikumbe," 1904–1907. The first reference to bosombi was on February 2, 1906.

86. "Njaso—Ikumbe," 5 June 1908, 30 July 1909.

87. On Grenfell's reprimand, see George Grenfell to John Weeks, Bolobo, 31 January 1898; John Weeks to the Commissaire Général, Monsembe, 8 November 1897; Governor General F. Fuchs to George Grenfell, n.d., all in Box A/20, BMSA. On Morel's campaign and Baynes's speech, see Marchal, *E. D. Morel,* I:26–27, 93–100, 124–25, 132–34.

88. Marchal, *E. D. Morel,* I:207; II:44–45, 91, 238–41, 415–16, 438; and Smith, *Yakusu,* 132. Elsewhere Smith argued that the Stanleyville-Lomani section of Province Orientale "suffered less" due to a "more enlightened" regime; "our neighbourhood has remained populous" (ibid., 9, 144–45). For Smith on Glave, see ibid., 55.

89. William Millman to My Dear Consul [Roger Casement], 6 August 1906, 7 August 1906, and 28 August 1906, all letters quoted in J. Butterworth, "Mokili in Congo," typescript, n.d. (ca. 1955), BMSA.

90. Millman to Casement, 7 August 1906, quoted in Butterworth, "Mokili," 178–79.

91. Millman to Casement, 28 August 1906, quoted in Butterworth, "Mokili," 179–80.

92. "So we joined an entry for the Gospel among the forest tribe of Yangole," sermon notes [of W. H. Ford?], in John F. Carrington Papers, Salisbury, U.K. (originals transferred to BMSA).

93. William Millman to Roger Casement, 7 August 1906 and 28 August 1906, quoted in Butterworth, "Mokili."

94. Marchal, *E. D. Morel,* II:45.

95. Saidi finally gave himself up and served his term after months in hiding, being released and back "amongst his people" just as Smith's book went to press (Smith, *Yakusu,* 24–29).

96. Letter from Rev. William Millman, 12 September 1908, quoted in Western Sub-Committee Book, no. 14, 18 November 1908, 39, BMSA.

97. "Native Church Funds," *YQN* 6 (December 1909): 7.

98. The reward offered for his capture was ineffective. Saidi came out of hiding in May and was set free again on November 10, 1910 ("Review of the Past Year," *YQN* 9 [December 1910]: 7–8).

99. "Taxation," *YQN* 12 (September 1911): 8.

100. Translation of Lokele text, *Mboli ya Tengai* 5 (April 1910), in John F. Carrington, "*Mboli ya Tengai* [Contents List]," John F. Carrington Papers, BMSA.

101. "Njaso—Ikumbe," 1910.

102. "Njaso—Ikumbe," 1910. Italics added. According to Tata Bafoya, a nyango in libeli was neither a woman nor necessarily kin, but an initiate shared food with this person forevermore. A Lokele research assistant of mine at Yakusu consistently translated the word *balimo* as *démons* or evil spirits. Bolimo means "spirit, ghost, the soul," according to incomplete, printed Lokele-English dictionary pages, 11, Printing Press Director's Office, Yakusu; see also Millman, *Vocabulary of Ekele,* 196 for spirit, and *bolimo obe* for "devil," 54.

103. "Njaso—Ikumbe," 1910. Bieka and yeka are part of Class 7/8 of Lokele (sing.: e-, y-; pl.: bi-, by-, y-); yeka may be used in singular or plural (Carrington, Sketch of Lokele Grammar, 8).

104. "A New Difficulty," *YQN* 7 (April 1910): 2.

105. "Taxation," *YQN* 4 (September 1911): 4. Paying taxes remained a sign of attaining "manhood" into the 1920s, and boys of about twelve were eager to pay; see W. H. Ennals, News Sheet, no. 19, 21 April 1923, BMSA. In 1911, the tax was ten shillings a year, which if teachers only received three pounds a year (three hundred and sixty-five pennies), would have amounted to one-sixth of their salary. Since missionaries were unwilling to "countenance the conceit" of schoolboys interested in receiving the "receipt cheque to wear and so pretend to be men," it would seem that state authorities did not require schoolboys to pay ("Taxation," 4).

106. John Whitehead, in [letter on trip on Lualaba steamer], *YQN* 14 (March 1912): 3.

107. Thiry, le receveur to Monsieur le Directeur, 15 December 1910, F. Fuchs Papers, MRAC.

108. William Millman, in "a note written in 1910," quoted in J. Butterworth, "Mokili in Congo," typescript, n.d. (ca. 1955), 177, BMSA.

109. W. Millman, "Missionary Medical Work on the Upper Congo," *BMS Annual Report,* December 1904, 605.

110. "Stapleton Memorial Hospital," *YQN* 6 (December 1909): 6.

111. "Church Matters," *YQN* (December 1910): 1–3.

112. "The Barter Store," *YQN* 48 (July 1921): 15.

113. "Events of the Quarter," *YQN* 8 (August 1910): 3; "Medical Work," *YQN* 8 (August 1910): 5; and "Njaso—Ikumbe," 31 December 1910. On the origins of this ironic African nickname for Stanley, which he himself translated as "breaker of rocks" and which was applied by extension to colonial (and postcolonial) state agents, see F. Bontinck, "Les deux Bula Matari," *Etudes Congolaises* 12, no. 3 (July–September 1969): 83–97.

114. H. Sutton Smith referred to a powerful, local, Lokele female "secret society" of 1908; see Smith, *Yakusu,* 28; and a Miss A. Wilkinson noted that they lost schoolgirls to a ritual of fattening and dancing after libeli ended in the mid-1920s. Missionaries accepted likiilo as relatively benign, though they did not name it; see A. Wilkinson, "The Ups and Downs of Girls' School Work," *YQN* 63 (July 1925): 10–11. Some people told me about a BaMbole variant of likiilo, and others told me about the BaMbole villages where likiilo is still practiced. Female initiation and fertility ritual have been absent from most ethnographies and histories of equatorial Africa since Audrey Richards' *Chisungu* (London: Faber and Faber, 1956), though this is changing. See Marie-Claude Dupré, "Comment être femme: un aspect du rituel Mukisi chez les Téké de la République Populaire du Congo," *Archives de Sciences Sociales des Religions* 46 (1978): 57–84; René Devisch, *Se recréer femme: Manipulation sémantique d'une situation d'infécondité chez les Yaka* (Berlin: Dietrich Reimer Verlag, 1984); and Filip De Boeck, "From Knots to Web: Fertility, Life-Transmission, Health, and Well-Being among the Aluund of Southwest Zaire" (Ph.D. diss., Katholieke Universiteit te Leuven, 1991). See, too, the remarkable study by Corinne A. Kratz, *Affecting Performance: Meaning, Movement, and Experience in Okriek? Women's Initiation* (Washington, D.C.: Smithsonian Institution Press, 1994). Likiilo, although it involved body marking (scarification), did not entail any genital cutting. Nor did libeli. The absence of clitoridectomy is not what kept missionaries relatively disinterested in likiilo, but rather, the fact that it was less linked to forms of political assertiveness and authority, and consequently, less threatening and disruptive.

115. These quotations come from field notes and interviews. Almost all of my interviews with some forty women in Yakusu, Yalolia, Yainyongo-Romée, and Ikongo included discussions of their likiilo experiences (or lack of them); see bibliography for a listing. Italics added.

116. The identification of "phases," as well as the use of the word, is mine. About six months after libeli in 1924, "three men from widely separated villages wrote out what they saw and gave their statements" to William Millman. His 1927 article is largely based on these statements, though it includes "information gained from various persons at different times during thirty years' sojourn in the country" (Millman, "Tribal Initiation," 368–69); see ibid., 369–77. I was unable to locate the original Lokele statements. John F. Carrington published an English translation of a Lokele account written by a literate 1924 initiate in the 1940s; see Carrington, "Initiation Language," 196–98. Perhaps lost in the process was a sense of how these rites may have been performed as hoax or farce. See Jan Vansina, "Initiation Rituals of the Bushong," *Africa* 25 (1956): 138–55; and André Droogers, *The Dangerous Journey: Symbolic Aspects of Boys' Initiation among the Wagenia of Kisangani, Zaire* (The Hague: Mouton, 1980).

117. Carrington's Lokele version states after an hour.

118. According to the Lokele text, everyone sat down quietly at this point, and the spirits taught the initiates the laws of libeli about quarreling, speaking and dancing, looking "beneath the

legs of a woman," generosity with food, and the importance of not laughing, speaking only the libeli language, and eating off the ground when returning to the village. Carrington, "Initiation Language," 196–97.

119. As opposed to much earlier, as indicated in Millman's version.

120. For these details, too, see Carrington, "Initiation Language," 197–98.

121. Among the BaMbole, food and drink during lilwa were served in "pots" that women usually used for intimate personal hygiene (Administrateur Territorial Lauwers, "Notes ethno-graphiques sur la peuplade des Bambole," Yanonge, 20 March 1922, in Archivalia De Cleene–De Jonghe, file no. 60, KADOC, Leuven).

122. Vansina, *Paths*, 188.

123. See John M. Janzen, "Toward a Historical Perspective on African Medicine and Health," *Beiträge zur Ethnomedezin, Ethnobotanik und Ethnozoologie* 8 (1983): 112.

124. Smith, *Yakusu*, 28.

125. "Manners and Costume: Dress," *YQN* 9 (December 1910): 4–6.

126. See Frederick A. Johnson, *A Standard Swahili-English Dictionary* (Oxford: Oxford University Press, 1939), 419, as opposed to the one by former BMS missionaries working in the Kasongo area: John Whitehead and L. F. Whitehead, *Manuel de Kingwana, le dialecte occidental de Swahili* (Wayika, Congo Belge: Mission de et à Wayika, 1928), 148.

127. Butterfield paraphrase of William Millman in J. Butterfield, "Mokili in Congo," n.d. (ca. 1955), 177, n. 1, BMSA.

128. "Manners and Customs: Dress," *YQN* 9 (December 1910): 6.

129. Ibid., 2; "Glory Be to His Name," *YQN* 21 (December 1913): 12; and "Servants of Jesus," *YQN* 26 (March 1915).

130. Barbara Ann Yates, "Knowledge Brokers: Books and Publishers in Early Colonial Zaire," *History in Africa* 14 (1987): 311–40, esp. 322–23. On the mission's literary production, 1900–1908, see Smith, *Yakusu*, 153–60. On the Lokele language, see John F. Carrington, "The Tonal Structure of Kele (Lokele)," *African Studies* (December 1943): 193–207; John F. Carrington, *Proverbes Lokele, Tokoko Twa Lokele* (Kisangani, 1973, polycopied manuscript); John F. Carrington Papers, BMSA; and Walter Henry Stapleton, *Comparative Handbook of Congo Languages* (Yakusu: n.p., 1903).

131. "Summary of Events of the Year," *YQN* 6 (December 1909): 1–2, 4; and "Our Native Magazine," *YQN* 17 (December 1912): 9; the French would have been calculated to attract young men. See also A. G. Mill, "The Radiance Spreads," *YQN* 152 (October 1955): 5–8.

132. "Njaso—Ikumbe," esp. 27 November 1914 and 27 May 1916.

2   Doctors and Airplanes

1. H. Sutton Smith, *Yakusu, the Very Heart of Africa: Being Some Account of the Protestant Mission at Stanley Falls, Upper Congo* (London: Carey Press, [1911?]), 205. Yakusu's missionaries may not have known that crocodiles were used in libeli medicines until the 1940s, when John Carrington took a research interest in libeli's history and esoteric language. Missionaries knew much earlier about initiates receiving a small wound "in the abdomen or in the small of the back . . . by which the attacking spirit . . . effected its entrance" (Smith, *Yakusu*,

66–67). On the contents of libeli medicines, see John F. Carrington, "The Initiation Language: Lokele Tribe," *African Studies* 6, no. 4 (1947): 197, including note 3. The ambivalent properties of these medicines is in keeping with John Janzen's findings: "Control of the agent that contributes to chaos, i.e. misfortune, possession, and the like, is the therapy which leads to health" (John M. Janzen, "Toward a Historical Perspective on African Medicine and Health," *Beiträge zur Ethnomidezin, Ethnobotanik und Ethnozoologie* 8 (1983): 112.

2. C. C. Chesterman, "Can You Pull a Crocodile Out with a Hook?" *YQN* 99 (October 1934): 13–17. On yaws, see Don R. Brothwell, "Yaws," in *The Cambridge World History of Human Disease,* ed. Kenneth F. Kiple (Cambridge: Cambridge University Press, 1993), 1096–1100; R. Mouchet, "Yaws and Syphilis among Natives in the Belgian Congo," *Kenya Medical Journal* 3 (1926–27): 242–45; A. Meheus, "Pian," in *Médecine et hygiène en Afrique centrale de 1885 à nos jours,* ed. P. G. Janssens, M. Kivits, and J. Vuylsteke (Brussels: Fondation Roi Baudouin, 1991), 1309–20; Kenneth F. Kiple, "Diseases of Sub-Saharan Africa to 1860," in *The Cambridge World History of Human Disease* (Cambridge: Cambridge University Press, 1993), 293–98; C. J. Hackett, "Yaws," in *Health in Tropical Africa during the Colonial Period,* ed. E. E. Sabben-Clare, D. J. Bradley, and K. Kirkwood (Oxford: Clarendon Press, 1980), 82–95; and Richard B. Sheridan, *Doctors and Slaves: A Medical and Demographic History of Slavery in the British West Indies, 1680–1834* (Cambridge: Cambridge University Press, 1985), 83–89, 214–15.

3. I have corrected Millman's spelling here from *libele;* William Millman, "The Tribal Initiation Ceremony of the Lokele," *International Review of Missions* 16 (1927): 377. Some people in the Stanleyville area called tertiary yaws or syphilis by the Lokele word for crocodile, *ngonde;* R. Mouchet, "Notes sur les dispensaires ruraux de la Province Orientale," *Annales de la Société Belge de la Médecine Tropicale* [hereafter ASBMT] 6 (1926): 146. At the time, Millman did not use the word fala, but rather leprosy in quotes, indicating that doctors diagnosed it as tertiary yaws. Millman wrote in 1907 that the breaking of any *bokili* or prohibition "would bring its own punishment in the form of some incurable skin disease—incurable until the white doctor cauterises it." See William Millman, "Religions without Scriptures: Among the Lokeles at Yakusu, Stanley Falls," *Missionary Herald,* 1907, 269. I have found no evidence of cauterization as a treatment for yaws in Africa prior to the use of arsenicals from 1910 and bismuth from circa 1918; see Hackett, "Yaws," 85. Leprosy, a disease that in "some of its dermatologic manifestations" resembles tertiary yaws and syphilis, was often confused with them; Allan M. Brandt, "Sexually Transmitted Diseases," in *Companion Encyclopedia of the History of Medicine,* vol. 1, ed. W. F. Bynum and Roy Porter (London: Routledge, 1993), 564. Such confusion was common among physicians on Caribbean slave plantations; see Kenneth F. Kiple, *The Caribbean Slave: A Biological History* (Cambridge: Cambridge University Press, 1984), 136–40.

4. Raymond E. Holmes, "A Surprise Visit to a District Dispensary," *YQN* 97 (April 1934): 11.

5. H. Roboam Likenyule, "Ende baina la Masiya. Kola losamo lofi loa Yesu," *Mboli ya Tengai* 324 (May 1934). Likenyule signed his letter "infirmier diplômé." Punctuation added for clarity.

6. Did missionaries learn more about relatively stable therapeutic aspects of libeli as their access to information and the lobe increased in the mid-1920s? The evidence suggests that the focusing on applying medicines to create back scars was not a new code in the 1924 round of libeli, though the special pills "which gives bravery" may well have been a new mimetic addition (see Millman, "Tribal Initiation Ceremony," 376).

7. W. H. Ennals, News Sheet no. 16, 23 December 1922, John F. Carrington Papers, Salisbury, U.K. (hereafter JFC Papers—Salisbury).

8. C. C. Chesterman, "Chasing the Terrors of Darkness," *YQN* 152 (October 1955): 12–13. On the soup incident, see also C. C. Chesterman, "Tropical Trail," Presidential Address to the Hunterian Society, 16 October 1967, 24, Phyllis Lofts Papers, Barton-on-Sea, U.K. (hereafter PL Papers). The evidence on this incident does not come from missionary sources alone; I also heard the story from Papa Lokangu, mission printer and lay historian, at Yakusu in 1989.

9. C. C. Chesterman, "How We Operate," *YQN* 66 (April 1926): 11.

10. C. C. Chesterman, "Yakusu Hospital Ltd.," *YQN* 51 (July 1922): 13–15. These renovations of the old Stapleton dispensary were distinct from the 1924 construction of a new hospital.

11. Bandombele [A. G. Mill], "What Are the Children Doing?" *YQN* 49 (November 1921), 12–13. The reference to "air-steamers that fly like birds" comes from a student essay in W. L. Chesterman, "A Few Quotations from Our Composition Class on the Subject of White People," *YQN* 78 (July 1929): 8–a [*sic*].

12. Bandombele, "What Are the Children Doing?"

13. BMS Yakusu Annual Medical Report, 1922, Hospital Director's Office, Yakusu (hereafter HDO, Yakusu; photocopies of full series given to BMSA by author). There was no mention of yaws in previous reports.

14. K. W. Todd, "Dreams Come True," *YQN* 70 (July 1927): 12; W. H. Ennals, News Sheet, no. 18, 18 March 1923, 81, JFC Papers—Salisbury. On the popularity of salvarsan injections for yaws elsewhere, see Terence Ranger, "Godly Medicine: The Ambiguities of Medical Mission in Southeast Tanzania, 1900–1945," *Social Science and Medicine* 15B (1981); and Marc Dawson, "The Anti-Yaws Campaign and Colonial Medical Policy in Kenya," *International Journal of African Historical Studies* 20 (1987): 417–37.

15. Maryinez Lyons, *The Colonial Disease: A Social History of Sleeping Sickness in Northern Zaire, 1900–1940* (Cambridge: Cambridge University Press), 99, 128–29. Their application was inconsistent, especially for women.

16. Ennals, News Sheet, no. 12, 27 October 1922, JFC Papers—Salisbury.

17. F. G. Spear, "Bewitched," *YQN* 54 (April 1923), 5–6; William Millman, "Another Point of View," *YQN* 54 (April 1923): 6; and "Referred to in Our Last Number," *YQN* 55 (July 1923): 7.

18. Millman, "Another Point of View," 8.

19. E. R. Millman, "Our Girls," *YQN* 43 (May 1919): 5.

20. "Developments in the Medical Mission," *YQN* 57 (January 1924): 19; and Charles E. Pugh, "The Coming of the Engine," *YQN* 57 (January 1924): 15–17.

21. On the rumors, see Chesterman, "Tropical Trail," 18. The Lofts note reads: "A Piece of Wood—once part of a tree of cruelty—which was turned into furniture for the hospital at Yakusu" (Typescript note, n.d., attached to piece of wood, PL Papers). On Zanzibari and Congo Independent State complicity in hangings in the region in the late-nineteenth century, see E. J. Glave, "Cruelty in the Congo Free State," *Century Magazine* 54, no. 32 (May–October 1897): 704–6. See also Jean-Luc Vellut, "La violence armée dans l'Etat Indépendant du Congo," *Cultures et développement* 16 (1984): 671–707.

22. Ennals, News Sheet, no. 24, 22 March 1924, JFC Papers—Salisbury.

23. For "social ostracism," see Mrs. Chesterman, "Yenga, Sunday Boy," *YQN* 59 (July 1924): b–c.

For "famine," see "Reaction," *YQN* 59 (July 1924): e. For "recrudescence" and 1,500, see "The Church," *YQN* 60 (October 1924): 3.

24. Millman, "Tribal Initiation," 364–80; and "Reaction," d. Once libeli began, the "state officers at that time . . . saw nothing that could be interfered with and vain were all our pleadings" (C. C. Chesterman, "The Swan Song of the Libeli," *YQN* 65 [January 1926]: 20).

25. Translation of Lokele text, *Mboli ya Tengai* 129 (August 1922), in John F. Carrington, "*Mboli ya Tengai* [Contents List]," John F. Carrington Papers, BMSA (hereafter JFC Papers—BMSA). While I was at Yakusu, missionaries bemoaned the high attendance at church on communion Sunday (once a month). They said that people came because they wanted to keep their "tickets to heaven" up to date; they wanted a signature on their membership card saying they had attended communion.

26. H. B. Parris, "Concerning the Collection," *YQN* 54 (April 1923): 13.

27. Ibid.; and "The Church," *YQN* 60 (October 1924): 3. On linginda and axhead circulation into the 1920s, see Colonel A. Bertrand, "Quelques notes sur la vie politique: le développement, la décadence des petites sociétés bantou du bas in central du Congo," *Revue de l'Institut de Sociologie de Bruxelles* 1 (1920): 77; Alfred Mahieu, *Numismatique du Congo, 1485–1924: instruments d'échange, valeurs monétaires, méreaux, médailles* (Brussels: Imprimerie Médicale et Scientifique, [1925?]), 120.

28. E. R. Millman, "To Stanley Falls to See the Prince," *YQN* 65 (January 1926): 7. The work in cleaning villages may have related to clearing bush as part of sleeping sickness campaigns; it was certainly colonial hygiene work.

29. A. G. Mill, "On Itineration," *YQN* 37 (December 1917): 3–4.

30. H. B. Parris, "Back to Yakusu, Voyage Jotting?" *YQN* 65 (January 1926): 4.

31. A. G. Mill, "The Big Push" *YQN* 45 (March 1920): 12; William Millman, "All in a Day's Work," *YQN* 50 (March 1922): 2–3; Charles E. Pugh, "Coming of the Engine," *YQN* 57 (January 1954): 15–17; and "Taking Stock," *YQN* 65 (January 1926): 3. All workers were men; 2,140 out of 2,613 church members were men.

32. A. G. Mill, "Lomami Days," *YQN* 73 (April 1928): 3–4; and W. H. Ford, "European Commerce and Native Character," *YQN* 74 (July 1928): 10.

33. "Clothes on the Congo," *YQN* 49 (November 1921): 10.

34. Thus, after some children showed Mrs. Pugh a path in 1920, "each of them received a little packet of salt, which was as dear to them as chocolates to an English child" (L. Gwendoline Pugh, "For the Children: Bessie," *YQN* 46 (September 1920): 3–6. A bag of imported salt supplemented a 1,500-franc bridewealth payment with missionary approval in 1925 (E. R. Millman, "Beauty and the Beast Mary," *YQN* 63 [July 1925]: 6–9). On BaMbole and Lokele chiefs, see Mrs. Chesterman, "First Impressions," *YQN* 44 (October 1921): 2–4; E. R. Millman, "To Stanley falls to See the Prince," *YQN* 65 (January 1926): 7–9; and E. R. Millman, "The News," *YQN* 75 (October 1928): 2–8. On domestics' names: C. C. Chesterman, "Essence of Yakusu," *YQN* 47 (1921): 9.

35. On Maypole dancing, see C. Ford, "From My Diary," *YQN* 70[a] (April 1927): 10; G. C. Ennals, "With the Little Ones," *YQN* 75 (October 1928): 15; "Prince Charles, Regent of Belgium Visits Yakusu," *YQN* 141 (September 1947): 2.

36. A. G. Mill, "Lomami Days," *YQN* 73 (April 1928): 3–4; Mrs. Mill, "The Struggle for Right

Living," *YQN* 82 (July 1930): 12–14; C. C. Chesterman, "Our First Forest Dispensary Revisited," *YQN* 85 (April 1931): 11; and "A Church Meeting: Held at Yasanga, Lomame [*sic*], in the Course of an Itineration by Mr. Parris," *YQN* 78 (July 1929): 12–13. On malinga (or *maringa*) music and dancing, see Phyllis M. Martin, *Leisure and Society in Colonial Brazzaville* (Cambridge: Cambridge University Press, 1995), 131–32, 136, 143. Other histories of music in colonial Zaire are available, but most neglect dance and the speed and itineraries by which these new forms of leisure arrived in rural areas; Michel Lonoh, *Essai de commentaire de la musique moderne* (Kinshasa: SEI/ANC, 1972); Sylvain Bemba, *Cinquante ans de musique du Congo-Zaïre (1920–1970)* (Paris: Présence Africaine, 1984); and Tchebwa Manda, *Terre de la chanson: la musique zaïroise hier et aujourd'hui* (Louvain-la-Neuve: Duculot, 1996).

37. "Neighbours," *YQN* 70[a] (April 1927): 11 (two issues of *YQN* carry the number seventy; this comes from the April issue, not its succeeding one of July 1927). Author not indicated, though the references to Chesterman's daughter, Heather Limengo, suggest that it was Chesterman. Great Physician idioms were ubiquitous in missionary discourse; see E. W. Barter, "How I Came to Yakusu," *YQN* 50 (March 1922): 7; and R. E. Holmes, "The Night Round," *YQN* 91 (October 1932): 16–17.

38. "A Review of the Year," *YQN* 92 (January 1933): 10.

39. K. C. Parkinson, "Boys' School," *YQN* 96 (January 1934): 5–6.

40. A. G. Mill, "Earthen Vessels," *YQN* 91 (October 1932): 9.

41. W. H. Ford, "African Dispersion," *YQN* 147[b] (September 1952): 2–3.

42. E. R. Millman, "Picking up the Gold and Silver," *YQN* 77 (April 1929): 2; and E. R. Millman, "Their First Tea Party," *YQN* 86 (July 1931): 2.

43. Rose E. Gee, "A Peep into a Nurse's Diary," *YQN* 21 (December 1913): 9.

44. Kendred Smith, "Yakusu Station," *Missionary Herald,* May 1901, 272; William Millman, "Missionary Medical Work on the Upper Congo," *Missionary Herald,* December 1904, 604–5; Rose E. G[ee], "Need for Medical Work at Yakusu," *YQN* 16 (September 1912): 4; Rose E. Gee, "A Peep into a Nurse's Diary," 8–10; and "Medical Work," *YQN* 18 (March 1913): 5.

45. Mill's basic medical training for missionaries at Livingstone College included bandaging wounds and extracting teeth; John N. Sinclair, "Our Storied Past: A Saga of Six Lives Molded into Three Families and Lived out on Four Continents" (Roseville, Minn., 1992, unpublished manuscript), 30. Chesterman extracted teeth for those not "frightened by the penny fee or the less terrible glint of the forceps" in 1921 (C. C. Chesterman, "The Hospital," *YQN* 48 [July 1921]: 12). On tooth pulling, see Paul Stuart Landau, "Explaining Surgical Evangelism in Colonial Southern Africa: Teeth, Pain, and Faith," *Journal of African History* 37 (1996): 261–81. Mill's clinical repertoire in 1916 and 1925 included treating cases of pneumonia, ulcers, and ascites, as well as lancing boils, buboes (yaws ulcers), and treating a hernia that he mistook for an abscess; Sinclair, "Our Storied Past," 103–4, 106. On 500 miles, see A. G. Mill, "Home Nursing," *YQN* 32 (September 1916): 4.

46. "Medical Work," *YQN* 8 (August 1910): 4; and "Nelly," *YQN* 11 (June 1911): 2–3.

47. Lyons, *Colonial Disease.*

48. See Etat Indépendant du Congo, *Recueil Mensuel des arrêtés, circulaires, instructions et ordres de service* (1906): 238–43. A 1917 circular stressed the importance of appreciating and collaborating with missionaries dedicated to sleeping sickness work: "Circulaire relative à la lutte

contre la maladie du sommeil," 7me Direction, no. 28, 19 May 1917, Congo Belge, *Recueil Mensuel des circulaires, instructions et ordres de service* (1917): 182. As late as 1923, a colonial doctor (or appropriate medical authority) was only required to inspect for sleeping sickness in a fifty-kilometer area around his residence; "Circulaire rappelant au personnel médical européen du Service de l'Hygiène l'obligation de la recherche systématique et du traitement des malades du sommeil," Hygiène no. 8, 8 March 1923, Congo Belge, *Recueil Mensuel* (1923): 23–27. See also Congo Belge, *Recueil Mensuel* (1909): 109–20.

49. "Circulaire prescrivant de ne rien négliger pour assurer l'exécution des mesures prophylacti-ques contre la maladie du sommeil," 2me Direction, no. 82, 25 June 1912, Congo Belge, *Recueil Mensuel* (1912): 257–59.

50. On the economics of atoxyl, see Jean-Luc Vellut, "La médecine européenne dans l'Etat Indé-pendant du Congo (1885–1908)," in *Analecta de réalisations médicales en Afrique centrale, 1885–1985*, ed. P. G. Janssens, M. Kivits, and J. Vuylsteke (Brussels: Fondation Roi Baudouin, 1991), 61–81.

51. Lyons, *Colonial Disease*, 80, 84, 184 (quotation from Todd, *Letters*, 12 July 1904, quoted in ibid., 84).

52. Ibid., 90, 108–9, 120, 188 (quotation from Todd, *Letters*, cited in ibid., 271 n. 35). For an excellent review of pharmaceuticals used, see ibid., 149, 152.

53. Alex G. Mill to Father, 7 December 1914, A. G. Mill Papers, in the private possession of John H. Sinclair, Roseville, Minn.; Sinclair, "Our Storied Past," 30, 62–63, 102; and "Sleeping Sickness," *YQN* 28 (September 1915): 6.

54. BMS, Yakusu Annual Medical Report, 1921, HDO, Yakusu.

55. C. C. Chesterman, "So Great Salvation: Hope for the Victims of Sleeping Sickness," *YQN* 59 (July 1924): f. Madness or "neurological degeneration with psychiatric disorders such as ner-vousness, irascibility, emotionalism, melancholia" were especially common in advanced cases of the disease (Lyons, *Colonial Disease*, 44). The use of white clay, a protective sign of closeness to ancestral spirits, suggests that kin remained active in the therapeutic process. On kaolin, see Jan Vansina, *Paths in the Rainforests: Toward a History of Political Tradition in Equatorial Africa* (Madison: University of Wisconsin Press, 1990), 291; Victor Turner, *The Forest of Symbols: Aspects of Ndembu Ritual* (Ithaca, N.Y.: Cornell University Press, 1967), 50, 65–66; and Piet Korse, "Le fard rouge et le kaolin blanc chez les Mongo de Basankoso et de Befale (Zaïre)," *Annales Aequatoria* 10 (1989): 10–39. There is no other evidence from Yakusu on the use of Twilight Sleep, an amnesia-producing analgesic used for women in childbirth labor, which "underlined the notion that . . . childbirth should take place in hospital" (Irvine Loudon, *Death in Childbirth: An International Study of Maternal Care and Maternal Mortality, 1800–1950* [Oxford: Oxford University Press, 1992], 348). See also Judith Walzer Leavitt, *Brought to Bed: Childbearing in America, 1750 to 1950* (New York: Oxford University Press, 1986), 128–41.

56. The Ilembo lazaret had an inner, palisaded "lock-up" for the advanced or "mad" cases by 1908; plate 10 in Lyons's book (also the cover photo) shows a chained "fou" at the Stanleyville lazaret in 1912 (Lyons, *Colonial Disease*, 112, 123).

57. C. C. Chesterman, "Tryparsamide in Sleeping Sickness," *Transactions of the Royal Society of Tropical Medicine and Hygiene* 16 (1922–23): 405 [hereafter *TRSTMH*]. See also C. C. Chester-man, in "Discussion," *TRSTMH* 40 (1947): 755.

58. *Daily Chronicle*, 10 July 1903, 6/5, as quoted in *Oxford English Dictionary*, 2d ed. (New York: Oxford University Press, 1989), 108.

59. "Circulaire prescrivant de ne rien négliger pour assurer l'exécution des mesures prophylactiques contre la maladie du sommeil," 2ème Direction, no. 82, 25 June 1912, Congo Belge, *Recueil Mensuel* (1912): 257–59.

60. Chesterman, "Discussion," 755. The case was that of Lisoi; Chesterman, "Tryparsamide in Sleeping Sickness," 405. An autobiographical sketch is in Chesterman, "Tropical Trail."

61. BMS Yakusu Annual Medical Report, 1921, HDO, Yakusu.

62. A. G. Mill, "Home Nursing," *YQN* 32 (September 1916): 4.

63. In 1949, it was still only 48 percent (BMS Yakusu Annual Medical Reports, 1921–49, HDO Yakusu). In 1937, BMS record keeping changed, and in that year statistics were kept both for males and females (509 versus 202), and for men, women, and children (429, 172, and 110 respectively), therefore showing that at least for 1937, adult women were as likely to be inpatients as were girls. See tables 1–3 in Nancy Rose Hunt, "Negotiated Colonialism: Domesticity, Hygiene, and Birth Work in the Belgian Congo" (Ph.D. diss., University of Wisconsin–Madison, 1992), 467–69.

64. The large proportion of female sleeping sickness patients in Chesterman's research reports ran counter to gender trends in medical care at Yakusu, within the colony, and in much of colonial Africa. As Rita Headrick and Megan Vaughan have argued, where colonial health care was voluntary, men were at least about twice as likely to be patients as women. See Rita Headrick, "The Impact of Colonialism on Health in French Equatorial Africa, 1880–1934" (Ph.D. diss., University of Chicago, 1987), 147, 549. See also Megan Vaughan, "Measuring Crisis in Maternal and Child Health: An Historical Perspective," in *Women's Health and Apartheid: The Health of Women and Children and the Future of Progressive Primary Health Care in Southern Africa*, ed. Marcia Wright, Zena Stein, and Jean Scandlyn (New York: Columbia University Press, 1988), 137. Why this was so has not been well elucidated. The military origins of colonial medical care were certainly part of the reason; this factor also fed the gendering of nursing and hospital spaces as male.

65. "Discussion," in C. C. Chesterman, "Some Results of Tryparsamide and Combined Treatment of Gambian Sleeping Sickness," *TRSTMH* 25 (1931–32): 437–38. Of the 268 patients treated, 82 (or 30.6 percent) were deemed cured; the sight of over 10 percent (27 out of 268) of the patients was affected. Chesterman thought "visual trouble must be expected to occur in at least 30 percent of second stage cases efficiently treated" (ibid., 433). Of the 248 cases where gender was indicated, 127 were women and girls. Most females were of childbearing age. Such a gender ratio differs from Lyons's more anecdotal, archival evidence; she argues that most women in northern Zaire successfully evaded sleeping sickness examinations through the 1920s, though a shift in official attitude on female participation seems to have surfaced in 1918 (Lyons, *Colonial Disease*, 86, 141, 187–88). Tryparsamide was a significant improvement over atoxyl and became one of the colony's drugs of choice; up to 30 percent of patients treated with atoxyl injections went blind (ibid., 120, 152).

66. C. C. Chesterman, "The Relation of Yaws and Goundou," *TRSTMH* 20 (1926–27): 554. On "boomerang leg" in Australia, see Brothwell, "Yaws," 1099; and C. J. Hackett, *Boomerang Leg and Yaws in Australian Aborigines* (London: Royal Society of Tropical Medicine and Hygiene,

1936). For photographs and a detailed study of such bone curvature in Uganda, see C. J. Hackett, *Bone Lesions of Yaws in Uganda* (Oxford: Blackwell, 1948).

67. C. C. Chesterman, in "Discussion" of C. J. Hackett, "The Clinical Course of Yaws in Lango, Uganda," *TRSTMH* 40 (1946): 206–27, esp. 224. See also Chesterman's comments in a discussion of Ellis B. Hudson, "Bejel: The Endemic Syphilis of the Euphrates Arab," *TRSTMH* 331 (1937): 41–42; and C. C. Chesterman and Kenneth W. Todd, "Clinical Studies with Organic Arsenic Derivatives in Human Trypanosomiasis and Yaws," *TRSTMH* 21 (1927–28): 227–32.

68. C. C. Chesterman in "Yaws: Discussion," *British Journal of Venereal Diseases* 4 (1928): 64. In hot, arid regions, endemic syphilis was often misread as venereally transmitted syphilis; see Megan Vaughan, *Curing Their Ills: Colonial Power and African Illness* (Stanford, Calif.: Stanford University Press, 1991), 137. "Syphilis was given a different name by the natives, and it ran a course different from yaws" (Chesterman, "Yaws: Discussion," 65). Many Congolese in the region called yaws *buba* (Sw.) or *congolie* (presumably after the colony). Unlike Europeans, they did not confuse it with syphilis, which they called *kaswende* (Sw.) or kassende; see, respectively, Mouchet, "Yaws and Syphilis," 245; and "Rapport médical de premier semestre," 1907, unpaged, in H (838) "Rapports sanitaires du District de l'Aruwimi," AA. On the local distinction between tertiary yaws and earlier manifestations of the disease, see Chesterman, "Yaws and Goundou," 554. On the historical confusion of yaws and syphilis, see Brothwell, "Yaws"; Mouchet, "Yaws and Syphilis"; and Megan Vaughan, "Syphilis in Colonial East and Central Africa: The Social Construction of an Epidemic," in *Epidemics and Ideas: Essays on the Historical Perception of Pestilence,* ed. Terence Ranger and Paul Slack (Cambridge: Cambridge University Press, 1992), 269–302. On the effects of yaws eradication on cross immunity from other treponemal diseases, see Hackett, "Yaws," 90; and Brothwell, "Yaws," 1097.

69. Chesterman, "Yaws: Discussion," 65; Alex G. Mill to Harold, 31 January 1915, A. G. Mill Papers, in the private possession of John H. Sinclair, Roseville, Minn.

70. Janzen, "Toward a Historical Perspective," 112.

71. Chesterman, "Yaws: Discussion," 64. Persistent secondary lesions included "crab yaws of the feet and granuloma remaining in the axilla or in the bend of the elbow, or other situations," and these could persist twenty to thirty years after the primary lesion. Chesterman never saw anyone suffering from tertiary lesions—"bony disease or deformity or ulcers of the skin"— who had had persistent secondary yaws (Chesterman, "Yaws: Discussion," 65). He wondered if persistent secondary yaws did not prevent tertiary yaws, and noted that local people's behavior followed this logic as they would hesitate to have their children treated until the "really florid eruption appears." He also implied that patients "with minimal lesions responded less favourably to treatment than did those with more florid lesions" (C. C. Chesterman, in "Discussion" of C. J. Hackett, "The Clinical Course of Yaws in Lango, Uganda," *TRSTMH* 40 [1946]: 224–25). Chesterman said he observed 30,000 cases of yaws during his fifteen years of service in the Congo (Chesterman, in "Discussion" of Ellis H. Hudson, "Bejel: The Endemic Syphilis of the Euphrates Arab," *TRSTMH* 31 [1937–38]: 41).

72. C. C. Chesterman, "A Congo Medical Itineration," *Missionary Herald,* 1924, 132.

73. "Reaction," *YQN* 59 (July 1924), d.

74. C. C. Chesterman, "The Swan Song of the Libeli," *YQN* 65 (January 1926): 20.

75. Tata Bafoya Bamanga, with Mama Tula, Yakusu, 25 November 1989. Quotations are from the former.

76. Ibid. Italics added. These feasts were a historically specific missionary strategy: "That time, when the whites came they were looking for people, yes, people in order to enter them into the church. . . . the doctors there, he came with his gun in the house. . . . he would call the people of the village, he would send hunters to the forest, they would kill animals. So they would come with these animals, they would cook and call the people of the village to come eat. That time the white people were just looking for people to start . . . the church" (Mama Tula, Yakusu, 25 November 1989).

77. W. H. Ennals and W. H. Ford organized Boy Scouts in 1924; see "The Prize Giving," *YQN* 57 (January 1924): 15; Alice Wilkinson, "The Welcome," *YQN* 57 (January 1924): 7; and Gladys Owen, "How We Arrived," *YQN* 57 (January 1924): 9. For explicit language about Boy Scout forest competitions providing a substitute for libeli, see W. H. Ford, "Camping in a Congo Forest," *YQN* 60 (October 1924): 6–7. For French as a parallel esoteric language, see Ford, "Camping"; and Carrington, "Initiation Language."

78. On the two rules and the "staggering figure," see "The Church," *YQN* 60 (October 1924): 3–5. The figure of 4,000 is in "Statistics in Round Figures," *YQN* 60 (October 1924): 1; and "Statistics," *YQN* 59 (July 1924): 1. These statistics do not give gender breakdowns; nor is it clear if women had to pay lifaefi. In 1923, away from the river in "the forest region," women accounted for just 1 percent of church membership (BMS, *Annual Report*, 1923, 53). In 1936, the total church membership was 3,532, only one-quarter of which was female (BMS, *Annual Report*, 1936, 31). On the number of teachers and "debarred from Communion," see Millman, "Tribal Initiation," 380. Another source states that one-tenth of church members—only some 400—broke the church rules of 1910 forbidding libeli; "Reaction," *YQN* 59 (August 1924): d–e.

79. E. R. M(illman), "One by One," *YQN* 64 (October 1925): 4–5. On confessions, see also "Seeking the Wayward," *YQN* 62 (April 1925): 9–10, a [*sic*]; C. C. Chesterman, "The Swan Song of the Libeli," *YQN* 65 (January 1926); and H. B. Parris, "A Riverside Lisongomi," *YQN* 66 (April 1926): 8–10. Church members dropped from 4,160 in 1924 to 2,547 in 1925, and did not rise above 4,100 again until 1930. There were 2,870 members in 1926. See T. B. Adam, *Africa Revisited: A Medical Deputation to the Baptist Missionary Society's Congo Field* (London: Baptist Missionary Society, 1931), 53.

80. On "enmity" and "goodwill," see C. C. C[hesterman], "The Result of Five Years' Anti-Sleeping Sickness Work," *YQN* 67 (July 1926): 8; on schools, see "Neighbours," *YQN* 70[a] (April 1927): 11; and Millman, "Tribal Initiation," 380.

81. On the dream, see K. C. Parkinson, "A Conversion," *YQN* 83 (October 1930): 12–13; on teachers, see Millman, "Tribal Initiation," 380; on hospital recruits, see BMS Yakusu Annual Medical Report, 1924, HDO, Yakusu; and Chesterman, "Yenga," *YQN* 59 (July 1924): b–c.

82. The reference uses the English word leprosy rather than *fala* ("Seeking the Wayward," *YQN* 62 [April 1925], 9–10, a [*sic*]). On confessions and the hospital, see Millman, "One by One," *YQN* 64 (October 1925), 5.

83. [Daniel Yaliole], "Lioi lia Yaliole Daniel," *Mboli ya Tengai* 183 (February 1927); and B. Phillipe Falanga, "Lifenyakani eoka ya libeli," *Mboli ya Tengai* 339 (March 1935).

84. On teachers as strangers, see especially [Isamoiso], "Lokasa loa M. Isamoiso wa Yangembe,"

Mboli ya Tengai 79 (December 1916); and [Victor Yenga], "Lokasa loa Victor Yenga," *Mboli ya Tengai* 291 (August 1931): 6–7. I have published the full Lokele texts (and English translations) of seven of these letters in Nancy Rose Hunt, "Letter-Writing, Nursing Men, and Bicycles in the Belgian Congo: Notes towards the Social Identity of a Colonial Category," in *Paths toward the Past: African Historical Essays in Honor of Jan Vansina*, ed. Robert W. Harms et al. (Atlanta, Ga.: African Studies Association, 1994), 187–210. On Lokele teachers as "missionaries to the forest people"—namely to Foma villages where evangelization expanded during the First World War, supported by the lifaefi of Lokele church members—see H. Lambotte, "Thoughts Suggested by a Picture of a Tank," *YQN* 37 (December 1917): 10. This had changed by 1922: "riverside Churches . . . scarcely pay their own expenses let alone help forest schools" (William Millman, "All in a Day's Work," *YQN* 50 [March 1922]: 2–4). Training for "forest teachers" had begun at Yaongama by 1922, whereas Lisase and Sindani, two river men "pioneered the work in the forest" over the previous decade (H. B. Parris, "Yaongama," *YQN* 57 [January 1924]: 22. One of every seven church members was an accredited teacher-evangelist in 1932, when money was scarce due to the depression (W. H. Ennals, "Yakusu Church," *YQN* 89 [April 1932]: 4). BaManga and Linja (BaMbole) men also became teachers in their regions, though Lokele evangelists were sent in at first, even if only briefly due to language barriers.

85. Lisoo first surfaced as a topic in a church meeting in 1912: "We learned with shame and regret and some people of the Church cut new Lisoo that came from the region of Basoko" ("Njaso—Ikumbe," 27 January 1912).

86. "Lokasa loa M. Isamoiso wa Yangembe," *Mboli ya Tengai* 79 (December 1916); and "Lokasa loa Tolanga wa Yalongolo," *Mboli ya Tengai* 87 (July 1917). Italics added.

87. Papa Boshanene, Yakusu, 24 February 1989; Baba Manzanza, Yainyongo-Romée, 16 September 1989; Tata Bafoya Bamanga, with Mama Tula, Yakusu, 25 November 1989; Mama Tula Sophie, Yakusu, 22 November 1989; Tata Bafoya Bamanga, with Mama Tula, Yakusu, 27 November 1989; Dipo Kesobe, with Baba Manzanza, Yainyongo-Romée, 13 December 1989; Lofanjola-Lisele (Pesapesa), Yainyongo-Romée, 29 December 1989; Dipo Kesobe, Tata Alikuwa, Baba Manzanza, and Liyaoto, Yainyongo-Romée, 29 December 1989; Liyaoto, Yainyongo-Romée, 30 December 1989; and Lofemba, Yainyongo-Romée, 31 December 1989 and 7 January 1990.

88. To evoke again the language of Claude Lévi-Strauss; see the introduction.

89. "Lokasa loa Lititiyo ende Baina," *Mboli ya Tengai* 130 (February 1930): 2. The term for "mixture of medicine" was *isasandu* and for horn was *liseke*, that is, a kanga's horn for mixing and holding medicine. The word for wealth was *bieto*. The word for applying medicine through cuts in the skin or cicatrization was ndotinya. The meaning of tokoli is unclear. *Kangasu*, "this kanga of ours," is a derogatory expression. The word used for medicine was either *tosandu* or *isasandu*, except where indicated as lisoo. The full Lokele text is in Hunt, "Letter-Writing," 194–95. Italics added; punctuation added for clarity.

90. On lemonade, see Mrs. Mill, "First Impressions," *YQN* 44 (October 1919): 4.

91. C. C. Chesterman, "The Swan Song of the Libeli," *YQN* 65 (January 1926): 19–22. On the role of Tata and the scale of villages involved in libeli of 1924 (thirty towns or villages, called "centres"), see Millman, "Tribal Initiation," 373.

92. Like David Apaka, another Congolese evangelist (and eventually pastor) whose life was threatened because he did not respect libeli secrets, who also "steadfastly declined to be intimidated" (W. H. Ford, "Bathsheba, David's Wife," *YQN* 103 [October 1935]: 4). For "most

trusted," see "Outpost Work," *YQN* 76 (January 1929): 20; for "sterling character," see "Joseph Lititiyo Appointed Overseer," *YQN* 80 (January 1930): 67; and for his influence, W. H. Ford, "The Pastor Hopes to Visit . . . ," *YQN* 80 (January 1930): 5.

93. "Seeking the Wayward," *YQN* 62 (April 1925): 9; and "Joseph Lititiyo Appointed Overseer," *YQN* 80 (January 1930).

94. C. C. Chesterman, "Vale Kaisala," *YQN* 78 (July 1929): d; and E. R. Millman, "Picking up the Gold and Silver," *YQN* 77 (April 1929): 2–6.

95. "Letters from Rev. H. Sutton Smith, of Yakusu," *Missionary Herald*, 1901, 437–39.

96. Mrs. Stapleton, "Work amongst the Girls," *Missionary Herald*, 1902, 248; and Smith, *Yakusu*, 213.

97. Ennals, News Sheet, no. 19, 21 April 1923, 87, JFC Papers—Salisbury.

98. E. R. Millman, "Picking up the Gold and Silver," *YQN* 77 (April 1929).

99. C. C. Chesterman, "Vale Kaisala," *YQN* 78 (July 1929).

100. "Joseph Lititiyo Appointed Overseer," *YQN* 80 (January 1930): 6–7. See also W. H. Ford, "Reapers," *YQN* 85 (April 1931): 8. The latter suggests that Lititiyo was appointed assistant missionary and native pastor in January 1931, and by April, as overseer of the entire Yaokanja district.

101. E. R. Millman, "Picking up the Gold and Silver," *YQN* 77 (April 1929). For the ritual death, see C. C. Chesterman, "Vale Kaisala," *YQN* 78 (July 1929). His life may also have embraced relations with Catholic missionaries, though this is not evident in his particular case.

102. On "as a boy," see "Letter to Dr. Charles Brown," *YQN* 96 (January 1934): 17; for Lititiyo's line, see E. R. Millman, "An Unposted Letter," *YQN* 80 (January 1930): 10; and Stanley Browne to Father, 4 November 1938, Stanley G. Browne Papers, Private Residence of Mrs. Stanley Browne, New Milton, U.K. (hereafter SGB Papers). I have nothing but such caricatured missionary evidence on cannibalism for this region, which is not to say that it might not have existed in some ritual and/or warrior practices. Local sorcery idioms certainly are through images of "bad people" stealing and consuming human bodily debris and parts.

103. [Joseph Lititiyo], "The Troubles of a General Superintendent," *YQN* 98 (July 1934): 2–3; and C. C. Chesterman, "Work of the Hospital," *YQN* 88 (January 1932): 13.

104. Nurse Lofts turned this occasion into a tourist exchange, buying to the astonishment of all onlookers, his "best 'go-to-palaver,' leopard skin hat" (Phyllis Lofts, "Native Aristocracy," *YQN* 70[b] ([July 1927]: 10). I infer from his dress and the dates that this was Lobanga.

105. C. C. Chesterman, "Vale Kaisala," *YQN* 78 (July 1929): d.

106. C. C. Chesterman, "The Swan Song of the Libeli," *YQN* 65 (January 1926). "*Limbekaote ayalifele liolo*" were the words of the song, sung in the esoteric libeli language; see Carrington, "Initiation Language," 206, where he translates *liolo* as man. Chesterman translated the words as "Each man has the care of his own flesh" and glossed: "Libeli secrets were to be guarded as one's skin." Man/flesh/skin: manhood and specifically phallus is likely more accurate. Lobanga felt castrated. Yakusu's missionaries interpreted the occasion as one that gave "his men verbal permission to tell, if they cared to, seeing that white men already knew, who the spirits were." After "the close of a palaver arranged by the district administrator"— to arraign these spirits?—Lobanga denied giving any such permission (Millman, "Tribal Initiation," 368).

107. C. C. Chesterman, "The Swan Song of the Libeli," *YQN* 65 (January 1926).

108. E. R. Millman, "Picking up the Gold and Silver," *YQN* 77 (April 1929).

109. C. C. Chesterman, "Vale Kaisala," *YQN* 78 (July 1929). Lobanga's cause of death is unclear. On market goods, see K. C. Parkinson, "A Lisongomi at Yaokombo," *YQN* 85 (April 1931): 6–8. On "last but one" and date, "Log Book," *YQN* 78[b] (July 1929): 14.

110. On chief rejections, see A. G. Mill, "The One Body," *YQN* 100 (January 1935): 12; on district length, see W. H. Ford, "Reapers," *YQN* 85 (April 1931); on the ordination, "Joseph Lititiyo Appointed Overseer," *YQN* 80 (January 1930); and [Joseph Lititiyo], "The Troubles of a General Superintendent," *YQN* 98 (July 1934): 2–3. Lititiyo was still "shepherd of [the] whole Yaokanja district covering some 57 villages" in 1954 (V. Mason, "Yaokanja Journey," *YQN* 150 [August 1954]: 11).

111. "Log Book," *YQN* 78[b] (July 1929): 14.

112. Libeli is distinctive in that it was never linked with male circumcision ritual along the Lokele stretch of the river as some earlier forms of what Vansina calls lilwa ritual were. The fobe (pl. of lobe) were much older than this new fashion in ritual practice, as were ideas of water spirits. It was logical to integrate libeli into these sacred places of powerful medicinal trees, which may have been as old as settlement; indeed, they would have influenced where these people, fleeing Ndiya's maelstrom in Isiko, settled. The word *ndiya* for water spirit is found to the north, too, especially up the Lindi. None of this is to suggest that people and ritual styles only moved in from the north. Vansina's reading of this river stretch as a border zone seems accurate. Specifically, Vansina uses H. Sutton Smith and Millman's accounts of libeli and Yakusu to argue that "tradition" died as Yakusu's missionaries and church elders ended libeli; see Vansina, *Paths.* I do not imagine any such sudden and complete rupture. Lobanga combined and resisted the specificities of this local interwar modernity in complex and shifting ways, and biomedicine, perhaps even evangelical medicine, was in the end key in the creolizing historical process that his biography concretizes.

113. "Several letters have mentioned the gibe that religion provides no meals, or wives or money. Some refer to the temporary confidence in the powers of Roman Catholic rosaries. Nor is the heckling confined to men; often women propose the puzzling questions that are passing through the minds of many" (William Millman, "Native Evangelists and the Changing Outlook," *YQN* 83 [October 1930]: 4–6).

114. Chiefs were also favoring "new cults" as a "counter movement to the Church" in 1928 ("Log Book," *YQN* 73 [April 1928]).

115. Eight penciled student essays about libeli, located in John F. Carrington's papers in Salisbury (JFC Papers—Salisbury), all carried the date of 17 September 1930; various clues in these papers makes me think that they were collected by the major teacher and writer on school affairs, W. H. Ford. The authors and sometimes titles are indicated here: Bofeka, "*Mboli ya libeli la lilimbi lia yao*" [News about Libeli and Its Cheating]; N. L. B. Daniel; Jean Falanga; Bofofe, [The Reason Why People Like Libeli]; L. Bosolongo; Baelogondi, [The Reason Why They Cling to Libeli]; and L. S. Bomboli, [About Libeli]. One essay not included in those I found was published in translation; see "From Our Student Essays: Why the Native Church Condemns the Secret Cult of Libeli," *YQN* 83 (October 1930): 13. A Yakoso woman, Mama Tula, told me about a woman who had been chained to a tree because she defied the authority of libeli. (Italics have been added to student essays.)

116. E. R. Millman, "Their First Tea Party," *YQN* 86 (July 1931): 2–5.

117. Student essays about libeli, JFC Papers—Salisbury.

118. Ibid. Italics added.

119. Anne Retel-Laurentin emphasizes a central African equation between sterility and sorcery; see Anne Retel-Laurentin, *Sorcellerie et ordalies* (Paris: Editions Anthropos, 1974). My discussions with infertile women at Yainyongo bear this out. Many had sought biomedical help. Since biomedicine had not worked, they read this as proof that someone had stolen some of their menstrual blood, or some other bodily secretion or part, to block their fertility.

120. E. R. M[illman], "The Prince Comes to Yakusu," *YQN* 65 (January 1926): 14–15, 17; and Phyllis Lofts, "Yakusu Alphabet," *YQN* 83 (October 1930): 8–9.

3   Dining and Surgery

1. Rose E. Gee, "First Experiences on the Congo," extract from *Missionary Herald,* August, n.d. (1911?), 269, in John F. Carrington Papers, Salisbury, U.K. (hereafter JFC Papers—Salisbury).

2. Mrs. Millman to Miss Bowser, 10 November 1930, Millman file, BMSA.

3. As in Mary Louise Pratt's book, *Imperial Eyes: Travel Writing and Transculturation* (London: Routledge, 1992).

4. I borrow the expression "topsy-turvy" from the book that became the Yakusu missionary bible on humor in "Congoland": Dan Crawford, *Thinking Black: Twenty-Two Years without a Break in the Long Grass of Central Africa* (London: Morgan and Scott, 1912).

5. Norbert Elias, *La civilisation des moeurs,* trans. Pierre Kamnitzer (1939; reprint, Paris: Calmann-Levy, 1973), 144, 179–83.

6. The idea that the Congo was "cannibal country" was long-standing in European cultural geographies, leading to a genre of travel literature bearing titles like the following: John H. Weeks, *Among Congo Cannibals: Experiences, Impressions, and Adventures during a Thirty Years' Sojourn amongst the Boloki and Other Congo Tribes* (London: Seeley Service and Co., 1913); and A. B. Lloyd, *In Dwarf Land and Cannibal Country* (London: T. Fisher Unwin, 1899). See, too, Thomas Richards, "Selling Darkest Africa," in *The Commodity Culture of Victorian England: Advertising and Spectacle, 1851–1914* (Stanford, Calif.: Stanford University Press, 1990). See also chapter 3, notes 58 and 140.

7. I borrow "not quite/not white" and its implications about colonial mimicry from Homi Bhabha, "Of Mimicry and Man: The Ambivalence of Colonial Discourse," *October* 28 (1984): 125–33.

8. C. C. Chesterman, "Chasing the Terrors of Darkness" *YQN* 152 (October 1955): 12; and Gladys Owen, "In the Ward," *YQN* 60 (October 1924): 14–15.

9. Gladys Owen, "I Was Blind and Now I Can See," *YQN* 63 (July 1925): 17–18; and W. H. Ennals, "Pictures of Life," *YQN* 71 (October 1927): 5–6. By 1926, stovaine, a local anesthetic administered by spinal, was also common (Gladys Owen, "Hospital Incidents," *YQN* 67 [July 1926]: 14–15).

10. C. C. Chesterman, "How We Operate," *YQN* 66 (April 1926): 10–12.

11. "Christmas at Yakusu," *YQN* 26 (March 1915): 11–12.

12. H. Sutton Smith, *Yakusu, the Very Heart of Africa: Being Some Account of the Protestant Mission at Stanley Falls, Upper Congo* (London: Carey Press, [1911?]). These nonconformist Protestant missionaries' cultural reference points ranged from Livingstone to Stanley, George Grenfell to Dan Crawford, and certainly extended to E. D. Morel and Roger Casement, though apparently not to Conrad. Their "heart" was the "poor, broken, bleeding Africa" described by Livingstone, while their station was located on the "fringe of the great gloomy forest" described by Stanley in *Darkest Africa* as full of cannibals.

13. "Christmas at Yakusu," *YQN* 26 (March 1915).

14. Crawford, *Thinking Black*, 416.

15. On "sight" and "tramping," see William J. W. Roome, *Tramping through Africa: A Dozen Crossings of the Continent* (New York: Macmillan, 1930), 176, 179; on Yakusu's colonial reputation, see A. Detry, *A Stanleyville* (Liège: Imprimerie La Meuse, 1912); and on Stanley's "fringe," Smith, *Yakusu*, xiii. On the nineteenth-century invention of the "dark continent," see Patrick Brantlinger, "Victorians and Africans: The Genealogy of the Myth of the Dark Continent," *Critical Inquiry* 12 (1985): 166–203.

16. Prince Albert, "Voyage au Congo belge par Cape Town," ca. 1909, Archives du Palais Royal, Brussels.

17. Relations between Protestant and Catholic missionaries in the Congo were often tense; see Ruth Slade Reardon, "Catholics and Protestants in the Congo," in *Christianity in Tropical Africa*, ed. C. G. Baëta (London: 1968), 83–100. Royal visits to Yakusu were instead expressions of bipartisanship. Prince Leopold III came in 1926, Albert returned as king accompanied by Queen Elizabeth in 1928, Princess Astrid came alone in 1933, and Prince Charles visited in 1947: see *YQN* 6 (December 1909); *YQN* 65 (January 1926); *YQN* 75 (October 1928); *YQN* 93 (April 1933); and *YQN* 141 (September 1947).

18. On "fairy tales" and "rehearsal," see G. C. Ennals, "With the Little Ones," *YQN* 75 (October 1928): 15–18; and on Dover Cliff, see "Yakusu Station," *YQN* 15 (June 1912): 5–6. These were especially Edith Millman's fairy tales: "the steamer Luxembourg is still moored at our beach near the steps which have been trodden by the feet of a King and Queen, of Princes and Dukes and a host of Lords and Ladies of high degree. The station is quiet. Not a drum is heard. A Princess is sleeping" (E. R. Millman, "The Royal Visit to Yakusu," *YQN* 93 [April 1933]: i).

19. On "at table," see M. Chesterman, "Jottings of the Junior," *YQN* 101 (April 1935): 12. On "the knife and fork doctrine," see John Howell, [BMS Kinshasa], "The Industrial Element in Missionary Methods," in Congo Missionary Conference, *Report of the General Conference of Missionaries of the Protestant Societies Working in Congoland* (Bolobo, 1904), 47; the exact reference reads: "Even the greatest enemy to a few fathoms of cloth and the knife and fork doctrine, has no desire to return to the customs of his forefathers" [hereafter CMC, *Report*].

20. On Saidi see Smith, *Yakusu*, 26 (date inferred from the table, 180–81). On Bonjoma see "Susanne: How She Came to School at Yakusu," *YQN* 31 (June 1916): 6. On Osinga see E. R. Millman, "Baendeleke, A Lokele Woman," *YQN* 27 (June 1915): 7–9.

21. W. L. Chesterman, "A Few Quotations from Our Composition Class on the Subject of White People," *YQN* 78 (July 1928): 8. See also A. Levare, *Le confort aux colonies* (Paris: Editions Larose, 1928); and Karen Tranberg Hansen, *Distant Companions: Servants and Employers in Zambia, 1900–1985* (Ithaca, N.Y.: Cornell University Press, 1989). On the etymology of "boy"

in French for domestic workers in Africa and Asia, see *Trésor de la langue française*, vol. 4 (Paris: Gallimard, 1985), 869–70.

22. W. H. Stapleton, "Quarterly Notes, No. 1, B.M.S. Yakusu, July 1904," *YQN* 28 (September 1915): 4.

23. K. C. Parkinson, "A Visitor and the School," *YQN* 78 (July 1929): 10–12; and CMC, *Report* (1904): 45–47. On industrial education, see also Barbara Ann Yates, "The Triumph and Failure of Mission Vocational Education in Zaire, 1879–1908," *Comparative Education Review* 20 (1976): 193–208.

24. On "self-reliance" see Barbara Ann Yates, "The Missions and Educational Development in Belgian Africa, 1876–1908" (Ph.D. diss., Columbia University, 1967), 239, 112. Charity, rather than building self-reliance, was more important in Catholic colonial conceptions. On "rudiments": BMS, Yakusu Annual Medical Report, 1954, Hospital Director's Office, Yakusu (hereafter HDO, Yakusu).

25. Howell, "Industrial Element," 44–47; CMC, *Report* (1907): 106, 115; and CMC, *Report* (1906): 75; and CMC, *Report* (1907): 115. On "Dandies" see CMC, *Report* (1907), 106.

26. On minstrelsy and urban dandy figures, see Jan Pieterse, *White on Black: Images of Africa and Blacks in Western Popular Culture* (New Haven, Conn.: Yale University Press, 1992), 134–35; Eric Lott, *Love and Theft: Blackface Minstrelsy and the American Working Class* (New York: Oxford University Press, 1993); and Michael Pickering, "Mock Blacks and Racial Mockery: The 'Nigger' Minstrel and British Imperialism," in *Acts of Supremacy: The British Empire and the Stage, 1790–1930*, ed. J. S. Bratton et al. (Manchester: Manchester University Press, 1991), 179–236, esp. 216, 228. Thanks to Joan Dayan for insights into "blackface rubrics." On blackface, colonial humor, and "petit nègre" figures, see also Kenneth W. Goings, *Mammy and Uncle Mose: Black Collectibles and American Stereotyping* (Bloomington: Indiana University Press, 1994); *Zaïre, 1885–1985: Cent ans de regards belges* (Brussels: CEC, 1985); Catherine M. Cole, "Reading Blackface in West Africa: Wonders Taken for Signs," *Critical Inquiry* 23 (1996): 183–215; Greg Dening, *Mr. Bligh's Bad Language: Passion, Power, and the Theatre on the Bounty* (Cambridge: Cambridge University Press, 1992); *Les cent aventures de la famille Mbumbulu* (Leopoldville: Presses de l'Imprimerie de l'Avenir, 1956); Révérend Père d'Hossche, *Les aventures de Mbope* (Leverville: Bibliothèque de l'Etoile, n.d.); and Richards, "Selling Darkest Africa." Also useful on humor are A. R. Radcliffe-Brown, "On Joking Relationships," in *Structure and Function in Primitive Society: Essays and Addresses* (Glencoe, Ill.: Free Press, 1952), 90–105; Mary Douglas, *Implicit Meanings: Essays in Anthropology* (London: Oxford University Press, 1975); Anne Hudson Jones, ed., *Images of Nurses: Perspectives from History, Art, and Literature* (Philadelphia: University of Pennsylvania Press, 1988); and Ruth Laub Coser, "Some Social Functions of Laughter: A Study of Humor in a Hospital Setting," *Human Relations* 12 (1959): 171–82.

27. Smith, *Yakusu*, 89–90; C. E. Pugh, "At Stanleyville," *YQN* 25 (December 1914): 9; "Letters from Rev. H. Sutton Smith of Yakusu," *Missionary Herald*, September 1901, 437; and Ernest E. Wilford, "Itinerating in the Yawembe District," *YQN* 11 (June 1911): 6–7. Itineration—to travel from place to place preaching—was a staple of the BMS lexicon, and part of evangelical missionary vocabularies in general, from at least the late–eighteenth century (*Oxford English Dictionary*, 2d ed. [New York: Oxford University Press, 1989], 149–50).

28. C. Ford, "From My Diary," *YQN* 69 (January 1927): 10.

29. L. Gwendoline Pugh, "A First Canoe Expedition," *YQN* 21 (December 1913): 5–7.

30. C. E. Pugh, "At Stanleyville," *YQN* 23 (December 1914): 9; and Pugh, "A First Canoe Expedition."

31. Smith, *Yakusu*, 90; and K. C. Parkinson, "Two Journeys," *YQN* 77 (April 1929): 9–12.

32. Patricia A. Turner, *Ceramic Uncles and Celluloid Mammies: Black Images and Their Influence on Culture* (New York: Anchor Books, 1994), 19; and especially, Pieterse, *White on Black*, 166–67.

33. Pugh, "A First Canoe Expedition."

34. S. G. Browne to his family, 30 December 1938, Stanley G. Browne Papers, New Milton, U.K. (hereafter SGB Papers). The lyrics are from Dick Best and Beth Best, eds., *Song Fest: Three Hundred Songs: Words and Music, including Folk Songs and Ballads, College Songs, Drinking Songs, Old Favorites, Parodies, Cowboy Songs, Chanties, Fiddle Tunes, Rounds, Spirituals, Etc.* (New York: Crown Publishers, 1945), 50–53.

35. A. G. Mill, "The Home within the Wilderness," *YQN* 103 (October 1935): 13–14. On links among the metaphor of "Heavenly Home" and "domesticated manliness" among nineteenth-century, middle-class evangelicals, see Leonore Davidoff and Catherine Hall, *Family Fortunes: Men and Women of the English Middle Class, 1780–1850* (London: Hutchinson, 1987). For this "domestic imaginary" in relation to codes of masculinity in colonial and military imaginaries, see Graham Dawson, *Soldier Heroes: British Adventure, Empire, and the Imagining of Masculinities* (London: Routledge, 1994), 63–64. Evangelical doctors, as we saw in chapter 2, drew on such codes of masculinity across "frontiers of domesticity" in and outside of Africa, suggesting that there was a questlike, masculine imaginary specific to tropical medicine.

36. CMC, *Report* (1918): 70.

37. "Infant Welfare, Yakusu," *YQN* 50 (March 1922): 4–6.

38. On shepherds, see CMC, *Report* (1904): 8; on "Fafa," see Smith, *Yakusu*, 80. For a domestic making his master "his adoptive *bwana*" [master] in a Belgian colonial memoir, see Mamba, *Les derniers crocos* (Brussels: Editions de l'Expansion Crocos, 1934), 89.

39. "The Other Side of the Screen," *YQN* 129 (July 1942): 13–14.

40. "The Elf's Progress," *YQN* 128 (April 1942): 13; *YQN* 133 (July 1943): 18; and *YQN* 134 (October 1943): 14.

41. L. Chesterman, "A Unique Dinner Party," *YQN* 52 (October 1922): 6–7.

42. E. R. Millman, "Their First Tea Party," *YQN* 86 (July 1931): 2–5.

43. The *YQN*, first published in 1908, was by 1915—with its pink cover, a floral, banana design, and anecdotal, whimsical vignettes of mission life—under the editorial control of the mission matriarch herself; indeed, Mrs. Millman's writing best typifies this style.

44. "Children Specially Supported," *YQN* 11 (March 1911): 6–7.

45. Ruth M. Slade, *English-Speaking Missions in the Congo Independent State (1878–1908)* (Brussels: ARSOM, 1958), 182.

46. Smith, *Yakusu*, 81; K. C. Parkinson, "A Visitor and the School," *YQN* 78 (July 1929): 10; Mrs. Millman to Miss Bowser, n.d., received 23 October 1935, Millman file, BMSA; and M. Chesterman, "The Junior Hopes to Visit England," *YQN* 105 (April 1936).

47. A missionary household was to become pulpit, laboratory, chapel, and school at Yakusu.

Compare Hansen, *Distant Companions,* 69; and "spatial and social segregation" in T. O. Beidelman, *Colonial Evangelism: A Socio-Historical Study of an East African Mission at the Grassroots* (Bloomington: Indiana University Press, 1982), 13, 70. On colonial bungalows, see "Africa, 1880–1940," in *The Bungalow: The Production of a Global Culture,* Anthony D. King (London: Routledge and Kegan Paul, 1984), 193–223.

48. Anne Summers, *Angels and Citizens: British Women as Military Nurses, 1854–1914* (London: Routledge and Kegan Paul, 1988), 3. See, too, Leonore Davidoff, "Mastered for Life: Servant and Wife in Victorian and Edwardian England," *Journal of Social History* 7 (1974): 406–28.

49. C. P. Williams, " 'Not Quite Gentlemen': An Examination of 'Middling Class' Protestant Missionaries from Britain, c. 1850–1900," *Journal of Ecclesiastical History* 31 (1980): 301–15. BMS Candidate Papers (missionary application files) as well as class antagonisms evident in private missionary letters suggest that most were of lower-middle-class backgrounds. Some were solidly middle class and some working class, however. Class competition could be fierce. Mrs. Millman objected to the arrival of single women missionaries in the 1920s; implicit in her objections were their working-class backgrounds. On the class backgrounds of some single women missionaries, see interview with Dorothy Daniel (raised in London's East End; a seamstress before her nurse training), Corse Staunton, 11 June 1991; and BMS Candidate Papers of Rose Gee (sample maker of ladies' underclothes before being trained as a nurse); Dorothy James (certified schoolteacher); E. N. Whitmore (attended the Horley Boarding School for Girls until age thirteen; father, a purser on a liner, had disappeared at the time of her birth); and Gertruida Reiling (daughter of a Dutch farmer), BMSA. Mrs. Millman also insisted on formal dress in white for tea at "the front" of her home on the riverbank. Some missionaries grew to hate the class airs that went with this obligatory daily ritual; some adored it. Nora Carrington, Salisbury, July 1990 and 8 June 1991; Mary Fagg, Thornham, 11–12 November 1990; Mali Browne, New Milton, 5 June 1991; and Dorothy Daniel, Corse Staunton, 11 June 1991. Class tensions seem to have increased with medicalization in the 1920s. The more well-to-do Chestermans (C. C. became a "Sir") arrived and built their "Chestermansion" with, as photos attest, a grand living room. Some of the tensions that swirled around the presence of the well-educated Brownes at Yakusu seem to have also related to class. (On the social origins of BMS missionaries in nineteenth-century Jamaica, see Catharine Hall, "White Visions, Black Lives: The Free Villages of Jamaica," *History Workshop Journal,* no. 36 [1993]: 100–132). For a sensitive, illuminating treatment on S. G. Browne and the 1950s controversy over his medical administration at Yakusu and within the BMS, see Brian Stanley, *The History of the Baptist Missionary Society, 1792–1992* (Edinburgh: T. and T. Clark, 1992), 356–63, 400.

50. [Mrs. Palmer], *Yalemba Monthly Letter,* 4 June 1924, BMSA.

51. Male nursing students included many previous missionary "boys." There were four out of five in 1935; seven out of thirteen in 1937; six out of seven in 1939; three out of seven in 1941; two out of twelve in 1943; one out of thirteen in 1945; seven out of twenty-three in 1947; five out of twenty-one in 1949; one out of four in 1951; three out of twenty-nine in 1953; six out of fifteen in 1955; and two out of twenty-one in 1957 (Student Record Cards, 1935–57, HDO, Yakusu).

52. The quotation is from Summers, *Angels and Citizens,* 47. See also Mary Poovey, *Uneven Developments: The Ideological Work of Gender in Mid-Victorian England* (London: Virago Press, 1989); Eva Gamarnikow, "Sexual Division of Labour: The Case of Nursing," in *Femi-*

nism and Materialism, ed. Annette Kuhn and AnnMarie Wolpe (London: Routledge and Kegan Paul, 1978), 96–213; and Pierre Guiral and Guy Thuillier, *La vie quotidienne des domestiques en France au XIXe siècle* (Paris: Hachette, 1978).

53. See, for example, A. F. Walls, " 'The Heavy Artillery of the Missionary Army': The Domestic Importance of the Nineteenth-Century Medical Missionary," in *The Church and Healing,* ed. W. J. Sheils (Oxford: Oxford University Press, 1982), 287–97.

54. On "boys" as injectionists, see Lloyd, *In Dwarf Land,* 208; and on the ambivalence of "boys," see Mamba, *Les derniers crocos.* The representation of master-servant relations changed with the arrival of Belgian women from the 1920s as masters and writers; compare Detry, *A Stanleyville;* and the books of Marie-Louise Comeliau. There was a sense of crisis over domestic help in the Belgian Africa of the 1950s when affording more than one became more difficult (two were still considered necessary for a couple posted *en brousse,* so that one could accompany the man on his travels). An advice manual for colonial women also encouraged discipline ("Be demanding"); cartoonlike pictures showed a lazy M. Molitor, asleep while ironing (*La femme au Congo: conseils aux partantes* [Brussels: n.p., (1958?)], 84–85).

55. Kathryn Hulme, *The Nun's Story* (London: Pan Books, 1956), 116, 114, 117. The arrival of these movie stars at Yakusu were the fairy tales of missionaries of the 1950s, much like Belgian royalty had been three decades before (Mali Browne, New Milton, 5 June 1991; and multiple photographs in the SGB Papers).

56. It will lead to a cross, therefore, among Dan Crawford, Mikhail Bakhtin, and what minstrelsy historian Eric Lott has called "love and theft." See Crawford, *Thinking Black,* 371; Mikhail Bakhtin, *Rabelais and His World,* trans. Hélène Iswolsky (Bloomington: Indiana University Press, 1984), 14, 79; and Lott, *Love and Theft.* On boy-to-nurse career patterns elsewhere, see Ralph A. Austen and Rita Headrick, "Equatorial Africa under Colonial Rule," in *History of Central Africa, Volume Two,* ed. David Birmingham and Phyllis Martin (London: Longman, 1983), 69. On nursing as a prestigious, though strained, position in colonial Zaire, see Willy De Craemer and Renée C. Fox, *The Emerging Physician: A Sociological Approach to the Development of a Congolese Medical Profession* (Stanford, Calif.: Hoover Institution on War, Revolution, and Peace, 1968); and Nancy Rose Hunt, "Letter-Writing, Nursing Men, and Bicycles in the Belgian Congo: Notes towards the Social Identity of a Colonial Category," in *Paths toward the Past: African Historical Essays in Honor of Jan Vansina,* ed. Robert Harms et al. (Atlanta, Ga.: African Studies Association Press, 1994). The gendering of nursing as male in much of sub-Saharan Africa prior to World War II needs comparative study. In most British colonies in sub-Saharan Africa, nurses were male until the Second World War, when explicit efforts began to regender the work as female; the same seems to have been the case for francophone Africa, at least in the Ivory Coast and French Equatorial Africa (AEF). Although nurse training for women and girls began only in the 1940s in most settings, they received training as midwives from the 1920s in Kenya, Uganda, and Sudan. See Ahmed Bayoumi, *The History of Sudan Health Services* (Nairobi: Kenya Literature Bureau, 1979); Danielle Domergue-Cloarec, *Politique coloniale française et réalités coloniales: La santé en Côte d'Ivoire, 1905–1958* (Paris: Académie des Sciences d'Outre-Mer, 1986); Gold Coast Colony, *The Training of Nurses in the Gold Coast* (Accra: Government Printing Department, 1947); Rita Headrick, *Colonialism, Health, and Illness in French Equatorial Africa, 1885–1935* (Atlanta, Ga.:

African Studies Association, 1994); Simon Ndirangu, *A History of Nursing in Kenya* (Nairobi: Kenya Literature Bureau, 1982); Ralph Schram, *A History of the Nigerian Health Services* (Ibadan, Nigeria: Ibadan University Press, 1971); and Megan Vaughan, *Curing Their Ills: Colonial Power and African Illness* (Stanford, Calif.: Stanford University Press, 1991). On nursing as female in South Africa, see Shula Marks, *Divided Sisterhood: Race, Class, and Gender in the South African Nursing Profession* (New York: St. Martin's Press, 1994).

57.   This was an immense genre, and many such schoolbooks are in local languages. See, for example, Charles Spire, *Conseils d'hygiène aux indigènes* (Brussels: Ministère des Colonies, 1922); William Millman, *Hygiène tropicale pour les écoles. Njaso ya Bosasu*, Fr. trans. Henri Anet (London: Bible Translation and Literature Society, 1921); E. R. Millman and William Millman, *A Mothercraft Manual for Senior Girls and Newly Married Women in Africa* (London: Carey Press for the Christian Literature Society, 1929); and the numerous *fichier* cards in the analytic card catalog at the Bibliothèque Africaine, Brussels. The table manners and cutlery tradition continues in manuals published by Zaire's Catholic press; see *Kujua Kuishi katika Watu Wengine* (Lubumbashi: Editions St.-Paul Afrique, 1989), 33–37. On the restructuring of Congolese space during sleeping sickness campaigns, see Maryinez Lyons, *The Colonial Disease: A Social History of Sleeping Sickness in Northern Zaire, 1900–1940* (Cambridge: Cambridge University Press, 1992).

58.   Quotation from Nicholas Thomas, "Sanitation and Seeing: The Creation of State Power in Early Colonial Fiji," *Comparative Studies in Society and History* 32 (1990): 149–70, esp. 160. On the early-nineteenth-century evangelical emphasis on moral hygiene and domestic purity, as well as twentieth-century social hygiene or eugenics in Britain, see Frank Mort, *Dangerous Sexualities: Medico-Moral Politics in England since 1830* (London: Routledge and Kegan Paul, 1987). This time lag in the circulation of ideas among metropole and colony indicates why quaint *YQN* vignettes about reformed cannibals may have found avid readers among British mission supporters, who were likely also active in metropolitan social hygiene (eugenic) movements directed at the urban poor. On such evangelical transpositions, see Jean Comaroff and John Comaroff, "Home-Made Hegemony: Modernity, Domesticity, and Colonialism in South Africa," in *African Encounters with Domesticity*, ed. Karen Tranberg Hansen (New Brunswick, N.J.: Rutgers University Press, 1992).

59.   On the word *soap*, see Georges Vigarello, *Le propre et le sale, L'hygiène du corps depuis le Moyen Age* (Paris: Seuil, 1985), 183. Quotations are from CMC, *Report* (1918): 70. The proximity of a British-operated, Huileries du Congo Belge (Unilever) soap-producing factory site to Yakusu likely increased this fascination with—and access to—soap. This site at Elisabetha (now Lokutu) was not far downriver, and Yakusu's missionaries had friendly ties with the British agents working there. On Unilever soap production and advertising, see Timothy Burke, *Lifebuoy Men, Lux Women: Commodification, Consumption, and Cleanliness in Modern Zimbabwe* (Durham, N.C.: Duke University Press, 1996).

60.   Norbert Elias quoted an 1859 English text to make this point in his *La civilisation des moeurs*, 144, 179–83.

61.   Davidoff, "Mastered for Life," 413; and Leonore Davidoff, "Class and Gender in Victorian England," in *Sex and Class in Women's History*, ed. Judith L. Newton, Mary P. Ryan, and Judith R. Walkowitz (London: Routledge and Kegan Paul, 1983), 23.

62. W. Holman Bentley, *Pioneering on the Congo* (London: Religious Tract Society, 1900), 287.

63. Walter Henry Stapleton, in *Missionary Herald*, May 1898, 261.

64. Mama Tula recalled that Salamo was from the riverain and Lokele village of Yafolo, adding that she learned this in class; Pastor Lofolata recalled her as being a girl from the Lokele-BaMbole or Foma village of Lolo (Tata Bafoya Bamanga, with Mama Tula, Yakusu, 25 November 1989; Mama Tula, Yakusu, 14 March 1989, from fieldnotes; and meeting with former Yakusu women students, organized by Mama Basuli Damali, Kisangani, 25 January 1990).

65. Roses were an important metaphor for domesticity at Yakusu, just as gardens were in Victorian England. Yakusu was renowned in Belgian circles for its rose gardens ("The Girls' School," *YQN* 34 [March 1917]: 10–11; Davidoff and Hall, *Family Fortunes*, 373; and Detry, *A Stanleyville*, 99). One missionary to the Congo commented, "We must teach these people to appreciate beauty. They call roses weeds" (see CMC, *Report* [1918]: 72).

66. On the colonial equation of slave woman with polygynous wife, see my "Noise over Camouflaged Polygamy, Colonial Morality Taxation, and a Woman-Naming Crisis in Belgian Africa," *Journal of African History* 32 (1991): 471–94.

67. Martin Green, "The Robinson Crusoe Story," in *Imperialism and Juvenile Literature*, ed. Jeffrey Richards (Manchester: Manchester University Press, 1989), 34–52, esp. 35; C. C. Chesterman, "My Man Sunday: How a Congo Houseboy Became a Conqueror of the Dread Diseases That Ravaged His People," *Reader's Digest* 51 (September 1947): 95–100; and W. L. Chesterman, "Yenga, Sunday Boy," *YQN* 59 (July 1924): 8b–c. For other Boy Sunday versions, see C. C. Chesterman, "Tropical Trail," Presidential Address to the Hunterian Society, 16 October 1967, 25, Lofts Papers, Barton-on-Sea; Raymond Holmes to Dr. Chesterman, 20 November 1941, Holmes file, BMSA; and Jessie Powell, "A Staff for Your Journey, Baptist Medical Missions, 1901–1951, A Pageant-Play," London, 1951, 48–65, Box H/57, BMSA.

68. Chesterman, "My Man Sunday"; and Powell, "A Pageant-Play."

69. Powell, "A Pageant-Play." A stock Belgian colonial hygiene/servant joke, for instance, which I heard from former Belgian colonials in 1988, was about a Congolese cook who peeled hard-boiled eggs with dirty hands, but tried to please his Madame by licking them clean.

70. E. Alexander Powell, *The Map That Is Half Unrolled: Equatorial Africa from the Indian Ocean to the Atlantic* (London: John Long, 1925). On European, especially francophone and Belgian humor, see, too, Pieterse, *White on Black*; *Zaïre, 1885–1985*; *Négripub: L'Image des Noirs dans la publicité* (Paris: Somogy, 1994); Yann Holo, "Les Représentations des africains dans l'imagerie enfantine," in *L'Autre et Nous: "Scènes et Types,"* ed. Pascal Blanchard et al. (Paris: Syros and ACHAC, 1995), 201–4; and (on comedic valet theatrical traditions) F. Ramirez and C. Rolot, *Histoire du cinéma colonial au Zaïre, au Rwanda, et au Burundi* (Tervuren: MRAC, 1985), esp. 348.

71. Patrick Brantlinger, "Victorians and Africans: The Genealogy of the Myth of the Dark Continent," *Critical Inquiry* 12 (1985): 218. I first heard about "thinking black"—the title of Dan Crawford's book—from Nora Carrington, a former Yakusu missionary, in 1990. She recalled two books that had been influential on her thinking. She criticized one, H. Sutton Smith's *Yakusu*, for denigrating Lokele and their canoes. She evoked Crawford's *Thinking Black* in speaking about cultural sensitivity, the need for missionaries to try to understand how Africans make sense of their worlds. Mrs. Carrington had joined her husband, John, at Yakusu in

the late 1930s, and they did not leave until the 1970s; they became part, therefore, of a post–Second World War and a postindependence generation of missionaries, some of whom were more self-consciously open to cultural relativism than those who had preceded them.

72. C. C. Chesterman, "Men or Animals?" *YQN* 93 (April 1930): 11.

73. Crawford, *Thinking Black*, 400, 111–12, 330, 334. The last quote, too, is from Crawford, 340; compare the 1916 quote regarding Chief Bonjoma in chapter 3, page 121.

74. Pieterse, *White on Black*, 114–19, esp. 119.

75. "Thinking black" references include Ennals, News Sheet, no. 16, 23 December 1922, JFC Papers—Salisbury; "Bible Schools," *YQN* 83 (October 1930), 1; "A Native Story," *YQN* 73 (April 1928): 20; and A. G. Mill, "Through a Glass Darkly," *YQN* 65 (January 1926): 22–24. See chapter 3, note 71.

76. John Carrington to Dear Friends, Yakusu Letter no. 3, 20 February 1940, JFC Papers, BMSA; and "Beginnings in the Bokumu," unsigned sermon notes [by W. H. Ford?], n.d., JFC Papers—Salisbury. The sermon notes are in English; they were written as a sermon for delivery in Britain during a missionary furlough.

77. Dening, *Mr. Bligh's Bad Language*, 266.

78. CMC, *Report* (1909): 33–35.

79. Smith, *Yakusu*, 80.

80. One senses a stiffening in master-servant relations in the 1950s as full-time servants replaced the earlier schoolboy system. Christmas gifts and other benefits became carefully regulated (Staff Meeting Minutes, 3 August 1949, 27 December 1949, 3 July 1950, 3 December 1953, District Pastor's Office, Yakusu).

81. "Answers to Correspondents," *YQN* 47 (January 1921): 15. Missionaries to the Congo were required to pay "all boys used as personal boys, house-boys, cooks, wash-boys, or garden-boys" out of their own pocket (Western Sub-Committee Minutes, 14 January 1896, Book no. 10, 88, BMSA; and W. H. Ennals, "Help in the Missionary Household," *YQN* 145 [February 1950]: 17–19).

82. Nora Carrington criticized the practice of missionary flogging at Yakusu (Nora Carrington, Salisbury, July 1990).

83. Ennals, "Help in the Missionary Household"; BMS, Yakusu Annual Medical Report, 1954, HDO, Yakusu; Nora Carrington, Salisbury, July 1990.

84. This spot was known in missionary memories as "the front." See note 49 above.

85. Tata Bafoya Bamanga, with Mama Tula, Yakusu, 27 November 1989. The Lokangu quotations come from my fieldnotes.

86. Papa Boshanene, Yakusu, 24 February 1989. The interview took place in the very house that had previously been the largest mission home, built originally for Dr. Chesterman, and known in mission circles as the "Chestermansion" (G. C. Ennals, "Wedding Bells," *YQN* 69 [January 1927]: 7).

87. Pastor Lofolata, Yalolia, 10 April 1989, from fieldnotes.

88. Tata Bafoya Bamanga, with Mama Tula, Yakusu, 27 November 1989.

89. E. R. Millman, "Their First Tea Party," *YQN* 86 (July 1931): 3–4; G. C. Wilkerson, "The First Lisongomi in the Bamangas," *YQN* 86 (July 1931): 9–11; K. C. Parkinson, "A Contrast: Two

Schools in the Fomas," *YQN* 97 (April 1934): 2–6; E. R. Millman, "A Man and His Wife," *YQN* 101 (April 1935): 2–3; and "At Easter Weekend," *YQN* 147[b] (September 1952): 11–14.

90. Tata Alikuwa, Yainyongo-Romée, 18 September 1989. Italics added.

91. All previous quotations are from Tata Tula, with Tula Rogier, Yakusu, 2 and 4 November 1989.

92. The expression is from 'Biyi Bandele-Thomas, *The Sympathetic Undertaker and Other Dreams* (London: Heinemann, 1991), 20.

93. E. R. Millman, "Getting Ready," *YQN* 65 (January 1926): 10; and E. R. Millman, "The Royal Visit to Yakusu," *YQN* 93 (April 1933).

94. Tata Bafoya Bamanga, with Mama Tula, Yakusu, 27 November 1989; and Tata Tula, with Tula Rogier, Yakusu, 2, 4 November 1989. Italics added.

95. CMC, *Report* (1921): 175. Unlike in other mission contexts, BMS missionaries working in the Congo were not able to keep their children with them. The maternal idiom had an emotional depth; see CMC, *Report* (1918): 109–15. Compare Patricia Grimshaw, " 'Christian Woman, Pious Wife, Faithful Mother, Devoted Missionary': Conflicts in Roles of American Missionary Women in Nineteenth-Century Hawaii," *Feminist Studies* 9 (1983): 489–521.

96. E. R. Millman, "The Visit of Governor and Madame Henry," *YQN* 40 (October 1918): 15. Company hawkers were selling soap in local markets by the mid-1930s (E. R. Millman, "Our Women," *YQN* 108 [January 1937]: 2–5). On "White Mama," see L. Gwendoline Pugh, "The Girls' School," *YQN* 48 (July 1921): 7–9.

97. CMC, *Report* (1911): 66–68, esp. 68; CMC, *Report* (1921): 180, 169–70. It is unlikely that Edith Millman also had housing for boys, though remaining missionary houses have old "boyeries" out back.

98. Mama Yaluani, Yainyongo-Romée, 1 October 1989; Mama Bokenge Limengo, with Mama Tula Sophie, Yakoso, 30 November 1989; Mama Machuli Georgine, Kisangani, 2 December 1989; Mama Asha Marguerite, Kisangani, 3 December 1989; Mama Machuli Bolendela, Kisangani, 3 December 1989; and meeting with former Yakusu women students, organized by Mama Damali Basuli, Kisangani, 25 January 1990. See also A. Bean, "The Fence," *YQN* 154 (December 1956): 5–8.

99. CMC, *Report* (1902): 78–79.

100. Mrs. Millman to Miss Bowser, n.d., received 5 December 1934, Millman file, BMSA; and Nancy Rose Hunt, " 'Single Ladies on the Congo': Protestant Missionary Tensions and Voices," *International Women's Studies Forum* 13 (1990): 395–403.

101. CMC, *Report* (1921): 179, 80.

102. Mama Machuli Bolendela, Kisangani, 3 December 1989. Italics added.

103. All previous quotes from ibid. People express the passage of time in Lokele, BaMbole, and Swahili with *teee, tiii,* and *ti ti ti,* varying the rhythm to enhance the story. Italics added.

104. L. M. Fagg, "The Training of Pupil-Midwives," *YQN* 149 (February 1953): 18.

105. Mama Machuli Georgine, Kisangani, 2 December 1989.

106. Mama Machuli Bolendela, Kisangani, 3 December 1989. She compared the world wars with the battle fought between BaTambatamba (Zanzibari) forces and Belgian-directed troops at the Romée River on May 22, 1893; see chapter 1. Italics added.

107. Mama Machuli Georgine, Kisangani, 2 December 1989. Italics added.

108. Davidoff, "Class and Gender," 21, 23.

109. Davidoff, "Mastered for Life," 413, 425.

110. Missionaries alone did not determine these pathways. The interests of local Congolese subjects were critical, especially since contact with mission life, and its associated clothing and food, seemed to pose risks to the fertility of women and their marriages in the early twentieth century. Although some chiefs turned over their daughters to the Millmans from 1916 so they would learn to iron and sew, the Lokele and their neighbors, as we shall see, considered contact with the sick more dangerous for females than for males. It is not clear who did laundry.

111. Mamiwata in popular paintings from Kisangani, like elsewhere in Zaire, entice with watches and alluring poses. Yet local people speak about Mamiwata as a water creature who drowns children in the river and causes infant convulsions that make them die (Tienebe-Mendierame Mangoni, "De quelques aspects de la pathologie mentale dans la sous-région de Kisangani: le cas des Lokele et des Wagenya [Contribution à l'Ethnopsychiatrie]" [Ph.D. diss., University of Kisangani, 1978]). Mamiwata as mermaid figures are likened to Bonama and Ndiya, just as the crocodiles swimming in the BaTambatamba's swimming hole and the deadly crocodile that Chesterman had shot in 1934 were. When Mamiwata mermaid figures were added as equivalents to preexisting rainbow and crocodile spirits is difficult to date, though the overlay is complete in postcolonial Congolese testimony. A Yakusu domestic servant became afraid of his Madami master, Mrs. Carrington, when she was outside combing her long hair one day, likely in the 1940s or 1950s (Nora Carrington, Salisbury, 8 June 1991). Local Zairians also told me that they wondered if the asexuality of unmarried missionary women was a hoax: "Didn't they hide their babies in Europe?"

112. A history of colonial toilets and toilet duties has yet to be written, though *who* performed such work for colonials is key to mapping the kinds of colonial deference rituals and gender imaging that I adumbrate here. See Bandele-Thomas's depiction of a night soil man in his novel, *Sympathetic Undertaker*.

113. C. C. Chesterman, "The Ba-infirmier," *YQN* 61 (January 1925): 5–9.

114. A. Bean, "The Fence," *YQN* 12 (December 1956): 5–8.

115. Daniel Miller, ed., *Unwrapping Christmas* (Oxford: Clarendon Press, 1993), 11.

116. The then all-male missionaries spoke of their determination, "though without a lady's presence," to not be without Christmas puddings and mincemeat (Smith, *Yakusu*, 249).

117. "Nelly," *YQN* 11 (June 1911): 2–3; and Ennals, Newssheet, 22 March 1924, 24c, JFC Papers—Salisbury. See, too, "Christmas at Yakusu," *YQN* 26 (March 1915): 1–12.

118. Claude Lévi-Strauss, "Father Christmas Executed," in *Unwrapping Christmas,* ed. Daniel Miller (Oxford, Clarendon Press, 1993), 41, 44.

119. "Christmas at Yakusu," 11.

120. Turkey is a recent addition to British Christmas dinners; see J. Pimlott, *An Englishman's Christmas: A Social History* (Atlantic Highlands, N.J.: Humanities Press, 1978).

121. Smith, *Yakusu*, 53–54.

122. Adam Kuper, "The English Christmas and the Family: Time Out and Alternative Realities," in *Unwrapping Christmas,* 157–75, esp. 160. On Christmas in the Caribbean, see Robert Dirks, "Slaves' Holiday," *Natural History* 84, 10 (1975): 82–86; "Festivals, Carnival, Holidays, and JanKanoo," in *After Africa: Extracts from British Travel Accounts and Journals of the*

Seventeenth, Eighteenth, and Nineteenth Centuries concerning the Slaves, Their Manners, and Customs in the British West Indies, Roger D. Abrahams and John F. Szwed, eds. (New Haven, Conn.: Yale University Press, 1983); "Christmas and Carnival on St. Vincent," in Roger D. Abrahams, *The Man-of-Words in the West Indies: Performance and the Emergence of Creole Culture* (Baltimore, Md.: Johns Hopkins University Press, 1983); and Robert Dirks, *The Black Saturnalia: Conflict and Its Ritual Expression on British West Indian Slave Plantations* (Gainesville: University Press of Florida, 1987). On Christmas in Britain and elsewhere, see Tony Bennett, ed., *Christmas: A Case Study,* vol. units 1/2 of *Popular Culture: Themes and Issues 1* (Milton Keynes, U.K.: Open University Press, 1981); and Miller, *Unwrapping Christmas.* A literature on hospital and military topsy-turvy Christmas meals—officers and/or doctors serving the common soldiers or nurses—is harder to come by, though these survive in the United Kingdom and Canada; see, for example, "The Christmas Entertainment: A New Idea for Hospitals," *Nursing Mirror and Midwives' Journal,* 21 November 1931, 151.

123. Bakhtin, *Rabelais,* 14, 79.

124. [C. C. Chesterman], "Christmas Condensed" *YQN* 50 (March 1922): 11–13.

125. Ennals, News Sheet, no. 17, 20 January 1923, 72, JFC Papers—Salisbury. In at least one year in the early 1920s, this "Party where Whites serve Blacks" was worthy of a photograph; the event was held on a mission lawn with wicker chairs arranged around several tables ("Party where Whites serve Blacks," Bush album no. 2, n.d., photograph collection, BMSA). Other photos in the same album carried dates of 1922. One photograph in the third Bush album, "Tea, Christmas Day—1922," showed all the missionaries outside, dressed in white, with two young Congolese girls present; another in the same album was of "Christmas sports and festivities—the greasy pole."

126. Ennals, News Sheet, no. 24, 22 March 1924, 24 b, JFC Papers—Salisbury.

127. Doris Moyles to My dear Friends, circular letter, 24 January 1937, JFC Papers—Salisbury; and John F. Carrington, "Christmas Greetings from Yakusu," circular letter, 23 December 1938, Box 1, John F. Carrington Papers, BMSA.

128. [C. C. Chesterman], "Christmas Condensed."

129. Stanley G. Browne, 31 December 1936, SGB Papers.

130. Ibid.

131. Stanley G. Browne to Father, 31 December 1937 [1938], SGB Papers.

132. Ibid.

133. Bakhtin, *Rabelais,* 12. On Bakhtin's "troublesome *folkloric* approach," see Peter Stallybrass and Allon White, *The Politics and Poetics of Transgression* (Ithaca, N.Y.: Cornell University Press, 1986), 26. On the troublesome word *folk* in African studies, see Karin Barber, "Popular Arts in Africa," *African Studies Review* 30 (1987): 1–78, 113–32.

134. I owe the insight on Africa as the lower half of the human body to a conversation with René Devisch in 1990. On gothic, "amorous bondage," see Joan Dayan, "Amorous Bondage: Poe, Ladies, and Slaves," *American Literature* 66 (1994): 239–73.

135. Bakhtin, *Rabelais,* 21, 411, 14.

136. "The Other Side of the Screen," *YQN* 129 (July 1942): 14.

137. A. G. Mill, "The Home within the Wilderness," *YQN* 103 (October 1935); and S. G. Browne, "Mrs. Ethel C. Mill," *YQN* 154 (December 1956): 14–15.

138. Natalie Zemon Davis, *Society and Culture in Early Modern France* (Stanford, Calif.: Stanford University Press, 1975), 103.

139. Henry Louis Gates Jr., *The Signifying Monkey: A Theory of Afro-American Literary Criticism* (New York: Oxford University Press, 1988).

140. Cannibalism was not an important theme in anglophone writing about Africa until the mid–nineteenth century (Brantlinger, "Victorians and Africans," 203). Henry Morton Stanley's writing, including *Through the Dark Continent* (1878; reprint, New York: Dover Publications, 1988) and *In Darkest Africa* (New York: Charles Scribner's Sons, 1890), helped popularize the theme. British Protestant missionary accounts of Congolese societies that would only trade ivory for people "they could eat," others that bought slaves and marketed them as cooked human flesh, and yet others horrified by the idea of strangers who ate human flesh are too pervasive to be dismissed as European whimsy. European fantasy, Congolese sorcery idioms, and the large semantic range of "eating" in Congolese languages were certainly at play in the conversations these writers report having had with Congolese. So, too, was a harsh history of raiding and trading of human strangers and unwanted persons as—the metaphor that riddles historical interpretation returns—meat. See, for example, Bentley, *Pioneering on the Congo*, 94–95, 101, 210–14, 254–63, 270–71. On Stanley's mixed reputation, see Felix Driver, "Henry Morton Stanley and His Critics: Geography, Exploration, and Empire," *Past and Present*, no. 133 (November 1991). Henry Ward's *Five Years with the Congo Cannibals* (London: Chatto and Windus, 1891) was a popular account in great demand; see Pieterse, *White on Black*, 117. Browne and his wife, Mali, served at Yakusu from the late 1930s through the late 1950s. They were fond of describing how Stanley Browne had been inspired to become a missionary after he read Bentley's *Pioneering in the Congo*, virtually required reading for BMS missionaries in the Congo. An incident when Bentley had entrusted a white baby to a "cannibal's" arms, only to watch the infant be returned safely if "a little grubby," was the inspirational episode for the young surgeon (whom we will meet again, especially in chapter 5). Mrs. Browne told me this story over breakfast in her home in England in 1990; Mali Browne, New Milton, 5 June 1991. The same account is in Browne's effusive biography (Sylvia Duncan and Peter Duncan, *Bonganga: Experiences of a Missionary Doctor* [London: Odhams Press, 1958]).

141. Among the best iconographic sources are Pieterse, *White on Black*; and *Zaïre, 1885–1985*; on advertising soap, chocolate, and bicycles, see *Négripub: L'Image des Noirs*.

142. On Bamboula figures, see Holo, "Les Représentations des africains dans l'imagerie enfantine."

143. On colonies as "places of excess," see Joan Dayan, "Paul Gilroy's Slaves, Ships, and Routes: The Middle Passage as Metaphor," *Research in African Literatures* 27 (1996): 8.

4 Nurses and Bicycles

1. Gladys C. Parris to Miss Bowser, Yaongama, 23 April 1932, in G. Owen file, BMSA.

2. Megan Vaughan, "Health and Hegemony: Representation of Disease and the Creation of the Colonial Subject in Nyasaland," in *Contesting Colonial Hegemony: State and Society in Africa and India*, ed. Dagmar Engels and Shula Marks (London: British Academic Press, 1994), 173.

3. Nicholas Thomas, *Entangled Objects: Exchange, Material Culture, and Colonialism in the Pacific* (Cambridge: Harvard University Press, 1991).

4. Gayatri Spivak, "Can the Subaltern Speak?" in *Marxism and the Interpretation of Culture,* ed. Cary Nelson and Lawrence Grossberg (Urbana: University of Illinois Press, 1988).

5. Ibid.

6. Carlo Ginzburg, *The Cheese and the Worms: The Cosmos of a Sixteenth-Century Miller* (Baltimore, Md.: Johns Hopkins University Press, 1980).

7. Jean-Luc Vellut, "La médicine européenne dans l'Etat Indépendant du Congo (1885–1908)," in *Analecta de réalisations médicales en Afrique centrale, 1885–1985,* ed. P. G. Janssens, M. Kivits, and J. Vuylsteke (Brussels: Fondation Roi Baudouin, 1991), 76; Terence Ranger, "Godly Medicine: The Ambiguities of Medical Mission in Southeast Tanzania, 1900–1945," *Social Science and Medicine* 15B (1981): 261–77; and Jean Comaroff, "The Diseased Heart of Africa: Medicine, Colonialism, and the Black Body," in *Knowledge, Power, and Practice: The Anthropology of Medicine and Everyday Life,* ed. Margaret Lock and Shirley Lindenbaum (Berkeley: University of California Press, 1993).

8. An early consideration investigated missionary medicine and maternal and infant welfare as a largely female, noncoercive domain (Deborah Gaitskell, "Women, Religion, and Medicine in Johannesburg between the Wars" (paper for the African History Seminar, School of Oriental and African Studies and Institute of Commonwealth Studies, University of London, 18 May 1983). Vaughan notes the high degree of "social engineering" involved in mission maternal and infant health work in Uganda (Vaughan, *Curing Their Ills: Colonial Power and African Illness* [Stanford, Calif.: Stanford University Press, 1991], 68). The record on midwifery and infant health initiatives and control is also different in Belgian Africa and British central Africa. Contrary to what Vaughan reports for the latter, the first major initiative in the Congo was by a mining company (not a mission community), and state welfare concerns began in the Congo during the interwar period (not after World War II); see Vaughan, *Curing Their Ills,* 65, 75.

9. The Belgian colonial *state,* as Jean-Luc Vellut has expressed it, "referred . . . only to an institution in the process of formation" (Vellut, "Articulations entre entreprises et Etat: Pouvoirs hégémoniques dans le bloc colonial belge [1908–1960]," in *Entreprises et entrepreneurs en Afrique [XIXe XXe siècles]* [Paris: l'Harmattan, 1983]: 51).

10. Bernard S. Cohn, *Colonialism and Its Forms of Knowledge: The British in India* (Princeton, N.J.: Princeton University Press, 1996).

11. W. Millman, "After Nearly Two Years," *YQN* 49 (November 1921): 1–3; E. R. Millman, "A Letter," *YQN* 49 (November 1921): 14; E. R. Millman, "Past and Present," *YQN* 57 (January 1924): 12; and W. H. Ennals, "A Highway Shall Be There," *YQN* 55 (July 1923): 2.

12. C. C. Chesterman, "A State Occasion," *YQN* 49 (November 1921): 3.

13. BMS Yakusu Annual Medical Report, 1921, Hospital Director's Office, Yakusu (hereafter HDO, Yakusu); and Maryinez Lyons, *The Colonial Disease: A Social History of Sleeping Sickness in Northern Zaire, 1900–1940* (Cambridge: Cambridge University Press, 1992).

14. The BMS was relieved that the state was willing to subsidize the costly drug expenses for sleeping sickness treatment; see MMA Committee Book, no. 7, 16 November 1920, 102–3, BMSA. On subsidy requirements for Assistance Médicale Indigène Bénévole, see Circulaire,

Hygiène no. 21, 7 September 1926, Congo Belge, *Recueil Mensuel des circulaires, instructions et ordres de service* (1926): 154–55.

15. "Hygiene and security of workers" legislation came into effect between 1921 and 1931 ("Considérations sur l'utilisation de la main-d'oeuvre au Congo belge," *Office International d'Hygiène Publique* 23 [1931]: 1627–51). Provincial variations are in Théodore Heyse, *Le Régime du Travail au Congo belge* (Brussels: Goemaere, Imprimeur du Roi, 1924). Some companies complained during the depression that state hygienic requirements were so expensive that they were seriously eroding their profits ("Personnel des Exploitations Agricoles," in "Rapport annuel sur la situation de l'agriculture," District de Stanleyville, RA/CB no. 8 [160], 1930, 25, AA).

16. BMS Yakusu Annual Medical Report, 1924, HDO, Yakusu.

17. C. C. Chesterman, "The Ba-infirmier," *YQN* 61 (January 1925): 5–9; and BMS Yakusu Annual Medical Report, 1929, HDO, Yakusu.

18. BMS Yakusu Annual Medical Reports, 1924–1929. These company dispensaries were listed as Yangambi (plantation), Traidiscore (industrial), Caefa (sawmill), and Belgika (plantation) (ibid., 1929). Chesterman explained to the BMS that these state- and company-subsidized dispensaries would not cost the mission society anything, and "will give us a very strong influence" (ibid., 1924).

19. C. C. Chesterman, "Resurgam," *YQN* 70[a] (April 1927): 2–3; and C. C. Chesterman, "Disciples of Aesculapius," *YQN* 77 (April 1929): 7–8. Grenfell went on to obtain the coveted "*assistant médical*" diploma, and by 1982, was living in Kinshasa. Before independence, he was *bourgemestre* of the Mangobo commune in Kisangani and *conseiller* of the Mouvement Nationale Congolaise, Lumumba Wing (MNC/L) in 1959; he served as a *député national* in 1960, a state minister in Patrice Lumumba's government, and as Président de la Province du Haut-Congo in June 1963 (see Benoît Verhaegen, "Preface," in *La vie de Disasi Makulo recueillie par son fils Makulo Akambu*, ed. Benoît Verhaegen, in *Notes, travaux, documents du CRIDE* 4 [Kisangani: Université de Kisangani, 1982]). This Disasi Makulo biography has been republished by Editions St. Paul, including as a Disasi Makulo comic book!

20. "Yakusu Boys at Government School in Stanleyville," *YQN* 72 (January 1928): 9; and K. C. Parkinson, "A Lisongomi at Yaokombo," *YQN* 85 (April 1931): 6–8.

21. Fifty had been founded by 1926, paid for by state, private, and *caisses de secteurs* funds; see R. Mouchet, "Notes sur les dispensaires ruraux de la Province Orientale," *ASBMT* 6 (1926): 145–60. Although a charitable organization was founded to help pay costs, the buildings continued to be paid for by the *caisse administrative des chefferies* funds in 1928. Maternities and midwives were envisaged; see A. de Meulemeester, "L'organisation des dispensaires ruraux de l'Oeuvre A.D.I.P.O. (Assistance aux Dispensaires Indigènes de la Province Orientale)," *Congo* 9 (1928): 1–12. When Médecin en Chef G. Trolli inspected some of these dispensaries, his "virulent" report created an uproar at the Ministry of Colonies, Brussels. He complained of a "gaspillage d'argent et bluff ridicule" (waste of money and ridiculous fraud), especially because Congolese were paying for the care received twice, once through the tax-produced customary *caisses* and again as patients. The ministry wanted the report suppressed, fearing the scandal that Trolli's words—"Nous trompons et volons l'Indigène" (We deceive the Native and steal from him)—might create ("Analyse du rapport Trolli," [1928?],

M.H. 45, H [4388] 35, "Hygiène en général," AA). On indirect rule in Province Orientale, see Crawford Young, *Politics in the Congo* (Princeton, N.J.: Princeton University Press, 1965), 130.

22. C. C. Chesterman, "A Call to Advance," *YQN* 94 (July 1933): 12–14.

23. BMS Yakusu Annual Medical Reports, 1934, 1948, HDO, Yakusu.

24. See A. Duren, "Quelques aspects de la vie médicale au Congo Belge," extract from *Le Scalpel* 2–5 (12, 19, 26 January and 2 February 1935); and G. Trolli, *Historique de l'assistance médicale aux indigènes du Congo Belge: Nouvelle méthode adoptée par FOREAMI, Résultats obtenus* (Brussels: Van Doosselaere, 1930). The founding of FOREAMI was critical in these shifts and this definition; see chapter 6.

25. W. H. Ennals, News Sheets, no. 22, 18 October 1923, and no. 24, 22 March 1924, John F. Carrington Papers, Salisbury, U.K. (hereafter JFC Papers—Salisbury).

26. C. C. Chesterman, "A Month's Joy Ride," *YQN* 95 (October 1933): 10.

27. BMS Yakusu Annual Medical Reports, 1935–1937, HDO, Yakusu; R. E. Holmes, "Medical Work in a Distant Tribe," *YQN* 104 (January 1936), 9–10; Stanley Browne to Harold, 25 March 1937, Stanley G. Browne Papers, New Milton, U.K. (hereafter SGB Papers); Stanley Browne to Dr. Chesterman, 27 January 1938; Stanley Browne to Dr. Chesterman, 25 November 1937; and Stanley Browne to Dr. Chesterman, 3 November 1937 (all Browne letters to Chesterman from S. G. Browne file, BMSA).

28. Edith Millman to Miss Bowser, 30 October 1933, Millman file, BMSA; and Stanley Browne to Harold, 25 March 1937, SGB Papers.

29. BMS Yakusu Annual Medical Report, 1927, HDO, Yakusu. Government grants paid for half of local expenditures in 1935, one third came from company payments and European patient fees, and approximately 17 percent came from Congolese patient fees and medicine sales (ibid., 1935).

30. For more on local shifts toward "foreign missions" and their effects on Yakusu's medical mission, see Nancy Rose Hunt, "Negotiated Colonialism: Domesticity, Hygiene, and Birth Work in the Belgian Congo" (Ph.D. diss., University of Wisconsin–Madison, 1992), chap. 3.

31. Stanley Browne to Ivy, 28 September 1938, SGB Papers; and R. E. Holmes, "Medical Work in a Distant Tribe," *YQN* 104 (January 1936).

32. R. E. Holmes, "The Building of Yaombole Dispensary," *YQN* 102 (July 1935): 16–18; and R. E. Holmes, "A Surprise Visit to a District Dispensary," *YQN* 97 (April 1934): 11–12.

33. C. C. Chesterman, "The Training and Employment of African Natives as Medical Assistants," *Proceedings of the Royal Society of Medicine* 25 (1931–1932), pt. 3:1067–76, esp. 1073.

34. Stanley Browne to Harold, 25 March 1937; and Stanley Browne to Father and all those left at 152, 6 September 1938 (both letters from SGB Papers).

35. R. E. Holmes, "Medical Work in a Distant Tribe," *YQN* 104 (January 1936). Some Turumbu (Olombo) sought their own dispensary, so they would no longer need to cross the river to reach one (W. H. Ennals, "The Visit of Mr. Hemmens of the Mission House to Our District," *YQN* 115 [October 1938]: 2–7, 23–25).

36. Stanley G. Browne, "The Training of Medical Auxiliaries in the Former Belgian Congo," *Lancet* 1 (19 May 1973): 1103–5.

37. Luise White, " 'They Could Make Their Victims Dull': Genders and Genres, Fantasies and Cures in Colonial Southern Uganda," *American Historical Review* 100 (1995): 1385 n. 24.

38. W. H. Ennals, "The Printed Page," *YQN* 76 (January 1929): 11–12; and W. H. Ennals, "The Year 1938 in Retrospect," *YQN* 117 (April 1939): 3. The assumption on readership dates to 1930 (W. H. Ennals, "Holding Forth the Word of Life," *YQN* 84 [January 1931]: 14–16).

39. Barbara Ann Yates, "Knowledge Brokers: Books and Publishers in Early Colonial Zaire," *History in Africa* 14 (1987): 321; William Millman, "Health Instruction in African Schools: Suggestions for a Curriculum," *Africa* 3 (1930): 484–99, esp. 489; and Browne, "Training of Medical Auxiliaries," 1104.

40. "A poetic conception of borrowing could also be a starting point for a rhetoric of lexical borrowing understood as a way of translating relationships of power and domination into discourse" (Johannes Fabian, "Scratching the Surface: Observations on the Poetics of Lexical Borrowing in Shaba Swahili," *Anthropological Linguistics* 24 [1982]: 39).

41. The term is, among others, Barbara Ann Yates's; see her "Knowledge Brokers."

42. [Filip Kwaita], "An Open Letter to the Home Church," *YQN* 77 (April 1929): 17–18.

43. R. E. Holmes, "Our Medical Work," *YQN* 92 (January 1933): 17–18. A prime example is a conversation between a Christian man and a kanga, written by a Yakusu teacher (see Baelongandi Joseph, Elève instituteur, "Tofenya" [Trouble], *Mboli ya Tengai* 217 [June 1930]). Punctuation has been added to *Mboli* translations for clarity.

44. C. C. Chesterman, "Disciples of Aesculapius," *YQN* 77 (April 1929): 8.

45. Labama H. Likenyule, "Lokasa loa Likenyule," *Mboli ya Tengai* 152 (August 1924): 2.

46. "Njaso ya Lisombo," *Mboli ya Tengai* 223 (1930): 7; and "Baenyeli ba basenji eoka ya likundu," *Mboli ya Tengai* 227 (1931). See, too, "Bewitching by the Ndoki: From a Native Preacher's Essay," *YQN* 85 (April 1931): 14.

47. Labama H. Likenyule, "Dispensaire Yasu nda Yaokombo" (Our Dispensary in Yaokombo), *Mboli ya Tengai* 295 (December 1931): 6.

48. Samwele Kamanga, "Bolimbi asotombolomo," *Mboli ya Tengai* 381 (May 1938): 6. Italics added.

49. Samwele Kamanga, "Lokasa loa Kamanga Samwele, Waluwa kenge etiwe," *Mboli ya Tengai* 310 (March 1935).

50. B. H. Tokwaulu, "Njaso ya Fengo," *Mboli ya Tengai* 193 (March 1928): 3–4.

51. B. John Siboko, "Fee ya Lisemoli lia Yeka Angene," *Mboli ya Tengai* 298 (March 1932): 6.

52. Ibid.

53. "Fetishism Again," *YQN* 27 (June 1915): 2–3; and "Extract from Diary of a Native Evangelist," *YQN* 34 (March 1917): 6–8. The same evangelist wrote to the priest asking him for soap.

54. W. H. Ennals, "The Open Book," *YQN* 72 (January 1928): 12–13.

55. "Lokasa loa Liita Infirmier," *Mboli ya Tengai* 213 (February 1930): 2. Italics added.

56. C. C. Chesterman, "Medical Itinerating on a Motor Bike," *YQN* 103 (October 1935): 17–19.

57. There were 947 bicycles in the Congo in 1925; 18,784 in 1929; 18,626 in 1933; 30,469 in 1937; and 52,206 in 1939. See Carlos Hauzeur de Fooz, *Un démi-siècle avec l'économie du Congo belge* (Brussels: n.p., 1957), 18. On the development of roads, use of Congolese labor, and road construction methods, see E. Devroey, *Le réseau routier au Congo belge et au Ruanda-Urundi* (Brussels: IRCB, 1939); and E. Devroey, *Nouveaux systèmes de pont métalliques pour les colonies et leur influence possible sur l'évolution des transports routiers au Congo belge et au Ruanda-Urundi* (Brussels: IRCB, 1947).

58. "Lokasa loa Victor Yenga," *Mboli ya Tengai* 291 (August 1931): 6–7.

59. Bamboli Cultuur Maatschappij (BCM) was founded in 1929 in Antwerp. By 1930, 979 hectares of BaMbole forest had been cleared and 755 planted with rubber and coffee. Concessions of 240 to 500 hectares were planned at Yahila, Yaleko, Yapehe, Yasendu, and Yatolema (*Recueil Financier* 37 [1930], t. 1:705). By 1938, Bamboli plantations were conspicuous, and factories for coffee, rubber, and palm oil were in place, as was a rice mill; by 1939, there were 1,770 hectares of coffee and rubber (*Recueil Financier* 47 [1940], t. 1:335–36). BCM hired its own doctor in 1948, which meant that Yakusu lost control of dispensaries at Yahila, Yaleko, Yapehe, Yasendu, Yaosenge, and Yatolema (BMS Yakusu Annual Medical Report, 1948, HDO, Yakusu).

60. BMS Yakusu Annual Medical Report, 1925, HDO, Yakusu; H. B. Parris, "Yaongama," *YQN* 57 (January 1924): 21–23; and Gladys Parris to Miss Bowser, 5 February 1936, G. Owen file, BMSA.

61. They appear in the colonial archival record as anonymous, practically trained personnel, often West African, working in state and company hospitals organized to care for equally unnamed, also male, Congolese workers (see Vellut, "La médecine européenne," 71, 75, 78–79).

62. The female category of accoucheuse was also institutionalized in the early 1920s. Male African nurses remained more numerous in the African medical profession than female midwives and nursing sisters in the Belgian Congo throughout the colonial period (see H. Vanderyst, "L'enseignement élémentaire médical pour indigènes, à tous ses degrés, au Congo belge," *L'aide médicale aux missions* 1 [15 October 1929]: 76–80; and Belgian Congo, *Rapports sur l'hygiène publique*, 1925, 1927–1947).

63. Jean Stengers, *Congo: Mythes et réalités, cent ans d'histoire* (Paris: Ducolot, 1989), 190.

64. Lyons, *Colonial Disease.*

65. Dr. Veroni, "Rapport . . . janvier–mars 1909," H (837), AA; Dr. Veroni, "Rapport . . . 1er trimestre 1910," H (837), AA; and Dr. Veroni, "Rapport sanitaire sur le 2 semestre de l'année 1910," H (841), AA.

66. Chef du Service Médical Commermeyer to Monsieur le Gouverneur Général, 16 June 1910, H (831), N 176, AA; and "Rapport sur l'hygiène publique," Province Orientale, 1913, 6, RA/CB (81) 1, AA.

67. "Ecoles pour infirmiers de couleur au Congo," 26 October 1920; "Ecoles de formation d'Assistants Médicaux Indigènes," 27 November 1920; and unsigned letter to Governor General, n.d.; all in H (4440) 697, AA.

68. M. Moeller, "Remarques," 16 October 1926, H (4348) 35, AA; and Ministre des Colonies Jasper to Governor General, 10 September 1928, H (4348) 35, M.H. 52, AA.

69. Dr. Veroni to Governor General, July 1909, H (837), AA; and Gouverneur Moeller, "Note concernant le rapport de M. le Médecin en Chef concernant le chef-lieu de Stanleyville et les dispensaires ruraux de district," 14 August 1928, H (4388) 35, M.H. 46, AA.

70. Dr. Veroni to Governor General, July 1909, H (837), AA.

71. C. C. Chesterman, *Manuel du dispensaire tropical,* trans. C. and R. Francotte (1929; reprint, London: United Society for Christian Literature, 1960). The Yakusu nursing school received official status in 1932, and began to be reimbursed for training government-hired nurses in 1937 (C. C. Chesterman to M. l'Administrateur Général des Colonies, 17 December 1937, H [4440] 698, "Ecoles d'Infirmiers et d'Assistants médicaux indigènes," AA).

72. E. R. Millman, "Picking up the Gold and Silver," *YQN* 77 (April 1929): 2.

73. E. R. Holmes, "The Medical Work," *YQN* 108 (January 1937): 14–16; and S. G. Browne, "A Successful Day," *YQN* 133 (July 1943): 7.

74. "Motifs donnés par les noirs pour ne pas s'engager à l'école des A.M.I., D'après une enquête faite à l'école primaire et professionelle," Stan[leyville], 3 September 1927, H (4388) 36, M.H. 76, AA.

75. Willy De Craemer and Renée C. Fox, *The Emerging Physician: A Sociological Approach to the Development of a Congolese Medical Profession* (Stanford, Calif.: Hoover Institution on War, Revolution, and Peace, 1968), 15–17.

76. Lyons, *Colonial Disease*. For a fascinating account on the appeal of itinerant medical work in the 1930s, see Duren, "Quelques aspects de la vie médicale." For an American perspective, see Charles A. Flood and William Sherman, "Medical Care in the Belgian Congo," *American Journal of Tropical Medicine* 24 (1944): 267–71.

77. Tata Alikuwa, Yainyongo-Romée, 26–27 December 1989. I collected tokwakwa tales in Yain-yongo often in spontaneous conversations on paths, in canoes, by fires, and before, during, and after more formal interviews, some of which included several people gathered around. There was no one in Yainyongo who did not know tokwakwa, and all adult men over forty knew about Mupendakula and Badjoko (see pages 187–88)—most women, too. Accounts about tokwakwa, Badjoko, and Mupendakula collected in Yakusu resemble those presented here. I quote here from eight transcribed and translated tapes; I also had a lengthy discussion about tokwakwa and Mupendakula with Mama Lisongomi and her daughter Marta one day. Details in the various conversations did vary, of course, as seen in the quotations included here. I regard these as a representative sample of tokwakwa public opinion in this village located at the ancient BaTambatamba site they remember as long ago theirs; the main themes are confirmed by Benoît Verhaegen and Rik Ceyssen's research. Italics added.

78. Lofanjola-Lisele (Pesapesa), Yainyongo-Romée, 29 December 1989. Italics added.

79. Lofemba, Yainyongo-Romée, 31 December 1989 and 7 January 1990. Italics added.

80. Tata Alikuwa, Yainyongo-Romée, 26–27 December 1989.

81. Lofanjola-Lisele (Pesapesa), Yainyongo-Romée, 29 December 1989. Italics added.

82. Ibid. Italics added.

83. Baba Manzanza, Yainyongo-Romée, 25 August 1989. Italics added.

84. Rik Ceyssens, "Mutumbula, mythe de l'opprimé," *Cultures et Développement* 7 (1975): 483–550; and the many essays of Luise White, including "Bodily Fluids and Usufruct: Controlling Property in Nairobi, 1917–1939," *Canadian Journal of African Studies* 24 (1990): 418–38; "Vampire Priests of Central Africa: African Debates about Labor and Religion in Colonial Northern Uganda," *Comparative Studies in Society and History* 35 (1993): 746–72; " 'They Could Make Their Victims Dull,' " 1379–402; and "Tsetse Visions: Narratives of Blood and Bugs in Colonial Northern Rhodesia, 1931–1939," *Journal of African History* 36 (1995): 219–45; and Jan Vansina, *Oral Tradition as History* (Madison: University of Wisconsin Press, 1985), 26.

85. Others have grappled with how to interpret such stories, yet the stories themselves have rarely been published. In his extraordinary compilation of historical and linguistic evidence, Rik Ceyssens only included one written—not performed—version, authored by a Congolese in a local language (Ceyssens, "Mutumbula").

86. All previous quotations from Tata Alikuwa and Bibi Bilefu Mari-Jeanne, Yainyongo-Romée, 6 January 1990. Italics added.

87. Bombolia Lisungi, Yainyongo-Romée, 8 January 1990. As in the Swahili, -*kumbatia* or clasp in the arms.

88. Tata Alikuwa and Bibi Bilefu Mari-Jeanne, Yainyongo-Romée, 6 January 1990.

89. Lofanjola-Lisele (Pesapesa), Yainyongo-Romée, 29 December 1989. Italics added.

90. Ibid. Italics added.

91. Ibid. Italics added.

92. Lofemba, Yainyongo-Romée, 31 December 1989 and 7 January 1990.

93. Vaughan, "Health and Hegemony," 200. See, too, on "the line between state and missionary medicine" not having been "always clearly drawn" (David Arnold, "Public Health and Public Power: Medicine and Hegemony in Colonial India," in *Contesting Colonial Hegemony: State and Society in Africa and India,* ed. Dagmar Engels and Shula Marks [London: British Academic Press, 1994], 135).

94. On Likenyule and Yenga working in the hospital alongside Lofoli, the hunter, see C. C. Chesterman, "Our Medical Department," *YQN* 84 (January 1931): 19–21.

95. René Maran, *Batouala* (1921; reprint, London: Heinemann, 1987), 31.

96. Baba Manzanza, Yainyongo-Romée, 25 August 1989.

97. See Benoît Verhaegen, "Kisangani pendant la deuxième guerre mondiale, 1939–1945," in *Le Congo belge durant la seconde guerre mondiale* (Brussels: Academie Royale des Sciences d'Outre-Mer, 1983); and Benoît Verhaegen, "Les violences coloniales au Congo belge," in *Cahiers d'actualité sociale* 4 (Kisangani: Presses Universitaires de Kisangani and Institut de Recherches Sociales Appliquées, 1987), esp. 19–24 (Declercq testimony).

98. On Badjoko's mixed reputation as an effective, harsh rubber tax collector, see David Northrup, *Beyond the Bend in the River: African Labor in Eastern Zaire, 1865–1940* (Athens: Ohio University Center for International Studies, 1988), 39. He was peddled in évolué publications of the 1950s as an important Congolese model ("Une figure historique: Joseph Badjoko," *Nos Images* 3, no. 25 [15 July 1950]). Bogumil Jewsiewicki tells me that he remains a popular hero in Kinshasa today. See also SOLO Ramazani, "Implantation des Topoke à Yanonge," *Cahiers du CRIDE* 65–66 (July–August 1982): 195–224; and Ch. Van de Lanoitte, *Sur les rivières glauques de l'Equateur* (Brussels: Iris, 1938): 194–201.

99. "Une figure historique."

100. Lofanjola-Lisele (Pesapesa), Yainyongo-Romée, 7 April 1989; "Njaso—Ikumbe," 7 September 1907; and (on his wife from Yakoso's Itale house) Mama Tula in interview with Tata Bafoya Bamanga, Yakusu, 25 November 1989.

101. G. C. Parris, "A Morning at Yalikina," *YQN* 95 (1933): 7.

102. "Une figure historique." On this grueling work and how to supervise it effectively, see Devroey, *Réseau routier au Congo belge.*

103. Mama Tula, in interview with Tata Bafoya Bamanga, Yakusu, 25 November 1989; and Baba Manzanza, Yainyongo-Romée, 25 August 1989.

104. For a marvelous analysis of culinary metaphors for reproductive processes in a Bamileke kingdom (where fetal movements are likened to a bubbling pot, a full-term fetus to cooked food, and giving birth to serving a carefully prepared and stirred meal, which has neither

stuck to the pot nor boiled over with miscarriage), see Pamela Feldman-Savelsburg, "Plundered Kitchens and Empty Wombs: Fear of Infertility in the Cameroonian Grassfields," *Social Science and Medicine* 39 (1994): 463–74. See, too, Eugenia Herbert, *Iron, Gender, and Power: Rituals of Transformation in African Societies* (Bloomington: Indiana University Press, 1993); and Carol Delaney, *The Seed and the Soil: Gender and Cosmology in Turkish Village Society* (Berkeley: University of California Press, 1991).

105.   Frank L. Lambrecht, *In the Shade of an Acacia Tree: Memoirs of a Health Officer in Africa, 1945–1959* (Philadelphia, Pa.: American Philosophical Society, 1991), 109–11; and P. G. Janssens, *La mortalité infantile aux Mines de Kilo; étude basée sur 1873 autopsies* (Brussels: IRCB, 1952). See also "Opportunities for Research in the Belgium Congo," *TRSTMH* 19 (1925–26): 185.

106.   Gladys Owen to Miss Bowser, 18 November 1929, Owen file, BMSA. There is almost no other evidence on autopsies at Yakusu. A "limited autopsy was allowed" on a young girl in 1922; see C. C. Chesterman, in "Discussion" *TRSTMH* 63 (1969): 5–92.

107.   Feldman-Savelsburg, "Plundered Kitchens."

108.   "Njaso ya Lisombo," *Mboli ya Tengai* 233 (1930): 7; and "Baenyeli ba basenji eoka ya likundu," *Mboli ya Tengai* 227 (1931).

109.   Gyan Prakash, "Science 'Gone Native' in Colonial India," *Representations* 40 (1992): 153–78.

110.   See, for example, Johannes Fabian, *Power and Performance: Ethnographic Explorations through Proverbial Wisdom and Theater in Shaba, Zaire* (Madison: University of Wisconsin Press, 1990).

111.   "A Letter from a Native Teacher to a Friend in England," *YQN* 36 (September 1917): 9–11.

112.   Ceyssens, "Mutumbula."

113.   Also the title of a caustic, satirical colonial newspaper.

114.   Prakash, "Science 'Gone Native,' " 168–69, 172.

115.   Baba Manzanza, Yainyongo-Roméе, 25 August 1989.

116.   As did Yanonge nurse, G. Etienne Nyama, "Lokasa loa Etienne Nyama," *Mboli ya Tengai* 314 (July 1933): 7; "Love to you who are reading and listening."

117.   "Children of classes" quotation from Tata Bafoya Bamanga, with Mama Tula, Yakusu, 27 November 1989. The other quotations are from Lofanjola-Lisele (Pesapesa), Yainyongo-Roméе, 29 December 1989.

118.   W. H. Ennals, News Sheet, no. 12, 27 October 1922, JFC Papers—Salisbury.

5   Babies and Forceps

1.   From 1945 to 1950, there were eight forceps deliveries; six were to remove stillborn fetuses, one baby died six hours after delivery, and one survived (Dorothy Daniel, birth register, 1945–1950, Dorothy Daniel Papers, Corse Staunton, U.K. [hereafter DD Papers]).

2.   Mary Fagg, Thornham, U.K., 12 November 1990.

3.   Mary Fagg, "God with Us," *YQN* 154 (December 1956): 4–5.

4.   Adrian Wilson, *The Making of Man-Midwifery: Childbirth in England, 1660–1770* (London: UCL Press, 1995), 85, 97, 99–101. See also Roy Porter, "A Touch of Danger: The Man-Midwife as Sexual Predator," in *Sexual Underworlds of the Enlightenment,* ed. G. S. Rousseau and Roy Porter (Chapel Hill: University of North Carolina Press, 1988), 206–32.

5. On therapeutic itineraries, see Marc Augé, "Introduction," Special Issue: "Interpreting Illness," *History and Anthropology* 2 (1985): 1–15; and John M. Janzen, *The Quest for Therapy in Lower Zaire* (Berkeley: University of California Press, 1978).

6. I compiled a complete record of the narrative textual accounts of 124 childbirth episodes, located in the station's quarterly newsletter and the private papers of the missionaries who worked at the station, as an appendix in Nancy Rose Hunt, "Negotiated Colonialism: Domesticity, Hygiene, and Birth Work in the Belgian Congo" (Ph.D. diss., University of Wisconsin–Madison, 1992), 426–66. A birth register itemizing the 281 cases that occurred during the period (1945–50) that Dorothy Daniel served at Yakusu and an obstetric operations register provided comparative points of reference (Dorothy Daniel, birth register, 1945–1950, DD Papers; and obstetrical operations register, 1953–1973, Maternity Ward, Yakusu).

7. My use of missionary sources is not unlike the way a historian of birth ritual in seventeenth-century England made exclusive use of the testimony of obstetricians to recover the perspectives and actions of parturients and women birth attendants. Adrian Wilson used these doctors' texts to reconstruct the "paths" by which they were called into birthing rooms; since such a "summoning" was in itself a "social act," related evidence gives historical entry to the social management of birth before the doctor was called (Wilson, "William Hunter and the Varieties of Man-Midwifery," in *William Hunter and the Eighteenth-Century Medical World*, ed. W. F. Bynum and Roy Porter [Cambridge: Cambridge University Press, 1985], 243–69).

8. E. R. Millman, "Among the Lokele Women and Children," *Missionary Herald*, April 1915, 251–53. This case seems to have been a turning point in mission policy on bridewealth; hereafter, the missionaries would insist on its payment to the bride's kin.

9. E. R. Millman, "A Bolt from the Blue and Some Babies," *YQN* 79 (October 1929): 12–14. On the veiled treatment of childbirth in Victorian novels, see John Hawkins Miller, " 'Temple and Sewer': Childbirth, Prudery, and Victoria Regina," in *The Victorian Family: Structure and Stresses,* ed. Anthony S. Wohl (London: Croom Helm, 1978), 23–43. Similar biblical imagery accompanied mission midwifery work elsewhere in east and central Africa (Megan Vaughan, *Curing Their Ills: Colonial Power and African Illness* [Stanford, Calif.: Stanford University Press, 1991], 67). See also "The House of Birth," *Nursing Mirror and Midwives' Journal* 51 (7 March 1931): 466; and V. M., "Welfare Work in Northern Rhodesia: 'The House of Life' at Mbereshi," *Nursing Mirror and Midwives' Journal* 55 (6 July 1935): 275–76.

10. One is a European case in which Congolese assisted. I have not included birth announcements in this thirteen. Of the 159 textual accounts collected on 124 (*not* 125) women's pregnancy and/or childbearing experiences, 19 were in mission publications, including 14 in the *Yakusu Quarterly Notes* (with one letter by a native evangelist) and one in *Mboli ya Tengai;* 12 were in hospital reports and data. The remainder were in missionary manuscripts, primarily private letters and the diary of Winifred Browne Burke; 78 separate entries on 53 cases were in this diary (see Hunt, "Negotiated Colonialism," 426–66; in this source, episode 33 should have been 32b).

11. How the lady/woman polarity encompassed empire is suggested by "the apocryphal story of the English mother who, when asked by her daughter how she should act on her wedding night, advised, 'Lie still and think of the Empire' " (Miller, " 'Temple and Sewer,' " 23–43, esp. 31, 32, 36). Miller does not give a source for this story.

12. Gladys Owen to Miss Bowser, 6 September 1929, Owen file, BMSA. British nurse-midwives shared delivery stories in their professional weekly, *Nursing Mirror and Midwives' Journal*. It is fair to speak of an adventure *genre* of these midwife tales from Africa. Most are stories of being called to assist in mud huts. Details of craniotomies and retained placentas were part of the genre; see "Old and New Methods in Zululand," *Nursing Mirror and Midwives' Journal* 51 (14 February 1931): 409; "Easy Labour for the Aborigines," *Nursing Mirror and Midwives' Journal* 51 (18 April 1931): 54; V. A. L., "A Night Adventure," *Nursing Mirror and Midwives' Journal* 51 (26 September 1931): 510; V. L., "Mission Work in South Africa," *Nursing Mirror and Midwives' Journal* 54 (14 April 1934): 32; I. H. J., "Night in a Mud Hut," *Nursing Mirror and Midwives' Journal* 55 (17 August 1935): 390; and M. B., "In Central Africa," *Nursing Mirror and Midwives' Journal* 55 (16 November 1935): 130.

13. Rose Gee, "A Peep into My Diary," *Missionary Herald* (1914): 220; C. C. Chesterman, "Chasing the Terrors of Darkness," *YQN* 152 (October 1955): 11–13, writing ca. December 1920; E. R. Millman, "What Christ is to the Women," *YQN* 92 (January 1933): 8–10; E. M. Lean, "And They Came to Him from Every Quarter," *YQN* 116 (January 1939): 20–21; A. D. Moyles, "From the Hospital," *YQN* 107 (October 1936): 11–14; S. G. Browne, "Sunshine and Shadow in the Topoke Forest," *YQN* 143 (October 1948): 2–6; and Mary Fagg, "God with Us," *YQN* 154 (December 1956): 4–5.

14. "Medical Work," *YQN* 8 (August 1910), 3–4.

15. Mrs. Mill, "The Struggle for Right Living," *YQN* 82 (July 1930): 12–14; C. C. Chesterman, "The Work of the Hospital," *YQN* 88 (January 1932): 13–15; and R. E. Holmes, "Our Medical Work," *YQN* 92 (January 1933): 17–18. For the complete texts of these thirteen episodes, see Hunt, "Negotiated Colonialism," Appendix Two (episodes 1, 3, 4, 6, 16, 22, 26, 27, 28, 32a, 35, 109, and 122), 426–65.

16. I draw on James C. Scott's notion of hidden and public transcripts here (Scott, *Domination and the Arts of Resistance: Hidden Transcripts* [New Haven, Conn.: Yale University Press, 1990]).

17. CMC, *Report* (1921): 179; and CMC, *Report* (1925): 36.

18. C. Mabie, "Medical Work among Women," CMC, *Report* (1911): 98. Protestant missionaries in Uganda and Malawi were similarly motivated (see Vaughan, *Curing Their Ills*).

19. C. C. Chesterman, *In the Service of the Suffering: Phases of Medical Missionary Enterprise* (London: Edinburgh House Press, 1940), 68.

20. Edith Millman to Miss Lockhart, n.d., received 21 February 1920, Millman file, BMSA.

21. Gladys Owen to Miss Bowser, 18 November 1929, Owen file, BMSA.

22. Phyllis Lofts, "Draft. July 1981. For Book on Medical Missionary Work," typescript, Phyllis Lofts Papers, Barton-on-Sea, U.K. (hereafter, PL Papers). "District work" was a British midwifery term for casework in private homes. British institutions hired midwives in domiciliary practice long after childbirth began to be medicalized (see Jane Lewis, *The Politics of Motherhood: Child and Maternal Welfare in England, 1900–1939* [London: Croom Helm, 1980], 128). Mary Fagg was a "district midwife," trained health visitor, and training midwife in England before going to the Congo in 1951; she had never held a midwifery position in a hospital (Fagg, Thornham, 11 November 1990).

23. Lofts, "Draft. July 1981," PL Papers.

24. Gladys Owen to Miss Bowser, 22 October 1929, Owen file, BMSA.

25. Gladys Owen to Miss Bowser, 31 March 1929, Owen file, BMSA. The story's structure—super-stitious medicine versus prayer—mirrors others. In 1937, Gladys (Owen) Parris met women manipulating leaves in a little black pot before they came to pray (G. C. Parris, "Women in the Congo Forest," YQN 109 [April 1937]: 6–7).

26. Lofts met Bolau in 1927 or 1928; Phyllis Lofts to Stanley Browne, 2 April 1981, PL Papers.

27. Phyllis Lofts, ["Many Were the Customs"], untitled typescript, ca. 1981, PL Papers. For an ethnographic account of a 1932 BaMbole birth, see Administrateur Territorial Lauwers, "Notes ethnographiques sur la peuplade des Bambole," Yanonge, 20 March 1922, in Archivalia DeCleene-De Jonghe, file no. 60, KADOC, Leuven.

28. Lofts, ["Many Were the Customs"].

29. Phyllis Lofts, "Adventures and Peradventures in Midwifery," ca. 1932, PL Papers. The text was written after the girl-nurses were in training at Yakusu (1930), and before Lofts's retirement from the mission field in 1934. In 1981, Lofts wrote Browne, "I made notes when she confided to me the various customs, traditions and treatments which witch-doctors and medicine-workers practised, and I wrote about them in an article published by the Nursing Mirror" (Phyllis Lofts to Stanley Browne, 2 April 1981, PL Papers). I was unable to locate the Nursing Mirror version in its 1930s' pages.

30. Gladys Owen to Miss Bowser, 6 September 1929, Owen file, BMSA.

31. E. R. Millman, "A Bolt from the Blue and Some Babies," YQN 79 (October 1929): 13.

32. Gladys Owen to Miss Bowser, 22 October 1929, Owen file, BMSA.

33. Gladys Owen to Miss Bowser, 6 September 1929, Owen file, BMSA. For a related incident, see M. B., "In Central Africa," Nursing Mirror and Midwives' Journal 55 (16 November 1935): 130.

34. Gladys Owen to Miss Bowser, 22 October 1929, Owen file, BMSA.

35. Phyllis Lofts, untitled longhand manuscript, n.d., PL Papers. On the use of bodily fluids in sorcery, see essays and letters in Mboli ya Tengai, 1920–1930.

36. E. R. Millman and William Millman, A Mothercraft Manual for Senior Girls and Newly Married Women in Africa (London: Carey Press for the Christian Literature Society, 1929), vii; and Gladys Owen to Miss Bowser, 18 November 1929, Owen file, BMSA.

37. Gladys Owen to Miss Bowser, 18 March 1930, Owen file, BMSA; and Gladys Owen, "Medical Work among Women and Babies," YQN 84 (January 1931): 21–22.

38. Lofts, ["Many Were the Custom"]. Also: "When we started the hospital we could train only boys: it was taboo in the villages for girls to take up nursing" (Phyllis Lofts, "A Journey into Faith," n.d., PL Papers). For the statistics, see Owen, "Medical Work."

39. On cultural differences between menstrual blood and the blood of childbirth, and parallels be-tween birthing and hunting elsewhere in central Africa, see Victor Turner, The Forest of Sym-bols: Aspects of Ndembu Ritual (Ithaca, N.Y.: Cornell University Press, 1967), 70, 77–78; Luc de Heusch, "Palm Wine, the Blood of Women, and the Blood of Beasts," in The Drunken King, or the Origin of the State, trans. Roy Willis (Bloomington: Indiana University Press, 1982), 144–86, esp. 168–69; and Filip De Boeck, "From Knots to Web: Fertility, Life-Transmission, Health, and Well-Being among the Aluund of Southwest Zaire" (Ph.D. diss., Katholieke Universiteit te Leuven, 1991).

40. Phyllis Lofts, "Cement Story," n.d., PL Papers.

41. On the history of this European idiom, see David Harley, "Historians as Demonologists: The Myth of the Midwife-Witch," *Social History and Medicine* 3 (April 1990): 1–26.

42. Phyllis Lofts to Stanley Browne, 2 April 1981, PL Papers. The personal conversion story of Bolau became Lofts's story, inscribed in speeches that she wrote in the 1970s. At Stanley Browne's request, Lofts submitted one version of her Bolau story for a book that he helped edit on medical missionary work. Her submission was not included (Stanley G. Browne, Frank Davey, and William A. R. Thomson, eds., *Heralds of Health: The Saga of Christian Medical Initiatives* [London: Christian Medical Fellowship, 1985]).

43. "From the Station Log-Book," *YQN* 122 (September 1940): 7. Bolau was listed as "native nurse" for 1932 and 1933, though these lists were not kept consistently. BMS Annual Medical Reports, 1932, 1933 Hospital Director's Office, Yakusu (hereafter HDO, Yakusu). A large plaque on a wall of the Yakusu hospital indicated that she received a midwife diploma in 1933.

44. Lofts, ["Many Were the Customs"].

45. A Dr. W. E. Davis trained two widows to be visiting midwives in the Lotumbe area from the late 1920s (Davis, *Caring and Curing in Congo and Kentucky* [North Middletown, Ky.: Erasmus Press, 1984], 79–81).

46. Lofts, ["Many Were the Customs"]; and Lofts, "Draft. July 1981."

47. Phyllis Lofts, untitled longhand manuscript, n.d., PL Papers.

48. Phyllis Lofts, "A More Excellent Way," *YQN* 90 (July 1932): 12–14. The article mentions "Singa," [sic] but erases the fact that it was an obstetric case.

49. Gladys [Owen] Parris to Miss Bowser, Yaongama, 23 April 1932, Owen file, BMSA.

50. Gladys [Owen] Parris to Miss Bowser, 23 April 1932, Yaongama, Owen file, BMSA; and H. B. Parris, "More Bambole Vignettes," *YQN* 111 (October 1937): 10–11.

51. Phyllis Lofts, "A More Excellent Way," *YQN* 90 (July 1932): 12–14.

52. Stanley G. Browne to Nellie, 23 August 1936, Stanley G. Browne Papers, New Milton, U.K. (hereafter SGB Papers). For published versions of the case, see A. D. Moyles, "From the Hospital," *YQN* 107 (October 1936): 11–14; and Sylvia Duncan and Peter Duncan, *Bonganga: Experiences of a Missionary Doctor* (London: Odhams Press, 1958), 35–39. Elsewhere in the colony, doctors were discovering that spinals were contraindicated in obstetric cases (J.-R. Kebers, "Les urgences anesthésiques en pathologie congolaise," Examen B/Médecins no. 236, Institute of Tropical Medicine [hereafter IMT], Antwerp, 1956).

53. Stanley G. Browne to Nellie, 23 August 1936, SGB Papers. The doctor's assumptions were in keeping with the thrust of infant welfare work in England; see, for example, Peter W. G. Wright, "Babyhood: The Social Construction of Infant Care as a Medical Problem in England in the Years around 1900," in *Biomedicine Examined*, ed. Margaret Lock and Deborah Gordon (Dordrecht, Netherlands: Kluwer Academic Publishers, 1988), 299–329.

54. Stanley G. Browne to Harold, 31 December 1936, SGB Papers.

55. Baba Manzanza, Yainyongo-Romée, 16 September 1989.

56. Among others, Mama Koto, Yaotoke, 20 March 1989 (from my fieldnotes).

57. Mama Malia Winnie, Kisangani, 4 December 1989.

58. Mrs. Ennals described Malia Winnie's mother as "a familiar figure through the years, little, wizened, working, never a professing Christian, living in the past" (G. Ennals, "The Long View," *YQN* 145 [February 1950]: 12–14). See, too, the "Litoi" sermon [by W. H. Ford?] John F.

Carrington Papers, Salisbury, U.K. In a 1982 letter, Malia Winnie Litoi used the name Wini-kolo Litoi Malia; see chapter 5, note 128.

59. Mama Malia Winnie, Kisangani, 4 December 1989.

60. Mama Malia Winnie, with Mama Damali Basenge and Mama Tula, Kisangani, 23 January 1990. The diploma date comes from the hospital school plaque at Yakusu. On Malia as a mother, see E. R. Millman, "What Christ Is to the Women," *YQN* 92 (January 1933): 8–10.

61. Tata Tula, with Tula Rogier, Yakusu, 2 and 4 November 1989. Malia Winnie and Tokolokaya were listed as the parents of one child born in Yakusu's maternity, and Tokolokaya was still listed as the father when Malia Winnie was in the maternity later for a miscarriage; Dorothy Daniel, birth register, 1945–1950, DD Papers.

62. Mama Malia Winnie, with Mama Damali Basenge and Mama Tula, Kisangani, 23 January 1990. Chesterman likely was involved from his London-based position as the head of the BMS Medical Missionary Association. Malia Winnie also associated the time she was called back to work with the aging of Bolau, then hospital midwife. "She became old, and they told Bolau, 'You, step down, Malia will stay.' So me, I came" (Mama Malia Winnie, Kisangani, 4 December 1989).

63. Mama Malia Winnie, with Mama Damali Basenge and Mama Tula, Kisangani, 23 January 1990. Tolombo is a local pronunciation of Olombo.

64. E. Muriel Lean, "Medical Pictures," *YQN* 125 (July 1941): 12–13; and E. Muriel Lean to Dr. Chesterman, 10 January 1942 [misdated, actually 10 January 1943], 10 May 1942, and 12 July 1943, Lean file, BMSA.

65. Mama Malia Winnie, Kisangani, with Mama Damali Basenge and Mama Tula, 23 January 1990.

66. Dorothy Daniel, Corse Staunton, 11 June 1991. Malia Winnie to Bosongo Bonganga, 30 August 1944, in "Aides-accoucheuses" file, HDO, Yakusu.

67. Dorothy Daniel, Corse Staunton, 11 June 1991; and Winnie Browne to Ivy [Winifred Browne Burke], 12 September 1940, SGB Papers. Daniel's birth register indicates that most women stayed at least seven days.

68. Dorothy Daniel, Corse Staunton, 11 June 1991. She attended Bloomsbury Trade School from age fourteen to sixteen, worked in ladies' tailoring from age sixteen to eighteen, and then began nursing training in about 1935. She was baptized in 1938 and joined the East London Tabernacle; Dorothy Daniel file, BMS Candidate Papers, BMSA.

69. Dorothy Daniel, Corse Staunton, 11 June 1991.

70. Ibid.

71. Ibid.

72. Lokele Examinations, 1940–1952, District Pastor's Office, Yakusu (hereafter DPO, Yakusa).

73. Dorothy Daniel, Corse Staunton, 11 June 1911.

74. Mama Malia Winnie, with Mama Damali Basenge and Mama Tula, Kisangani, 23 January 1990. With thanks to Tim Johnson for helping me sort out how an ectopic removal entailed taking a "chunk out of the uterus."

75. When a leaf quivers in an eerie, contrary way, a healer knows that the plant is the right one; Nora Carrington, Salisbury, 8 June 1991. Her botanist husband, John, studied local medicines and healers, as many of his manuscripts show (John F. Carrington Papers, BMSA).

76. Mama Malia Winnie, Kisangani, 4 December 1989. Italics denote speaker's emphasis. Likely

drawing on her subsequent experience in Catholic hospitals in Kisangani, Malia Winnie sometimes referred to unmarried missionary nurses at Yakusu as nuns or *ba-soeurs*.

77. Ibid. Italics added. She agreed with local beliefs that if the woman in labor entered the river, the baby would hurry to come out. This had been the case with her first baby (Mama Malia Winnie, with Mama Damali Basenge and Mama Tula, Kisangani, 23 January 1990).

78. Mama Malia Winnie, with Mama Damali Basenge and Mama Tula, Kisangani, 23 January 1990.

79. Mama Malia Winnie, Kisangani, 4 December 1989.

80. Winifred Browne, diary, 1 January 1942, Winifred Browne Burke Papers, Godalming, U.K. (hereafter WBB Papers); and Nora Carrington, Salisbury, 8 June 1991.

81. Dorothy Daniel, Corse Staunton, 11 June 1991.

82. Mama Malia Winnie, Kisangani, 4 December 1989.

83. Men tend to be called in only if the wife does not confess; otherwise they are not present. A 1932 colonial description of a BaMbole birth suggests that the husband was there and his anger could increase the amount of wealth (thirty to fifty francs worth) that each adulterer owed him (Lauwers, "Notes ethnographiques").

84. A theme I develop at length in Nancy Rose Hunt, "Noise over Camouflaged Polygamy, Colonial Mortality Taxation, and a Woman-Naming Crisis in Belgian Africa," *Journal of African History* 32 (1991): 471–94.

85. Stanley G. Browne to Nellie, 23 August 1936, SGB Papers.

86. Stanley G. Browne to Nellie and Everybody, 4 January 1937, SGB Papers.

87. E. Muriel Lean, "Our New Maternity Ward—Behind the Scenes," *YQN* 122 (September 1940): 3.

88. Papa Boshanene, Yakusu, 24 February 1989.

89. Mama Malia Winnie, with Mama Damali Basenge and Mama Tula, Kisangani, 23 January 1990. The earliest evidence on an intravenous infusion for an obstetric case (an ectopic pregnancy) is from 1937 (Stanley G. Browne to Ivy, 20 May 1937, SGB Papers).

90. Mama Malia Winnie, Kisangani, 4 December 1989.

91. The woman was admitted after three days in labor. The first child had been stillborn, and this one was in the posterior position. A cesarean section was performed, and a stillborn fetus was removed. Daniel, birth register, 1945–1950, case no. 240, DD Papers.

92. Stanley G. Browne to Father, Nellie, and All, 16 June 1943, SGB Papers. His sister's diary confirms that at least one of these was a "destructive operation" (Winifred Browne, diary, Yakusu, 4 June 1943, WBB Papers).

93. Stanley G. Browne to Father, Nellie, and All, 17 June 1942, SGB Papers. Browne did not specifically identify this case as an embryotomy as he did for another case where the "girls in training" observed in April 1943.

94. Gladys Owen to Miss Bowser, 22 October 1929, Owen file, BMSA. Embryotomies and craniotomies (the surgical destruction of the fetus and especially the head to permit vaginal extraction) figured as moral questions that divided birth practitioners over whose life was most important, that of the mother or that of the fetus. In the United States, Catholic priests argued strongly against craniotomies from the 1880s on (Judith Walzer Leavitt, "The Growth of Medical Authority: Technology and Morals in Turn-of-the-Century Obstetrics," *Medical Anthropology Quarterly* 1 [1987]: 230–55).

95. Laura Briggs, "Fair Fruit and Foul: Discourses of Race in Nineteenth-Century Obstetrics and

Gynecology" (paper presented to the American Studies Association, Nashville, Tenn., 28–31 October 1994).

96. Through podalic version (Wilson, *Making of Man-Midwifery,* 20, 24 [n. 25]; see also Wilson, "William Hunter," 85, 97, 99–101). Craniotomies were favored more and lasted longer among Protestant, Anglo-Saxon doctors, because such surgery represented a viable alternative to the risk that a cesarean section posed to maternal life. Catholic doctors—whether in the United States, in Europe, or in the Belgian Congo—did not perform embryotomies once cesareans were defensible. By the middle of the nineteenth century, French obstetricians were more likely to perform cesareans than English practitioners, who, more concerned for maternal life than infant life or infant baptism, would resort to craniotomy; embryotomies became exceptional in France in the second half of the nineteenth century, but did not decline in England until the 1900s. As the turn-of-the-century debate among American Catholics demonstrates, the contrast at work was largely a religious one. See Ornella Moscucci, *The Science of Woman: Gynaecology and Gender in England, 1800–1929* (Cambridge: Cambridge University Press, 1990), 141–42; Jacques Gélis, *La sage-femme ou le médecin: Une nouvelle conception de la vie* (Paris: Fayard, 1988), 346–48; and Leavitt, "Growth of Medical Authority."

97. As they certainly did in April 1943 when a second twin died in utero (Stanley G. Browne to Father and All, 30 April 1943), sGB Papers.

98. Tata Tula, with Tula Rogier, Yakusu, 2 and 4 November 1989. Italics added.

99. Ibid. This makes one wonder about Adrian Wilson's leap in logic about seventeenth-century British women's terror of craniotomies (Wilson, *Making of Man-Midwifery,* 50).

100. Dorothy Daniel, Corse Staunton, 11 June 1991. One C-section, although she didn't recall it, is listed in her birth register of 283 cases. Dorothy Daniel, birth register, case no. 240, 14 March 1950, DD Papers.

101. Dorothy Daniel, Corse Staunton, 11 June 1991.

102. See G. Valcke, "Note," *ASBMT* 14 (1934): 432–33.

103. Personal communication to author from Mary Fagg, 31 May 1989. Blood transfusions are one of the factors that contributed to the decline in the maternal mortality associated with cesarean sections in the post-1945 period (see Dyre Trolle, *The History of the Caesarean Section* [Copenhagen: Reitzel, 1982], 68–69).

104. Mary Fagg to Dear Friends, 28 May 1954, Fagg prayer letters file, BMSA.

105. "Towards Health and Wholeness, the 1955 Chapter in the Story of B.M.S. Medical Work," medical pamphlet from "Pamphlets, Mostly Medical, All Fields," Box H/56, BMSA.

106. Both mothers survived; one of the babies died (Mary Fagg to Dear Friends, 13 March 1956, Fagg prayer letters file, BMSA; and Mary Fagg to Dear Friends, 15 June 1957, Fagg prayer letters file, BMSA).

107. Neither symphysiotomies nor vacuum extraction came into play at Yakusu in this period, although they were being hailed in the rest of the colony in the late 1950s.

108. On the availability of sulfonamides, see Irvine Loudon, *Death in Childbirth: An International Study of Maternal Care and Maternal Mortality, 1800–1950* (Oxford: Oxford University Press, 1992).

109. BMS Yakusu Annual Medical Report, 1946, HDO, Yakusu.

110. Personal communication from Mary Fagg, 31 May 1989.

111. G. Brun, "L'embryotomie cervicale dans les présentations transversales," *Maroc Médical* 50, no. 536 (June 1970): 395–96; John B. Lawson, "Embryotomy for Obstructed Labour," *Tropical Doctor* 4 (1974): 188–91; C. C. Ekwempu, "Embryotomy Versus Caesarean Section," *Tropical Doctor* 8 (1978): 195–97; and J. Y. Obed, "Fetal Decapitation: The Application and Safety of the Stout Embryotomy Scissors," *Tropical Doctor* 24 (1994): 139–40.

112. Personal communication from Mary Fagg, 31 May 1989.

113. Dorothy Daniel, birth register, 1945–1950, DD Papers.

114. Ibid.

115. Obstetrical operations register, 1953–1959, Maternity Ward, Yakusu. The register did not list C-sections, likely because these cases were transferred to the main operating theater.

116. On not confusing "compassion" for maternal life with the apparent "cruelty" of the method, I draw on Wilson, *Making of Man-Midwifery*, 20.

117. The "suite" of available instrumental interventions at Yakusu during this period was not unlike that of a seventeenth-century doctor's in England, where a medical man was also not called on to save babies' lives, but mothers' lives. In each setting, calls came late and craniotomies were often the only chance of saving a mother's life. The absence of cesareans is only part of what unites these practices from disparate eras. Their emergency-oriented character is the key commonality. A seventeenth-century English doctor was summoned, however; he made house calls (see Wilson, *Making of Man-Midwifery*, 49–51). Forceps were used regularly at Yakusu, suggesting that they were preferred to embryotomy instruments when feasible. On forceps deliveries, see Stanley G. Browne to Ivy, 24 May 1936, SGB Papers; and Winifred Browne, diary, Yakusu, 25–29 January 1943 (live delivery) WBB Papers. Embryotomy procedures and instruments continue to be included in midwife manuals, primarily for "midwives in remote areas of developing countries," as it is assumed that except in cases of hydrocephaly or other gross fetal malformation, conditions liable to obstruct labor can be diagnosed during pregnancy or resolved by a cesarean section (Margaret F. Myles, *A Textbook for Midwives* [Edinburgh: Churchill Livingstone, 1972], 647–51).

118. On the prevalence of station women, see Gladys Owen to Miss Bowser, 18 November 1929, Owen file, BMSA; Gladys Owen to Miss Bowser, 18 March 1930, Owen file, BMSA; and Mali Browne to Father, Nellie, and Ivy, 22 July 1941, SGB Papers.

119. Winifred Browne, diary, Yalemba and Yakusu, 1942–1944, WBB Papers; and Dorothy Daniel, birth register, 1945–1950, DD Papers.

120. Of the 280 births recorded in Daniel's register, 17 percent (forty-five) were from the Yakoso village, 13 percent (thirty-seven) were from the Yakusu mission station, and 8 percent (twenty-three) and 4 percent (eleven) were from the nearby villages of Yatumbo and Yawenda respectively (Dorothy Daniel, birth register, 1945–1950, DD Papers).

121. E. R. Millman, "What Christ Is to the Women," *YQN* 92 (January 1933): 8–10.

122. W. H. Ford, "The Pastor Hopes to Visit," *YQN* 80 (January 1930): 3–5.

123. In 1899, when the society investigated the question, the Yakusu church saw "no reason for refusing membership to a polygamist provided no new marriage is contracted after conversion." Moreover, Mr. Millman's opinion in 1899 was: "When one of many wives is converted . . . she should not be instigated to leave her home" (William Millman to Mr. Baynes, 7 November 1899, in "Correspondence on Polygamy" file, ca. 1898–1919, Box A/61, BMSA). A woman named Bangala was excluded from membership because she married Badjoko who

was already married on September 7, 1906. On October 8–9, 1908, the Yakusu church decided that a Christian woman whose husband took a second wife would not be permitted to take communion until she had left him; see "Ikumbe sha Etanda la Bekumi" [Yakusu Church Elders Minute Book], 1904–1933, esp. 7 September 1906 and 8–9 October 1908, DPO, Yakusu. Yakusu baptism candidates interpreted biblical stories accordingly: "Nicodemus had a lot of wives and Jesus said that unless he got rid of all his wives he could not enter the Kingdom of heaven!" (Gladys Parris to Miss Bowser, 17 May 1933, Owen file, BMSA).

124. Chesterman claimed infant mortality was as high as 500 infants for every 1,000 in the region at large; pneumonia and diarrhea exacerbated the frequent attacks of malaria to which infants were subject during their first two years of life. Between 1924 and 1935, among the over 1,000 infants who attended the Yakusu baby clinic for weekly doses of quinine, infant mortality was less than 150 (C. C. Chesterman, "Blackwater Fever in a Negro Child," *Lancet* 7 [1935]: 554). It remained as high as 10 to 15 percent in the district in 1939 (Chesterman, "Blackwater Fever," 554; Raymond Holmes, "Medical Report," *YQN* 117 [April 1939]: 28).

125. "'Why We Do Not Believe' (Told to Our Native Evangelists)," *YQN* 19 (June 1913): 11. Concerns about the effect of infertility and infant mortality on marriage continued (E. R. Millman, "What Christ Is to the Women," *YQN* 92 [January 1933]: 8–10). The problem of "venereal disease and childless marriages" was discussed by the Yakusu Station Committee in 1947, when "it was agreed that no effective legislation can be made" (Station Committee Minutes, 29 June 1947, DPO, Yakusu.

126. Basuwa of Yatolema, "In Sorrows Many: A Letter from a Native Evangelist," *YQN* 103 (October 1935): 20.

127. Tata Alikuwa, Yainyongo-Romée, 18 September 1989. The "hardships attending pregnancy and child-rearing in native communities contribute in some measure to the continuance of polygamy" (Millman and Millman, *Mothercraft Manual,* vii). The loss of one nurse, Liita Pierre, from the church membership made some missionaries pause: "His wife was barren, and he could not face the jeers and recriminations of his neighbours and members of his family. So he married another wife . . . and was put out of work and out of the Church. . . . He wants to follow Jesus, and does his best to help with the work of the church. . . . What would you do in a case like this?" (Stanley Browne to Father and All, 23 January 1939, SGB Papers).

128. Malia Winnie was "thrilled with her slip" that Lofts sent her in 1954 (Mali to Phyllis in margin of Stanley G. Browne to Phyllis Lofts, 29 November 1954, PL Papers). Malia Winnie "died with crying" when her "White teacher and Mama" died; she put on a scarf that Lofts had given her and had her photograph taken with flowers in her hand as if she had been at the funeral (Malia Winnie to Miss Lofts, 5 July 1968, PL Papers; and Winikolo Litoi Maria to Mama and Bosongo Carrington, 26 August 1982, PL Papers).

129. Duncan and Duncan, *Bonganga;* and P. Thompson, *Mister Leprosy* (London: Hodder and Stoughton, 1980).

130. E. R. Millman, "Mothercraft on the Congo," *YQN* (April 1930): 8–11.

131. The dearth of material and infant care information in Yakusu's doctor's annual reports implies that this was not a major mission agenda, insofar as these male missionaries defined them (BMS Yakusu Annual Medical Reports, 1921–1960, HDO, Yakusu).

132. Tata Tula, with Tula Rogier, Yakusu, 2 and 4 November 1989. Italics added.

133. Mama Lifaefi Bangala, Yakoso, 24 November 1989. On saliva in lilembu rituals among the Lokele, see Mulyumba wa Mamba Itongwa, "Quelques données sur le rôle de la salive dans les sociétés traditionelles de l'Afrique noire," *Revue Zaïroise de psychologie et de pédagogie* 4, no. 1 (1975): 127–34. Italics added.

134. Mama Tula in Mama Lifaefi Bangala interview, Yakoso, 24 November 1989. Italics added.

135. Briggs, "Fair Fruit and Foul," 7.

136. Mary Fagg, Thornham, 11 November 1990. On Browne and cannibals, see chapter 3, note 140.

137. Craniotomies were not exclusively practiced on women of African descent, though at least in the United States, the horrors of craniotomies *for doctors* became associated with black skin and its ready availability for surgical study (Briggs, "Fair Fruit and Foul"). The links between race and gynecology are more commonly made in reference to fistula surgery and the career of Dr. J. Marion Sims. Generally credited as a founding father of American gynecology due to his perfection of fistula repair techniques in the 1840s, Sims was a slave-owning plantation doctor in Alabama at the time; "the availability of slave women as specimens for surgical experimentation allowed Sims to take the steps necessary to originate American gynecology" (Deborah Kuhn McGregor, *Sexual Surgery and the Origins of Gynecology: J. Marion Sims, His Hospital, and His Patients* [New York: Garland Publishing, 1989], 37, 40). Irvine Loudon dates a shift in the tendency to perform craniotomies rather than cesareans to the 1900s in the United Kingdom (based on data from a London hospital where, from 1890 to 1899, 21 percent of the contracted pelvis cases were handled by craniotomy and 5 percent by cesarean, whereas from 1900 to 1909, 29 percent of such cases were handled by cesarean and only 5 percent by craniotomy) (Loudon, *Death in Childbirth*, 135–36).

138. Dorothy Daniel, birth register, 1945–1950, DD Papers.

139. Stanley G. Browne to Harold, 31 December 1936, SGB Papers; J. R. Lomby, *The Cambridge Bible for Schools and Colleges: The First Book of Kings* (Cambridge: University Press, 1894), 1, Kings, iii, vv. 16–28.

6   Colonial Maternities

1. Marie-Louise Comeliau, *Blancs et noirs: Scènes de la vie congolaise* (Paris: Charles Dessart, 1942), 166–72, esp. 166–67, 169.

2. Ibid., 166. On the Swahili term *bwana*, see Johannes Fabian, with Kalundi Mango and with linguistic notes by W. Schicho, *History from Below: The 'Vocabulary of Elisabethville' by André Yav; Texts, Translations, and Interpretive Essay* (Amsterdam: John Benjamins Publishing Company, 1990), 133.

3. I quote here from Jane Jenson, "Gender and Reproduction: Or, Babies and the State," *Studies in Political Economy* 20 (1986): 9–45. On maternalist policies in Europe and its colonies, see also Seth Koven and Sonya Michel, "Womanly Duties: Maternalist Politics and the Origins of Welfare States in France, Germany, Great Britain, and the United States, 1880–1920," *American Historical Review* 95 (1990): 1076–108; Gisela Bock and Pat Thane, eds., *Maternity and Gender Policies: Women and the Rise of the European Welfare States, 1880s–1950s* (London: Routledge, 1991); Anna Davin, "Imperialism and Motherhood," *History Workshop* 5 (Spring

1978): 9–66; Frederick Cooper, "From Free Labor to Family Allowances: Labor and Society in Colonial Discourse," *American Ethnologist* 16 (1989): 745–65; and Ann Laura Stoler, *Race and the Education of Desire: Foucault's "History of Sexuality" and the Colonial Order of Things* (Durham, N.C.: Duke University Press, 1995).

4. On pronatalism in the Force Publique, see Bryant P. Shaw, "*Force Publique, Force Unique:* The Military in the Belgian Congo, 1914–1939" (Ph.D. diss., University of Wisconsin–Madison, 1984), 269–70, 277. On the major copper mining company, Union Minière du Haut-Katanga, see Nancy Rose Hunt, " 'Le bébé en brousse': European Women, African Birth Spacing, and Colonial Intervention in Breast Feeding in the Belgian Congo," *International Journal of African Historical Studies* 21 (1988): 401–32.

5. Who read Belgian colonial novels and memoirs? The reading public seems to have been limited to a Belgian colonial one, whether resident in Belgium or the Congo; the class, religious, and linguistic range among this "popular" readership would have been considerable. For an excellent analysis of the genre by Belgian authors who wrote in French, see Pierre Halen, *Le petit belge avait vu grand: une littérature coloniale* (Brussels: Labor, 1993). The archaic word *matrone* suggests a midwife who "exercises illegally the work of a midwife or who practices abortions" (*Trésor de la langue française* [Paris: Gallimard, 1985]). Sometimes, if frightened of sorcery, a worker's wife would give birth in the forest (Comeliau, *Blancs et noirs,* 59).

6. Raymond Holmes to Dr. Chesterman, 18 November 1939, Holmes file, BMSA.

7. E. R. Millman, "The Royal Visit to Yakusu," *YQN* 93 (April 1933): iv.

8. Maurist Dony, *Mashauri kwa Mama wa Kongo* (Brussels: FBEI, n.d.).

9. Stanley G. Browne, "The Medical Work," *YQN* 112 (January 1938), 25–28; C. C. Chesterman, "Sometime Medical Missionary at Yakusu," *YQN* 166 (July 1936), 2–7; BMS Western Sub-Committee, book no. 18, 6 November 1935, BMSA; and Stanley G. Browne to Father and All, 10 September 1936, Stanley G. Browne Papers, New Milton, U.K. (hereafter SGB Papers).

10. Holmes to Chesterman, 18 November 1939, Holmes file, BMSA.

11. E. M. Lean, "Our New Maternity Ward: Behind the Scenes," *YQN* 122 (September 1940): 1–2.

12. The literature here is ever growing. For a good bibliography and essays on Australia, Britain, Burma, Canada, Malaya, the Netherlands, and South Africa, see Valerie Fildes, Lara Marks, and Hilary Marland, eds., *Women and Children First: International Maternal and Infant Welfare, 1870–1945* (London: Routledge, 1992). See, too, Rima D. Apple, "Constructing Mothers: Scientific Motherhood in the Nineteenth and Twentieth Centuries," *Social History of Medicine* 8 (1995): 161–78, esp. note 44.

13. BMS Yakusu Annual Medical Report, 1939, Hospital Director's Office, Yakusu (hereafter HDO, Yakusu).

14. Read, too, here: specific localization. It is not necessarily multiple or mixed "metropoles" that created the multiple "metropolitanizations" of maternity in the Congo; engagements with local situations and practices would have been equally as important (Nancy Rose Hunt, "Introduction," *Gender and History* 8 [1996]: 323–37).

15. See, for example, V. Barthélémi, "Etude sur la syphilis au Congo belge," Examen B/Médecins no. 16a, Institute of Tropical Medicine, Antwerp, 1921 (hereafter IMT). See also "Rapports sanitaires du district de l'Aruwimi," H (838), AA.

16. Dr. Veroni to M. le Gouverneur Général, 4 January 1909, H (841), AA.

17. "Rapport sur l'hygiène de 3ème trimestre," 1906, H (834), AA.

18. Dr. Veroni to M. le Gouverneur Général, 4 January 1909, H (841), AA.

19. "Rapport sur l'hygiène de 3ème trimestre," 1906, H (834), AA; and "Rapport Médical du 2ème semestre," District de l'Aruwimi, 1909, H (838), AA.

20. Mme Van den Perre, president of the Gouttes de Lait de Saint-Gilles in Belgium, founded the Ligue under the Belgian queen's patronage (Mme Van der Kerken, "Les oeuvres sociales et humanitaires au Congo Belge," in *Congrès Colonial National*, Ve session, no. 15, 1941, 8). On the Kisantu clinic, see Léon Guebels, *Relation complète des travaux de la Commission Permanente pour la Protection des Indigènes* (Brussels: Editions J. Duculot, n.d. [1952?]), 130. See also Hunt, " 'Le bébé en brousse,' " 402–3.

21. Davin, "Imperialism and Motherhood." The Belgian church took the lead in the Catholic drive against birth control in western Europe in 1909 (Ron J. Lesthaeghe, *The Decline of Belgian Fertility, 1800–1970* [Princeton, N.J.: Princeton University Press, 1977], 135–39). See, too, Lucien Garot, *Médecine sociale de l'enfance et oeuvres de protection du premier âge* (Liège: Editions Desoer, 1946); and Camille Jacquart, *La mortalité infantile dans les Flandres* (Brussels: Albert Dewit, 1907).

22. Godelieve Masuy-Stroobant, *Les déterminants individuels et régionaux de la mortalité infantile: La Belgique d'hier et d'aujourd'hui* (Louvain-la-Neuve: CIACO, 1983), 80–81.

23. [Belgium], *Congrès Colonial National*, [IIème] (Brussels: Imprimerie Lesigne, 1926), 157–58. The Ligue's work was met, however, with "skepticism" and "disdain" by some doctors, missionaries, and colonial officials until the early 1920s, when doctors and missionaries began applauding the Ligue's work, and the state agreed to subsidize it (Hunt, " 'Le bébé en brousse,' " 403–4). For Province Orientale, see R. Mouchet, "La natalité et la mortalité infantile dans la Province Orientale," *ASBMT* 6 (1926): 165–74.

24. Dr. Veroni, "Rapport sanitaire sur le 2ème semestre," 1910, H (841), AA; and "Circulaire réglementant la situation des femmes des travailleurs de l'Etat," Intérieur no. 43/a, 21 July 1903, in Etat Indépendant du Congo, *Recueil Mensuel des arrêtés, circulaires, instructions et ordres de service* (1903): 98–99.

25. Commissaire Général de Meulemeester to M. le Gouverneur Général, 14 January 1909, H (830), doc. N/116, AA. The state would approve a temporary exemption for a former soldier with five children, one still breast-feeding, for instance, but otherwise found exemptions wanting in economic benefits; Ministre Renkin to M. Le Gouverneur Général, 25 March 1909, H (830), AA; and Ministre Renkin to M. le Gouverneur Général, 25 April 1910, H (830), AA.

26. F. Houssiau, "Quelques considérations sur la pratique médicale au Congo belge principalement à Léopoldville," Examen B/Médecins no. 1, IMT, 1912, 38. Only 723 (4.4 percent) were children; ibid., 1, 38. In 1926, the Léopoldville (Est) native hospital had 192 beds for men and 48 for women and children; A. Staub, "Rapport résumant des observations concernant le service de chirurgie à Léopoldville de juillet 1925 à juillet 1926," Examen B/Médecins no. 47, IMT, 1926, 2.

27. Dr. Veroni, "Rapport sur l'hygiène et les conditions sanitaires de Stanleyville," June 1908–February 1909, H (841), AA. See, too, Jean-Luc Vellut, "Matériaux pour une image du blanc dans la société coloniale du Congo belge," in *Stéréotypes nationaux et préjugés raciaux aux XIXe et XXe siècles*, ed. Jean Pirotte (Leuven: Editions Nauwelaerts, 1982).

28. A. Detry, *A Stanleyville* (Liège: Imprimerie La Meuse, 1912): 119–59; and Dr. Veroni, "Rapport sur l'hygiène et les conditions sanitaires de Stanleyville," June 1908–February 1909, H (841), AA.

29. Alfred Corman, *Annuaire des missions catholiques au Congo belge* (Brussels: Albert Dewit, 1924), 7–8, chart at 200–201.

30. The "first white woman to enter the Congo valley" was Miss Bosson, financée of Henry Craven of the London-based Livingstone Inland Mission; she sailed from England in December 1878. Other missionary women continued to arrive, especially after the American Baptist Missionary Union assumed charge in 1884, sending single women as well, including an African American Miss Fleming in 1884 (Fanny E. Guinness, *The New World of Central Africa, with a History of the First Christian Mission on the Congo* [London: Hodder and Stoughton, 1890]: 197, 200, 444 [photo], 453). The first BMS woman missionary in the lower Congo was Mrs. Thomas (Minnie) Comber, who arrived in June 1879 but died within three months; others did not come until 1886, including the first single woman missionary. George Grenfell returned to the Congo from Cameroon in 1880 with his Jamaican wife, Rose, and their daughter, Patience Elizabeth. Grenfell had been expelled from the BMS in 1878 for having impregnated Miss Rose Edgerley, then the Jamaican housekeeper of their church in Victoria, Cameroon (Brian Stanley, *The History of the Baptist Missionary Society, 1792–1992* [Edinburgh: T. and T. Clark, 1992], 119–20, 125). Patience Elizabeth went on to become a single woman missionary teacher at Yakusu before dying there in 1899 (*Missionary Herald*, May 1899, 268; August 1899; and May 1900, 263–65).

31. "La femme blanche au Congo," Institut de Solvay, Travaux du Groupe d'Etudes coloniales, no. 4, extract from *Bulletin de la Société Belge d'Etudes Coloniales* 5 (May 1910): 8–10.

32. Émile Zola, *Fécondité* (Paris: Librairie Charpentier et Fasquelle, 1899); discussed in Michael S. Teitelbaum and Jay M. Winter, *The Fear of Population Decline* (Orlando, Fla.: Academic Press, 1985), 23–28.

33. Pierre Daye, *Problèmes Congolais* (Brussels: Ecrits, 1943): 28–30. On Empire Day, see Anne Bloomfield, "Drill and Dance as Symbols of Imperialism," in *Making Imperial Mentalities: Socialisation and British Imperialism,* ed. J. A. Mangan (Manchester: Manchester University Press, 1990), 74–95. On the contributions of Colonial Days to the Ligue's income, see Ligue pour la Protection de l'Enfance noire au Congo Belge, *Rapports Annuels*, 1929–1930, 7; 1936–1937, 12. By 1936–37, a bridge tournament and ball were four times as important to the Ligue's income as the Colonial Days (ibid.).

34. Depopulation and a low birthrate became dominant themes in a vast colonial demographic literature. For an excellent annotated bibliography of the same, see Anne Retel-Laurentin, *Infécondité en Afrique noire: Maladies et conséquences sociales* (Paris: Masson, 1974), 141–88. Historians tend to agree that equatorial Africa, particularly the forest region of the French and Belgian Congo, bore some of the worst population catastrophes in Africa during the late nineteenth and early twentieth centuries; see Steven Feierman, "Struggles for Control: The Social Roots of Health and Healing in Modern Africa," *African Studies Review* 28 (1985): 85–93. Attempts to assess the extent of depopulation in the Congo have been riddled by the original, problematic calculations of Henry Morton Stanley; see William Roger Louis and Jean Stengers, *E. D. Morel's History of the Congo Reform Movement* (London: Oxford University Press, 1968), 252–56.

35. For this argument, see David Voas, "Subfertility and Disruption in the Congo Basin," in *African Historical Demography,* vol. 2 (Edinburgh: Centre of African Studies, University of Edinburgh, 1981), 777–99. For other perspectives, see Anatole Romaniuk, *La fécondité des populations congolaises* (Paris: Mouton, 1967), 129–70; Retel-Laurentin, *Infécondité en Afrique noire;* and Bogumil Jewsiewicki, "Toward a Historical Sociology of Population in Zaire," *African Population and Capitalism,* ed. Dennis Cordell and Joel W. Gregory (Boulder, Colo.: Westview Press, 1987), 271–79. Depopulation was a major subject within "red rubber" inquiries.

36. The eugenic society was an organization of primarily Free Mason doctors, affiliated with the lay University of Brussels. An excellent source on family allocation legislation and the Ligue des Familles Nombreuses remains D. V. Glass, *Population: Policies and Movements in Europe* (Oxford: Oxford University Press, 1940). On the religious and ideological characteristics of eugenics (or especially from 1930, "social hygiene") in Belgium, see W. De Raes, "Eugenetika in de Belgische medische wereld tijdens het interbellum," *Revue belge d'Histoire contemporaine* 20 (1989): 399–464. See also Chris Vandenbroeke, "Démographie: La dualité de la norme et des faits," in *Les années trente en Belgique: la séduction des masses* (Brussels: CGER, 1994), 125–37, 342; and V. Cocq and Fr. Mercken, "L'assistance obstétricale au Congo belge (y compris le Ruanda-Urundi)," *Gynécologie et Obstétrique* 31, no. 4 (1935): 457.

37. From the late 1880s, Leopold II promised close Congo Free State support to Belgian Catholic missionaries who went to his colony. With the exception of a four-year period during and just after World War I when one non-Catholic Liberal, Louis Franck, served as Minister of the Colonies in Brussels, almost all subsequent Ministers of the Colonies belonged to the Catholic Party until the mid-1950s. Big business, though under some Liberal influence, was nationalist in orientation, and thus, willing to make agreements with Belgian Catholic missions for the provision of Congolese social and medical welfare. Roman Catholic missions, therefore, had major control over schools and state hospitals in the Congo from 1925 to 1955.

38. In so doing, Union Minière broke with South African mining practice (where only whites were skilled workers) and closely followed the recommendations of a special commission's report on the Congo's "social question" in 1924; for greater detail, see Hunt, " 'Le bébé en brousse.' " On "trinity" logic—capital, church, state—in the Congo, see Crawford Young, *Politics in the Congo* (Princeton, N.J.: Princeton University Press, 1965); but compare Jean-Luc Vellut, "Articulations entre entreprises et Etat: Pouvoirs hégémoniques dans le bloc colonial belge (1908–1960)," in *Entreprises et entrepreneurs en Afrique (XIXe et XXe siècles)* (Paris: l'Harmattan, 1983).

39. Hunt, "Le bébé en brousse."

40. In Léopold Flion, "Cercles d'Etudes coloniales de l'Université de Bruxelles: Femmes et enfants blancs au Congo, au point de vue médical," *Bruxelles-Médical* 8 (1927–1928): 529–31.

41. Pierre Daye, "Au Congo il faut des femmes blanches," [1924], in *Problèmes Congolais* (Brussels: Ecrits, 1943): 145–46.

42. As late as 1924, one of the first colonial doctors, Dryepondt, insisted that tolerating "discreet concubinage" was very different than "favoring debauchery." Yet ménagères became disreputable, while the fate of their métis offspring became an indelicate issue. Some argued that it was these "irregular unions" that were bad, not their "fertility." Others, like Dryepondt, pointed to the infertility of these Congolese "housekeepers" (Dr. Dryepondt, "La question des

métis au Congo Belge: Causerie faite au Cercle Africaine à Bruxelles," 1 July 1924, AI 14 [4674], "Mulâtres. Avant 1940," AA). The early colonial medical focus on male hygiene made clear the links among venereal disease, sterility, and miscarriages; the same concerns emerged from some of the doctors' first experiences with obstetrics in the colony. See, for example, Barthélémi, "Etude sur la syphilis." Doctors, aware of the effects of gonorrhea and syphilis on miscarriages and newborns, noted that ménagères were rarely mothers (Rapport sur l'hygiène de 3ème trimestre, 1906, H [834], AA). One traveler who remarked on "the ménagère" as "an institution of the Congo" noted: "there are no half-breed children; the ménagères with the help of witch-doctors see to that. . . . But whatever the cause, the result tends to simplify the future problem of the Congo" (Hermann Norden, *Fresh Tracks in the Belgian Congo: From Its Uganda Border to the Mouth of the Congo* [Boston: Small, Maynard, and Company, 1924], 180–83). Everyone did not see the future as so simple: children of mixed race in the Congo posed dilemmas. Neither welcomed by whites nor blacks, they were "malcontents," while the girls tended to be in "toilette criarde, cherchant aventure" (loud clothes, looking for adventure) ("La femme blanche au Congo," 7). See also "Rapports sanitaires du district de l'Aruwimi," H (838), AA. Curiously, métis daughters were among the first Congolese women to be persuaded to perform bodily nursing and midwifery work. Two took midwife exams at Boma's school in 1916; and one "dame mulâtresse, digne sous tous rapports" (mulatto lady, respectable from all points of view) was studying at Brussels' Ecole de Médicine Tropicale in 1931 (she failed an exam, though it was hoped that she would pass when she took it again) ("Ecole des Accoucheuses Indigènes à Boma, Rapport et Statistiques sur l'Année 1926," RA/CB [82] 3, "Rapports Médicaux des différents missions"; and Directeur Général to Madame Watry-Ponselle, Union des Femmes Coloniales, 3 February 1931, H [4389] 56, document N/978, AA).

43. Hunt, "Le bébé en brousse." Not all European women were Belgian, but by the 1920s, efforts were underway to nationalize the colonial presence. See also the special issue "Femmes coloniales au Congo belge," of *Enquêtes et Documents d'Histoire Africaine* 7 (1987). Concerns about the effects of the tropical climate on white women's hormones and fertility surged again during the war, when most Belgian women could at best take four-month holidays in South Africa; J. Lambillon proposed comparative research on missionary nuns, though he admitted this would be "difficult and delicate" (J. Lambillon, "Note au sujet des troubles endocriens de la femme européenne durant les années de guerre au Congo belge," *ASBMT* 27 [1947]: 95–104, esp. 103).

44. G. Trolli, "Le Service Médical au Congo belge," Annexe no. 31, in Congo Belge, *Rapport sur l'hygiène publique*, 1925, 76–79.

45. Congo Belge, *Rapport sur l'hygiène publique*, 1925, 22.

46. At least in Province Orientale, where the numbers of normal European births increased from 1930 (see RA/CB (151) 1, Province Orientale, Service Médical, Rapport Technique Annuel, 1931). A royal decree of 30 October 1931 required employers to give medical care to the wives of all white employees under contract (Cocq and Mercken, "L'assistance obstétricale au Congo belge," 442).

47. Annexe au Rapport Annuel, 1915, RA/CB (81) 4, AA; and Annexe au Rapport Annuel, 1915, RA/CB (81) 3, AA; and Congo Belge, *Rapport sur l'hygiène publique*, 1925, 15; 1929, 36; and 1940, 59–60.

48. Jean-Luc Vellut, "Les Belges au Congo (1885–1960)," in *La Belgique, Sociétés et cultures depuis 150 Ans, 1830–1980*, ed. Albert d'Haenens (Brussels: Ministère des Affaires Etrangères, 1980), 262. Twenty-one more congregations of nuns came to the Congo during the same period, 1915 to 1928 (J. Van Wing and V. Goeme, *Annuaire des Missions Catholiques au Congo Belge et au Ruanda-Urundi* [Brussels: L'Edition Universelle, 1949]).

49. Her pregnancy and birth were complicated by malaria; afterward, she did not hesitate to entrust her baby to a "boy" (Margaret Sally Eulick, *White Mother in Africa* [New York: Richard R. Smith, 1939], 14, 18–19, 93–107). By 1928, there was a hospital for whites with two rooms organized as a maternity, though no maternity care was provided for Congolese women. Each doctor took care of twenty-five to thirty Europeans and two to three thousand Congolese workers. See H. Gillet, "Le service médical des Sociétés minières du Kasai (Champs diamantifères du Kasai)," *ASBMT* 8 (1928): 233–49.

50. Flion, "Cercles d'Etudes," 529–31.

51. Mrs. Mill, "The Struggle for Right Living," *YQN* 82 (July 1930): 12–14. C. C. Chesterman, "The Work of the Hospital," *YQN* 88 (January 1932): 13–15; and R. E. Holmes, "Our Medical Work," *YQN* 92 (January 1933): 17–18. In 1924, the Yakusu hospital sent a bill to the state for thirty days of private maternity nursing "rendered by Mademoiselle Owen to Madame Ringoet in connection with her confinement." An annotation indicated that the bill was the first of its type, and that if the state refused to pay, the bill should be canceled (Bill for services, Yakusu Hospital, 30 October 1924, in dossier no. 6, "Gouvernement G," HDO, Yakusu.

52. *Mboli ya Tengai* 217 (1930); and Gladys Owen to Miss Bowser, 27 February 1931, Owen file, BMSA.

53. Mrs. Millman to Miss Bowser, n.d. [ca. 1931], Millman file, BMSA; Gladys Owen to Miss Bowser, 27 February 1931, Owen file, BMSA; and Gladys Parris to Miss Bowser, 3 June 1937, Owen file, BMSA.

54. Dr. Holmes to Dr. Chesterman, 18 November 1939, R. Holmes file, BMSA; and BMS Yakusu Annual Medical Report, 1949, HDO, Yakusu.

55. Winifred Browne diary, Yakusu, 22 November 1943, Winifred Browne Burke Papers, Godalming (hereafter WBB Papers), and Stanley G. Browne to Father, Nellie, and All, 1 December 1943, SGB Papers.

56. Dorothy Daniel, birth register, 1945–1950, Dorothy Daniel Papers, Corse Staunton. See also E. Muriel Lean to Dr. Chesterman, 10 January 1942, Lean file, BMSA.

57. Dr. Barlovatz to Dr. Browne, 14 July 1948; 29 July 1948; 20 August 1948; 23 August 1948; 26 August 1948; and Wednesday, Twenty Hrs., n.d., in dossier no. 16, "Territoire Yangambi," HDO, Yakusu.

58. Mary Fagg to Dear Friends, 15 June 1957, Fagg prayer letters, BMSA. See also Mary Fagg, Thornham, 11 November 1990.

59. Hunt, "Le bébé en brousse." Compare Masuy-Stroobant, *Les déterminants individuels*.

60. Jean-Marie Habig, "Enseignement médical pour coloniaux, 2ème partie, Psychopathologie de l'Européen et du Noir" (Ligue Coloniale Belge, Cours Coloniaux de Bruxelles, Brussels, 1944, unpublished manuscript), 10–11 [available in the Bibliothèque Africaine, Brussels].

61. Jean-Marie Habig, *Vivre en Afrique centrale: Santé, hygiène, morale* (Brussels: L'Edition Universelle, 1952), 251, 256.

62. C. Debroux, "Comportement démographique de la population européenne après la seconde guerre mondiale," *Enquêtes et Documents d'Histoire Africaine* 7 (1987): 5–14, esp. 10. Debroux argues that the medical and social selection of those going to the colony was an important factor in the difference.

63. Masuy-Stroobant, *Les Déterminants individuels.*

64. In Flion, "Cercles d'Etudes," 529–31.

65. Cocq and Mercken, "L'assistance obstétricale au Congo belge," 481; "Mesures à prendre en faveur des enfants indigènes qui perdent leur mère au moment de leur naissance ou peu de temps après," Secrétariat Général no. 3, 5 February 1925, Congo belge, *Recueil Mensuel* (1925): 30; and "Circulaire réglementant l'organisation et le fonctionnement des diverses formations sanitaires du service de la Colonie," Hygiène no. 16, 17 June 1926, Congo Belge, *Recueil Mensuel* (1926): 91–107, esp. 95.

66. "Ecole des Accoucheuses Indigènes à Boma, Rapport et Statistiques sur l'Année 1926," RA/CB (82) 3, "Rapports Médicaux des différents missions," AA; and Croix-Rouge du Congo, *Rapport Annuel*, 1927, 19–20.

67. Séance du 31 janvier 1929 de "Pour la Protection de la Femme Indigène," F.P. (2612) no. 945, "Personnel noir. Protection des femmes indigènes," AA.

68. G. Fronville, "Six années de pratique chirurgicale chez les noirs du Katanga," Examen B/Médecins no. 44, IMT, 1926, 86, 95, 98.

69. E. Rebuffat, "Contribution a l'étude de relèvement de la natalité au Congo belge," Examen B/Médecins no. 48a, IMT, 1927.

70. Cocq and Mercken, "L'assistance obstétricale au Congo belge," 454. See also Shaw, "Force Publique, Force Unique," 278–83.

71. Fronville, "Six années de pratique chirurgicale," 86.

72. He did not indicate how he handled this childbirth presentation. Dr. Grossule, "Rapport médical," District de l'Aruwimi, 2e semestre 1907, H (838), "Rapports sanitaires du district de l'Aruwimi," AA.

73. Houssiau, "Quelques considérations à Léopoldville." Vesicovaginal fistulas, rare in Europe but common in African practice, were usually of obstetric origin; on thirty-three cases, see P. Valcke, "Les fistules vésico-vaginales en pratique rurale," Examen B/Médecins no. 301, IMT, 1959.

74. C. Pulieri, "Rapport sur les observations d'Afrique," Examen B/Médecins no. 2, IMT, 1912, 3.

75. Cocq and Mercken, "L'assistance obstétricale au Congo belge." Paul Weindling notes that a unifying force among these diverse political ideologies and the historical expressions to which they gave rise was the new phenomenon of transnational technocrats, especially the emergence of demographers and their skills in population, fertility, and cohort analysis (Weindling, "Fascism and Population in Comparative European Perspective," in *Population and Resources in Western Intellectual Traditions*, ed. Michael S. Teitelbaum and Jay M. Winter [Cambridge: Cambridge University Press, 1989], 102–21). On interwar positive eugenics in Belgium, see De Raes, "Eugenetika."

76. Cocq and Mercken, "L'assistance obstétricale au Congo belge," esp. 496. The transposition of the ideas emanating from social Catholic population movements in Belgium to the colony was an easy passage in political terms. The Ministry of Colonies was controlled largely by the Catholic Party from the mid-1920s to the mid-1950s, as close missionary ties and ministerial

appointments testified. In Belgium, however, both secular and ecclesiastical milieus tended to be pronatalist and favor social hygiene, though anticlerical, neo-Malthusian (pro–birth control) groups were also active. The latter orientation rarely found its way to the colony, where there was moral panic over the thought that Congolese women used abortifacients, and where by the 1950s, some Belgian doctors may have been imprisoned for providing clandestine abortions within their private European practices.

77. R. Van Nitsen, *L'Hygiène des travailleurs noirs dans les camps industriels du Haut-Katanga* (Brussels: IRSC, 1933).

78. Hunt, " 'Le bébé en brousse.' "

79. FOREAMI, *Rapport annuel,* 1931. See also G. Trolli, *Historique de l'assistance médicale aux indigènes du Congo belge: Nouvelle méthode adoptée par FOREAMI, Résultats obtenus* (Brussels: Van Doosselaere, 1930).

80. On FOREAMI, see A. Duren, "Quelques aspects de la vie médicale au Congo belge," extract from *Le Scalpel* 2–5 (12, 19, 26 January and 2 February 1935); Trolli, *Historique de l'assistance médicale aux indigènes du Congo belge;* and FOREAMI, *Rapports annuels,* 1931–1955.

81. Province Orientale, Service de l'Hygiène, "Rapport Annuel," 1922, 29, RA/CB (149) 4, AA.

82. Madeleine Migeon, *La faute du soleil! Eve en Afrique* (Brussels: Editions de l'Expansion Belge, n.d.), 240–41, 179. By 1940, the government was no longer hiring lay nurses ("Cours de Puericulture," Caisse no. 337, in H 4457 [779], AA).

83. Le Directeur Général to Monsieur l'Administrateur Général, 8 December 1932, H 4493 (1128), Oeuvres de l'Enfance, Consultations de Nourissons, 1931–1956, AA. Of the thirteen congregations in 1923, six had arrived in the 1890s and two in the 1910s (Alfred Corman, *Annuaire des missions,* 1924, 7–8, chart at 200–201; Corman, *Annuaire des missions,* 1935, 11–13, 380, 386; Fr. de Meeus and D. R. Steerberghen, *Les Missions religieuses au Congo belge* [Antwerp: Editions Zaïre, 1947], unpaged charts; and Marie-Joseph Lory, *Face à l'avenir: L'église au Congo belge et au Ruanda-Urundi* [Tournai: Casterman, 1958], 204–5).

84. Christian charity as practiced by female religious orders was long defined to include medical works, such as nursing work in hospitals (Jacques Léonard, "Femmes, religion et médecine: Les religieuses qui soignent, en France au XIXe siècle," *Annales: Economies, Sociétés, Civilisations* 32 [1977]: 887–907). Yet pregnant women were explicitly excluded as patients from many Belgian hospitals until the early nineteenth century, where "nursing sisters" were also in short supply (see Paul Bonenfant, *Le problème du paupérisme en Belgique à la fin de l'Ancien Régime,* mémoire, Classe des Lettres et des Sciences Morales et Politiques, vol. 35 [Brussels: Académie Royale de Belgique, 1934], 183). (Although there was a maternity hospital in medieval Louvain; see Walter John Marx, *The Development of Charity in Medieval Louvain* [Yonkers, N.Y.: self-published, 1936], 73–74.) Rather, local Catholic churches tended to have married, older women with midwifery skills act as parish midwives. These village women would, in alliance with local priests, handle baptisms in emergencies, and conduct the kind of morality control work (paternity confessions) that was thought necessary in the case of unmarried and widowed parturients. Protestant midwives, meanwhile, were the subject of prosecutions because they did not baptize (see Mireille Laget, "Childbirth in Seventeenth- and Eighteenth-Century France: Obstetrical Practices and Collective Attitudes," in *Medicine and Society in France,* ed. Robert Forster and Orest Ranum [Baltimore, Md.: Johns Hopkins University Press, 1980], 144–46). On Belgian obstetric practice and legislation, see Roger Darquenne, "L'obstétrique

aux XVIIIe et XIXe siècles," in *Ecoles et livres d'école en Hainaut du XVIe au XIXe siècle* (Mons, Belgium: Editions Universitaires de Mons, 1971), 184–312. On bastardy confessions and paternity claims in eighteenth-century Maine, see Laurel Thatcher Ulrich, *A Midwife's Tale: The Life of Martha Ballard, Based on Her Diary, 1785–1812* (New York: Knopf, 1990), 147–61. On adultery confessions and how they were carried into colonial maternity wards in the Central African Republic, see Anne Retel-Laurentin, *Sorcellerie et ordalies* (Paris: Editions Anthropos, 1974), 188–93.

85. And this after the governor general's proposal of replacing the Franciscaines in Stanleyville with either the Soeurs Chanoinesses de St-Augustin or the Soeurs Charité de Gand was not pursued (Inspecteur Général to Monsieur le Ministre, 28 December 1925; Inspecteur Général to M. l'Inspecteur Général, Chef de Service, 3 May 1926; Secrétaire Général to M. le Gouverneur Général, 11 March 1927; and Projet de Convention entre le Ministre des Colonies et la Révérende Mère Supérieure des Franciscaines Missionaires de Marie, 1 January 1927). By the end of 1927, the European lay personnel at the African hospital in Stanleyville had been replaced entirely by the nursing nuns. The agreement was annotated, changing the wording "laïque accoucheuse diplômée" to read "agrégée accoucheuse diplômée" (Rapport d'Inspection de Stanleyville, March 1928, by Dr. Trolli, 3). All documents are in H [4393], Hôpital de Stanleyville, AA.

86. Fr. Mercken, "L'assistance obstétricale missionaire au Congo belge," *L'Aide Médicale aux Missions* 7 (October 1935): 71.

87. L. Mottoulle, "Maternités noires et religieuses blanches au Congo belge," *Revue Coloniale Belge* 4, no. 106 (1 March 1950): 160–61; Corman, *Annuaire des missions*, 1924, 7–8, chart at 200–201; Corman, *Annuaire des missions*, 1935, 11–13, 380, 386; de Meeus and Steerberghen, *Les missions religieuses au Congo belge*, unpaged charts; and Lory, *Face à l'avenir*, 204–5. There were 60 Belgian congregations (26 francophone and 34 Flemish, according to the language used to indicate headquarter addresses), 2 Dutch, 2 French, and 1 congregation from Luxembourg in 1949. Their size varied from 4 to 228 nuns; 14 congregations had only 4 to 10 nuns present in the Congo, 33 congregations had 11 to 25 nuns present, 9 had 26 to 44 nuns, and 3 had 53 to 88 nuns. Thirty-eight percent of the 1951 nuns belonged to the 4 largest orders (with 162 to 228 members each), 3 of which had headquarters in Flanders and 1, the Soeurs Franciscaines, a French-language address in Brussels. See Van Wing and Goeme, *Annuaire des Missions Catholiques*, 12–13, 17–24, 636–38. On the histories, maternity sites, and nuns' names and credentials of these 65 congregations, see ibid.

88. "Since Our Last Issue," *YQN* 49 (November 1921): 6; C. C. Chesterman, "Developments in the Medical Mission," *YQN* 57 (January 1924), 19; and Ligue pour la Protection de l'Enfance noire au Congo Belge, *Rapport Annuel*, 1925–1926, 46–47.

89. G. C. Owen, "A District Baby Clinic," *YQN* 85 (April 1931), 9–11; C. C. Chesterman, "The Work of the Hospital," *YQN* 88 (January 1932), 13–15. I take the vocabulary of "global cultural flows" from Arjun Appadurai (see his *Modernity at Large: Cultural Dimensions of Globalization* [Minneapolis: University of Minnesota Press, 1996]).

90. BMS Yakusu Annual Medical Reports, 1929–1959, HDO, Yakusu.

91. "In the absence of a State ruling for wives of teachers in the district who may have babies, it was agreed that it should be recommended to the Consistoire that the Church be responsible

for the payment of these allowances" (Staff Committee Minutes, 27 December 1946, District Pastor's Office, Yakusu).

92. Ordinary budgets for medical services constituted about 10 percent of the total Belgian Congo budget annually from 1946 (this amount ranged from about 200 million Congolese francs in 1946 to about 1.2 billion francs in 1957). From 1950, extraordinary budgets for construction of medical services in connection with a ten-year plan amounted to about another 300 million francs per year. In addition, the FBEI was spending about 150 million francs a year beginning in 1949 on medical equipment for rural areas (Belgium, Office de l'Information et des Relations Publiques pour le Congo Belge et le Ruanda-Urundi, *Health in Belgian Africa* [Brussels: Inforcongo, 1958], 16–17).

93. Yakusu's district did not precisely coincide with the Isangi *territoire*, but it came close. Isangi territoire was relatively prolific. Sterility was a much larger problem in the Opala territoire, where only 17,785 women out of 33,148 were fertile (2,434 out of 5,184 of those ages twenty-five to twenty-nine) in the mid-1950s as opposed to 30,029 women out of 38,753 (4,308 out of 5,144 in the twenty-five- to twenty-nine-year cohort) in the Isangi territoire. Women of the Isangi territoire tended to have 3.10 live births in their lifetime, whereas those of the Opala territoire tended to only have 1.66 live births (Th. Verheust, "Enquête démographique par sondage, 1955–1957—Province Orientale, District de Stanleyville—District du Haut-Uélé," *Cahiers du CEDAF* 22 [1978], 32, 36). These territorial distinctions suggest an ethnic (Lokele of Isangi versus BaMbole of Opala) contrast in infertility rates.

94. Mama Malia Winnie, Kisangani, 4 December 1989.

95. Mary Fagg to Dear Friends, 13 March 1956, Fagg prayer letter file, BMSA.

96. "Together with God," 1956, 20–22, from "Pamphlets, Mostly Medical, All Fields," Box H/56, BMSA.

97. Mary Fagg, "The Training of Pupil-Midwives," *YQN* 149 (February 1953): 18.

98. Mary Fagg to Dear Friends, 15 June 1957, Fagg prayer letter file, BMSA.

99. Mary Fagg to Dear Friends, February 1958, Fagg prayer letter file, BMSA. Fagg commented on the morality problems several times; see also Mary Fagg to Dear Friends, 7 August 1955; 15 August 1956; 5 July 1957, Fagg prayer letter file, BMSA.

100. Mary Fagg to Dear Friends, 31 March 1959, Fagg prayer letter file, BMSA.

101. Missionary interpretations of Malia Winnie were continually colored by their (limited) knowledge of her difficult marriage: "She has had a hard life, remaining faithful to this weak and wayward husband of hers, never giving up hope that one day her prayers for him will be answered and he will overcome" (G. Ennals, "The Long View," *YQN* 145 [February 1950]: 14). Tokolokaya was dismissed from the medical service in 1949 for drinking at Yalemba: "His wife, Malia Winnie, who independently of her husband holds work in the Hospital, has stated that she wishes to remain in the work at Yakusu and will not follow her husband. It was agreed to allow her to remain at Yakusu in the work. Her husband will be allowed to live with her. Malia is to make a public statement in front of the deacons that she has decided voluntarily to do this" (Station Council Minutes, 16 January 1949, District Pastor's Office, Yakusu). By the end of the year, Tokolokaya had "repented" and was readmitted to church fellowship and hospital employment (ibid., 27 December 1949).

102. Mama Malia Winnie, Kisangani, 4 December 1989.

103. Mama Noel Dickie, Kisangani, 23 January 1990.

104. Mama Loséa Martine, Kisangani, 4 December 1989.

105. Mama Machuli Georgine, Kisangani, 2 December 1989.

106. E. Muriel Lean to Dr. Chesterman, 10 May 1942, Lean file, BMSA.

107. It was agreed that the girls "must leave 10 fr. per month in their books until [the] end [of] 2 years' training" (Winnie Browne, diary, Yakusu, 1 January 1944, WBB Papers).

108. Winnie Browne, diary, Yakusu, 29 January 1944, WBB Papers.

109. Staff Meeting Minutes, 27 December 1948, District Pastor's Office, Yakusu (hereafter DPO, Yakusu).

110. Dr. A. Aretti, BIARO, to Dr. Browne, 5 March 1956, 29 March 1956, 4 July 1956; R. Mommens and R. Wauters, BIARO, to Dr. Browne, 6 October 1956; and Dr. F. Van Mierlo to Médecin-Directeur de l'Ecole des aides-accoucheuses, Mission B.M.S. à Yakusu, 22 August 1956 (all in dossier no. 31, "Inspection Médicale Scolaire," HDO, Yakusu).

111. Mama Machuli Georgine, Kisangani, 3 December 1989; and group interview with Yakusu-trained nurses and midwives, Kisangani, 29 April 1989.

112. R. Holmes, "The Building of the Yaombole Dispensary," YQN 102 (July 1935): 16–18. In a 1941 letter, Browne reviewed the careers of several nurses, including a few husband-wife teams; he noted that "even our 'cast-offs' do very good in various spheres" (Stanley G. Browne to Dr. Chesterman, 20 November 1941, Browne file, BMSA).

113. E. Muriel Lean to Dr. Chesterman, dated 10 January 1942 [actually 1943], Lean file, BMSA.

114. Station Committee Minutes, 29 June 1948, DPO, Yakusu.

115. "Together with God," 1956, 21–22, from "Pamphlets, Mostly Medical, All Fields," Box H/56, BMSA.

116. Mary Fagg to Dear Friends, 15 August 1956, Fagg prayer letter file, BMSA.

117. BMS Yakusu Annual Medical Reports, 1951–1957, HDO, Yakusu; see also Hunt "Negotiated Colonialism," tables 4–6, 470–72.

118. Janson Baofa to Monsieur le Médecin-agréé, Yangonde, 17 October 1956, in dossier no. 36, "Correspondance des Infirmiers," HDO, Yakusu.

119. Madeleine Lititiyo to Dr. Browne, Yangonde, 13 January 1957; Bosongo Bonganga Browne to Aide-Accoucheuse Madeleine, 15 January 1957; Madeleine Lititiyo to Doctor Browne, 2 July 1957. All letters, written in Lokele, are in "Aides-Accoucheuses" file, HDO, Yakusu.

120. The first five nuns arrived in Yanonge in 1939; this nursing congregation was founded the year before in Luxembourg ("Soeurs de Sainte-Elisabeth," 1938–1964 file, in Chancellerie offices, Procure Catholique, Kisangani). Information on this maternity hospital proved difficult to trace (personal communication from Soeur Jeanne Bosko, Maison Mère des Soeurs de Sainte-Elisabeth to author, 17 April 1990). Three of the Soeurs de Sainte-Elisabeth of Luxembourg were killed by the BaSimbas in Kisangani in 1964. No nuns ever returned to Yanonge, nor was the hospital director able to locate any written documentation. Papa Tika Kalokola, Bonama Yaya, Mama Monsanyembo, with Yenge Ituku and Lofanjola-Lisele (Pesapesa), Yanonge, 6 September 1989; Mama Monsanyembo (Mosa), Yanonge, 15 November 1989. Such "waiting homes," fashionable again under the new "Safe Motherhood" campaigns of the 1990s, were fairly standard fare in the Congo by the 1950s.

121. There were 456 births (including 5 dystocial) at the Yanonge maternity hospital in 1956, and

419 (including 13 dystocial) in 1957 (BMS Yakusu Annual Medical Report, 1956, 1957, HDO, Yakusu). Yakusu's church-supported dispensaries delivered only 14 percent of the pregnancies observed (39 out of 270), Yakusu's company dispensaries (all Belgika by the 1950s) delivered 50 percent (68 out of 137) of the births, and Yakusu's state dispensaries (including Yanonge and Yangonde) administered 60 percent (933 out of 1,549). For these and other statistics, see the tables in Nancy Rose Hunt "Negotiated Colonialism: Domesticity, Hygiene, and Birth Work in the Belgian Congo" (Ph.D. diss., University of Wisconsin–Madison, 1992).

122. Shangazi Angelani, Yainyongo-Romée, 21 September 1989.

123. E. Muriel Lean, "Our New Maternity Ward—Behind the Scenes," *YQN* 122 (September 1940): 3. Statistics on baby clinics and birth confinements at Yakusu date from 1937, the year the new ward's foundation was laid; BMS Yakusu Annual Medical Report, 1937, BMSA.

124. Young, *Politics in the Congo*, 131, 133.

125. Masuy-Stroobant, *Les Déterminants individuels.*

126. Anatole Romaniuk, "The Demography of the Democratic Republic of Congo," in *The Demography of Tropical Africa,* William Brass et al. (Princeton, N.J.: Princeton University Press, 1968), 248–49. On postwar social legislation to encourage large families, including family allocation and tax exemption laws, see Ghu-Gha Bianga, "La politique démographique au Congo belge," *Population* 33 (1978): 189–94. The birthrate also rose in this period.

127. Young, *Politics in the Congo*, 230, 231.

128. "Chronique de la vie indigène," *La Voix du Congolais* 11, no. 109 (April 1955): 376.

129. Tejaswini Niranjana, *Siting Translation: History, Post-Structuralism, and the Colonial Context* (Berkeley: University of California Press, 1992); and Nicholas Thomas, *Entangled Objects: Exchange, Material Culture, and Colonialism in the Pacific* (Cambridge: Harvard University Press, 1991).

130. Mama Monsanyembo (Mosa), Yanonge, 15 November 1989.

131. Ibid.

132. Ibid.

133. Papa Tika Kalokola, Bonama Yaya, Mama Monsanyembo, with Yenge Ituku and Lofanjola-Lisele (Pesapesa), Yanonge, 6 September 1989.

134. Papa Boshanene, Yakusu, 24 February 1989.

135. Mama Elisa Shanana and Bibi Alimo Singili, Yakoso, 23 November 1989.

136. Papa Boshanene, Yakusu, 24 February 1989. Matabish signifies gift, tip, even bribe.

137. Dorothy James file, Candidate Papers, BMSA.

138. Gladys Owen, "Part of a Morning's Work," *YQN* 58 (April 1924): 2; and Gordon Spear, "The Hospital," *YQN* 53 (January 1923): 3.

139. "Thanks!" *YQN* 84 (January 1931): 24; G. C. Ennals, "The Happiest Time of the Year," *YQN* 85 (April 1931): 4–5; and "Thanks!" *YQN* 86 (July 1931): 7.

140. Winifred Browne to Ivy, 12 September 1940, SGB Papers.

141. E. Muriel Lean to Dr. Chesterman, 10 May 1942, Lean file, BMSA.

142. J. D. Moore, "Mondays and Tuesdays at Two," *YQN* 149 (February 1953): 16–17.

143. Mary Fagg to Dear Friends, 15 June 1957, Fagg prayer letter file, BMSA.

144. See Maurist Dony, *Mashauri kwa Mama wa Kongo* (Brussels: FBEI, n.d. [1953?]).

145. The arrival of First World public health care is Jean-Luc Vellut's argument; see his "Détresse matérielle et découvertes de la misère dans les colonies belges d'Afrique centrale, ca. 1900–1960," in *La Belgique et l'étranger aux XIXe et XXe siècles*, ed. Michel Dumoulin and Eddy Stols (Louvain-la-Neuve: Nauwelaerts, 1987).

146. Inforcongo Photographs, Photothèque, Section Historique, MRAC.

147. Kathryn Hulme, *The Nun's Story* (London: Pan Books, 1956), 117–18.

148. "Chronique de la vie indigène," *La Voix du Congolais* 139 (October 1957): 807; and "Chronique de la vie indigène," *La Voix du Congolais* 9, no. 88 (July 1953): 481. The subsequent issue exhibited a photo of a "practical baby crib" (*La Voix du Congolais* 10, no. 94 [January 1954]: 44). It is possible that maternity care was discussed so often because the subject was not censored by colonial authorities; it was not a subject of feature articles in the journal.

149. For *Tintin au Congo,* see Hergé, *Les aventures de Tintin: Reporter du Petit "Vingtième" au Congo* (1931; reprint, Tournai, Belgium: Casterman, 1982); and Hergé, *Les aventures de Tintin: Tintin au Congo* (1946; reprint, Paris-Tournai: Casterman, 1974). For Mbumbulu cartoons, see *Nos Images,* esp. "Les aventures de la famille Mbumbulu," *Nos Images,* Sw. ed., 8, no. 124, 20 November 1955, 19. See, too, Nancy Rose Hunt, "*Tintin au Congo* and Its Colonial and Post-Colonial Reformulations," paper presented at the "Images and Empires" conference, Yale University, 14–16 February 1997.

150. G. Valcke, "Note," *ASBMT* 14 (1934): 432–33.

151. Notably, A. Duboccage, "La natalité chez les Bakongo dans ses rapports avec la gynécologie," *ASBMT* 9 (1929): 265–74; P. Guillot, "Quelques cas gynécologiques et actes opératoires qu'ils ont provoqués chez les noirs du Congo," *Bulletin de la Société de Pathologie Exotique* 23 (1930): 205–9; and A. Duboccage, "Notes cliniques du service gynécologique de la FOMULAC [Fondation Médicale de l'Université de Louvain au Congo] à Kisantu," *ASBMT* 14 (1934): 421–33.

152. Dr. Vander Elst, "Six mois de gynécologie à l'Hôpital des Noirs de Léopoldville," *Bruxelles-Médical* 26 (1946): 1312–13.

153. Previously, obstetrics and gynecology were embraced within doctors' reports on colonial surgery. See Staub, "Rapport résumant des observations concernant la chirurgie"; G. Linaro, "Les affections chirurgicales plus communes des indigènes de l'Equateur," Examen B/Médecins no. 36, IMT, 1926; Fronville, "Six années de practique chirurgicale," 23–24; R. Thémelin, "Thèse présentée pour l'examen B," Examen B/Médecins no. 70a–b, IMT, 1930; and J. P. Valcke, "Six années de practique chirurgicale au Congo," Examen B/Médecins no. 81, IMT, 1934, 3–4.

154. The literature is substantial, and particularly can be followed in colonial doctors' IMT exams (available at the Institute in Antwerp), and the *ASBMT*; other colonial medical journals and *Bruxelles-Médical* are additional sources. One of the major obstetrician authors was J. Lambillon, who took an interest in the growth of eclampsia among city women in the post–World War II period; see his "Contribution à l'étude du problème obstétrical chez l'autochtone du Congo belge" (Thèse d'Agrégation de l'Enseignement Supérieur, Université Catholique de Louvain, Brussels, 1950); and his "Evolution de la pathologie obstétricale en Afrique centrale de 1935 à 1960," *ASBMT* 44 (1964): 487–92.

155. Duboccage, "La natalité chez les Bakongo."

156. G. Platel and Yv. Vandergoten, "Réflexions sur les résultats obtenus par une consultation des nourrissons au Mayombe (Congo belge)," *ASBMT* 20 (1940): 297–333, esp. 312–14. Their objection to Catholicism was most evident in their defense of polygyny as a practice that women favored because it diminished their workloads (ibid., 313–14).

157. Ibid. Italics added.

158. Gouverneur Général Jungers to M. le Gouverneur, 3 March 1949, H 4493 (1128), "Oeuvres de l'Enfance. Consultations de nourrissons," AA.

159. See especially his unpublished report about his study journey (photocopy in the possession of the author was located in the old colonial provincial library in Kisangani) (Marc Vincent, "Mission d'Information," [OREAMI, (Brussels?), 1957 polycopied report]). His formal recommendations were less detailed and less critical; see Marc Vincent, *Les problèmes de protection maternelle au Congo belge et au Ruanda-Urundi* (Brussels: FOREAMI, 1959).

160. J. Lambillon, "Evolution du problème obstétrical à Léopoldville," *Académie Royale des Sciences Coloniales, Bulletin des Séances* 3 (1957): 1390–91.

161. Ibid., 1403–8. A decade earlier, a Dr. Perin from Kimvula in the lower Congo preferred forceps deliveries. He thought that embryotomies were too risky due to the retention of fetal debris (though he had performed one once for a shoulder presentation with an engaged arm); he considered C-sections too dangerous in this "native milieu," where what counted was maternal life (F. Perin, "Etude du bassin obstétrical chez la femme noire," *Recueil de Travaux de Sciences Médicales au Congo Belge* 3 [January 1945]: 32–42). Dr. Staub had thirty-six normal and seventeen dystocial cases in 1925–26 in Leopoldville; he performed cesareans on three Congolese women (one died), and a craniotomy on a European woman with a stillborn fetus (the woman died). Dr. Fronville handled thirty-two births from 1921 to 1925; six were dystocial, and he performed one C-section. Dr. Thémelin handled thirty normal and eight abnormal Congolese cases, and fifteen normal and six abnormal European cases, in his work at Kamina for the BCK railroad company (Compagnie du chemin de fer du Bas-Congo au Katanga) in 1930; no cesareans were performed. Among the five C-sections that Valcke performed, three women survived and two—both Europeans—died (Staub, "Rapport résumant des observations concernant la chirurgie"; Fronville, "Six années de practique chirurgicale," 23–24; Thémelin, "Thèse présentée"; and Valcke, "Six années"). On the dangers of cesareans in colonial practice, see Perin, "Etude du bassin obstétrical chez la femme noire," 32–42, esp. 41.

162. J.-R. Kebers, "Les urgences anesthésiques en pathologie congolaise," Examen B/Médecins no. 236, IMT, 1956, 23–73. Dyre Trolle, *The History of the Caesarean Section* (Copenhagen: Reitzel, 1982), 78. More detailed research would be required to know how exceptional Bukavu's statistics were; there are hints in the literature that nutritional improvements in the postwar period increased fetus size considerably, especially affecting women from ethnic groups where body size is small. Cases of disproportion in childbirth (big baby, small mother) continue to be more frequent in the Yakusu region among the smaller Komo women. On Bukavu, see also H. Peene, "Etude radiométrique de 100 bassins de femmes de race Bashi," Examen B/Médecins no. 272, IMT, 1958.

163. Vincent, "Mission d'Information"; and Vincent, *Les problèmes de protection maternelle*.

164. E. Muriel Lean to Dr. Chesterman, 10 May 1942, Lean file, BMSA.
165. Mama Komba Lituka, Yakoso, 24 November 1989.
166. Ibid. Mama Josephine Koto received her Yakusu diploma in 1956 and then worked for four years (1957–60). She recalled working with Likenja Katheline and Machuli Georgine, who had received their diplomas in 1956 and 1953, at the state hospital in Isangi (Mama Josephine Koto, untaped interview, Yaokombo, 1989; and from "List of Yakusu-trained Midwives, 1930–1963," plaque mounted on an office wall, Yakusu Hospital).
167. Winifred Browne to Dad, 27 September 1940, SGB Papers; and E. D. M. White, "A Typical Wednesday," YQN 150 (August 1954): 17–18. On postnatal seclusion practices elsewhere in the forest, see Hélène Pagezy and Anne Marie Subervie, *Sida et modification des comportements sexuels: le cas des reclusions de longue durée chez les Mongo du sud du Zaïre*, Rapport final de contrat ANRS, Projet no. 90085, 1990–1992 (Aix-en-Province and Paris: CNRS and ANRS, 1992).
168. E. D. M. White, "A Typical Wednesday," YQN 150 (August 1954): 17.
169. "Luckily she has a conscience that pricks her. She has been helping me to clean out the store and I had a cupboard open and was then called away. I never thought of sending her out until I came back, but in that short time she stole six vests. I shouldn't have known if she hadn't come round at night with them" (E. Muriel Lean to Dr. Chesterman, 10 May 1942, Lean file, BMSA).
170. Baba Manzanza, Yainyongo-Roméé, 16 September 1989.
171. Mama Kumbula Wayinoko Rosa, Yainyongo-Roméé, 10 November 1989.
172. Mama Lifoti Anastasia Anna, Yainyongo-Roméé, 10 November 1989.
173. Tata Bafoya Bamanga, with Mama Tula, Yakusu, 25 November 1989. Italics added.

7   Debris

1. Mama Malia Winnie, Kisangani, 4 December 1989; and Mama Malia Winnie with Mama Damali Basenge and Mama Tula, Kisangani, 23 January 1990.
2. Group interview with Yakusu-trained midwives, Mamas Asha Marguerite, Machuli Bolendela, Machuli Georgine, and Loséa Martine, and Yakusu-trained nurses, Loolo Libata and Lombale-Botowato, Kisangani, 29 April 1989.
3. The proportion of women giving birth in maternity hospitals or clinics in 1982 was 92 percent in Kinshasa, 80 percent in Lubumbashi, 73 percent in Kananga, and 45 percent in Kisangani. See Ngondo a Iman Pitshandenge, "Mortalité et morbidité infantiles et juvéniles dans les grandes villes du Zaïre en 1986–1987," *Zaïre-Afrique* 31, no. 251 (January 1991): 49–60, esp. 57; and Mwanalessa Kikassa, "Planification familiale, fécondité et santé familiale au Zaïre: Rapport sur les résultats d'une enquête régionale sur la prévalence contraceptive en 1982–1984," *Zaïre-Afrique* 25, no. 200 (December 1985): 597–615. Both articles cite the same source; where the other 20 percent of Kisangani women were giving birth is unclear.
4. Group interview, with Yakusu-trained midwives and nurses, Kisangani, 29 April 1989. Italics added. All subsequent quotations in chapter 7 are from my fieldnotes of 1989–90; the chapter is generally written in the past tense, given the tumultuous events that have affected the region since this time.

5. See, particularly, Meredeth Turshen, "The Impact of Economic Reforms on Women's Health and Health Care in Sub-Saharan Africa," in *Women in the Age of Economic Transformation: Gender Impact of Reforms in Post-Socialist and Developing Countries*, ed. Nahid Aslanbeigui, Steven Pressman, and Gale Summerfield (London: Routledge, 1994), 77–94.

6. Data from Kinshasa from the late 1980s point to the gap between delivery costs at a basic state hospital and the Cliniques Universitaires serving a middle class; one charged the equivalent of eight dollars for a delivery, the other sixty. Further, attitudes and access to biomedical care, like the risks of getting seriously sick, are class phenomena in Zaire, as is demonstrated by stark differences in seroconversion and AIDS incidence among pregnant women with HIV and their offspring in these two Kinshasa hospitals serving distinct socioeconomic populations (Robert W. Ryder et al., "Perinatal Transmission of the Human Immunodeficiency Virus Type 1 to Infants of Seropositive Women in Zaire," *New England Journal of Medicine* 320 [22 June 1989]: 1637–42; and Robert W. Ryder and Susan E. Hassig, "The Epidemiology of Perinatal Transmission of HIV," *AIDS* 2, suppl. 1 [1988]: S83–89).

7. Health care fees are difficult to study because there were overlapping practices, which were rarely enunciated as policy and changed often. People usually insisted that they did not pay for medical care, and especially for obstetric care in the colonial period, though the evidence indicates that nostalgia may have led to some forgetting here. The Baptist Missionary Society believed in patient fees for all but the destitute, and Yakusu's missionaries were collecting them from early in the century. Moreover, Yakusu's hospital received patients who had traveled long distances, avoiding free care at state hospitals, to pay at Yakusu, particularly for surgery. Since Yakusu's missionaries were also running a health network for local companies, required by legislation of the early 1920s, they were providing free health care for workers and eventually their families. Additionally, hygiene legislation required that treatment for major epidemic diseases be free. Thus, from the 1910s, as we saw, sleeping sickness care provided by Yakusu's missionaries was free of charge, leading in part to its local disparagement. The list of applicable diseases in this epidemic category had soared by the time of the mass vaccination campaigns of the 1950s. Province Orientale did have its own network of rural dispensaries by the 1920s, and in this case, there was a notion of cost recovery, not through user fees but rather through user taxation. The budgets for these dispensaries came from those monies collected as taxes by customary chiefs, which then became part of customary rule funds (R. Mouchet, "Notes sur les dispensaires ruraux de la Province Orientale," *ASBMT* 6 [1926]: 145–60).

8. Rhonda Smith, USAID, and Melinda Moore, then head of research at the (also USAID-funded) Ecole de Santé Publique, untaped discussions with author, Kinshasa, 23 January 1989.

9. Franklin C. Baer, untaped discussion with author, SANRU, Kinshasa, January 1989.

10. Glenn Rogers, "Child Survival Strategy" (USAID, May 1987, unpublished manuscript), 9. See also Franklin C. Baer, "The Primary Health Care Strategy in Zaire" (SANRU, Kinshasa, ca. 1985, unpublished manuscript); and Ricardo A. Bitran et al., "Etude sur le financement des zones de santé au Zaire, juin–octobre 1986, USAID/Kinshasa" (Resources for Child Health Project, Contract no. DPE-5927-C-00-5068-00, Arlington, VA., 1986, unpublished report).

11. Abstracts for: PD-BAK-141, Project Paper, 1981; PD-AAP-481, Audit Report, 1984; PD-BAT-220, Project Evaluation Summary, 1984; and PD-AAU-429, Project Paper, 1985. Quotations from abstracts for: XD-BBF-376-A, Special Evaluation, 1986; PD-AAW-579, Audit

Report, 1987; PN-ABD-548, AID-Supported Study, 1989; PN-AAX-244, Special Evaluation, 1990; and PD-ABE-094, Project Evaluation Summary, 1992. These abstracts of USAID reports on Zaire were kindly sent by the Agency for International Development/Center for Development Information and Evaluation/Development Information Services Clearinghouse (AID/CDIE/DISC) Development Information System, USAID, Washington, D.C. Karawa and Nyankunde are American medical missions, and links between them and SANRU headquarters were strong. Yakusu was on the books and clearly receiving funds, though Baer had not received recent annual reports; thus, Yakusu data were not integrated into the reports that he shared with me.

12. Papa Tika Kalokola, Bonama Yaya, Mama Monsanyembo, with Yenge Ituku and Lofanjola-Lisele (Pesapesa), Yanonge Hospital, 6 September 1989.

13. Just a couple days after Stanleyville came under popular army control on August 5, 1964, some of their rebel soldiers, known as Simba, occupied the Yakusu mission while yelling "Simba" war cries and "mai Lumumba mai." Despite their almost immediate execution of the Yakusu hospital director, Pierre Lifenya, Yakusu's missionaries coexisted with the Simba and hospital work went on. The missionaries remained untouched, even after the Stanleyville rebel regime's "white umbrella" policy led to the seizing of Belgian and American nationals as hostages to use as a shield against aerial bombardment. The missionaries were evacuated the day after the Belgian-American parachute operation known as "Dragon Rouge" began in the Lumumbist capital of Stanleyville on November 26, 1964. The zone between Kisangani and Opala remained insecure for months, likely until well after Mobutu came to power on November 25, 1965. Simba, meaning lion in Swahili, was the name given to popular army or rebel troops in the eastern Congo from June 1964 on. For a detailed account of the Yakusu mission occupation and evacuation, see Dr. James Taylor, "Our Last Days at Yakusu (Before the Evacuation)," *Baptist Times,* 17 December 1964, 8–9. On rebel symbolism and its Lumumba specificity in northeastern Congo, see Crawford Young, "Rebellion and the Congo," in *Protest and Power in Black Africa,* ed. Robert I. Rotberg and Ali A. Mazrui (New York: Oxford University Press, 1970), 969–1011.

14. Lombale used the French word *bleu.* Whether he meant natural indigo dyes or a commercial laundering agent is unclear, though given the rest of his testimony, the former is more likely.

15. The 1970s and 1980s's historiographical focus on rebelling peasantries in African studies partly helps explain the fact that richly detailed local histories of this rebellion have not been written. All I had to say was the word *history,* and people wanted to share, first and foremost, their autobiographical memories of this harrowing period of "war" and flight.

16. Mary Fagg, Thornham, 12 November 1990.

17. Papa Tika Kalokola, Bonama Yaya, Mama Monsanyembo, with Yenge Ituku and Lofanjola-Lisele (Pesapesa), Yanonge Hospital, 6 September 1989. Italics added.

18. Mama Monsanyembo (Mosa), Yanonge, 15 November 1989. Italics added.

19. Bagoma Loula from Yakusu accompanied me to Yalengi, six villages upriver from Yakusu, on March 4, 1989. Three TBAs, Bichainwe, Boyale, and Ilowo, had been trained partly by Evans and partly at weekly antenatal clinics at Yakusu. They had handled eight births in the health center since January, and most years there were about twenty-five. Parturients returned immediately to their homes. Antenatal fees cost 150 zaires and births 500 zaires (200 of which

went to the TBAS) at Yalengi, whereas a birth cost 1000 zaires at Yakusu if a woman had not followed antenatal care there.

20. Susan Chalmers, in English, Yakusu, 26–27 November 1989.

21. Having more women than men in the church was normal, according to the regional pastor, Mokili (named after Mr. Millman); about 70 percent of members were women (fieldnotes, Yanonge, 4 April 1989).

22. There is huge variation in the region regarding placenta burial or river disposal. Both are considered appropriate, protective practices, though forest peoples were more likely to do the former and riverain the latter.

23. As we saw in chapter 1, the value attached to light skins cannot be attached to ancient—and continuing—color categories alone. White (kaolin or pemba, cassava powder, milk powder), red (camwood or shele, palm oil), and black (charcoal) remained central in reproductive ritual as they were in the days of libeli and likiilo. Mothers wanted to give birth to pale babies and lighten their own skin during periods of seclusion. These lighter-skinned babies were called *basongo* (white people); their skin coloring was compared to mine. I also knew one woman without a husband who used chemical lighteners on her skin.

24. At Yakusu, ergometrine was routinely administered in 1989–90. Dr. Mairi Burnett, the obstetrician and gynecologist then at Yakusu, explained that in the West, it is given even earlier. Evans's ideas about the matter seem to have influenced local practice; thus, usually one waits until the placenta has come out. A textbook located at Yakusu indicated that it was common practice in the early 1970s in the United Kingdom in order to prevent trapping the placenta inside due to spasm of the lower uterine (see Margaret F. Myles, *A Textbook for Midwives* [Edinburgh: Churchill Livingstone, 1972], 325).

25. When I later discussed what I had witnessed with Susan Chalmers, a missionary nurse at Yakusu, she said that she knew about this nurse, and they had seen some of the consequences of his malpractice at Yakusu. She also said that the practice of fundal pressure would never occur in the United Kingdom, but imagined that Belgian nuns in remote colonial sites may have practiced it. She added that she could see why such an extreme measure was used—even though it poses serious risks for uterine rupture—in situations where instrumental interventions were not available (Susan Chalmers, in English, Yakusu, 26–27 November 1989). The critical missing technology was a vacuum extractor (ventouse); its use can be taught to midwifery practitioners with limited skills and experience. It also has rendered forceps virtually obsolete, and could have been as high a SANRU priority as TBA training.

26. The cost of a SANRU birth was lower if a woman regularly attended kilo. This was the practice at Yakusu, and likely in all SANRU centers under their jurisdiction.

27. Among the Lele, this sex pollution is called *hanga* (see Mary Douglas, *The Lele of the Kasai* [London: Oxford University Press, 1963]). Likewise, sanga is not limited to the time of pregnancy and troubles with childbearing. A husband can get sanga anytime his wife is adulterous. A related disorder concerns the newborn; if a mother is adulterous when breast-feeding, the baby will drink her lover's semen and die. If she sleeps with her own husband, the child will not walk well.

28. A practice also mentioned in V. Cocq and Fr. Mercken, "L'assistance obstétricale au Congo belge (y compris le Ruanda-Urundi)," *Gynécologie et Obstrétrique* 31, no. 4 (1935).

29. The only time I was ever referred to as Madami was with such interpretations of affliction.

30. Saliva is an important way of extending blessings in the region.

31. Lofanjola-Lisele (Pesapesa), Yainyongo-Romée, 7 April 1989. Italics added.

32. Ibid.

33. Rhonda Smith, USAID, untaped discussion with author, Kinshasa, 23 January 1989.

34. Rogers, "Child Survival Strategy," 9. See also Baer, "Primary Health Care Strategy"; and Bitran et al., "Etude sur le financement des zones de santé."

35. Ricardo Bitran, "A Household Health Care Demand Study in the Bokoro and Kisantu Zones of Zaire, Vol. 2, Utilization Patterns" (Resources for Child Health Project, Contract no. DPE-5927-C-00-5068-00, Arlington, Va., n.d., draft manuscript).

36. Each of forty-one of sixty-seven SANRU health zones was divided into nine to forty-three health sections in 1989 (in a country mapped out to contain, ideally, 306 zones of 100,000 persons with twenty health sections each). Instead, the population per section ranged from 2,259 to 19,864 persons. Although SANRU signaled the percentage of sections per zone with maternities (8 to 100 percent), the more salient fact is that the average population served per maternity in 1987 ranged from 7,481 to as low as sixty-eight persons (not women)! What is striking, therefore, is the density of maternity structures per capita in some regions, a legacy of colonial construction projects (and perhaps subsequent outmigration). Only two of these forty-one zones had maternity structures serving more than about 6,000 persons; twenty-two zones had maternities serving 1,000 persons or less each, and twelve of these zones an average of 500 persons or less per maternity ("Pourcentage des aires de santé de la ZSR avec service de maternité selon rapport 1987" [a computer-generated data report], SANRU Office Records, Kinshasa).

37. E. E. Evans-Pritchard, *Witchcraft, Oracles, and Magic among the Azande* (1937; reprint, Oxford: Oxford University Press, 1985), 80.

38. They moved in flight upriver—to near (likely the new) Yatuka and Bokuma (eventually Tata Tula's Belgika post)—when Belgian armed forces arrived to fight with BaTambatamba near the Romée in 1893. They moved back downriver, just upriver from the current site, after a Yakusu doctor—Browne?—insisted that the village be relocated for hygiene reasons (*filaires*). And they moved continually for about two years when they were on the run and living in scattered, uneasy forest settlements as BaSimba fought battles in their midst.

39. People could tell me exactly how many such ngbaka there used to be per "clan" (bokulu) and the name of the big men who originally constructed them. They also told me how these "clans" were organized in space and the households that lived side by side. The time when the village was relocated for hygiene reasons was circa 1938 to 1942. Since everyone dispersed for two years of hiding in the forest between 1964 and 1966, many people left for Kisangani. Those households that remain no longer reside together spatially as, in Jan Vansina's terminology, one house.

40. It is possible that similar kinds of suspension of customary food sharing and moral justice came into play in the past, when Lokele, for example, went to trade and offer wives among more powerful strangers, whether up the Lindi among the Mba or at Zanzibari strongholds and slave-worked farms. Yet the asili/kizungu dichotomy is so near to the colonial division of space into customary and extracustomary zones, and the lexeme so tied to colonial disrup-

tion, that even though older, especially Zanzibari, dichotomies are lurking within it, the colonial division of justices, moralities, and living arrangements reinforced the strong bush/ civilization divide. Extracustomary referred to urban, industrial, plantation, state, military, or mission work spaces where customary law and rule did not apply, and many workers and sometimes whole households moved among these zones.

41. As Lingala entered local vocabularies, Mobutu speeches, and *animation* songs, Zairians spoke and sang more about *kobota elengi*, often an elaborate, extravagant festivity among the urban middle- and upper-classes. It is comparable to the kind of celebration that followed the *wale* of a woman who gave birth in an *eelo* or *likwakulu*, Pesapesa explained one day. It is the fête of coming out of wale: "If you come out of a wale, but now in kizungu, thus coming out of the maternité, then they do a fête of kobota. They call it in Lingala: kobota elengi."

42. Compensation of midwives was similar among the Shambaa of East Africa in 1918, and this was still the case in the late 1970s (Steven Feierman, "Popular Control over the Institutions of Health: A Historical Study," in *The Professionalisation of Medicine*, ed. Murray Last and G. L. Chavanduka [Manchester: Manchester University Press, 1986], 211–12). In Zambia among the Luvale in the early 1970s, women were choosing hospital births to avoid popular midwives' fees, comparable in 1970–72 to bridewealth (see Anita Spring, "Women's Rituals and Natality among the Luvale of Zambia" [Ph.D. diss., Cornell University, 1976], 161).

43. Bernard Hours, *L'Etat sorcier: Santé publique et société au Cameroun* (Paris: Editions l'Harmattan, 1985), 160.

44. "In some local carving, though, the belly is distended because it contains the fetish. The stick is accepted by Zaïrois as the stick of the chief. While the chief holds the stick off the ground the people around him can speak; when the chief sets his stick on the ground, the people fall silent and the chief gives his decision" (V. S. Naipaul, "A New King for the Congo," *New York Review of Books* 22, no. 11, 26 June 1975, 19).

45. "Il est protegé, il se cache dedans elle, et ne peut pas mourir."

46. I follow closely and quote from Lieve Joris in her *Back to the Congo* (London: Macmillan, 1992), 89. On these themes, see also Michael G. Schatzberg, *The Dialectics of Oppression in Zaire* (Bloomington: Indiana University Press, 1988).

Departures

1. Kathleen Stewart, "On the Politics of Cultural Theory: A Case for 'Contaminated' Cultural Critique," *Social Research* 58 (1991): 395–412, esp. 411.

2. An expression taken from Jennifer Beinart, "Darkly through a Lens: Changing Perceptions of the African Child in Sickness and Health, 1900–1945," in *In the Name of the Child: Health and Welfare, 1880–1940*, ed. Roger Cooter (London: Routledge, 1992), 220–36, esp. 236.

3. Michel de Certeau, *The Practice of Everyday Life*, trans. Steven Rendall (Berkeley: University of California Press, 1984), xvii. The original reads: "tente de repérer les types d'*opérations* qui caractérisent la consommation . . . et de reconnaître en ces pratiques d'appropriation les indicateurs de la créativité qui pullule là même où disparaît le pouvoir de se donner un langage propre" (Michel de Certeau, *L'invention du quotidien: I. Arts de faire*, ed. Luce Girard [Paris: Gallimard, 1990], xliii). A *parole* vs. *langue* distinction (or speech/consumption

versus system of signs/lexemes/objects) remains active in this poststructural formulation that might have been better translated into English as "where practice ceases to have an exclusive language."

4. Not only operational and exegetical, but also positional as elaborated by Victor Turner in his "Ritual Symbolism, Morality, and Social Structure among the Ndembu," in *The Forest of Symbols: Aspects of Ndembu Ritual* (Ithaca, N.Y.: Cornell University Press, 1967), 48–58. In earlier writing, Turner insisted that dominance is never total, but rather "situational," even "episodic," even though "history is very often crystallized in dominant ritual symbols" (Victor Turner, *Chihamba, the White Spirit* [Manchester: Manchester University Press, 1962], 70, 74).

5. In the Lokele region, including Kisangani, these images are called "Inakwame" or "It's stuck." See T. K. Biaya, "L'impasse de crise zaïroise dans la peinture populaire urbaine, 1970–1985," in *Art et politiques en Afrique noire/Art and Politics in Black Africa* (Ottawa: Canadian Association of African Studies and Sofi Press, 1989), 95–120; and Bogumil Jewsiewicki, "Painting in Zaire: From the Invention of the West to the Representation of Social Self," in *Africa Explores: Twentieth Century African Art*, ed. Susan Vogel (New York: Center for African Art, 1991), 130–51.

6. H. Sutton Smith, *Yakusu, the Very Heart of Africa: Being Some Account of the Protestant Mission at Stanley Falls, Upper Congo* (London: Carey Press, [1911?]), 34 (see also inset photograph of wind motor model, 28–29). The model prams and dispensary contests were included in Mrs. Browne's scrapbooks and memories (Mali Browne, New Milton, 5 June 1991).

7. Like every history for that matter. "A truly total history would cancel itself out—its product would be nought. . . . History is . . . never history, but history-for. It . . . inevitably remains partial—that is, incomplete—and this is itself a form of partiality. . . . We need only recognize that history is a method with no distinct object. . . . As we say of certain careers, history may lead to anything, provided you get out of it" (Claude Lévi-Strauss, *The Savage Mind* [Chicago, Ill.: University of Chicago Press, 1970], 257–58, 262).

GLOSSARY

All words are part of local Lokele and Kimbole speech among Lokele and Foma (BaMbole), though many are loanwords from French, Swahili (often local Kingwana orthography), and English. The latter derivations are indicated, where possible.

abacost. From the French "à bas costumes" or "down with suits." A Mao-like Mobutu suit, proper male gear for the middle and upper classes in *authenticité* Zaire.

accoucheuse [Fr.]. Midwife with biomedical training.

Arabisé [Fr.]. See *BaNgwana* and *BaTambatamba.*

asili [Sw.]. Natural, local, customary, traditional.

authenticité [Fr.]. Authenticity; specially refers to the "authenticity" policy of Mobutu's Zaire.

avion [Fr.]. Airplane.

baekesi (sing. *boekesi*). Teacher-evangelists.

ba-infirmiers [Fr.]. Lokele-ization of nurses. See *infirmier.*

balimo (sing. *bolimo*). Spirits; ancestral spirits.

BaNgwana [Sw.]. Muslim, Zanzibari persons, presumably freeborn and of partial Arab descent. Officially called *Arabisés.* Compare *BaTambatamba.*

basenji [Sw., *washenzi*]. Uncivilized persons; pagans; heathens; savages. Compare *kisenji.*

basongo (sing. *bosongo*). White people.

BaTambatamba. Local Zanzibari-influenced people, not necessarily of Arab or Swahili descent. Followers of BaNgwana from Maniema and beyond. Officially called *Arabisés.* Compare *BaNgwana.*

batshuaka. Strangers; non-"Lokele." Lokele consider Mba, Komo, and Bali as strangers, but not Wagenia, Olombo, and Foma.

bayomba. Maternal kin.

bieka (sing. *yeka*). Wealth or bounty. In the plural, usually food (many things of wealth); in the singular, *yeka,* usually thing (of wealth).

boekesi. See *baekesi.*

boi [Fr./Sw.]. "Boy." Domestic servant.

bokulu. Ya-prefaced village section claiming descent from a single ancestor. "Clan" (colonial and local usage). "House" in Jan Vansina's lexicon.

bolaya [Sw.]. Derived from *Ulaya* or Europe. Imitation, European-manufactured axhead or *shoka*, used for currency. Introduced ca. 1902 and tended to supplant *tondo* as currency.

bonama. Menacing phantom of sky or water. Often used for rainbow. Also called *monama.*

Bonganga. White doctor. Derived from *nganga* [Sw.], healer.

bosombi. Colonial tax; until *lifaefi* was adopted instead, the term was also used for church offering.

bowai. Period of female seclusion that commences immediately after marriage and continues for several months, often through the woman's first pregnancy. Final male seclusion period of *libeli.*

cabinet [Fr.]. Water closet; used to refer to bathing and toilet enclosures that tend to be large enough to also be used for childbirth.

dispensaire [Fr.]. Dispensary.

eelo. Forest clearing used for judicial and ritual matters, including childbirth.

l'Etat [Fr.]. The State.

évolué (pl. *évolués*) [Fr.]. Literally, evolved person(s). Francophone African colonial elite.

fala. Crippling, bone-altering disease and/or skin ulcers. Thought to have been caused by breaking a prohibition or a *lilwa* curse. Sometimes translated as leprosy, though from the 1920s more often as tertiary yaws.

falanga [Fr./Sw.]. Francs; money. Name of 1910 round of *libeli.*

fobe (pl. of *lobe*). Sacred groves of medicinal trees. Sites for *libeli.*

fonoli. Form of sorcery, perhaps quite recent, that is found along the river in the Congo. Usually involves disappeared, buried people who live on as invisible slaves after their corpses are thought buried, and do a live, rich person's work.

infirmier [Fr.]. Nurse.

hôpitalo [Fr./Sw.]. Hospital or dispensary.

kalasi [Eng./Sw.]. Class; school.

kanga. Healer; religious specialist; "witchdoctor."

kasa (pl. of *lokasa*). Leaves, papers, documents, books.

kelekele. Thank you.

kilo [Fr./Sw.]. Kilogram; baby-weighing station; baby clinic.

kisenji [Sw.]. In the manner of *basenji.*

kumi. Patriarch; house leader; chief; big man.

kwaya. Modern, jazz-associated dance.

langue [Fr.]. Language; system of signs. Compare *parole.*

libeli. Lilwa-associated male initiation rites as practiced among the Lokele and Foma.

lichecha. Special, pampered, protected child.

lieme. An older, three-to-four-month-old pregnancy or fetus that moves within the mother.

lifaefi. Gift(s); church offering(s).

likenja. Bride given as a gift to effect a truce, an alliance, and/or trading rights.

likiilo. Female puberty ritual of seclusion, fattening, and dancing as practiced among the Lokele and Foma.

lilembu. Ceremony to send good blessings to someone and neutralize ill will. Frequently involves spitting saliva and smearing palm oil. Common after childbirth to neutralize the effects of touching the blood of childbirth.

lilwa. Male initiation rites among BaMbole and other *Ya*-lancers of the region. Associated with cuts, oaths, and cursing gestures.

linganda. Lance used in paying bridewealth. Sometimes written as *liganda.* Same as *ngbele.*

lisole. An early pregnancy that does not move within the mother and whose *kisila* gas can be dangerous.

lisoo. Charm, medicine.

lobe (pl. *fobe*). Sacred grove of medicinal trees. Site for *libeli.*

lokasa (pl. *kasa*). Leaf, paper, document, book.

lokele or *Lokele.* A mollusk shell associated with *ndiya* water spirit (thus *lokele lya ndiya*); a ceremony of alliance using this shell; the ethnic and linguistic term for the fishing people of the Upper Congo and Lower Lomami and their language.

lokwamisa. Affliction of delayed or blocked birth; prolonged or obstructed labor.

lopangu. Fenced-in enclosure, often attached to a house. Not unlike a *cabinet* enclosure.

malinga. Modern, jazz-associated dance.

Mamiwata. A mermaid figure.

matabish. Gift, tip, bribe.

mbotesa. Midwife; popular midwife with no hospital or hygiene training.

ménagère [Fr.]. Housewife. In the Congo, a white man's Congolese concubine.

mutumbula. Tale(s) about anthropophagic activities, especially of Europeans, found in central Africa, especially the Congo.

muzungu [Sw.]. White person. Compare *basongo*; *wazungu.*

ndembu. Medicinal mixture in salve form.

ndimo. Bad water creature; bad person turned into a water-living creature; crocodile-man.

ndiya (also, *Ndiya*). Water spirit, sometimes used as proper noun.

ndotinya. To cut (especially to cut a judicial decision or skin).

ndotinya lilwa. To cut *libeli* scars, oaths, and medicines.

ngbele. Lance used in paying bridewealth. Same as *linganda.*

nyango. Mother; in *libeli,* initiate guide, "sponsor," or "mother."

opération [Fr.]. Operation, surgery.

parole [Fr.]. Speech. Compare *langue.*

pemba. White chalk, kaolin.

shele. Camwood powder.

shoka [Sw.]. Small iron axhead(s) used as currency. From ca. 1902, manufactured in Europe.

tokwakwa. Tale(s) about anthropophagic activities, especially of Europeans. A genre of *mutumbula* specific to the Kisangani-Opala region, including the Yakusu district.

tondo. Small iron axhead locally crafted and etched, also known as *shoka,* six to ten inches long. Currency form. Compare *bolaya.*

tosumbe. Form of dancing, considered obscene by the Yakusu church.

ventouse [Fr.]. Vacuum extractor used in obstetrics.

wale. Postnatal seclusion period.

wazungu [Sw.]. White people. Compare *basongo*; *muzungu.*

Ya-. Village or house toponym, indicating the people of. Thus Yakoso: the people of Koso.

BIBLIOGRAPHY

Archives and Manuscripts

Belgium

Katholiek Documentatie en Onderzoekscentrum (KADOC). Leuven.
  Archivalia N. De Cleene and Ed. de Jonghe.
  Photothèque.
Ministère des Affaires Etrangères et de Commerce Extérieur. Archives Africaines (AA). Brussels.
  Fonds: Affaires Indigènes (AI); Hygiène (H); FOREAMI (FOR);
    and Rapports Annuels, Congo Belge (RA/CB).
Musée Royal de l'Afrique Centrale (MRAC). Tervuren.
  Section Historique:
    Collection des Films Inforcongo; Papiers G. Fivé; Papiers F. Fuchs;
      and Photothèque.
  Section Ethnographique:
    Collection of money objects; Dossiers ethnographiques; and Photothèque.
Palais Royal. Archives. Brussels.
  Prince Albert, "Voyage au Congo belge par Cape Town," ca. 1909, dossier 75.

United Kingdom

Stanley G. Browne (SGB) Papers. Private Residence of Mrs. Stanley Browne. New Milton, U.K.
Winifred Browne Burke (WBB) Papers. Private Residence. Godalming, U.K.
John F. Carrington Papers. Private Residence of Mrs. John F. Carrington. Salisbury, U.K. (Note: These papers, loaned to me by Mrs. Carrington and cited as the JFC Papers—Salisbury, have been transferred to BMSA, Regent's Park College, Oxford, where presumably they will be added to the Carrington Papers.)
Dorothy Daniel (DD) Papers. Private Residence. Corse Staunton, U.K.
Mary L. Fagg Papers. Private Residence. Thornham, Hunstanton.

Phyllis Lofts (PL) Papers. Private Residence of David and Gillian Lofts. Barton-on-Sea.
Regent's Park College. Oxford.
  Baptist Missionary Society Archives (BMSA).
  Mboli ya Tengai, 1910–60.
  Yakusu Quarterly Notes (YQN), 1909–60.
  John F. Carrington (JFC) Papers.
Rhodes House Library. Oxford.
  Stanley G. Browne: "Links with the Past." 1940. Mss. Afr. S. 1277.
Sudan Archives. University of Durham. Durham.
  Misses Wolff Papers.

Congo (Democratic Republic)

Archives Régionales du Haut-Zaïre. Kisangani.
Centre Aequatoria. Bamanya.
  Fonds Hulstaert.
  Fonds Boelaert.
Chancellerie Offices, Procure Catholique. Kisangani.
  "Soeurs de Sainte-Elisabeth" file, 1938–1964.
Yakusu Mission Station. Yakusu.
  Hospital Director's Office (HDO)
    BMS Yakusu Annual Medical Reports, 1921–1960.
    Hospital Records.
  Medical School Director's Office. Medical Training School Records.
  District Pastor's Office (DPO):
    Yakusu Church Records.
    "Njaso—Ikumbe." [Yakusu Church Minutes Logbook.]
  Printing Press Director's Office: Yakusu Printing Press Records.

Interviews

Swahili (Kingwana) was the primary language of my field research and interviewing in Upper Zaire. All interviews, unless otherwise mentioned, were in Swahili. With the exception of two interviews in Lokele and one in Kimbole (noted below), I did not use an interpreter, though a research assistant was usually present. I became proficient in local Swahili (as opposed to standard Swahili, as used in Tanzania and learned at the University of Wisconsin–Madison and a summer institute in coastal Kenya) by studying Lokele. I acquired a rich Lokele vocabulary related to childbirth, medicines, sorcery, and healing, and was able to follow the general contents of a Lokele conversation. Because of the late-nineteenth-century BaTambatamba (Zanzibari) presence, especially at Yainyongo, as well as an important Catholic presence at the nearby state post of Yanonge, Swahili has remained the principal lingua franca and language of instruction in state and Catholic schools. Swahili was the language of choice among children at Yainyongo-Romée during my stay; most adults used it about 40 percent of the time.

Most interviews were individualized. Sometimes research assistants also contributed, as did kin and friends who came to watch and listen. In Yainyongo-Romée, I also recorded numerous sessions of storytelling, women's songs, *totofu* music (children's music on simulated instruments), and drumming, as well as actual childbirth scenes; these are not included here. Nor can such a listing do justice to the myriad informal conversations that I had, the many others that I overheard, and the knowledge that seeped in as I listened, observed, and took part in daily life.

Interviews are listed by location and then chronologically. Women are indicated by the honorifics of Mama, Bibi, or Shangazi; names are listed as they were given to me by the interviewee. Untaped interviews are indicated by an asterisk (*) rather than by tape number. Mama Tula Sophie, Tula Rogier, and Bibi Bilefu Mari-Jeanne assisted me with interviews. Tula Rogier and Mota Moya transcribed about 80 percent of the interviews, although I often returned directly to my tapes to verify transcriptions, as well as to recall context and tone. I owe this work to the wise and dedicated labor of these assistants and the generous sharing of life, memories, knowledge, and laughter of all those listed below.

Congo (Democratic Republic)
Ikongo

> Mama Machuli Ofomale Atiwani, 14 November 1989 (41a–b).
>
> Mama Somboli, 14 November 1989 (41a).
>
> Mama Somboli, 11 January 1990 (100a–b).

Kisangani

> Group interview with Yakusu-trained midwives, Mamas Asha Marguerite, Machuli Bolen-dela, Marjorie Georgine, and Loséa Martine, and Yakusu-trained nurses, Loolo Libata and Lombale-Botowato, 29 April 1989 (11a–b).
>
> Mama Machuli Georgine, 2 December 1989 (54–55a).
>
> Mama Asha Marguerite, 3 December 1989 (55a–b).
>
> Mama Machuli Bolendela, 3 December 1989 (55b–56).
>
> Mama Loséa Martine, 4 December 1989 (57a–b).
>
> Mama Malia Winnie Litoi, 4 December 1989 (58–59a).
>
> Mama Damali Basuli, 23 January 1990 (101a–b).
>
> Mama Ilondo Elisa, 23 January 1990 (103a–b).
>
> Mama Malia Winnie Litoi, with Mama Damali Basenge and Mama Tula, 23 January 1990 (102a–b).
>
> Mama Noel Dickie, 23 January 1990 (101b–102a).
>
> Erik Weli Lissa and Mama Lifetu Marie-Peggy, 24 January 1990 (103b–104a).
>
> Meeting with former Yakusu women students, organized by Mama Basuli Damali, 25 January 1990 (104b–105).

Yainyongo-Romée

> Lofanjola-Lisele (Pesapesa), 7 April 1989 (6a–b).
>
> Mama Sila and Mama Yaluani, 7 April 1989 (6b–7a).
>
> Baba Manzanza, 25 August 1989 (18a).
>
> Mama Lisongomi and Bibi Marta, 30 August 1989 (20a–b).

Shangazi Maria Yaonge, 7 September 1989 (22b).

Liyaoto-Batokale, 9 September 1989 (23a–b).

Mama Sila, 10 September 1989 (24a).

Baba Manzanza, 16 September 1989 (25b–26a).

Tata Alikuwa, 18 September 1989 (26a–b).

Mama Biliama, with Bibi Bilefu Mari-Jeanne, 18 September 1989 (27a).

Shangazi Angelani, 21 September 1989 (27b–28a).

Mama Botelnanyele Machuli in Lokele, with Mama Balasi Marta, 21 September 1989 (28a–b).

Mama Afeno Susana, 22 September 1989 (28b–29a).

Mama Bolaiti Coletta, 28 September 1989 (29a).

Mama Machozi, 28 September 1989 (29b).

Mama Baelo and Mama Nyota, 1 October 1989 (30a–b).

Mama Yaluani, 1 October 1989 (31b–32a).

Mama Yenga Chaus and Bibi Balasi Marta, 1 October 1989 (31a–b).

Mama Komata and Mama Posho Busungu, 2 October 1989 (32b–33a).

Bibi Viviane and Mama Viviane, 4 November 1989 (37a–b).

Mama Afeno and Mama Posho Busunga, with Mama Tika, 9 November 1989 (38a–b).

Mama Bafeta Liseko, 10 November 1989 (39b–40a).

Mama Kumbula Wayinoko Rosa, 10 November 1989 (38b–39a).

Mama Lifoti Anastasia Anna, 10 November 1989 (39a–b).

Mama Bakita Monique, 13 November 1989 (40b).

Mama Tika, 15 November 1989 (41a–b, 42a–b).

Bibi Bolaiti Coletta, 13 December 1989 (62a).

Dipo Kesobe, with Baba Manzanza, 13 December 1989 (63a–b).

Mama Biliama and Bibi Alphonsine, 14 December 1989 (64a–b).

Mama Lisongomi, 19 December 1989 (67b–68).

Tata Alikuwa and Bosunga, 20 December 1989 (68b–69).

Mama Sila, 22 December 1989 (73a–b).

Tata Kango, 23 December 1989 (74a–b).

Tata Mwanamuke Bisato Bola, in Kimbole, with Bibi Bilefu Mari-Jeanne, 24 December 1989 (75a–b).

Tata Alikuwa, 26–27 December 1989 (80a–b).

Avion, 28 December 1989 (83a–b).

Dipo Kesobe, Tata Alikuwa, Baba Manzanza, and Liyaoto, 29 December 1989 (87a).

Lofanjola-Lisele (Pesapesa), 29 December 1989 (84–85).

Liyaoto, 30 December 1989 (87a–88a).

Lofemba, 31 December 1989 and 7 January 1990 (96–97).

Tata Alikuwa and Bibi Bilefu Mari-Jeanne, 6 January 1990 (93–94).

Bibi Bilefu Mari-Jeanne and Bibi Amelia, 8 January 1990 (90).

Bombolia Lisungi, 8 January 1990 (97b).

Mama Lisongomi, 10 January 1990 (99a).

Mama Sila, 10 January 1990 (99a–b).

Mama Sila and Shangazi Angelani, 10 January 1990 (91b).

Mama Sila, 11 January 1990 (100b–101a).

Yainyongo-Topoke

Mama Ongowino Susana, 23 September 1989 (29a).

Yakoso

Mama Bichainwe Miliama, 3 March 1989 (4a).
Mama Botono Bertha, with Mama Tula, 23 November 1989 (44a).
Mama Elisa Shanana and Bibi Alimo Singili, 23 November 1989 (44a–b).
Mama Liyalanyongo, 23 November 1989 (44b–45a).
Mama Bachalonge and Tata Bangombe Kilongose, 24 November 1989 (46b).
Mama Komba Lituka, 24 November 1989 (46a).
Mama Lifaefi Bangala, 24 November 1989 (46a).
Mama Bokenge Limengo, with Mama Tula Sophie, 30 November 1989 (52–53).
Tata Botakawae Lifofa, 30 November 1989 (53b).

Yakusu

Mama Tula Sophie, February 1989 (1b).
Papa Boshanene, 24 February 1989 (2a).
Mama Tula Sophie, 8 August 1989 (12–13a).
Mama Tula Sophie, 17 August 1989 (14a–b).
Tata Tula, with Tula Rogier, 2 November 1989 (35a–b).
Tata Tula, with Tula Rogier, 4 November 1989 (36a–b).
Mama Tula Sophie, 22 November 1989 (42–43).
Papa Lokangu, 24 November 1989 (45a–b).
Tata Bafoya Bamanga, with Mama Tula, 25 November 1989 (46b–47).
Susan Chalmers, in English, 26–27 November 1989 (48–50).
Tata Bafoya Bamanga, with Mama Tula, 27 November 1989 (51–52a).

Yalenge

Mama Bichainwe, Mama Boyate, and Mama Ilowa, 4 March 1989 (5a).

Yalolia

Mama Lituka Masitaki, in Lokele, with Lituka Bisilenge, 11 April 1989 (8a–b).
Pasteur Lofolata-Liende and Botelanyele-Lingoso, 12 April 1989 (8b).
Pasteur Lofolata-Liende, with Mama Pasteur Baseko-Lofolata Nace and Mama Lituka-Biselenge,
    13 April 1989 (10a–b).

Yalolimela

Yenga-Bokowa, Ile Yaolimela (Bertha), 25 February 1989 (3a).

Yanonge

Papa Tika Kalokola, Bonama Yaya, Mama Monsanyembo, with Yenge Ituku and Lofanjola-Lisele
    (Pesapesa), Yanonge Hospital, 6 September 1989 (22a).
Mama Monsanyembo (Mosa), 15 November 1989 (41b).
Mama Sila, 5 January 1990 (91a).

Yatomba (forest behind)

Linda Tososola and Papa Lomata, 19 August 1989 (16a–b).

United Kingdom

Nora Carrington, Salisbury, 8 June and July 1990 (*).
Mary Fagg, Thornham, 11 November 1990 (107).
Mary Fagg, Thornham, 12 November 1990 (*).
Mali Browne, New Milton, 5 June 1991 (108, *).
David and Gillian Lofts, Barton-on-Sea, 6–8 June 1991 (*).
Nora Carrington, Salisbury, 8 June 1991 (*).
Dorothy Daniel, Corse Staunton, 11 June 1991 (*).
Margaret Pitt, North Harrow, 16 June 1991 (*).
Winifred Browne Burke, Godalming, 17 June 1991 (109).

Books, Articles, Theses, and Papers

Abrahams, Roger D. *The Man-of-Words in the West Indies: Performance and the Emergence of Creole Culture.* Baltimore, Md.: Johns Hopkins University Press, 1983.

Abrahams, Roger D., and John F. Szwed, eds. *After Africa: Extracts from British Travel Accounts and Journals of the Seventeenth, Eighteenth, and Nineteenth Centuries concerning the Slaves, Their Manners, and Customs in the British West Indies.* New Haven, Conn.: Yale University Press, 1983.

Adam, T. B. *Africa Revisited: A Medical Deputation to the Baptist Missionary Society's Congo Field.* London: Baptist Missionary Society, 1931.

Adams, Mark B. *The Wellborn Science: Eugenics in Germany, France, Brazil, and Russia.* Oxford: Oxford University Press, 1990.

Annales de la Société Belge de la Médecine Tropicale. Antwerp, 1920–1960.

Appadurai, Arjun. "Disjuncture and Difference in the Global Cultural Economy." *Public Culture* 2 (1990): 1–24.

Appiah, Kwame Anthony. *In My Father's House: Africa in the Philosophy of Culture.* New York: Oxford University Press, 1992.

Apple, Rima D. "Constructing Mothers: Scientific Motherhood in the Nineteenth and Twentieth Centuries." *Social History of Medicine* 8 (1995): 161–78.

Arnold, David. "Public Health and Public Power: Medicine and Hegemony in Colonial India." In *Contesting Colonial Hegemony: State and Society in Africa and India,* edited by Dagmar Engels and Shula Marks. London: British Academic Press, 1994.

Augé, Marc. "Introduction." Special Issue: "Interpreting Illness." *History and Anthropology* 2 (1985): 1–15.

Austen, Ralph A., and Rita Headrick. "Equatorial Africa under Colonial Rule." In *History of Central Africa,* edited by David Birmingham and Phyllis Martin. Vol. 2. London: Longman, 1983.

Baer, Franklin C. "The Primary Health Care Strategy in Zaire." Bureau du Projet Santé Rurale (SANRU), Kinshasa, ca. 1985. Unpublished manuscript.

——. "The Role of the Church in Managing Primary Health Care in Zaire." SANRU Project

USAID/DSP/ECZ 660-107, Office of Project Santé Rurale (SANRU), Kinshasa, ca. 1988. Unpublished paper.

Bakhtin, Mikhail. *Rabelais and His World*, translated by Hélène Iswolsky. Bloomington: Indiana University Press, 1984.

Bandele-Thomas, 'Biyi. *The Sympathetic Undertaker and Other Dreams*. London: Heinemann, 1991.

Baptist Missionary Society. *Annual Reports*. 1923–1936.

Barber, Karin. "Popular Arts in Africa." *African Studies Review* 30 (1987): 1–78, 113–32.

Barthélémi, V. "Etude sur la syphilis au Congo belge." Examen B/Médecins no. 16a, IMT, 1921.

Bayart, Jean-François. *L'Etat en Afrique: La politique du ventre*. Paris: Fayard, 1989.

Bayoumi, Ahmed. *The History of Sudan Health Services*. Nairobi: Kenya Literature Bureau, 1979.

Beidelman, T. O. "Witchcraft in Ukaguru." In *Witchcraft and Sorcery in East Africa*, edited by John Middleton and E. H. Winter. London: Routledge and Kegan Paul, 1963.

——. *Colonial Evangelism: A Socio-Historical Study of an East African Mission at the Grassroots*. Bloomington: Indiana University Press, 1982.

——. *Moral Imagination in Kaguru Modes of Thought*. Bloomington: Indiana University Press, 1986.

Beinart, Jennifer. "Darkly through a Lens: Changing Perceptions of the African Child in Sickness and Health, 1900–1945." In *In the Name of the Child: Health and Welfare, 1880–1940*, edited by Roger Cooter. London: Routledge, 1992.

[Belgium]. *Congrès Colonial National*, [IIème]. Brussels: Imprimerie Lesigne, 1926.

Belgium. Office de l'Information et des Relations Publiques pour le Congo Belge et le Ruanda-Urundi. *Health in Belgian Africa*. Brussels: Inforcongo, 1958.

Bell, Heather. "Midwifery Training and Female Circumcision in the Inter-War Anglo-Egyptian Sudan." *Journal of African History* 39 (1998): 298–312.

Bella, Hassan. "Sudanese Village Midwives: Six Decades of Experience with Part-Time Health Workers." In *Advances in International Maternal and Child Health*, edited by D. B. Jelliffe and E. F. P. Jelliffe. Vol. 4. Oxford: Clarendon Press, 1984.

Bemba, Sylvain. *Cinquante ans de musique du Congo-Zaïre (1920–1970)*. Paris: Présence Africaine, 1984.

Bennett, Tony, ed. *Christmas: A Case Study*. Vol. units 1/2 of *Popular Culture: Themes and Issues I*. Block 1. Milton Keynes, U.K.: Open University Press, 1981.

Bentley, W. Holman. *Pioneering on the Congo*. London: Religious Tract Society, 1900.

Bernard. "Une société chez les Babali." *Congo* 2 (1922): 349–53.

Berrera, Guilia. *Dangerous Liaisons: Colonial Concubinage in Eritrea, 1890–1941*. PAS Working Paper no. 1. Evanston, Ill.: Program of African Studies, Northwestern University, 1996.

Bertrand, Colonel A. "Quelques notes sur la vie politique, le développement, la décadence des petites sociétés bantou du bassin central du Congo." *Revue de l'Institut de Sociologie de Bruxelles* 1 (1920): 75–91.

Best, Dick, and Beth Best, eds. *Song Fest: Three Hundred Songs: Words and Music, including Folk Songs and Ballads, College Songs, Drinking Songs, Old Favorites, Parodies, Cowboy Songs, Chanties, Fiddle Tunes, Rounds, Spirituals, Etc.* New York: Crown Publishers, 1945.

Beti, Mongo. *Perpetua and the Habit of Unhappiness*. London: Heinemann, 1978.

Bhabha, Homi. "Of Mimicry and Man: The Ambivalence of Colonial Discourse." *October* 28 (1984): 125–33.

Bianga, Ghu-Gha. "La politique démographique au Congo belge." *Population* 33 (1978): 189–94.

Biaya, T. K. "L'Impasse de crise zaïroise dans la peinture populaire urbaine, 1970–1985." In *Art et politiques en Afrique noire/Art and Politics in Black Africa*. Ottawa: Canadian Association of African Studies and Safi Press, 1989.

Bibeau, Giles. "La communauté musulmane de Kisangani." In *Kisangani, 1876–1976: Histoire d'une ville*, edited by Benoît Verhaegen. Kinshasa: Presses Universitaires du Zaïre, 1975).

Biebuyck, Daniel P. *Lega Culture: Art, Initiation, and Moral Philosophy among a Central African People*. Berkeley: University of California Press, 1973.

———. "Sculpture from the Eastern Zaire Forest Regions: Mbole, Yele, and Pere." *African Arts* 10 (1976): 54–61, 99–100.

Bitran, Ricardo A. "A Household Health Care Demand Study in the Bokoro and Kisantu Zones of Zaire, Vol. 2, Utilization Patterns." Resources for Child Health Project, Contract no. DEP-5927-C-00-5068-00, Arlington, Va., n.d. Draft manuscript.

Bitran, Ricardo A., et al. "Etude sur le financement des zones de santé au Zaïre, juin–octobre 1986, USAID/Kinshasa." Resources for Child Health Project, Contract no. DPE-5927-C-00-5068-00, Arlington, Va., 1986. Unpublished report.

Bloomfield, Anne. "Drill and Dance as Symbols of Imperialism." In *Making Imperial Mentalities: Socialisation and British Imperialism*, edited by J. A. Mangan. Manchester: Manchester University Press, 1990.

Boddy, Janice. "Remembering Amal: On Birth and the British in Northern Sudan." In *Pragmatic Women and Body Politics*, edited by Margaret Lock and Patricia A. Kaufert. Cambridge: Cambridge University Press, 1998.

Bock, Gisela, and Pat Thane, eds. *Maternity and Gender Policies: Women and the Rise of the European Welfare States, 1880s–1950s*. London: Routledge, 1991.

Bolya, Paul. "Etude ethnographique des coutumes des Mongo, La naissance, Chapitre III." *La Voix du Congolais* 140 (November 1950).

Bonenfant, Paul. *Le problème du paupérisme en Belgique à la fin de l'Ancien Régime*. Mémoire, Classe des Lettres et des Sciences Morales et Politiques, vol. 35. Brussels: Académie Royale de Belgique, 1934.

Bontinck, F. "Les deux Bula Matari." *Etudes Congolaises* 12, no. 3 (July–September 1969): 83–97.

Brandt, Allan M. "Sexually Transmitted Diseases." In *Companion Encyclopedia of the History of Medicine*, edited by W. F. Bynum and Roy Porter. Vol. 1. London: Routledge, 1993.

Brantlinger, Patrick. "Victorians and Africans: The Genealogy of the Myth of the Dark Continent." *Critical Inquiry* 12 (1985): 166–203.

Brausch, Georges. *Belgian Administration in the Congo*. London: Oxford University Press, 1961.

Breckenridge, Carol, ed. *Consuming Modernity: Public Culture in a South Asian World*. Minneapolis: University of Minnesota Press, 1995.

Briggs, Laura. "Fair Fruit and Foul: Discourses of Race in Nineteenth-Century Obstetrics and Gynecology." Paper presented at the American Studies Association, Nashville, Tenn., 28–31 October 1994.

Brothwell, Don R. "Yaws." In *The Cambridge World History of Human Disease*, edited by Kenneth F. Kiple. Cambridge: Cambridge University Press, 1993.

Browne, Stanley G. "The Training of Medical Auxiliaries in the Former Belgian Congo." *Lancet* 1 (19 May 1973): 1103–5.

Browne, Stanley G., Frank Davey, and William A. R. Thomson, eds. *Heralds of Health: The Saga of Christian Medical Initiatives.* London: Christian Medical Fellowship, 1985.

Brun, G. "L'embryotomie cervicale dans les présentations transversales." *Maroc Médical* 50, no. 536 (June 1970): 395–96.

Buell, Raymond Leslie. *The Native Problem in Africa.* 2 vols. 1928. Reprint, London: Frank Cass, 1965.

Burke, Timothy. *Lifebuoy Men, Lux Women: Commodification, Consumption, and Cleanliness in Modern Zimbabwe.* Durham, N.C.: Duke University Press, 1996.

Burns, Catherine Eileen. "Reproductive Labors: The Politics of Women's Health in South Africa, 1900 to 1960." Ph.D. diss., Northwestern University, 1994.

Cambier, René. "Note de la carte des campagnes antiesclavagistes." In *Atlas général du Congo et du Ruanda-Urundi.* Vol. 14. Brussels: ARSOM, 1948–60.

Carrington, John F. "The Tonal Structure of Kele (Lokele)." *African Studies* 3 (December 1943): 193–207.

———. "The Initiation Language: Lokele Tribe." *African Studies* 6, no. 4 (1947): 196–207.

———. "Lilwaakoi—a Congo Secret Society." *Baptist Quarterly* 12, no. 8 (1947): 237–44.

———. *A Comparative Study of Some Central African Gong-Languages.* Brussels: IRCB, 1949.

———. *Talking Drums of Africa.* London: Carey Kingsgate Press, 1949.

———. *Proverbes Lokele, Tokoko twa Lokele.* Kisangani, 1973. Polycopied manuscript.

———. "Sketch of Lokele Grammar (Missionaries of Yakusu)." Salisbury, U.K., 1984. Unpublished manuscript.

Les cent aventures de la famille Mbumbulu. Leopoldville: Presses de l'Imprimerie de l'Avenir, 1956.

Ceulemans, P. *La question arabe et le Congo (1883–1892).* Brussels: ARSC, 1958.

Ceyssens, Rik. "Mutumbula, mythe de l'opprimé." *Cultures et développement* 7 (1975): 483–550.

Chesterman, C. C. "Tryparsamide in Sleeping Sickness." *TRSTMH* 16 (1922–23): 405.

———. "The Relation of Yaws and Goundou." *TRSTMH* 20 (1926–27): 554.

———. In "Yaws: Discussion." *British Journal of Venereal Diseases* 4 (1928): 64.

———. *Manuel du dispensaire tropical,* translated by C. and R. Francotte. 1929. Reprint, London: United Society for Christian Literature, 1960.

———. "Some Results of Tryparsamide and Combined Treatment of Gambian Sleeping Sickness." *TRSTMH* 25 (1931–32): 415–44.

———. "The Training and Employment of African Natives as Medical Assistants." *Proceedings of the Royal Society of Medicine* 25 (1931–1932), pt. 3:1067–76.

———. "Blackwater Fever in a Negro Child." *Lancet* 7 (1935): 554.

———. In "Discussion" of Ellis H. Hudson, "Bejel: The Endemic Syphilis of the Euphrates Arab." *TRSTMH* 31 (1937–38): 41–42.

———. *In the Service of the Suffering: Phases of Medical Missionary Enterprise.* London: Edinburgh House Press, 1940.

———. In "Discussion" of C. J. Hackett, "The Clinical Course of Yaws in Lango, Uganda." *TRSTMH* 40 (1946): 206–27.

———. "The Contribution of Protestant Missions to the Health Services of the Congo." *ASBMT,* Supplément: "Liber Jubilaris J. Rhodhain" (December 1947): 37–46.

——. In "Discussion." *TRSTMH* 40 (1947): 755.

——. "My Man Sunday: How a Congo Houseboy Became a Conqueror of the Dread Diseases That Ravaged His People." *Reader's Digest* 51 (September 1947): 95–100.

——. In "Discussion." *TRSTMH* 63 (1969): 5–92.

Chesterman, C. C., and Kenneth W. Todd. "Clinical Studies with Organic Arsenic Derivatives in Human Trypanosomiasis and Yaws." *TRSTMH* 21 (1927–28): 227–32.

Cocq, V., and Fr. Mercken. "L'assistance obstétricale au Congo belge (y compris le Ruanda-Urundi)." *Gynécologie et Obstétrique* 31, no. 4 (1935): 401–513.

Cohen, David William. "Doing Social History from Pim's Doorway." In *Reliving the Past: The Worlds of Social History,* edited by Oliver Zunz. Chapel Hill: University of North Carolina Press, 1985.

Cohn, Bernard S. "The Census, Social Structure, and Objectification in South Asia." In *An Anthropologist among the Historians and Other Essays.* Delhi: Oxford University Press, 1987.

——. *Colonialism and Its Forms of Knowledge: The British in India.* Princeton, N.J.: Princeton University Press, 1996.

Cole, Catherine M. "Reading Blackface in West Africa: Wonders Taken for Signs." *Critical Inquiry* 23 (1996): 183–215.

Colwell, A. Stacie C. "Morphing the Body Collective: Subtexts and Sequelae of Colonial Population Studies." Paper presented to Fortieth Annual Meeting of the African Studies Association, Columbus, Ohio, 13–16 November 1997.

Comaroff, Jean. "The Diseased Heart of Africa: Medicine, Colonialism, and the Black Body." In *Knowledge, Power, and Practice: The Anthropology of Medicine and Everyday Life,* edited by Margaret Lock and Shirley Lindenbaum. Berkeley: University of California Press, 1993.

Comaroff, Jean, and John Comaroff. "Home-Made Hegemony: Modernity, Domesticity, and Colonialism in South Africa." In *African Encounters with Domesticity,* edited by Karen Tranberg Hansen. New Brunswick, N.J.: Rutgers University Press, 1992.

Comeliau, Marie-Louise. *Blancs et Noirs: Scènes de la vie congolaise.* Paris: Charles Dessart, 1942.

——. *Demain, coloniale!* Antwerp: Editions Zaïre, 1945.

Congo Belge. *Rapport sur l'hygiène publique.* 1925–1947.

Congo Belge. *Recueil Mensuel des circulaires, instructions et ordres de service.* 1908–1959.

Congo Belge. Direction Générale des Services Médicaux. *Rapport Annuel.* 1948–1958.

Congo Belge. Service de l'Hygiène. *Conseils d'hygiène aux indigènes.* Brussels: n.p., 1926.

Congo Missionary Conference. *Reports of the General Conference of Missionaries of the Protestant Societies Working in Congoland.* 1902. 1904. 1906. 1907. 1909. 1911. 1918. 1921. 1924.

Conrad, Joseph. *Heart of Darkness,* edited by D. C. R. A. Goonetilleke. Peterborough, Ontario: Broadview Literary Texts, 1995.

"Considérations sur l'utilisation de la main-d'oeuvre au Congo belge." *Office International d'Hygiène Publique* 23 (1931): 1627–51.

Cook, Albert. "Note on Dr. Mitchell's Paper on the Causes of Obstructed Labour in Uganda." *East African Medical Journal* 15 (October 1938): 215–19.

Cookey, S. J. S. *Britain and the Congo Question, 1885–1913.* London: Longmans, Green, and Co., 1968.

Coombes, Annie E. *Reinventing Africa: Museums, Material Culture, and Popular Imagination.* New Haven, Conn.: Yale University Press, 1994.

Cooper, Frederick. "From Free Labor to Family Allowances: Labor and Society in Colonial Discourse." *American Ethnologist* 16 (1989): 745–65.

Coquery-Vidrovitch, Catherine, Alain Forest, and Herbert Weiss, eds. *Rébellions-révolutions au Zaïre, 1963–1965.* 2 vols. Paris: l'Harmattan, 1987.

Corman, Alfred. *Annuaire des missions catholiques au Congo belge.* Brussels: Albert Dewit, 1924.

———. *Annuaire des missions catholiques au Congo belge.* Brussels: l'Edition Universelle, 1935.

Coser, Ruth Laub. "Some Social Functions of Laughter: A Study of Humor in a Hospital Setting." *Human Relations* 12 (1959): 171–82.

Crawford, Dan. *Thinking Black: Twenty-Two Years without a Break in the Long Grass of Central Africa.* London: Morgan and Scott, 1912.

Crine, B. "La structure sociale des Foma (Haut-Zaïre)." *Cahiers du CEDAF* 4 (1972).

Croix-Rouge du Congo. *Rapports Annuel.* 1927. 1930. 1932. 1934. 1936. 1938. 1940–1945.

Crowder, Michael. *The Flogging of Phineas McIntosh: A Tale of Colonial Folly and Injustice, Bechuanaland 1933.* New Haven: Yale University Press, 1988.

Darquenne, Roger. "L'obstétrique aux XVIIIe et XIXe siècles." In *Ecoles et livres d'école en Hainaut du XVIe au XIXe siècle.* Mons, Belgium: Editions Universitaires de Mons, 1971.

Davidoff, Leonore. "Mastered for Life: Servant and Wife in Victorian and Edwardian England." *Journal of Social History* 7 (1974): 406–28.

———. "Class and Gender in Victorian England." In *Sex and Class in Women's History,* edited by Judith L. Newton, Mary P. Ryan, and Judith R. Walkowitz. London: Routledge and Kegan Paul, 1983.

Davidoff, Leonore, and Catherine Hall. *Family Fortunes: Men and Women of the English Middle Class, 1780–1850.* London: Hutchinson, 1987.

Davin, Anna. "Imperialism and Motherhood." *History Workshop* 5 (spring 1978): 9–66.

Davis, Natalie Zemon. *Society and Culture in Early Modern France.* Stanford, Calif.: Stanford University Press, 1975.

———. "The Shapes of Social History." *Storia della Storiographia* 17 (1990): 28–34.

Davis, W. E. *Caring and Curing in Congo and Kentucky.* North Middletown, Ky.: Erasmus Press, 1984.

Dawson, Graham. *Soldier Heroes: British Adventure, Empire, and the Imagining of Masculinities.* London: Routledge, 1994.

Dawson, Marc. "The Anti-Yaws Campaign and Colonial Medical Policy in Kenya." *International Journal of African Historical Studies* 20 (1987): 417–37.

Dayan, Joan. "Amorous Bondage: Poe, Ladies, and Slaves." *American Literature* 66 (1994): 239–73.

———. "Paul Gilroy's Slaves, Ships, and Routes: The Middle Passage as Metaphor." *Research in African Literatures* 27 (1996): 8.

Daye, Pierre. "Au Congo il faut des femmes blanches." 1924. In *Problèmes congolais.* Brussels: Ecrits, 1943.

De Boeck, Filip. "From Knots to Web: Fertility, Life-Transmission, Health, and Well-Being among the Aluund of Southwest Zaire." Ph.D. diss., Katholieke Universiteit te Leuven, 1991.

Debroux, C. "Comportement démographique de la population européenne après la seconde guerre mondiale." *Enquêtes et Documents d'Histoire Africaine* 7 (1987): 5–14.

de Certeau, Michel. *The Practice of Everyday Life,* translated by Steven Rendall. Berkeley: University of California Press, 1984.

———. *L'invention du quotidien: I. Arts de faire,* edited by Luce Giard. Paris: Gallimard, 1990.

De Craemer, Willy, and Renée C. Fox. *The Emerging Physician: A Sociological Approach to the Development of a Congolese Medical Profession.* Stanford, Calif.: Hoover Institution on War, Revolution, and Peace, 1968.

de Heusch, Luc. *The Drunken King, or the Origin of the State,* translated by Roy Willis. Bloomington: Indiana University Press, 1982.

De Jonghe, E. "Formations récentes de sociétés secrètes au Congo belge." *Africa* 9 (1936): 56–63.

Delaney, Carol. *The Seed and the Soil: Gender and Cosmology in Turkish Village Society.* Berkeley: University of California Press, 1991.

Delathuy, A. M. *Jezuiten in Kongo met zwaard en kruis.* Berchem: EPO, 1986.

Delcommune, A. *Vingt années de vie africaine. Récits de voyages, d'aventures et d'exploration au Congo belge (1874–1893).* Vol. 1. Brussels: Larcier, 1922.

De Mahieu, Wauthier. *Qui a obstrué la cascade: Analyse sémantique du rituel de la circoncision chez les Komo du Zaïre.* Cambridge: Cambridge University Press, 1985.

de Meeus, Fr., and D. R. Steerberghen. *Les Missions religieuses au Congo belge.* Antwerp: Editions Zaïre, 1947.

de Meulemeester, A. "L'organisation des dispensaires ruraux de l'Oeuvre A.D.I.P.O. (Assistance aux Dispensaires Indigènes de la Province Orientale)." *Congo* 9 (1928): 1–12.

Dening, Greg. *Mr. Bligh's Bad Language: Passion, Power, and the Theatre on the Bounty.* Cambridge: Cambridge University Press, 1992.

De Raes, W. "Eugenetika in de Belgische medische wereld tijdens het interbellum." *Revue belge d'Histoire contemporaine* 20 (1989): 399–464.

de Saint Moulin, Léon. "What Is Known of the Demographic History of Zaire since 1885?" In *Demography from Scanty Evidence: Central Africa in the Colonial Era,* edited by Bruce Fetter. Boulder, Colo.: Lynne Rienner, 1990.

Detry, A. *A Stanleyville.* Liège: Imprimerie La Meuse, 1912.

Devisch, René. *Se recréer femme: Manipulation sémantique d'une situation d'infécondité chez les Yaka.* Berlin: Dietrich Reimer Verlag, 1984.

Devroey, E. *Le réseau routier au Congo belge et au Ruanda-Urundi.* Mémoire. Brussels: IRCB, 1939.

———. *Nouveaux systèmes de pont métalliques pour les colonies et leur influence possible sur l'évolution des transports routiers au Congo belge et au Ruanda-Urundi.* Mémoire. Brussels: IRCB, 1947.

d'Hossche, Révérend Père [Mupe Doshi, pseud.]. *Les aventures de Mbope.* Leverville: Bibliothèque de L'Etoile, n.d.

Dirks, Robert. "Slaves' Holiday." *Natural History* 84 (1975): 82–86.

———. *The Black Saturnalia: Conflict and Its Ritual Expression on British West Indian Slave Plantations.* Gainesville: University Press of Florida, 1987.

Domergue-Cloarec, Danielle. *Politique coloniale française et réalités coloniales: La santé en Côte d'Ivoire, 1905–1958.* Paris: Académie des Sciences d'Outre-Mer, 1986.

Dony, Maurist. *Mashauri kwa Mama wa Kongo.* Brussels: FBEI, [1953?].

Douglas, Mary. *The Lele of the Kasai.* London: Oxford University Press, 1963.

———. *Implicit Meanings: Essays in Anthropology.* London: Oxford University Press, 1975.

Driver, Felix. "Henry Morton Stanley and His Critics: Geography, Exploration, and Empire." *Past and Present* 133 (November 1991): 134–66.

Droogers, André. *The Dangerous Journey: Symbolic Aspects of Boys' Initiation among the Wagenia of Kisangani, Zaire.* The Hague: Mouton, 1980.

Duboccage, A. "La natalité chez les Bakongo dans ses rapports avec la gynécologie." *ASBMT* 9 (1929): 265–74.

——. "Notes cliniques du service gynécologique de la FOMULAC à Kisantu." *ASBMT* 14 (1934): 421–33.

Duncan, Sylvia, and Peter Duncan. *Bonganga: Experiences of a Missionary Doctor.* London: Odhams Press, 1958.

Dupré, Georges. *Un ordre et sa destruction.* Paris: ORSTOM, 1982.

——. *Les naissances d'une société: Espace et historicité chez les Beembé du Congo.* Paris: ORSTOM, 1985.

Dupré, Marie-Claude. "Comment être femme: un aspect du rituel Mukisi chez les Téké de la République Populaire du Congo." *Archives de Sciences Sociales des Religions* 46 (1978): 57–84.

Duren, A. "Quelques aspects de la vie médicale au Congo belge." Extract from *Le Scalpel* 2–5 (12, 19, 26 January and 2 February 1935).

Ekwempu, C. C. "Embryotomy versus Caesarean Section." *Tropical Doctor* 8 (1978): 195–97.

Elias, Norbert. *La civilisation des moeurs,* translated by Pierre Kamnitzer. 1939. Reprint, Paris: Calmann-Levy, 1973.

Erny, P. "Placenta et cordon ombilical dans la tradition africaine." *Psychopathologie africaine* 5 (1969): 139–48.

Etat Indépendant du Congo. *Recueil Mensuel des arrêtés, circulaires, instructions et ordres de service.* 1903–1907.

Eulick, Margaret Sally. *White Mother in Africa.* New York: Richard R. Smith, 1939.

Evans-Pritchard, E. E. *Witchcraft, Oracles, and Magic among the Azande.* 1937. Reprint, Oxford: Oxford University Press, 1985.

Fabian, Johannes. "Scratching the Surface: Observations on the Poetics of Lexical Borrowing in Shaba Swahili." *Anthropological Linguistics* 24 (1982): 14–50.

——. *Language and Colonial Power: The Appropriation of Swahili in the Former Belgian Congo, 1880–1938.* Berkeley: University of California Press, 1986.

——. *Power and Performance: Ethnographic Explorations through Proverbial Wisdom and Theater in Shaba, Zaire.* Madison: University of Wisconsin Press, 1990.

Fabian, Johannes, with Kalundi Mango and with linguistic notes by W. Schicho. *History from Below: The 'Vocabulary of Elisabethville' by André Yav; Texts, Translations, and Interpretive Essay.* Amsterdam: John Benjamins Publishing Company, 1990.

Feeley-Harnik, Gillian. *The Lord's Table: Eucharist and Passover in Early Christianity.* Philadelphia: University of Pennsylvania Press, 1981.

——. "Finding Memories in Madagascar." In *Images of Memory: On Remembering and Representation,* edited by Susanne Küchler and Walter Melion. Washington, D.C.: Smithsonian Institution Press, 1991.

Feierman, Steven. "Struggles for Control: The Social Roots of Health and Healing in Modern Africa." *African Studies Review* 28 (1985): 73–147.

——. "Popular Control over the Institutions of Health: A Historical Study." In *The Professionalisation of Medicine,* edited by Murray Last and G. L. Chavanduka. Manchester: Manchester University Press, 1986.

Feierman, Steven, and John M. Janzen, eds. *The Social Basis of Health and Healing in Africa.* Berkeley: University of California Press, 1992.

Feldman-Salvesburg, Pamela. "Plundered Kitchens and Empty Wombs: Fear of Infertility in the Cameroonian Grassfields." *Social Science and Medicine* 39 (1994): 463–74.

La femme au Congo: conseils aux partantes. Brussels: n.p., [1958?].

"La femme blanche au Congo." Institut Solvay, Travaux du Groupe d'Etudes coloniales, no. 4. Extract from *Bulletin de la Société belge d'Etudes coloniales* 5 (May 1910).

"Femmes coloniales au Congo belge." Special Issue: *Enquêtes et Documents d'Histoire africaine* 7 (1987).

Fildes, Valerie, Lara Marks, and Hilary Marland, eds. *Women and Children First: International Maternal and Infant Welfare, 1870–1945.* London: Routledge, 1992.

Flion, Léopold. "Cercles d'Etudes coloniales de l'Université de Bruxelles: Femmes et enfants blancs au Congo, au point de vue médical." *Bruxelles-Médical* 8 (1927–1928): 529–31.

Flood, Charles A., and William Sherman. "Medical Care in the Belgian Congo." *American Journal of Tropical Medicine* 24 (1944): 267–71.

Ford, John. *The Role of Trypanosomiases in African Ecology: A Study of the Tsetse Fly Problem.* Oxford: Clarendon Press, 1971.

FOREAMI. *Rapports annuel.* 1931. 1933. 1934. 1935. 1936. 1948. 1950. 1954. 1955.

Foster, W. D. *The Church Missionary Society and Modern Medicine in Uganda: The Life of Sir Albert Cook, K.C.M.G., 1870–1951.* Newhaven, East Sussex: Newhaven Press, 1978.

Foucault, Michel. *Discipline and Punish: The Birth of the Prison.* New York: Vintage, 1979.

———. *History of Sexuality.* New York: Vintage Books, 1985.

Fronville, G. "Six années de pratique chirurgicale chez les noirs du Katanga." Examen B/Médecins no. 44, IMT, 1926.

Gaitskell, Deborah. "Women, Religion, and Medicine in Johannesburg between the Wars." Paper for the African History Seminar, School of Oriental and African Studies and Institute of Commonwealth Studies, University of London, 18 May 1983.

———. " 'Getting Close to the Hearts of Mothers': Medical Missionaries among African Women and Children in Johannesburg between the Wars." In *Women and Children First: International Maternal and Infant Welfare, 1870–1945,* edited by Valerie Fildes, Lara Marks, and Hilary Marland. London: Routledge, 1992.

Gamarnikow, Eva. "Sexual Division of Labour: The Case of Nursing." In *Feminism and Materialism,* edited by Annette Kuhn and AnnMarie Wolpe. London: Routledge and Kegan Paul, 1978.

Garot, Lucien. *Médecine sociale de l'enfance et oeuvres de protection du premier âge.* Liège: Editions Desoer, 1946.

Gates, Henry Louis, Jr. *The Signifying Monkey: A Theory of Afro-American Literary Criticism.* New York: Oxford University Press, 1988.

Geldformen und Zierperlen der Naturvölker. Führer durch das Museum für Völkerkunde und Schweizerische. Basel: Museum für Volkskunde, 1961.

Gélis, Jacques. *La sage-femme ou le médecin. Une nouvelle conception de la vie.* Paris: Fayard, 1988.

Gillet, H. "Le service médical des Sociétés minières du Kasai (Champs diamantifères du Kasai)." ASBMT 8 (1928): 233–49.

Ginsburg, Faye D., and Rayna Rapp, eds. *Conceiving the New World Order: The Global Politics of Reproduction.* Berkeley: University of California Press, 1995.

Ginzburg, Carlo. *The Cheese and the Worms: The Cosmos of a Sixteenth-Century Miller.* Baltimore, Md.: Johns Hopkins University Press, 1980.

Glass, D. V. *Population: Policies and Movements in Europe*. Oxford: Oxford University Press, 1940.

Glassman, Jonathon. *Feasts and Riot: Revelry, Rebellion, and Popular Consciousness on the Swahili Coast, 1856–1888*. Portsmouth, N.H.: Heinemann, 1995.

Glave, E. J. "Cruelty in the Congo Free State." *Century Magazine* 54, no. 32 (May–October 1897): 699–715.

Goings, Kenneth W. *Mammy and Uncle Mose: Black Collectibles and American Stereotyping*. Bloomington: Indiana University Press, 1994.

Gold Coast Colony. *The Training of Nurses in the Gold Coast*. Accra: Government Printing Department, 1947.

Gosse, J. P. "Les méthodes et engins de pêche des Lokele." *Bulletin Agricole du Congo Belge* 2 (1961): 335–85.

Green, Martin. "The Robinson Crusoe Story." In *Imperialism and Juvenile Literature*, edited by Jeffrey Richards. Manchester: Manchester University Press, 1989.

Grewal, Inderpal, and Caren Kaplan, eds. *Scattered Hegemonies: Postmodernity and Transnational Feminist Practices*. Minneapolis: University of Minnesota Press, 1994.

Grimshaw, Patricia. " 'Christian Woman, Pious Wife, Faithful Mother, Devoted Missionary': Conflicts in Roles of American Missionary Women in Nineteenth-Century Hawaii." *Feminist Studies* 9 (1983): 489–521.

Guebels, Léon. *Relation complète des travaux de la Commission Permanente pour la Protection des Indigènes*. Brussels: Editions J. Duculot, [1952?].

Guillot, P. "Quelques cas gynécologiques et actes opératoires qu'ils ont provoqués chez les noirs du Congo." *Bulletin de la Société de Pathologie Exotique* 23 (1930): 205–9.

Guinness, Fanny E. *The New World of Central Africa, with a History of the First Christian Mission on the Congo*. London: Hodder and Stoughton, 1890.

Guiral, Pierre, and Guy Thuillier. *La vie quotidienne des domestiques en France au XIXe siècle*. Paris: Hachette, 1978.

Guyer, Jane I. "Wealth in People and Self-Realization in Equatorial Africa." *Man* 28 (1993): 243–65.

———. "Wealth in People, Wealth in Things—Introduction." *Journal of African History* 36 (1995): 83–90.

———. *Money Matters: Instability, Values, and Social Payments in the Modern History of West African Communities*. Portsmouth, N.H.: Heinemann, 1995.

Guyer, Jane I., and Samuel M. Eno Belinga. "Wealth in People as Wealth in Knowledge: Accumulation and Composition in Equatorial Africa." *Journal of African History* 36 (1995): 91–120.

Habig, Jean-Marie. "Enseignement médical pour coloniaux, 2ème partie, Psychopathologie de l'Européen et du Noir." Ligue Coloniale Belge, Cours Coloniaux de Bruxelles, Brussels, 1944. Unpublished manuscript.

———. *Vivre en Afrique centrale: Santé, hygiène, morale*. Brussels: l'Edition Universelle, 1952.

Hackett, C. J. *Boomerang Leg and Yaws in Australian Aborigines*. London: Royal Society of Tropical Medicine and Hygiene, 1936.

———. *Bone Lesions of Yaws in Uganda*. Oxford: Blackwell, 1948.

———. "Yaws." In *Health in Tropical Africa during the Colonial Period*, edited by E. E. Sabben-Clare, D. J. Bradley, and K. Kirkwood. Oxford: Clarendon Press, 1980.

Halen, Pierre. *Le petit belge avait vu grand: une littérature coloniale*. Brussels: Labor, 1993.

Hall, Catharine. "White Visions, Black Lives: The Free Villages of Jamaica." *History Workshop Journal*, no. 36 (1993): 100–132.

Hannerz, Ulf. *Cultural Complexity: Studies in the Social Organization of Meaning.* New York: Columbia University Press, 1992.

Hansen, Karen Tranberg. *Distant Companions: Servants and Employers in Zambia, 1900–1985.* Ithaca, N.Y.: Cornell University Press, 1989.

Harley, David. "Historians as Demonologists: The Myth of the Midwife-Witch." *Social History and Medicine* 3 (April 1990): 1–26.

Hauzeur de Fooz, Carlos. *Un démi-siècle avec l'économie du Congo belge.* Brussels: n.p., 1957.

Headrick, Rita. "The Impact of Colonialism on Health in French Equatorial Africa, 1880–1934." Ph.D. diss., University of Chicago, 1987.

———. *Colonialism, Health, and Illness in French Equatorial Africa, 1885–1935.* Atlanta, Ga.: African Studies Association, 1994.

Herbert, Eugenia. *Iron, Gender, and Power: Rituals of Transformation in African Societies.* Bloomington: Indiana University Press, 1993.

Hergé. *Les aventures de Tintin: Reporter du Petit 'Vingtième' au Congo.* 1931. Reprint, Tournai, Belgium: Casterman, 1982.

———. *Les aventures de Tintin: Tintin au Congo.* 1946. Reprint, Paris-Tournai: Casterman, 1974.

Heyse, Théodore. *Le Régime du Travail au Congo belge.* Brussels: Goemaere, Imprimeur du Roi, 1924.

Holo, Yann. "Les Représentations des africains dans l'imagerie enfantine." In *L'Autre et Nous: "Scènes et Types,"* edited by Pascal Blanchard et al. Paris: Syros and ACHAC, 1995.

Horn, David G. *Social Bodies: Science, Reproduction, and Italian Modernity.* Princeton, N.J.: Princeton University Press, 1994.

Hours, Bernard. *L'Etat sorcier: Santé publique et société au Cameroun.* Paris: Editions l'Harmattan, 1985.

Houssiau, F. "Quelques considérations sur la pratique médicale au Congo belge principalement à Léopoldville." Examen B/Médecins no. 1, IMT, 1912.

Hulme, Kathryn. *The Nun's Story.* London: Pan Books, 1956.

Hunt, Nancy Rose. " 'Le bébé en brousse': European Women, African Birth Spacing, and Colonial Intervention in Breast Feeding in the Belgian Congo." *International Journal of African Historical Studies* 21 (1988): 401–32.

———. " 'Single Ladies on the Congo': Protestant Missionary Tensions and Voices." *International Women's Studies Forum* 13 (1990): 395–403.

———. "Noise over Camouflaged Polygamy, Colonial Morality Taxation, and a Woman-Naming Crisis in Belgian Africa." *Journal of African History* 32 (1991): 471–94.

———. "Negotiated Colonialism: Domesticity, Hygiene, and Birth Work in the Belgian Congo." Ph.D. diss., University of Wisconsin–Madison, 1992.

———. "Letter-Writing, Nursing Men, and Bicycles in the Belgian Congo: Notes towards the Social Identity of a Colonial Category." In *Paths toward the Past: African Historical Essays in Honor of Jan Vansina,* edited by Robert W. Harms et al. Atlanta, Ga.: African Studies Association Press, 1994.

———. Review of *Milk, Honey, and Money,* by Christopher C. Taylor. *International Journal of African Historical Studies* 28 (1995): 458–61.

———. "Introduction." *Gender and History* 8 (1996): 323–37.

——. *"Tintin au Congo* and Its Colonial and Post-Colonial Reformulations." Paper presented at the "Images and Empires" conference, Yale University, 14–16 February 1997.

Inchi Yetu. Yakusu and Stanleyville: Librairie de la B.M.S., 1952.

Itongwa, Mulyumba wa Mamba, "Quelques données sur le rôle de la salive dans les sociétés traditionelles de l'Afrique noire." *Revue Zaïroise de psychologie et de pédagogie* 4, no. 1 (1975): 127–34.

Jacquart, Camille. *La mortalité infantile dans les Flandres.* Brussels: Albert Dewit, 1907.

Janssens, P. G. *La mortalité infantile aux Mines de Kilo; étude basée sur 1873 autopsies.* Brussels: IRCB, 1952.

Janzen, John M. *The Quest for Therapy in Lower Zaire.* Berkeley: University of California Press, 1978.

——. "Toward a Historical Perspective on African Medicine and Health." *Beitrâge zur Ethnomedizin, Ethnobotanik und Ethnozoologie* 8 (1983): 99–138.

——. *Ngoma: Discourses of Healing in Central and Southern Africa.* Berkeley: University of California Press, 1992.

Janzen, John M., and Steven Feierman, eds. "The Social History of Disease and Medicine in Africa." Special Issue of *Social Science and Medicine* 13B, no. 4 (1979).

Jenson, Jane. "Gender and Reproduction: Or, Babies and the State." *Studies in Political Economy* 20 (1986): 9–45.

Jewsiewicki, Bogumil. "Toward a Historical Sociology of Population in Zaire." In *African Population and Capitalism,* edited by Dennis Cordell and Joel W. Gregory. Boulder, Colo.: Westview Press, 1987.

——. "Painting in Zaire: From the Invention of the West to the Representation of the Social Self." In *Africa Explores: Twentieth Century African Art,* edited by Susan Vogel. New York: Center for African Art, 1991.

Jewsiewicki, Bogumil, ed. *Art pictural zaïrois.* Sillery, Quebec: Septentrion, 1992.

Jhala, Violet. "The Development of Maternal and Child Welfare Work in Colonial Malawi." Paper presented at the Women in Africa Seminar Series, Department of Extra-Mural Studies, London University, 3 June 1985.

Johnson, Frederick. *A Standard Swahili-English Dictionary.* Oxford: Oxford University Press, 1939.

Johnston, Sir Harry. *George Grenfell and the Congo.* 2 vols. London: Hutchinson and Co., 1908.

Jones, Anne Hudson, ed. *Images of Nurses: Perspectives from History, Art, and Literature.* Philadelphia: University of Pennsylvania Press, 1988.

Jones, Colin. "Montpellier Medical Students and the Medicalisation of Eighteenth-Century France." In *Problems and Methods in the History of Medicine,* edited by Roy Porter and Andrew Wear. London: Croom, 1987.

Joris, Lieve. *Back to the Congo.* London: Macmillan, 1992.

Kalala, Nkudi. "Identité et Société: Les fondements d'une marginalité. Le cas des Mbole." Ph.D. diss., UNAZA, Campus de Kisangani, 1977.

——. "Le Lilwaakoy des Mbole du Lomami. Essai d'analyse de son symbolisme." *Les Cahiers du CEDAF* 4 (1979).

Kebers, J.-R. "Les urgences anesthésiques en pathologie congolaise." Examen B/Médecins no. 236, IMT, 1956.

Keim, Curtis A. "The Mangbetu Worldview under Colonial Stress: *Nebeli.*" In *African Reflections: Art from Northeastern Zaire,* edited by Enid Schildkrout and Curtis A. Keim. Seattle: University of Washington Press, 1990.

Kikassa, Mwanalessa. "Planification familiale, fécondité et santé familiale au Zaïre. Rapport sur les résultats d'une enquête régionale sur la prévalence contraceptive en 1982–1984." *Zaïre-Afrique* 25, no. 200 (December 1985): 597–615.

King, Anthony D. *The Bungalow: The Production of a Global Culture.* London: Routledge and Kegan Paul, 1984.

Kiple, Kenneth F. *The Caribbean Slave: A Biological History.* Cambridge: Cambridge University Press, 1984.

——, ed. *The Cambridge World of Human Disease.* Cambridge: Cambridge University Press, 1993.

Korse, Piet. "Le fard rouge et le kaolin blanc chez les Mongo de Basankoso et de Befale (Zaïre)." *Annales Aequatoria* 10 (1989): 10–39.

Koven, Seth, and Sonya Michel. "Womanly Duties: Maternalist Politics and the Origins of Welfare States in France, Germany, Great Britain, and the United States, 1880–1920." *American Historical Review* 95 (1990): 1076–108.

Koven, Seth, and Sonya Michel, eds. *Mothers of a New World: Maternalist Politics and the Origins of Welfare States.* New York: Routledge, 1993.

Kratz, Corinne A. *Affecting Performance: Meaning, Movement, and Experience in Okiek? Women's Initiation.* Washington, D.C.: Smithsonian Institution Press, 1994.

Kujua Kuishi katika Watu Wengine. Lubumbashi: Editions St.-Paul Afrique, 1989.

Kuper, Adam. "The English Christmas and the Family: Time out and Alternative Realities." In *Unwrapping Christmas,* edited by Daniel Miller. Oxford: Clarendon Press, 1993.

Laget, Mireille. "Childbirth in Seventeenth- and Eighteenth-Century France: Obstetrical Practices and Collective Attitudes." In *Medicine and Society in France,* edited by Robert Forster and Orest Ranum. Baltimore, Md.: Johns Hopkins University Press, 1980.

Lambillon, J. "Note au sujet des troubles endocriens de la femme européenne durant les années de guerre au Congo belge." *ASBMT* 27 (1947): 95–104.

——. "Contribution à l'étude du problème obstétrical chez l'autochtone du Congo belge." Thèse d'Agrégation de l'Enseignement Supérieur, Université Catholique de Louvain, Brussels, 1950.

——. "Evolution du problème obstétrical à Léopoldville." *Académie Royale des Sciences Coloniales, Bulletin des Séances* 3 (1957): 1389–410.

——. "Evolution de la pathologie obstétricale en Afrique centrale de 1935 à 1960." *ASBMT* 44 (1964): 487–92.

Lambin, Francis. *Congo Belge, publié sous les auspices du Ministère des Colonies et du Fonds Colonial de Propagande Economique et Sociale.* Brussels: Editions Cuypers, 1948.

Lambrecht, Frank L. *In the Shade of an Acacia Tree: Memoirs of a Health Officer in Africa, 1945–1959.* Philadelphia, Pa.: American Philosophical Society, 1991.

Landau, Paul Stuart. *The Realm of the Word: Language, Gender, and Christianity in a Southern African Kingdom.* Portsmouth, N.H.: Heinemann, 1995.

——. "Explaining Surgical Evangelism in Colonial Southern Africa: Teeth, Pain, and Faith." *Journal of African History* 37 (1996): 261–81.

Lawson, John B. "Embryotomy for Obstructed Labour." *Tropical Doctor* 4 (1974): 188–91.

Lawson, John B., and D. B. Stewart. *Obstetrics and Gynaecology in the Tropics and Developing Countries.* London: Edward Arnold, 1967.

Leavitt, Judith Walzer. *Brought to Bed: Childbearing in America, 1750 to 1950.* New York: Oxford University Press, 1986.

———. "The Growth of Medical Authority: Technology and Morals in Turn-of-the-Century Obstetrics." *Medical Anthropology Quarterly* 1 (1987): 230–55.

Lejeune-Choquet, Adolphe. *Histoire militaire du Congo.* Brussels: Alfred Castaigne, 1906.

Léonard, Jacques. "Femmes, religion et médecine: Les religieuses qui soignent, en France au XIXe siècle." *Annales: Economies, Sociétés, Civilisations* 32 (1977): 887–907.

Lesthaeghe, Ron J. *The Decline of Belgian Fertility, 1800–1970.* Princeton, N.J.: Princeton University Press, 1977.

Levare, A. *Le confort aux colonies.* Paris: Editions Larose, 1928.

Lévi-Strauss, Claude. *The Savage Mind.* Chicago: University of Chicago Press, 1970.

———. "Father Christmas Executed." In *Unwrapping Christmas,* edited by Daniel Miller. Oxford: Clarendon Press, 1993.

Lewis, Jane. *The Politics of Motherhood: Child and Maternal Welfare in England, 1900–1939.* London: Croom Helm, 1980.

Ligue pour la Protection de l'Enfance noire au Congo Belge. *Rapports Annuel.* 1925–1926. 1928–1929. 1929–1930. 1936–1937. 1937–1938. 1938–1939. 1946–1947. 1947–1948. 1948–1949. 1949–1951.

Likaka, Osumaka. "Rural Protest: The Mbole against Belgian Rule, 1897–1959." *IJAHS* 27 (1994): 589–617.

Linaro, G. "Les affections chirurgicales plus communes des indigènes de l'Equateur." Examen B/Médecins no. 36, IMT, 1926.

Lloyd, A. B. *In Dwarf Land and Cannibal Country.* London: T. Fisher Unwin, 1899.

Lokomba, Baruti. "Structure et fonctionnement des institutions politiques traditionnelles chez les Lokele (Haut-Zaïre)." *Cahiers du CEDAF* 8 (1972).

———. "Kisangani centre urbain et les Lokele." In *Kisangani, 1876–1976: Histoire d'une ville,* edited by Benoît Verhaegen. Kinshasa: Presses Universitaires du Zaïre, 1975.

Lonoh, Michel. *Essai de commentaire de la musique moderne.* Kinshasa: SEI/ANC, 1972.

Lonsdale, John, and Bruce Berman. *Unhappy Valley: Conflict in Kenya and Africa.* London: James Curry, 1992.

Lory, Marie-Joseph. *Face à l'avenir. L'église au Congo Belge et au Ruanda-Urundi.* Tournai: Casterman, 1958.

Lott, Eric. *Love and Theft: Blackface Minstrelsy and the American Working Class.* New York: Oxford University Press, 1993.

Loudon, Irvine. *Death in Childbirth: An International Study of Maternal Care and Maternal Mortality, 1800–1950.* Oxford: Oxford University Press, 1992.

Louis, William Roger, and Jean Stengers. *E. D. Morel's History of the Congo Reform Movement.* London: Oxford University Press, 1968.

Lumby, J. R. *The Cambridge Bible for Schools and Colleges: The First Book of Kings.* Cambridge: University Press, 1894.

Lyons, Maryinez. *The Colonial Disease: A Social History of Sleeping Sickness in Northern Zaire, 1900–1940.* Cambridge: Cambridge University Press, 1992.

——. "The Power to Heal: African Medical Auxiliaries in Colonial Belgian Congo and Uganda." In *Contesting Colonial Hegemony: State and Society in Africa and India,* edited by Dagmar Engels and Shula Marks. London: British Academic Press, 1994.

Mabie, C. "Medical Work among Women." *Congo Missionary Conference,* 1911.

MacGaffey, Janet, with Vwakyanakazi Mukohya et al. *The Real Economy of Zaire.* Philadelphia: University of Pennsylvania, 1991.

MacGaffey, Wyatt. *Modern Kongo Prophets: Religion in a Plural Society.* Bloomington: Indiana University Press, 1983.

Mahieu, Alfred. *Numismatique du Congo, 1485–1924: instruments d'échange, valeurs monétaires, méreaux, médailles.* Brussels: Imprimerie Médicale et Scientifique, [1925?].

Mamba. *Les derniers crocos.* Brussels: Editions de l'Expansion Crocos, 1934.

Manda, Tchebwa. *Terre de la chanson: la musique zaïroise hier et aujourd'hui.* Louvain-la-Neuve: Duculot, 1996.

Mangoni, Tienebe-Mendierame. "De quelques aspects de la pathologie mentale dans la sous-région de Kisangani: le cas des Lokele et des Wagenya (Contribution à l'Ethnopsychiatrie)." Ph.D. diss., University of Kisangani, 1978.

Maran, René. *Batouala.* 1921. Reprint, London: Heinemann, 1987.

Marchal, Jules. *E. D. Morel contre Léopold II: L'Histoire du Congo, 1900–1910.* 2 vols. Paris: l'Harmattan, 1996.

Marks, Shula. *Divided Sisterhood: Race, Class, and Gender in the South African Nursing Profession.* New York: St. Martin's Press, 1994.

Martens, Ludo. *Une femme du Congo.* Brussels: EPO, 1991.

Martin, Phyllis M. *Leisure and Society in Colonial Brazzaville.* Cambridge: Cambridge University Press, 1995.

Marx, Walter John. *The Development of Charity in Medieval Louvain.* Yonkers, N.Y.: self-published, 1936.

Masuy-Stroobant, Godelieve. *Les Déterminants individuels et régionaux de la mortalité infantile: La Belgique d'hier et d'aujourd'hui.* Louvain-la-Neuve: CIACO, 1983.

Mboli ya Tengai. Yakusu, 1910–1960.

McGregor, Deborah Kuhn. *Sexual Surgery and the Origins of Gynecology: J. Marion Sims, His Hospital, and His Patients.* New York: Garland Publishing, 1989.

Meheus, A. "Pian." In *Médecine et hygiène en Afrique centrale de 1885 à nos jours,* edited by P. G. Janssens, M. Kivits, and J. Vuylsteke. Brussels: Fondation Rôi Baudouin, 1991.

Meillassoux, Claude. "Essai d'interprétation du phénomène économique dans les sociétés traditionelles." *Cahiers d'etudes africaines* 4 (1960): 38–67.

Mercken, Fr. "L'assistance obstétricale missionaire au Congo belge." *L'Aide Médicale aux Missions* 7 (October 1935): 68–72.

Migeon, Madeleine. *La faute du soleil! Eve en Afrique reportage.* Brussels: Les Editions de l'Expansion Belge, 1931.

Miller, Daniel, ed. *Unwrapping Christmas.* Oxford: Clarendon Press, 1993.

Miller, John Hawkins. "'Temple and Sewer': Childbirth, Prudery, and Victoria Regina." In *The Victorian Family: Structure and Stresses,* edited by Anthony S. Wohl. London: Croom Helm, 1978.

Millman, E. R., and William Millman. *A Mothercraft Manual for Senior Girls and Newly Married Women in Africa*. London: Carey Press for the Christian Literature Society, 1929.

Millman, William. *Hygiène tropicale pour les écoles. Njaso ya Bosasu*, French translation by Henri Anet. London: Bible Translation and Literature Society, 1921.

——. *Vocabulary of Ekele: The Language Spoken by the Lokele Tribe Living between Yanjali and Stanleyville*. Yakusu: BMS, 1926.

——. "The Tribal Initiation Ceremony of the Lokele." *International Review of Missions* 16 (1927): 364–80.

——. "Health Instruction in African Schools: Suggestions for a Curriculum." *Africa* 3 (1930): 484–500. *Missionary Herald*. London, 1896–1924.

Mitchell, J. Clyde. *The Kalela Dance: Aspects of Relationships among Urban Africans in Northern Rhodesia*. Rhodes-Livingstone Paper 27. Manchester: Manchester University Press, 1959.

Mitchell, J. P. "On the Causes of Obstructed Labour in Uganda." *East African Medical Journal* 15 (September 1938): 177–89.

——. "On the Causes of Obstructed Labour in Uganda." *East African Medical Journal* 15 (October 1938): 205–14.

Morel, E. D. *Red Rubber: The Story of the Rubber Slave Trade Flourishing on the Congo in the Year of Grace, 1906*. 1906. Reprint, New York: Haskell House, 1970.

Mort, Frank. *Dangerous Sexualities: Medico-Moral Politics in England since 1830*. London: Routledge and Kegan Paul, 1987.

Moscucci, Ornella. *The Science of Woman: Gynaecology and Gender in England, 1800–1929*. Cambridge: Cambridge University Press, 1990.

Mottoulle, L. "Maternités noires et religieuses blanches au Congo belge." *Revue Coloniale Belge* 4, no. 106 (1 March 1950): 160–61.

Mouchet, R. "La natalité et la mortalité infantile dans la Province Orientale." *ASBMT* 6 (1926): 165–74.

——. "Notes sur les dispensaires ruraux de la Province Orientale." *ASBMT* 6 (1926): 145–60.

——. "Yaws and Syphilis among Natives in the Belgian Congo." *Kenya Medical Journal* 3 (1926–27): 242–45.

Mulyumba, wa Mamba Itongwa. "Quelques données sur le rôle de la salive dans les sociétés traditionelles de l'Afrique noire." *Revue zaïroise psychologie et de pédagogie* 4 (1975): 127–34.

Munzombo, Kambale, and Shanga Minga. "Une société secrète au Zaïre: les hommes-crocodiles de la zone d'Ubundu." *Africa* (Rome) 42 (1987): 226–38.

Myles, Margaret F. *A Textbook for Midwives*. Edinburgh: Churchill Livingstone, 1972.

Naipaul, V. S. "A New King for the Congo." *New York Review of Books* 22, no. 11, 26 June 1975, 19.

Ndirangu, Simon. *A History of Nursing in Kenya*. Nairobi: Kenya Literature Bureau, 1982.

Négripub: L'image des noirs dans la publicité depuis un siècle. Paris: Somogy, 1994.

Ngamilu Awiry, Romain B. *L'Aviation civile et militaire zaïroise: Aperçu historique*. Braine-l'Alleud, Belgium: J. M. Collet, 1993.

Niranjana, Tejaswini. *Siting Translation: History, Post-Structuralism, and the Colonial Context*. Berkeley: University of California Press, 1992.

Norden, Hermann. *Fresh Tracks in the Belgian Congo: From Its Uganda Border to the Mouth of the Congo*. Boston: Small, Maynard, and Company, 1924.

Northrup, David. *Beyond the Bend in the River: African Labor in Eastern Zaire, 1865–1940*. Athens: Ohio University Center for International Studies, 1988.

Nos Images. Leopoldville, 1948–55.

Nursing Mirror and Midwives' Journal. 1931–1935.

Obed, J. Y. "Fetal Decapitation: The Application and Safety of the Stout Embryotomy Scissors." *Tropical Doctor* 24 (1994): 139–40.

Obenga, e Théophile. "Naissance et puberté en pays Kongo au XVIIe siècle." *Cahiers congolais d'anthropologie et d'histoire* 9 (1984): 19–30.

"Opportunities for Research in the Belgian Congo." *TRSTMH* 19 (1925–26): 185.

Oxford English Dictionary. 2d ed. New York: Oxford University Press, 1989.

Pagezy, Hélène, and Anne Marie Subervie. *Sida et modification des comportements sexuels: le cas des reclusions de longue durée chez les Mongo du sud du Zaïre*. Rapport final de contrat ANRS, Projet no. 90085, 1990–1993. Aix-en-Provence and Paris: CNRS and ANRS, 1992.

Peene, H. "Etude radiométrique de 100 bassins de femmes de race Bashi." Examen B/Medécins no. 272, IMT, 1958.

Perin, F. "Etude du bassin obstétrical chez la femme noire." *Recueil de Travaux de Sciences Médicales au Congo Belge* 3 (1945): 32–42.

Pickering, Michael. "Mock Blacks and Racial Mockery: The 'Nigger' Minstrel and British Imperialism." In *Acts of Supremacy: The British Empire and the Stage, 1790–1930*, edited by J. S. Bratton et al. Manchester: Manchester University Press, 1991.

Pieterse, Jan. *White on Black: Images of Africa and Blacks in Western Popular Culture*. New Haven, Conn.: Yale University Press, 1992.

Pimlott, J. *An Englishman's Christmas: A Social History*. Atlantic Highlands, N.J.: Humanities Press, 1978.

Pishandenge, Ngondo a Iman. "Mortalité et morbidité infantiles et juvéniles dans les grandes villes du Zaïre en 1986–1987." *Zaïre-Afrique* 31, no. 251 (January 1991): 49–60.

Platel, G., and Yv. Vandergoten. "Réflexions sur les résultats obtenus par une consultation des nourrissons au Mayombe (Congo belge)." *ASBMT* 20 (1940): 297–333.

Pons, Valdo. *Stanleyville: An African Urban Community under Belgian Administration*. Oxford: Oxford University Press, 1969.

Poovey, Mary. *Uneven Developments: The Ideological Work of Gender in Mid-Victorian England*. London: Virago Press, 1989.

Porter, Roy. "A Touch of Danger: The Man-Midwife as Sexual Predator." In *Sexual Underworlds of the Enlightenment*, edited by G. S. Rousseau and Roy Porter. Chapel Hill: University of North Carolina Press, 1988.

Powell, E. Alexander. *The Map That Is Half Unrolled: Equatorial Africa from the Indian Ocean to the Atlantic*. London: John Long, 1925.

Prakash, Gyan. "Science 'Gone Native' in Colonial India." *Representations* 40 (1992): 153–78.

Pratt, Mary Louise. *Imperial Eyes: Travel Writing and Transculturation*. London: Routledge, 1992.

Prins, Gwyn. "But What Was the Disease? The Present State of Health and Healing in African Studies." *Past and Present* no. 124 (August 1989): 159–79.

Prost, Antoine. "Catholic Conservatives, Population, and the Family in Twentieth-Century France." In *Population and Resources in Western Intellectual Traditions*, edited by Michael S. Teitelbaum and Jay M. Winter. Cambridge: Cambridge University Press, 1989.

Pulieri, C. "Rapport sur les observations d'Afrique." Examen B/Médecins no. 2, 1912.

Quiggin, A. Hingston. *A Survey of Primitive Money: The Beginnings of Currency.* 1949. Reprint, London: Metheun, 1979.

Racine, Aimée, and Eugène Dupréel. *Enquête sur les conditions de vie des familles nombreuses en Belgique.* Paris: Libraire du Recueil Sirey, 1933.

Radcliffe-Brown, A. R. "On Joking Relationships." In *Structure and Function in Primitive Society: Essays and Addresses.* Glencoe, Ill.: Free Press, 1952.

Rafael, Vicente L. *Contracting Colonialism: Translation and Christmas Conversion in Tagalog Society under Early Spanish Rule.* Durham, N.C.: Duke University Press, 1993.

Raikes, Alanagh. "Women's Health in East Africa." *Social Science and Medicine* 28 (1989): 447–59.

Ramirez, F., and C. Rolot, *Histoire du cinéma colonial au Zaïre, au Rwanda, et au Burundi.* Tervuren: MRAC, 1985.

Ranger, Terence. *Dance and Society in Eastern Africa, 1890–1970: The Beni Ngoma.* Berkeley: University of California Press, 1975.

——. "Godly Medicine: The Ambiguities of Medical Mission in Southeast Tanzania, 1900–1945." *Social Science and Medicine* 15B (1981): 261–77.

Rebuffat, E. "Contribution à l'étude de relèvement de la natalité au Congo belge." Examen B/Médecins no. 48, IMT, 1927.

Retel-Laurentin, Anne. *Infécondité en Afrique noire: Maladies et conséquences sociales.* Paris: Masson, 1974.

——. *Sorcellerie et ordalies.* Paris: Editions Anthropos, 1974.

Richards, Audrey. *Chisungu.* London: Faber and Faber, 1956.

Richards, Thomas. *The Commodity Culture of Victorian England: Advertising and Spectacle, 1851–1914.* Stanford, Calif.: Stanford University Press, 1990.

Roberts, Allan. "'Like a Roaring Lion': Tabwa Terrorism in the Late Nineteenth Century." In *Banditry, Rebellion, and Social Protest in Africa,* edited by Donald Crummey. London: James Currey, 1986.

Rogers, Glenn. "Child Survival Strategy." Kinshasa, May 1987. Unpublished USAID manuscript.

Romaniuk, Anatole. *La fécondité des populations congolaises.* Paris: Mouton, 1967.

——. "The Demography of the Democratic Republic of Congo." In *The Demography of Tropical Africa,* by William Brass et al. Princeton, N.J.: Princeton University Press, 1968.

Roome, William J. W. *Tramping through Africa: A Dozen Crossings of the Continent.* New York: Macmillan Company, 1930.

Rosaldo, Renato. *Ilongnot Head-Hunting, 1883–1974: A Study in Society and History.* Stanford, Calif.: Stanford University Press, 1980.

Rouvroy, V. "Le 'Lilwa' (District de l'Aruwimi. Territoire des Bambole)." *Congo* 1 (1929).

Ryder, Robert W., and Susan E. Hassig. "The Epidemiology of Perinatal Transmission of HIV." *AIDS* 2, suppl. 1 (1988): S83–89.

Ryder, Robert W., et al. "Perinatal Transmission of the Human Immunodeficiency Virus Type 1 to Infants of Seropositive Women in Zaire." *New England Journal of Medicine* 320 (22 June 1989): 1637–42.

Sabakinu, Kivilu. "Population et santé dans le processus de l'industrialisation du Zaïre." *Canadian Journal of African Studies* 18 (1984): 94–98.

Saer, Juan José. *The Witness,* translated by Margaret Jull Costa. London: Serpent's Tail, 1990.

Sahlins, Marshall. *Islands of History.* Chicago: University of Chicago Press, 1985.

Saile, Wawima Tshosomo. "Les Lokele et le grand commerce sur le fleuve de la fin du XIXe siècle au début du XXe siècle." Mémoire en Histoire, UNAZA, Campus de Lubumbashi, 1974.

Sargent, Carolyn Fishel. *Maternity, Medicine, and Power: Reproductive Decisions in Urban Benin.* Berkeley: University of California Press, 1989.

Schatzberg, Michael G. *The Dialectics of Oppression in Zaire.* Bloomington: Indiana University Press, 1988.

Schmeltz, J. D E., and J. P. B. de J. de Jong. *Ethnographisch Album van het Stroomgebied van den Congo.* Haarlem: H. Kleinmann and Co., 1904–1916.

Schneider, William H. *Quality and Quantity: The Quest for Biological Regeneration in Twentieth-Century France.* Cambridge: Cambridge University Press, 1990.

Schram, Ralph. *A History of the Nigerian Health Services.* Ibadan, Nigeria: Ibadan University Press, 1971.

Scott, James C. *Domination and the Arts of Resistance: Hidden Transcripts.* New Haven, Conn.: Yale University Press, 1990.

Shaw, Bryant P. "Force Publique, Force Unique: The Military in the Belgian Congo, 1914–1939." Ph.D. diss., University of Wisconsin–Madison, 1984.

Sheridan, Richard B. *Doctors and Slaves: A Medical and Demographic History of Slavery in the British West Indies, 1680–1834.* Cambridge: Cambridge University Press, 1985.

Sheriff, Abdul. *Slaves, Spices, and Ivory in Zanzibar: Integration of an East African Commercial Empire into the World Economy, 1770–1873.* Athens: Ohio University Press, 1987.

Sinclair, John N. "Our Storied Past: A Saga of Six Lives Molded into Three Families and Lived out on Four Continents." Roseville, Minn., 1992, unpublished manuscript.

Slade [Reardon], Ruth M. *English-Speaking Missions in the Congo Independent State (1878–1908).* Brussels: ARSOM, 1958.

———. "Catholics and Protestants in the Congo." In *Christianity in Tropical Africa,* edited by C. G. Baëta. London: Oxford University Press, 1968.

Smith, H. Sutton. *Yakusu, the Very Heart of Africa: Being Some Account of the Protestant Mission at Stanley Falls, Upper Congo.* London: Carey Press, [1911?].

Solo, Ramazani. "Implantation des Topoke à Yanonge." *Cahiers du CRIDE* 65–66 (July-August, 1982): 195–224.

Soloway, Richard. *Demography and Degeneration: Eugenics and the Declining Birthrate in Twentieth-Century Britain.* Chapel Hill: University of North Carolina Press, 1990.

Spire, Charles. *Conseils d'hygiène aux indigènes.* Brussels: Ministère des Colonies, 1922.

Spivak, Gayatri. "Can the Subaltern Speak?" In *Marxism and the Interpretation of Culture,* edited by Cary Nelson and Lawrence Grossberg. Urbana: University of Illinois Press, 1988.

Spring, Anita. "Women's Rituals and Natality among the Luvale of Zambia." Ph.D. diss., Cornell University, 1976.

Stallybrass, Peter, and Allon White. *The Politics and Poetics of Transgression.* Ithaca, N.Y.: Cornell University Press, 1986.

Stanley, Brian. *The History of the Baptist Missionary Society, 1792–1992.* Edinburgh: T. and T. Clark, 1992.

Stanley, Henry Morton. *Through the Dark Continent: Or, the Sources of the Nile, around the Great*

Lakes of Equatorial Africa, and down the Livingstone River to the Atlantic Ocean. 2 vols. 1878. Reprint, New York: Dover Publications, 1988.

——. *The Congo and the Founding of Its Free State: A Story of Work and Exploration.* New York: Harper and Brothers, 1885.

——. *In Darkest Africa.* New York: Charles Scribner's Sons, 1890.

Stapleton, Walter Henry. *Comparative Handbook of Congo Languages.* Yakusu: n.p., 1903.

Staub, A. "Rapport résumant des observations concernant le service de chirurgie à Léopoldville de juillet 1925 à juillet 1926." Examen B/Médecins no. 47, IMT, 1926.

Stengers, Jean. *Congo: Mythes et réalités, cent ans d'histoire.* Paris: Ducolot, 1989.

Stewart, Kathleen. "On the Politics of Cultural Theory: A Case for 'Contaminated' Cultural Critique." *Social Research* 58 (1991): 395–412.

Stoler, Ann Laura. *Race and the Education of Desire: Foucault's "History of Sexuality" and the Colonial Order of Things.* Durham, N.C.: Duke University Press, 1995.

Stones, R. Y. "On the Causes of Obstructed Labour in Uganda." *East African Medical Journal* 15 (October 1938): 219–20.

Summers, Anne. *Angels and Citizens: British Women as Military Nurses, 1854–1914.* London: Routledge and Kegan Paul, 1988.

Summers, Carol. "Intimate Colonialism: The Imperial Production of Reproduction in Uganda, 1907–1925." *Signs* 16 (1991): 787–807.

Swantz, Lloyd W. "The Role of the Medicine Man among the Zaramo of Dar es Salaam." Ph.D. diss., University of Dar es Salaam, 1972.

Taussig, Michael. *Mimesis and Alterity: A Particular History of the Senses.* New York: Routledge, 1993.

Taylor, Christopher C. *Milk, Honey, and Money: Changing Concepts in Rwandan Healing.* Washington, D.C.: Smithsonian Institution Press, 1992.

Teitelbaum, Michael S., and Jay M. Winter. *The Fear of Population Decline.* Orlando, Fla.: Academic Press, 1985.

——, eds. *Population and Resources in Western Intellectual Traditions.* Cambridge: Cambridge University Press, 1989.

Thomas, Lynn M. " '*Ngaitana* (I will circumcise myself)': The Gender and Generational Politics of the 1956 Ban on Clitoridectomy in Meru, Kenya." *Gender and History* 8 (1966): 338–63.

Thomas, Nicholas. "Sanitation and Seeing: The Creation of State Power in Early Colonial Fiji." *Comparative Studies in Society and History* 32 (1990): 149–70.

——. *Entangled Objects: Exchange, Material Culture, and Colonialism in the Pacific.* Cambridge, Mass.: Harvard University Press, 1991.

Thompson, P. *Mister Leprosy.* London: Hodder and Stoughton, 1980.

Trésor de la langue française. Paris: Gallimard, 1985.

Trolle, Dyre. *The History of the Caesarean Section.* Copenhagen: Reitzel, 1982.

Trolli, G. *Historique de l'assistance médicale aux indigènes du Congo Belge: Nouvelle méthode adoptée par FOREAMI, Résultats obtenus.* Brussels: Van Doosselaere, 1930.

——. *Exposé de la législation sanitaire du Congo belge et du Ruanda-Urundi.* Brussels: n.p., 1938.

Trolli, Laure. "Les femmes coloniales et l'enfance noire." *Bulletin de l'Union Coloniale* 17, no. 112 (February 1940): 33–34.

Turner, Patricia A. *Ceramic Uncles and Celluloid Mammies: Black Images and Their Influence on Culture.* New York: Anchor Books, 1994.

Turner, Victor. *Chihamba, the White Spirit.* Manchester: Manchester University Press, 1962.

———. *The Forest of Symbols: Aspects of Ndembu Ritual.* Ithaca, N.Y.: Cornell University Press, 1967.

———. *The Drums of Affliction.* Oxford: Clarendon Press and International African Institute, 1968.

Turshen, Meredeth. "The Impact of Economic Reforms on Women's Health and Health Care in Sub-Saharan Africa." In *Women in the Age of Economic Transformation: Gender Impact of Reforms in Post-Socialist and Developing Countries,* edited by Nahid Aslanbeigui, Steven Pressman, and Gale Summerfield. London: Routledge, 1994.

Ulrich, Laurel Thatcher. *A Midwife's Tale: The Life of Martha Ballard, Based on Her Diary, 1785–1812.* New York: Knopf, 1990.

United States Agency for International Development. *AID/CDIE/DISC Development Information System.* Abstracts on "USAID Reports—Health in Zaire (including SANRU)." Washington, D.C., 1976–1994.

———. *Santé pour tous: SANRU II, Projets de Soins de Santé Primaires en Milieu Rural.* USAID Project Data Report on 660-0107, Basic Rural Health II, 19 August 1985.

Valcke, G. "Note." *ASBMT* 14 (1934): 432–33.

Valcke, J.P. "Six années de pratique chirurgicale au Congo." Examen B/Médecins no. 81, IMT, 1934.

Valcke, P. "Les fistules vésico-vaginales en pratique rurale." Examen B/Médecins no. 30, IMT, 1959.

Van de Lanoitte, Ch. *Sur les rivières glauques de l'Equateur: Troise années en brousse congolaise.* Brussels: Iris, 1938.

Vandenbroeke, Chris. "Démographie: La dualité de la norme et des faits." In *Les années trente en Belgique: la séduction des masses.* Brussels: CGER, 1994.

Vander Elst, Dr. "Six mois de gynécologie à l'Hôpital des Noirs de Léopoldville." *Bruxelles-Médical* 26 (1946): 1312–13.

Van der Kerken, Mme. "Les Oeuvres sociales et humanitaires au Congo Belge." In *Congrès Colonial National,* Ve session, no. 15, 1940.

Vanderyst, H. "L'enseignement élémentaire médical pour indigènes, à tous ses degrés, au Congo belge." *L'aide médicale aux missions* 1 (15 October 1929): 76–80; 2 (15 January 1930): 16–17; 2 (15 July 1930): 15–16; and 3 (15 July 1931): 60–61.

Van Haute-De Kimpe, Bernadette. "The Mbole and Their Lilwa Sculptures." *Africa Insight* 15, no. 4 (1985): 288–97.

Van Nitsen, R. *L'hygiène des travailleurs noirs dans les camps industriels du Haut-Katanga.* Brussels: IRCB, 1933.

Van Onselen, Charles. "Reactions to Rinderpest in Southern Africa, 1896–1897." *Journal of African History* 8 (1972): 474–88.

Vansina, Jan. "Initiation Rituals of the Bushong." *Africa* 25 (1956): 138–55.

———. *Oral Tradition as History.* Madison: University of Wisconsin Press, 1985.

———. *Paths in the Rainforests: Toward a History of Political Tradition in Equatorial Africa.* Madison: University of Wisconsin Press, 1990.

Van Wing, J., and V. Goeme. *Annuaire des Missions Catholiques au Congo Belge et au Ruanda-Urundi.* Brussels: L'Edition Universelle, 1949.

Vaughan, Megan. "Measuring Crisis in Maternal and Child Health: An Historical Perspective." In *Women's Health and Apartheid: The Health of Women and Children and the Future of Progressive Primary Health Care in Southern Africa,* edited by Marcia Wright, Zena Stein, and Jean Scandlyn. New York: Columbia University Press, 1988.

———. *Curing Their Ills: Colonial Power and African Illness.* Stanford, Calif.: Stanford University Press, 1991.

———. "Syphilis in Colonial East and Central Africa: The Social Construction of an Epidemic." In *Epidemics and Ideas: Essays on the Historical Perception of Pestilence,* edited by Terence Ranger and Paul Slack. Cambridge: Cambridge University Press, 1992.

———. "Health and Hegemony: Representation of Disease and the Creation of the Colonial Subject in Nyasaland." In *Contesting Colonial Hegemony: State and Society in Africa and India,* edited by Dagmar Engels and Shula Marks. London: British Academic Press, 1994.

Vellut, Jean-Luc. "Les Belges au Congo (1885–1960)." In *La Belgique, Sociétés et cultures depuis 150 Ans, 1830–1980,* edited by Albert d'Haenens. Brussels: Ministère des Affaires Etrangères, 1980.

———. "Matériaux pour une image du blanc dans la société coloniale du Congo belge." In *Stéréotypes nationaux et préjugés raciaux aux XIXe et XXe siècles,* edited by Jean Pirotte. Leuven: Editions Nauwelaerts, 1982.

———. "Articulations entre entreprises et Etat: Pouvoirs hégémoniques dans le bloc colonial belge (1908–1960)." In *Entreprises et entrepreneurs en Afrique (XIXe et XXe siècles).* Paris: l'Harmattan, 1983.

———. "La violence armée dans l'Etat Indépendant du Congo." *Cultures et développement* 16 (1984): 671–707.

———. "Détresse matérielle et découvertes de la misère dans les colonies belges d'Afrique centrale, ca. 1900–1960." In *La Belgique et l'étranger aux XIXe et XXe siècles,* edited by Michel Dumoulin and Eddy Stols. Louvain-la-Neuve: Editions Nauwelaerts, 1987.

———. "La médecine européenne dans l'Etat Indépendant du Congo (1885–1908)." In *Analecta de réalisations médicales en Afrique centrale, 1885–1985,* edited by P. G. Janssens, M. Kivits, and J. Vuylsteke. Brussels: Fondation Roi Baudouin, 1991.

Vellut, Jean-Luc, Florence Loriaux, and Françoise Morimont. *Bibliographie historique du Zaïre à l'époque coloniale (1880–1960): Travaux publiés en 1960–1996.* Louvain-la-Neuve and Tervuren: Centre d'Histoire de l'Afrique and MRAC, 1996.

Verhaegen, Benoît. "Kisangani pendant la deuxième guerre mondiale, 1939–1945." In *Le Congo belge durant la seconde guerre mondiale.* Brussels: ARSOM, 1983.

———. "Les violences coloniales au Congo belge." In *Cahiers d'actualité sociale* 4. Kisangani: Presses Universitaires de Kisangani and Institut de Recherches Sociales Appliquées, 1987.

Verhaegen, Benoît, ed. *La vie de Disasi Makulo recueillie par son fils Makulo Akambu.* In *Notes, travaux, documents du CRIDE* 4. Kisangani: Université de Kisangani, 1982.

Verheust, Th. "Enquête démographique par sondage, 1955–1957—Province Orientale, District de Stanleyville—District du Haut-Uélé." *Cahiers du CEDAF* 22 (1978).

Vigarello, Georges. *Le propre et le sale, L'hygiène du corps depuis le Moyen Age.* Paris: Seuil, 1985.

Vincent, Marc. "Mission d'Information." [Brussels?]: OREAMI, 1957. Polycopied report.

———. *Les problèmes de protection maternelle au Congo belge et au Ruanda-Urundi.* Brussels: FOREAMI, 1959.

Voas, David. "Subfertility and Disruption in the Congo Basin." In *African Historical Demography.* Vol. 2. Edinburgh: Centre of African Studies, University of Edinburgh, 1981.

La Voix du Congolais. Leopoldville, 1945–1960.

Vulhopp, Tilla. *Une politique des familles nombreuses en Belgique.* Louvain: Editions de la Société d'Etudes Morales, Sociales et Juridiques, 1928.

Walls, A. F. "'The Heavy Artillery of the Missionary Army': The Domestic Importance of the Nineteenth-Century Medical Missionary." In *The Church and Healing,* edited by W. J. Sheils. Oxford: Oxford University Press, 1982.

Ward, Henry. *Five Years with the Congo Cannibals.* London: Chatto and Windus, 1891.

Weeks, John H. *Among Congo Cannibals: Experiences, Impressions, and Adventures during a Thirty Years' Sojourn amongst the Boloki and Other Congo Tribes.* London: Seeley Service and Co., 1913.

Weindling, Paul. *Health, Race, and German Politics between National Unification and Nazism, 1870–1945.* Cambridge: Cambridge University Press, 1989.

——. "Fascism and Population in Comparative European Perspective." In *Population and Resources in Western Intellectual Traditions,* edited by Michael S. Teitelbaum and Jay M. Winter. Cambridge: Cambridge University Press, 1989.

White, Luise. "Bodily Fluids and Usufruct: Controlling Property in Nairobi, 1917–1939." *Canadian Journal of African Studies* 24 (1990): 418–38.

——. "Vampire Priests of Central Africa: African Debates about Labor and Religion in Colonial Northern Uganda." *Comparative Studies in Society and History* 35 (1993): 746–72.

——. "'They Could Make Their Victims Dull': Genders and Genres, Fantasies and Cures in Colonial Southern Uganda." *American Historical Review* 100 (1995): 1379–402.

——. "Tsetse Visions: Narratives of Blood and Bugs in Colonial Northern Rhodesia, 1931–1939." *Journal of African History* 36 (1995): 219–45.

Whitehead, John, and L. F. Whitehead. *Manuel de Kingwana, le dialecte occidental de Swahili.* Wayika, Congo Belge: Mission de et à Wayika, 1928.

Williams, C. P. "'Not Quite Gentlemen': An Examination of 'Middling Class' Protestant Missionaries from Britain, c. 1850–1900." *Journal of Ecclesiastical History* 31 (1980): 301–15.

Wilson, Adrian. "William Hunter and the Varieties of Man-Midwifery." In *William Hunter and the Eighteenth-Century Medical World,* edited by W. F. Bynum and Roy Porter. Cambridge: Cambridge University Press, 1985.

——. *The Making of Man-Midwifery: Childbirth in England, 1660–1770.* London: UCL Press, 1995.

Wilson, Monica. *Communal Rituals of the Nyakyusa.* London: Oxford University Press, 1959.

Wome, Bokemo. "Recherches ethno-pharmacognosiques sur les plantes médicinales utilisées en médecine traditionelle à Kisangani (Haut-Zaïre)." Ph.D. diss., Université Libre de Bruxelles, 1985.

Wright, Peter W. G. "Babyhood: The Social Construction of Infant Care as a Medical Problem in England in the Years around 1900." In *Biomedicine Examined,* edited by Margaret Lock and Deborah Gordon. Dordrecht, Netherlands: Kluwer Academic Publishers, 1988.

Yakusu Quarterly Notes. Yakusu, 1910–1960.

Yates, Barbara Ann. "The Missions and Educational Development in Belgian Africa, 1876–1908." Ph.D. diss., Columbia University, 1967.

——. "The Triumph and Failure of Mission Vocational Education in Zaire, 1879–1908." *Comparative Education Review* 20 (1976): 193–208.

——. "Knowledge Brokers: Books and Publishers in Early Colonial Zaire." *History in Africa* 14 (1987): 311–40.

Yoka, Lye M. "Mythologie de l'argent-monnaie à Kinshasa. Culte de la débrouille." Paper presented to the Colloque " 'L'argent, feuille morte?' l'Afrique centrale avant et après le désenchantement de la modernité," Katholieke Universiteit Leuven, Leuven, Belgium, 1996.

Young, Crawford. *Politics in the Congo.* Princeton, N.J.: Princeton University Press, 1965.

——. "Rebellion and the Congo." In *Protest and Power in Black Africa,* edited by Robert I. Rotberg and Ali A. Mazrui. New York: Oxford University Press, 1970.

Young, Robert. *Colonial Desire.* London: Routledge, 1995.

Zaïre, 1885–1985: Cent ans de regards belges. Brussels: CEC, 1985.

Zola, Émile. *Fécondité.* Paris: Librairie Charpentier et Fasquelle, 1899.

INDEX

Nancy Rose Hunt is Assistant Professor in the Departments
of History and Obstetrics and Gynecology at the
University of Michigan.

Library of Congress Cataloging-in-Publication Data
Hunt, Nancy Rose.
A colonial lexicon; of birth ritual, medicalization, and mobility
in the Congo / Nancy Rose Hunt.
    p.   cm. — (Body, Commodity, Text)
Includes bibliographical references (p.   ) and index.
ISBN 0-8223-2331-1 (cloth : alk. paper). —
ISBN 0-8223-2366-4 (paper : alk. paper)
1. Birth customs—Congo (Democratic Republic).   2. Birth
customs—Religious aspects.   3. Childbirth—Religious
aspects—Christianity.   4. Yakusu (Mission : Congo)—History.
5. Protestant churches—Missions—Congo (Democratic
Republic)—History.   6. Congo (Democratic Republic)—Social
life and customs.   I. Title.
GT2465.C74H85   1999
392.1′2′096751—dc21   99-26315